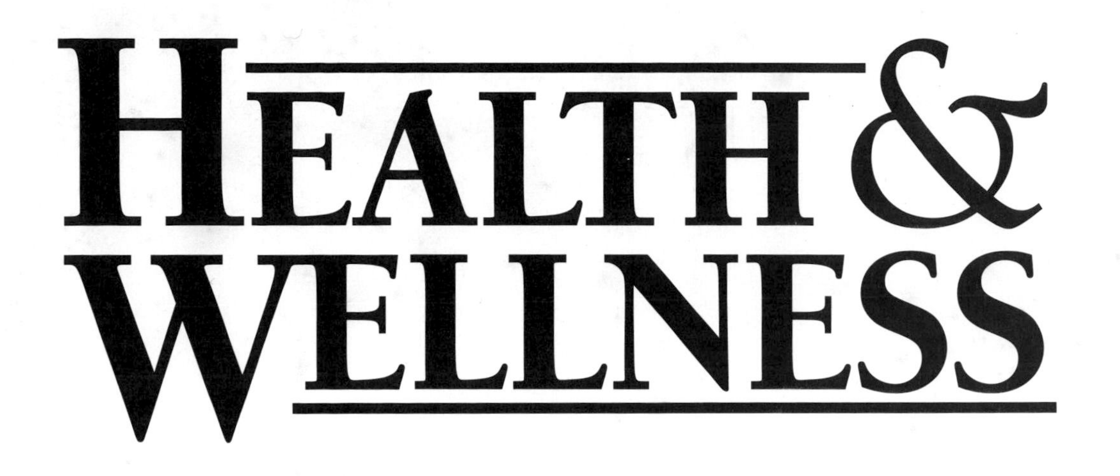
Health & Wellness

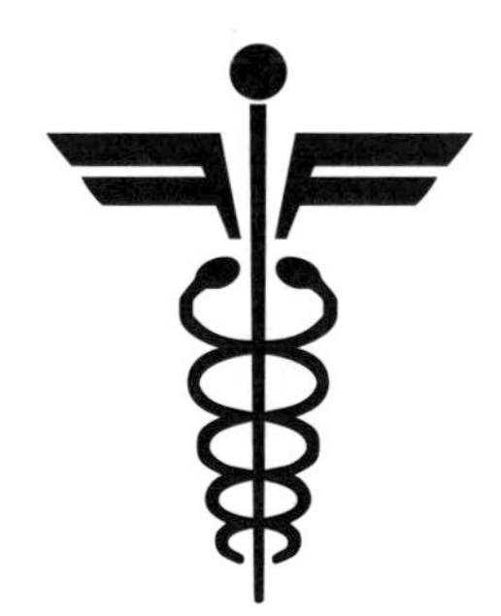

SW

Published In 1999
THE SOUTHWESTERN COMPANY
Nashville, TN

Health and Wellness
Manufactured under the direction of FRP™—a division of Southwestern/Great American, Inc.
Nashville, Tennessee

**Sourcing**
Sharon Dean

**Production Director**
Mark Sloan

**Production Coordinator**
George McAllister

**Digital Prepress Coordinator**
Donna Bailey

**Production**
Waller Digital

**Sales Directors**
Creig Soeder Roy Loftin
Dave Causer Fred Prevost
Jeff Hawley

ISBN # 0-87197-4797



Printed in the United States of America.

**Library of Congress Cataloging-in-Publication Data**
The medical advisor home edition,
by the editors of Time-Life Books.
p. cm.
Includes bibliographical references
and index.
ISBN 0-7835-5250-5 (softcover)
1. Medicine, Popular—Encyclopedias. 2. Alternative medicine
Encyclopedias. I. Time-Life Books.
RC81.A2M38 1997
616—dc21 97-10717 CIP



First printing. Printed in U.S.A.
School and library distribution by
Time-Life Education,
P.O. Box 85026, Richmond,
Virginia 23285-5026.



---

**The textual and visual descriptions of medical conditions and treatment options in this book should be considered as a reference source only; they are not intended to substitute for a healthcare practitioner's diagnosis, advice, and treatment. Always consult your physician or a qualified practitioner for proper medical care.**

**Before using any drug or natural medicine mentioned in this book, be sure to check with your healthcare practitioner, and check the product packaging or other reliable source of information for any warnings or cautions. You should keep in mind that herbal remedies are not as strictly regulated as drugs.**

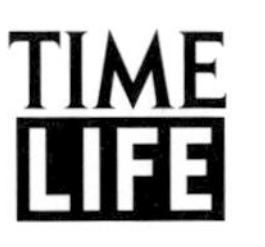


By the Editors of
TIME-LIFE BOOKS
Alexandria, VA

# LEG PAIN

*Read down this column to find your symptoms. Then read across.*

| SYMPTOMS | AILMENT/PROBLEM |
| --- | --- |
| ◆ leg pain following an injury, but you can move your leg. | ◆ Soft-tissue injury |
| ◆ leg pain following an injury, and you cannot move your leg or walk; severe pain even at rest. | ◆ Fracture or dislocation |
| ◆ pain and swelling after excessive athletic or other physical activity. | ◆ Overuse injury |
| ◆ aching in your legs with ankle or foot swelling, especially after long periods of standing; possibly, prominent dark blue blood vessels in your legs and feet. | ◆ Varicose veins |
| ◆ cramping pain in calves, thighs, feet, or hips when walking or exercising that stops with rest; muscle fatigue. | ◆ Peripheral vascular disease (blocked arteries and other venous or arterial problems) |
| ◆ shooting or burning pain in your buttocks and down the back of one leg; worsens with coughing, sneezing, bending, or lifting. | ◆ Sciatica |
| ◆ a throbbing or burning sensation beneath the skin of your leg; a red, warm, tender, cordlike vein is visible. | ◆ Superficial phlebitis |
| ◆ pain and swelling throughout your leg, especially when your foot is flexed. | ◆ Deep phlebitis |
| ◆ persistent, severe pain in one area of your leg; fever above 100°F; general feeling of malaise; tender or red area over a bone in your leg. | ◆ Bone infection |

| WHAT TO DO | OTHER INFO |
| --- | --- |
| ◆ Try RICE: rest, ice (cubes wrapped in a thin cloth), compression (not-too-tight bandage), elevation (with pillows). *(See Sprains and Strains.)* | ◆ Strenuous use of affected muscles should be avoided until the pain is gone. |
| ◆ **Call your doctor now.** See Athletic Injuries and Emergencies/First Aid: Fractures and Dislocations. | ◆ In addition to conventional treatment the homeopathic remedy Arnica may be initially helpful to reduce swelling and bruising. |
| ◆ See Athletic Injuries. Curtail or stop the activity that caused injury. | ◆ Overuse injuries of the leg include shin splints and tendonitis. |
| ◆ Wear elastic support stockings and take an anti-inflammatory painkiller such as ibuprofen. Medical treatment options include laser therapy, chemical injection, and surgery. | ◆ The cause is damage to valves in the veins, resulting in poor circulation in your legs. Deep varicose veins are less common but may cause serious circulatory problems. |
| ◆ Call your doctor. See Circulatory Problems, Atherosclerosis, and Heart Disease. Treatment depends on the cause; it may include medication to improve blood flow or bypass surgery. | ◆ Stopping smoking, improving your diet, and exercising regularly may be helpful. |
| ◆ See your doctor. Treatment may include muscle relaxants, analgesics, and/or physical therapy. | ◆ Acupuncture treatments may relieve mild or acute sciatica. Chiropractic manipulation may be able to reduce pressure on the nerve. |
| ◆ See Phlebitis. To ease the pain, lie down and prop your legs up 6 to 12 inches above the level of your heart. Apply a heating pad or moist warm pack to the swollen area. | ◆ Your doctor may suggest compression support stockings, aspirin to reduce inflammation, and if an infection is found, an antibiotic. |
| ◆ **Call your doctor now.** You may need to be hospitalized for tests and anticoagulation treatment. See Phlebitis. | ◆ The danger is that a clot in a deep vein can break away and lodge in a lung (pulmonary embolism), a potentially fatal complication. |
| ◆ **Call your doctor now.** See Infections. Treatment typically includes antibiotics. | ◆ Infection may occur after a wound, fracture, or other injury. |

# LEUKEMIA

## SYMPTOMS

Many types of leukemia produce no obvious symptoms in early stages. Eventually symptoms may include any of the following:

- anemia and related symptoms, such as fatigue, pallor, and a general feeling of illness.
- a tendency to bruise or bleed easily, including bleeding from the gums or nose, or blood in the stool or urine.
- susceptibility to infections such as sore throat or bronchial pneumonia, which may be accompanied by headache, low-grade fever, mouth sores, or skin rash.
- swollen lymph nodes, typically in the throat, armpits, or groin.
- loss of appetite and weight.
- discomfort under the left lower ribs (caused by a swollen spleen).

In advanced stages, symptoms may include sudden high fever, confusion, seizures, inability to talk or move limbs, and an altered state of consciousness.

## CALL YOUR DOCTOR IF:

- you experience any of the symptoms described above and cannot readily explain their occurrence. Your blood cell count should be tested.
- you experience unexplained bleeding, high fever, or a seizure. You may need emergency treatment for **acute leukemia.**
- you are in remission from leukemia and notice signs of recurrence, such as infection or easy bleeding. You should have a follow-up examination.

Leukemia is cancer of the blood. Unlike other cancers, leukemia does not produce tumors but results in rampant overproduction of cancerous white blood cells. Leukemia—the term derives from the Greek words for "white" and "blood"—is often considered a disease of children, yet it actually affects far more adults. It is more common in men than women, and in Caucasians than African Americans; almost 30,000 cases are diagnosed in the United States each year.

The term "life-giving" often applied to blood is no exaggeration. Suspended in its liquid plasma are disease-fighting white cells, wound-stanching platelets, and red cells that carry oxygen to every part of the body. Every day hundreds of billions of new blood cells are produced in the bone marrow—most of them red cells. In people with leukemia, however, the body starts producing more white cells than it needs. Many of the extra white cells do not mature normally, yet they tend to live well beyond their normal life span.

Despite their vast numbers, these leukemic cells are unable to fight infection the way normal white blood cells do. As they accumulate, they interfere with vital organ functions, including the production of healthy blood cells. Eventually the body does not have enough red cells to supply oxygen, enough platelets to ensure proper clotting, or enough normal white cells to fight infection, making people with leukemia anemic and susceptible to bruising, bleeding, and infection.

Cases of leukemia are classified as acute or chronic. Cancer cells in **acute leukemias** start multiplying before they develop beyond their immature stage. **Chronic leukemias** progress more slowly, with cancer cells developing to full maturity. Leukemias are further classified according to the type of white blood cell involved. Under a microscope, two main types of white blood cells are easily distinguishable: Myeloid cells contain tiny particles or granules; lymphoid cells usually do not.

**Acute lymphocytic,** or **lymphoblastic, leukemia (ALL),** sometimes called childhood leukemia, is the most common type of cancer in children; **acute myelogenic leukemia (AML)** is the most common form of leukemia in adults. Without treatment, acute leukemias are usually fatal within months. Treatment effectiveness varies with the type and stage of the disease, but the younger the patient, the greater the chances of remission. In leukemia, remission means that no more cancerous cells can be detected and bone marrow appears normal. Adult patients treated for **ALL** have an 80 to 90 percent chance of attaining remission; about 40 percent of those who do so survive at least another five years, with a chance of a full cure. Patients treated for **AML** have a 60 to 70 percent chance of remission; about 20 percent of those survive at least three years, with a possibility of a full cure.

Chronic leukemias tend to affect middle-aged adults. **Chronic lymphocytic leukemia (CLL)** is the most benign, slowly progressing type. It can be controlled effectively with medication, and may require no treatment in its early stages. **Chronic myelogenic leukemia (CML)** is more aggressive. Since it is difficult to prevent this disease from escalating to an acute phase even with treatment, average survival time is about four years. Each of these four main types of leukemia can be divided into many subtypes. Other, rare, forms of the disease include **hairy cell, prolymphocytic, megakaryocytic, basophilic,** and **eosinophilic** leukemia.

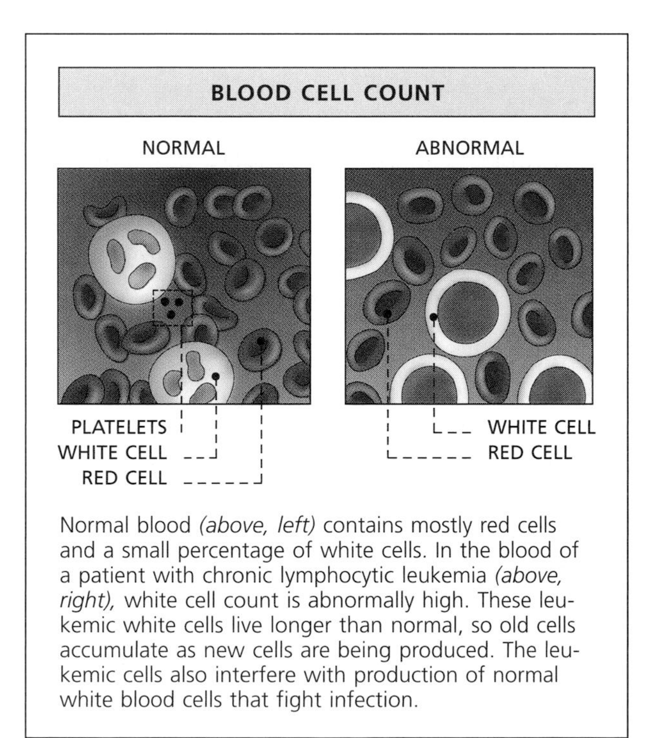


Normal blood *(above, left)* contains mostly red cells and a small percentage of white cells. In the blood of a patient with chronic lymphocytic leukemia *(above, right),* white cell count is abnormally high. These leukemic white cells live longer than normal, so old cells accumulate as new cells are being produced. The leukemic cells also interfere with production of normal white blood cells that fight infection.

## CAUSES

No one knows exactly what causes leukemia, but some people seem genetically predisposed to the disease. Chromosome abnormalities are associated with leukemia and with a preleukemic disease called myelodysplasia. Nine out of ten people with **CML,** for example, have an abnormal chromosome called the Philadelphia chromosome in their blood cells. This chromosome is an acquired abnormality; it is neither inherited nor passed on to one's children. Chromosome abnormalities associated with congenital disorders such as Down syndrome strongly correlate with certain types of leukemia, and at least one virus in the same family as the human immunodeficiency virus (HIV) has been associated with a rare form of the disease.

Environmental factors seem to influence the risk of developing leukemia. Tobacco smokers are more prone to certain leukemias than nonsmokers. Research also suggests that prolonged exposure to radiation, various chemicals in home and work environments, and low-frequency electromagnetic fields may be associated with leukemia—but there is no definitive proof.

### DIAGNOSTIC AND TEST PROCEDURES

Because many types of leukemia show no obvious symptoms early on, the disease may be diagnosed incidentally during a physical examination or as a result of routine blood tests. If a patient has enlarged lymph nodes, swollen gums, an enlarged liver or spleen, significant bruising, or a small pinpoint rash, the doctor should suspect leukemia. A blood test showing an abnormal white cell count is usually adequate for a tentative diagnosis. To confirm the diagnosis and identify the specific type, the patient will have a needle biopsy of bone marrow from a pelvic bone and a test for cancer cells. In the case of **CML,** DNA tests will check for the Philadelphia chromosome.

### CANCER IN CHILDREN

Having leukemia—or any other cancer—is scary, whether you're a child or an adult. But cancer is

### Coping with Chemotherapy

*Cancer patients who receive chemotherapy tend to experience unpleasant side effects. This is a particular concern for leukemia sufferers, since chemotherapy is essential to their treatment. Fortunately, medication can help relieve side effects to an encouraging degree, as can various complementary therapies.*

*The method doesn't matter as long as it works. Acupuncture has traditionally been used to relieve the pain and discomfort of many illnesses, including cancer. Any of several relaxation techniques—including massage, yoga, qigong, meditation, or progressive muscle relaxation—may help subdue the pain and nausea frequently experienced after chemotherapy. Others find relief in hobbies, listening to music, or simply reading a good book.*

*To control nausea that may occur in anticipation of chemotherapy, adults may find help in biofeedback training, while children often respond well to various kinds of distraction or to hypnotherapy.*

not necessarily a death sentence, and all people with cancer deserve to live their lives fully and richly. If your child gets cancer, the best thing you can do is remember he's a child first and a cancer patient second.

Attitudes can be surprisingly contagious. Don't pretend the disease doesn't exist; this won't fool you or your child, and it won't help you face the questions and emotions generated by cancer. Try to have a sense of optimism and good humor. Encourage friends, family, and others in your child's life to act normally and help him live a normal life. This means nurturing without coddling, and empathizing without being either overly protective or overly lenient. If your family needs help coping with cancer, see the Appendix for a list of organizations to contact.

While you are caring for this special child, don't forget his siblings—they need you, too. And when you're feeling overwhelmed, remember that chances are better than even that your child will recover.

## TREATMENT

While the reported incidence of leukemia has not changed much since the 1950s, more people are surviving longer, thanks mainly to advances in chemotherapy. Childhood leukemia **(ALL),** for example, represents one of the most dramatic success stories of cancer treatment: Some 90 percent of children diagnosed with the disease attain remission, and more than half are cured completely. The five-year survival rate for all patients with **ALL** has risen from 4 percent in the 1960s to more than 50 percent in the 1990s.

### CONVENTIONAL MEDICINE

For **acute leukemia,** the immediate goal of treatment is remission. The patient undergoes aggressive chemotherapy in a hospital for several weeks and is kept in sterile isolation and cleansed constantly to reduce the chance of infection. Since acute leukemia patients have extremely low counts of healthy blood cells, they are usually given blood and platelet transfusions to boost their natural immune function and to help stop bleeding. They may also receive drugs to combat infection and to reduce nausea and vomiting that may occur as side effects of the chemotherapy.

People with **ALL** are likely to attain satisfactory remission after several weeks of aggressive chemotherapy in a hospital. To keep the disease under control, they will continue receiving low-dose chemotherapy and possibly radiation therapy for a month or more to eliminate residual cancer traces. At home they will receive an on-and-off maintenance protocol for months or even years. Since **AML** does not respond as well to chemotherapy, the best chance of lasting remission or cure depends on successful bone marrow transplantation, which requires a willing donor with compatible tissue type and genetic characteristics—usually a family member.

A bone marrow transplant has three stages: preparation, operation, and recovery. First, the patient's cancerous white blood cell count is brought under control—usually by chemotherapy but possibly by leukopheresis, a mechanical process that separates cancer cells from the blood. During the operation stage, the patient's bone marrow is destroyed by intensive chemotherapy to avoid rejection of new marrow. The patient then receives about one tablespoon of donor marrow. Recovery is the most dangerous stage: Until the donor marrow cells start producing new blood, the patient is left with virtually no white blood cells, making death by infection a strong possibility. Once the donor marrow multiplies sufficiently—usually in two to six weeks—the outlook for long-term remission and sometimes a complete cure is good. Bone marrow transplantation is still both expensive and risky, but it offers the best chance of remission and cure for **AML** and recurring cases of **ALL.**

Since **CLL** generally affects older people and progresses slowly, conventional treatment tends to be conservative. As long as symptoms are absent, the disease requires no treatment. If swelling appears in lymph nodes and other organs, CLL can usually be controlled for years with oral chemotherapy. Many people with CLL lead basically normal lives and die of unrelated causes.

Oral chemotherapy can effectively control symptoms of **CML** for several years before the disease becomes acute. CML sufferers may survive longer if they receive interferon, a naturally occurring protein that can kill or slow the growth of cancerous cells. Because most cases of CML eventually advance to an acute phase despite treatment, some doctors advise bone marrow transplantation during the chronic phase.

In addition to using standard treatments, some doctors are experimenting with immunological ones. The hope is that interferon or other so-called biologic response modifiers will either kill leukemic cells or restore their normal form and function. Scientists are investigating other methods of killing cancer cells without harming normal cells, including use of the experimental drug interleukin and identifying specific antibody proteins that target cancer cells so they can be destroyed by injections of radioactive substances.

For more information on chemotherapy, radiation, and other treatments, see Cancer.

## COMPLEMENTARY THERAPIES

Realistically, there is no acceptable substitute for conventional cancer treatment. While many alternative therapies are being incorporated into mainstream medical care, none is a proven cancer cure. Alternative therapies may improve the quality of a cancer patient's life but are best viewed as potential complements to, not replacements for, conventional care.

The best complementary therapies are those that help control the pain, discomfort, and anxiety of cancer and its treatment. Stress-reducing exercises—along with certain vitamins, nutrients, and herbal remedies that may enhance immune function—can be particularly beneficial. For more information on complementary therapies, see Cancer.

## AT-HOME CARE

- To lessen the chance of the nausea that may result from chemotherapy, eat light snacks throughout the day rather than large meals.
- To reduce the chance of infection, avoid people who are obviously sick; wash your hands well before eating and before and after going to the toilet; take a warm shower or bath daily, and pat rather than rub yourself dry.
- If you cut or scratch yourself, follow thorough antiseptic procedures. If you develop signs of infection—fever, chills, sore throat, cough, swollen or reddened skin—get medical treatment immediately.
- Leukemia patients prone to bleeding because of a low platelet count should not use medications containing aspirin; it may inhibit clotting. ■

L

# LICE

## SYMPTOMS

- **head lice:** intense itching on the scalp, especially behind the ears and at the nape of the neck.
- **body lice:** unexplained scratch marks on the body, hives, eczema, and red pimples on the shoulders or torso.
- **pubic lice:** continual itching around the pubic area, and perhaps a rash.

## CALL YOUR DOCTOR IF:

- you need help getting rid of lice or if scratching has led to infection.

Lice are tiny parasites that live on human beings and feed on blood. They seldom cause serious medical problems, but they are both annoying and contagious. Every four hours or so, a louse bites into a tiny blood vessel for a meal. You don't feel the initial bites, because lice inject an anesthetic. However, the bites later begin to itch, and your scratching can lead to infection.

**Head lice** *(Pediculus humanus capitis)* are about the size of a sesame seed and can be easily seen, although they hide quickly in response to light. Their eggs, called nits, are barely visible, whitish ovals cemented to hair shafts. Head lice are extremely contagious, especially among schoolchildren. They afflict an estimated 6 to 12 million children in the United States. Twice as many girls as boys get head lice, not because of greater hair length, but because girls have more physical contact with one another and share more personal articles (hats, clothing, combs, headphones) that can transmit head lice. Head lice are rare among African Americans, possibly because the shafts of their hair have a shape that lice cannot grasp easily.

**Pubic lice** *(Phthirius pubis)* are yellow-gray insects found in the pubic region and transmitted by sexual contact. The size of a pinhead, they are slightly translucent and barely visible against light-colored skin. They are also called crab lice, or crabs, because of their shape and the crablike claws with which they cling to hair. Eggs can barely be seen as tiny white particles glued so firmly to hair shafts that they are not removed by normal washing.

**Body lice** *(Pediculus humanus corporis)* are nearly identical in appearance to head lice but are more difficult to find. When not feeding, they tend to hide in the seams of clothing and folds of bedding. Signs of their presence are scratch marks, hives, or small red pimples, usually on the shoulders, torso, or buttocks. If the lice are not treated, rashes or welts may develop.

## CAUSES

Contrary to common belief, lice are not related to poor hygiene. In fact, head lice are thought to prefer clean hair to dirty hair. Lice live successfully all over the world, wherever people gather in close proximity, as in schools.

## TREATMENT

The goal of treatment is to remove all lice and nits. This usually requires repeated efforts, because a few adults may escape by hiding in clothing or bedding, and eggs are difficult to kill.

### CONVENTIONAL MEDICINE

To get rid of **head lice,** the most common treatment is to kill the adults with an insecticidal shampoo and to clear out the nits with a special fine-toothed comb. The safest and most effective preparation is permethrin cream rinse, available over the counter. For best results, follow the directions exactly. Other family members should be treated; about 60 percent of infected children have relatives who carry lice.

To avoid spreading the lice, infected children should be kept home from school until they are treated. Wash all clothing, towels, and bed linens in hot, soapy water, and dry in a hot dryer. You can also sterilize bedding or other items by placing them in a plastic bag for 14 days; the nits will hatch in about a week and die of starvation. Combs, brushes, and barrettes can be disinfected by soaking in hot, soapy water for 10 minutes.

For those who prefer to avoid the use of insecticides, try a "combing only" technique. Wash the hair with ordinary shampoo and conditioner and leave wet. With a fine-toothed comb, stroke slowly outward from the roots through one lock of hair at a time. Lice will land on the back of the comb, get caught between the teeth, or fall off. Space at least 30 strokes over the head. Repeat every three days. Because newborn lice do not lay eggs for the first week, all the lice should disappear after about two weeks of combing.

**Pubic lice** can be treated with over-the-counter medications containing pyrethrins (natural insecticides). Your sexual partners will also have to be treated. Crabs are sometimes found on eyelashes or eyebrows; to remove them, use an ophthalmic ointment such as physostigmine.

To treat **body lice,** wash the entire body with soap and water. If this is not effective, you may have to use an insecticidal preparation, which usually kills all the lice. Wash all clothing and bedding in hot water and dry in a hot dryer. Store clothes for two weeks in plastic bags or place them in dry heat of 140°F for three to five days.

### ALTERNATIVE CHOICES

Several alternative treatments may make it easier to get rid of lice.

#### AROMATHERAPY

For treatment of head lice, wash the hair and rinse slowly with 6 drops each of essential oils of rosemary *(Rosmarinus officinalis)* and red thyme *(Thymus vulgaris)* mixed in a pint of warm water. You may substitute this combination with 12 drops of essential oil of lavender *(Lavandula officinalis).* Dry the hair naturally (not with a blow dryer), then comb with a fine-toothed comb. For prevention, soak your comb in water with 10 drops of essential oil of red thyme, and comb hair thoroughly.

#### HOMEOPATHY

Depending on symptoms, a practitioner may prescribe various remedies, such as Psorinum (30c), for children who are afflicted with head lice.

## PREVENTION

Preventing reinfestation is as important as initial treatment. This is especially true for **head lice,** which spread quickly from head to head. If you discover lice on your child, notify school or day-care authorities at once, since classmates are likely to be infected. Talk with your children and their friends to be sure they understand the risks. You may be reluctant to talk about this subject with strangers, but head lice are a social ailment that can only be dealt with socially. ■

# LIVER CANCER

## SYMPTOMS

Liver cancer usually has no initial symptoms, but may eventually cause:

- pain, swelling, or tenderness in the upper right section of the abdomen.
- yellowing of the skin and whites of the eyes, as in jaundice.
- itching all over the body.
- swollen legs.

In the advanced stage, symptoms may include fever, appetite and weight loss, nausea, vomiting, fatigue, general weakness, and loss of sexual drive.

## CALL YOUR DOCTOR IF:

- you develop symptoms that suggest liver cancer. Although the symptoms may be related to another liver disorder or some other ailment, it's best not to let them go undiagnosed for more than a few weeks. Early detection of cancer ensures better response to treatment.

L

The liver continuously filters blood that circulates through the body, converting nutrients and drugs absorbed in the digestive tract into ready-to-use chemicals. It also removes toxins and other chemical waste products from the blood and readies them for excretion. Because all the blood in the body must pass through it, the liver is unusually accessible to cancer cells traveling in the bloodstream. Ironically, while the liver can cleanse the body of ingested or internally produced poisons, it cannot cleanse itself of cancer.

Most liver cancer is **secondary**, meaning the malignancy originated elsewhere in the body—usually the colon, lung, or breast. **Primary liver cancer**, which starts in the liver, accounts for about 2 percent of cancers in the United States but up to half of all cancers in some undeveloped countries, mainly because of the prevalence of hepatitis, a contagious virus that predisposes a person to liver cancer. Worldwide, primary liver cancer strikes twice as many men as women and is most likely to affect people over 50.

## CAUSES

Primary liver cancer tends to occur in livers damaged by congenital defects or diseases such as hepatitis B and C, and cirrhosis. More than half of all people diagnosed with primary liver cancer have cirrhosis, and those who suffer from hemochromatosis, or iron overload, are at even greater risk. Various carcinogens are associated with primary liver cancer, including some cholesterol-lowering drugs, certain herbicides, and such chemicals as vinyl chloride and arsenic. Male hormones—androgens or steroids—taken by some athletes can cause benign liver tumors and may promote liver cancer. Aflatoxins, a type of plant mold, are also implicated *(box, right)*.

### DIAGNOSTIC AND TEST PROCEDURES

Screening for early detection of primary liver cancer is not performed routinely but should be considered by people at high risk for the disease. To diagnose liver cancer, a doctor must rule out other causes of the symptoms. Blood studies that

## Clean out your cupboard

*Research shows a clear link between aflatoxins in the food supply and the incidence of primary liver cancer. Food grown in some parts of tropical Africa harbors aflatoxins, a potent carcinogen produced by a fungus in the soil. But aflatoxins are not unique to Africa—they may be lurking in the peanut butter that has been on your shelf for the past five years. Aflatoxins develop naturally in many foods—seeds, grains, rice, and nuts—as they age, especially under humid conditions. To avoid contamination, keep dry food in airtight containers and store in a cool place. Discard any food that becomes moldy, soft, rancid, or shriveled, or whose package expiration date has passed.*

measure tumor markers—substances elevated in the presence of a particular cancer—can aid diagnosis. Ultrasound and CT scans may reveal existing tumors, but only a biopsy will distinguish a benign tumor from a malignant one.

## TREATMENT

Any liver cancer is difficult to cure. **Primary liver cancer** is rarely detectable early, when it is most treatable. **Secondary liver cancer** is hard to treat because it has already spread. Also, the liver's complex network of blood vessels makes surgery difficult. Most therapy concentrates on making patients feel better and perhaps live longer.

### CONVENTIONAL MEDICINE

Patients with early-stage tumors that can be removed surgically have the best chance of being cured. Unfortunately, most liver cancers are inoperable at diagnosis, either because the cancer is too advanced or the liver is too diseased to permit surgery. In some patients, radiation or chemotherapy reduces their tumors to operable size. After surgery, chemotherapy or low-dose radiation may help kill remaining cancer cells. Patients in remission must be monitored closely for potential recurrence. A few patients may be eligible for a liver transplant; although the procedure is risky, it offers some chance of cure.

Advanced liver cancer has no standard curative treatment. Chemotherapy and low-dose radiation may control the cancer's spread and ease pain. Most patients receive strong painkilling medication along with drugs to relieve nausea and swelling or to improve appetite. People with advanced liver cancer may choose to join clinical trials testing new approaches to treatment. Such studies include freezing tumor cells to kill them; using biological agents such as interferon or interleukin 2 to stimulate immune cells into attacking cancer more vigorously; and delivering lethal agents directly to cancer cells through synthetic proteins designed to target specific tumors. *(See Cancer for more information on treatments.)*

### COMPLEMENTARY THERAPIES

Pain is a frequent but manageable consequence of advanced liver cancer. Complementary therapies that may prove beneficial include **massage, relaxation** techniques, **body work, biofeedback, hypnotherapy,** and **acupuncture.**

## PREVENTION

- If you risk exposure to hepatitis, get immunized against hepatitis B.
- Drink alcohol only in moderation.
- If you work around chemicals linked to liver cancer, follow safety guidelines to avoid unnecessary contact.
- Before taking iron supplements, check with a doctor to make sure you really need them.
- Do not use anabolic steroids unless medically necessary.

# LOU GEHRIG'S DISEASE

## SYMPTOMS

- in the early stages, increasing weakness in one limb, especially in a hand.
- difficulty in walking; clumsiness with the hands; impaired speech.
- as the disease progresses, weakening of other limbs, perhaps accompanied by twitching, muscle cramping, and exaggerated, faster reflexes.
- problems with chewing, swallowing, and breathing; drooling may occur.
- rippling of the muscle fibers, called fasciculations, under the skin.
- eventual paralysis.

## CALL YOUR DOCTOR IF:

- you have any of the symptoms above; Lou Gehrig's disease requires professional medical care.

Lou Gehrig's disease—named after the baseball player who died in 1941, and clinically known as amyotrophic lateral sclerosis, or ALS—is an incurable, degenerative neurological disorder. For reasons that are not understood, the nerve cells of the brain and spinal cord that control voluntary muscle movement gradually deteriorate. As a result, muscles waste away, ultimately leading to paralysis and death, usually in two to five years. The only nerve cells affected are the motor neurons; sensory and intellectual functioning remains normal throughout. Pain does not accompany the disease at any stage.

ALS is relatively rare: About 5,000 new cases are diagnosed in the U.S. each year. It almost always strikes after the age of 40, and it afflicts more men than women.

## CAUSES

Though the cause of ALS is unknown, genetic inheritance plays a role in 5 to 10 percent of cases. Some researchers believe that so-called familial ALS (that is, inherited ALS) is caused by a defective gene that prevents the body from producing a normal amount of an enzyme called superoxide dismutase (SOD). This enzyme helps neutralize free radicals, highly reactive oxygen molecules produced during metabolism and capable of damaging body tissues. Researchers speculate that defects in protective enzymes may also account for noninherited ALS, and that environmental toxins may be a factor.

Some evidence suggests that the disease may be triggered by exposure to heavy metals, animal hides, or fertilizers. In addition, viral infection and severe physical trauma have been implicated as causative factors. Other theorists link ALS to a phenomenon called excitotoxicity, in which the nerve cells that control movement are so relentlessly stimulated by glutamate, a neurotransmitter, that they eventually die.

### DIAGNOSTIC AND TEST PROCEDURES

A neurologist will administer an electromyogram (EMG) to test for nerve damage. Additional tests

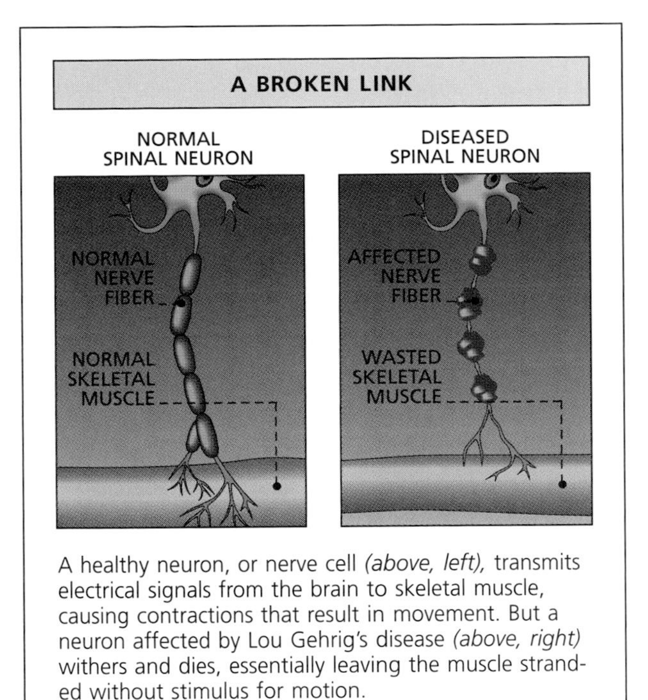

A healthy neuron, or nerve cell *(above, left)*, transmits electrical signals from the brain to skeletal muscle, causing contractions that result in movement. But a neuron affected by Lou Gehrig's disease *(above, right)* withers and dies, essentially leaving the muscle stranded without stimulus for motion.

can rule out muscular dystrophy, multiple sclerosis, spinal cord tumors, or other diseases.

## TREATMENT

Although no treatment slows or halts the progression of the disease, various drugs and devices are available to help control symptoms and make living with ALS easier.

### CONVENTIONAL MEDICINE

Physical therapy can improve circulation and help prolong muscle use in the early stages of ALS. In addition, various medications may be prescribed as the disease progresses. Baclofen relieves stiffness (spasticity) in the limbs and throat. Muscle decline and weight loss can be slowed with nutritional supplements called branched chain amino acids (BCAAs). Quinine or phenytoin will ease cramps. Tricyclic antidepressants can help control excess saliva production—one of the symptoms of ALS.

A highly controversial experimental therapy involves synthetic forms of an insulin-like nerve growth factor called cell-derived neurotrophic factor; it may protect motor neurons and stimulate the regeneration of damaged cells.

### ALTERNATIVE CHOICES

#### ACUPUNCTURE

Acupuncture may temporarily reduce swallowing difficulties and may also alleviate the depression that can come from coping with ALS.

#### CHIROPRACTIC

Spinal manipulation may relieve back problems for ALS patients who, forced by their condition to remain seated for long periods of time, may experience back and shoulder pain.

#### NUTRITION AND DIET

Perhaps because of swallowing difficulties, people with ALS are often malnourished and may benefit from vitamin supplements; liquid forms will probably be easier to take than tablets.

Tests indicate that some neuromuscular symptoms may be relieved by 200 to 1,200 IU of vitamin E with thiamine (vitamin $B_1$) each day. Some evidence suggests that supplements of coenzyme Q10, a protein catalyst, may slow the nerve-tissue atrophy that comes with ALS.

In addition, the amino acids leucine, isoleucine, and valine may help ALS patients maintain muscle strength and prolong walking ability.

### AT-HOME CARE

As their condition deteriorates, ALS patients will need assistance from a caregiver, but mechanical and electronic devices can prolong mobility and independence. Portable computers and voice amplifiers can make communicating easier. Food processors will reduce hard-to-chew foods into easy-to-swallow portions. A walker or self-propelled wheelchair will enable the patient to get around. A respirator can ease breathing difficulties, and a self-suctioning device can help the patient deal with increased saliva secretions and difficulty in swallowing. ■

L

# LUMPS

*Read down this column to find your symptoms. Then read across.*

| SYMPTOMS | AILMENT/PROBLEM |
|---|---|
| Check with your doctor about any new or unusual lump for which there is no explanation; such lumps may be a sign of cancer. | |
| ◆ one or more red, pus-filled nodules ranging from one-quarter to one inch in diameter on the face, buttocks, neck, or armpits; may last two weeks or sometimes longer. | ◆ Boil |
| ◆ a lump that may or may not be painful and that usually is in the upper and outer region of the breast. | ◆ Benign cyst (may come and go with hormone fluctuations such as those of the menstrual cycle); possibly, cancerous tumor (may dimple or crease the skin above it or cause the nipple to turn inward or itch) |
| ◆ a lump beneath the skin, especially in the areas of the groin and abdomen; may be tender; you may feel an aching, heavy sensation when you sit down. | ◆ Hernia |
| ◆ one or more painless lumps or swellings most likely in the neck, armpits, or groin. | ◆ Perhaps swollen lymph nodes caused by the presence of infection somewhere in your body; potentially a sign of Hodgkin's disease or other lymphoma |
| ◆ swelling, especially in the neck, armpits, or groin, that is accompanied by fatigue, fever, and sore throat. | ◆ Mononucleosis |
| ◆ a painful enlargement of the salivary glands (located between the ear and jaw) accompanied by chills, headaches, tiredness, and fever. | ◆ Mumps |
| ◆ a small, flesh-colored or whitish lump with enlarged blood vessels, or a firm, wartlike lump that grows gradually, especially in areas exposed to the sun. | ◆ Perhaps only a wart but potentially basal cell carcinoma or squamous cell carcinoma |
| ◆ a painless lump in a testicle; most common in young and middle-aged men. | ◆ Perhaps a benign cyst but potentially a cancerous tumor |

| WHAT TO DO | OTHER INFO |
| --- | --- |
| ◆ Apply hot compresses to bring a boil to a head more quickly . Clean and bandage a ruptured boil until the area heals. Do not squeeze or lance a boil on your own. | ◆ Boils are the result of staph infection. Herbal therapies such as echinacea (*Echinacea* spp.) and goldenseal *(Hydrastis canadensis)* may help fight infection. |
| ◆ See Breast Cancer; Breast Problems. Always check with your doctor about new or unusual lumps. | ◆ Milk ducts can become swollen during phases of your menstrual cycle, causing cysts; caffeine can aggravate this condition. |
| ◆ Call your doctor. You will probably need surgery to repair the rupture. | ◆ Don't be misled by size. The tinier opening of a small rupture is more apt to cut off circulation to the protruding tissue—a serious condition. |
| ◆ Call your doctor without delay for a diagnosis. An infection may need treatment with antibiotics. | ◆ Accompanying symptoms in the case of lymphoma can include fever, loss of appetite, sweats, general feeling of poor health, and sometimes itching. |
| ◆ Call your doctor to confirm the diagnosis. Rest in bed, and return to normal activity gradually. | ◆ Certain vitamins and some herbal and homeopathic therapies may speed recovery, possibly by boosting the immune system. |
| ◆ In a child, mumps calls for bed rest and acetaminophen for pain. In a teenage or adult male, it should be checked by a doctor because of a slight risk of sterility. | ◆ The testicles may become swollen in a teenage or adult male with mumps. |
| ◆ See Skin Cancer and the Visual Diagnostic Guide. | ◆ Almost all forms of skin cancer are related to sunlight exposure, so limit sun exposure and wear sunscreen. |
| ◆ See Testicle Problems; Testicular Cancer. | ◆ Men should examine their testicles regularly by gently rolling the skin between their fingers to check for lumps. Testicular cancer is highly curable if caught early. A benign cyst may form if the tube that sperm pass through—the epididymis—is clogged. |

# LUNG CANCER

## SYMPTOMS

In its early stages, lung cancer normally has no symptoms. When symptoms start to appear, they are usually caused by blocked breathing passages or the spread of cancer to other parts of the body. Symptoms can include:

- chronic, hacking, raspy coughing, sometimes with blood-streaked sputum—the so-called smoker's cough.
- recurring respiratory infections, including bronchitis or pneumonia.
- shortness of breath, wheezing, persistent chest pain.
- hoarseness.
- swelling of the neck and face.
- pain and weakness in the shoulder, arm, or hand.
- if cancer has spread beyond the lungs: fatigue, weakness, loss of weight and appetite, intermittent fever, severe headaches, and body pain.

## CALL YOUR DOCTOR IF:

- you develop any symptoms that suggest lung cancer, especially chronic cough, blood-streaked sputum, wheezing, hoarseness, or recurrent lung infection. You should have a thorough pulmonary examination.

Although lung cancer is the leading cause of cancer death in the United States, it is also one of the most preventable kinds of cancer. At least 4 out of 5 cases are associated with cigarette smoking, and the cause-and-effect relationship has been documented. During the 1920s, large numbers of men began to smoke cigarettes, presumably in response to increased advertising. Twenty years later, the incidence of lung cancer in men climbed sharply. In the 1940s, significantly more women became smokers. Twenty years later, there was a similar dramatic increase in lung cancer among women.

Lung tumors almost always start in the spongy, pinkish gray walls of the bronchi—the tubular, branching airways of the lungs. More than 20 types of malignant tumors that originate in the lung itself—primary lung cancer—have been identified. The major types are **small cell lung cancer** and **nonsmall cell lung cancer.** The more common nonsmall variety is further divided into **squamous cell carcinoma, adenocarcinoma,** and **large cell carcinoma.**

**Squamous cell carcinoma** usually starts in cells of the central bronchi, the largest branches of the bronchial tree. It is the most common type of lung cancer in men and in smokers; it is the easiest to detect early, since its distinctive cells are likely to show up in tests of sputum samples. It also tends to be most responsive to treatment because it spreads relatively slowly.

**Adenocarcinoma**—the most common type of lung cancer in women and nonsmokers—tends to originate along the outer edges of the lungs in the small bronchi or smaller bronchioles. Adenocarcinoma often spreads to spaces between the lungs and the chest wall, and its typical location makes early detection difficult.

**Large cell carcinomas** are a group of cancers with large, abnormal-looking cells that tend to originate along the outer edges of the lungs. They are the least common of the nonsmall cell lung cancers.

**Small cell lung cancer** is the most aggressive form of the disease; it is also called oat cell cancer because, under a microscope, its cells resemble oat grains. Like squamous cell carcinoma, this cancer usually originates in the central bronchi.

It spreads quickly, often before symptoms appear, making it particularly threatening.

More than 170,000 people in the U.S. are diagnosed with lung cancer each year, most between the ages of 40 and 70. Only 1 percent of lung cancer patients are younger than 30, and only about 10 percent are older than 70. The overall five-year survival rate for lung cancer is improving and now stands at about 15 percent. An individual cancer sufferer's prognosis will vary according to the type of lung cancer involved, the person's overall health, and the status of the cancer at the time of diagnosis.

## CAUSES

As with any cancer, each person's genetic pattern influences susceptibility to lung cancer. The fact that lung cancer runs in some families suggests that a predisposition can be inherited. Additionally, certain genetic traits have been identified that make some people more susceptible than others to carcinogens like those found in tobacco smoke.

Nonetheless, anyone who smokes one pack of cigarettes daily is 20 times more likely than a nonsmoker to develop lung cancer. For people who smoke more than two packs a day, the risk more than triples. Breaking the smoking habit reduces risk significantly, yet former smokers are always slightly more susceptible than nonsmokers. Secondhand tobacco smoke can also cause lung cancer, giving nonsmokers who live or work with smokers a somewhat higher lung cancer risk than those in smoke-free environments.

Carcinogens other than those found in tobacco or tobacco smoke can also cause lung cancer if inhaled in quantity over time. However, experts disagree about how much exposure to specific carcinogens is dangerous. Workers who are exposed on a daily basis to asbestos, silica, mineral dusts, coal dust, arsenic, or the radioactive gas radon *(see the box on page 561)* are much more likely than the average person to develop lung cancer, especially if they are smokers.

Lung tissue that has been scarred by disease or infection, such as scleroderma or tuberculosis, is most susceptible to tumor growth. Because of a high incidence of lung cancer among people who eat large amounts of dietary fat and cholesterol, some researchers speculate that diet may also influence lung cancer risk.

**TUMORS IN THE LUNGS**

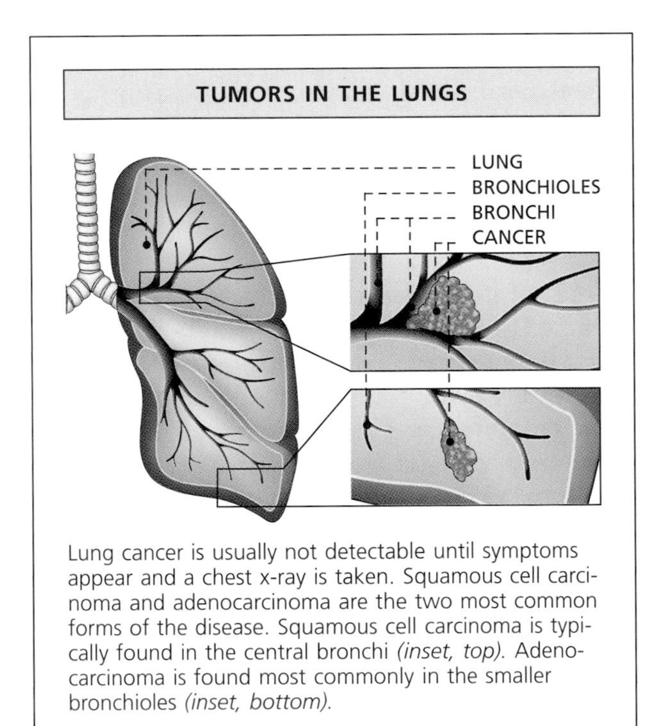


Lung cancer is usually not detectable until symptoms appear and a chest x-ray is taken. Squamous cell carcinoma and adenocarcinoma are the two most common forms of the disease. Squamous cell carcinoma is typically found in the central bronchi *(inset, top)*. Adenocarcinoma is found most commonly in the smaller bronchioles *(inset, bottom)*.

### DIAGNOSTIC AND TEST PROCEDURES

If a routine physical examination reveals swollen lymph nodes above the collarbone, a mass in the abdomen, weak breathing, abnormal sounds in the lungs, or dullness when the chest is tapped, your doctor may suspect a lung tumor. Some lung cancers produce abnormally high blood levels of certain hormones or substances such as calcium. If a person shows such evidence and no other cause is apparent, a doctor should consider lung cancer.

Once a malignant tumor begins to cause symptoms, it is usually visible on an x-ray. Occasionally a tumor that has not yet begun to cause symptoms is spotted on a chest x-ray taken for another purpose. A CT scan of the chest may be ordered for a more detailed examination. While examinations of sputum or lung fluid may reveal fully developed cancer cells, diagnosis is usually confirmed through a biopsy. With the patient lightly anesthetized, the doctor guides a thin, lighted tube through the nose and down the air passages to the site of the tumor, where a tiny tissue sample can be removed. If the biopsy confirms cancer, other tests will determine the type of cancer and how far it has spread. Nearby lymph nodes can be tested for cancer cells, while imaging techniques such as CT scans and bone scans can detect tumors elsewhere in the body.

Because sputum examinations and chest x-rays have not proved particularly effective in detecting small tumors characteristic of early lung cancer, annual chest x-rays for lung cancer screening are not recommended by the American Cancer Society, the National Cancer Institute, or the American College of Radiology.

## TREATMENT

If the cancer can be successfully removed surgically, the patient has an excellent chance of surviving at least one year, and usually a better than 50 percent chance of living at least five years. The challenge comes in detecting lung cancer early enough to make surgery possible. See Cancer for more specific information on treatments such as chemotherapy and radiation therapy.

### CONVENTIONAL MEDICINE

The decision to perform surgery is based not only on the type of lung cancer and how far it has spread but also on the patient's overall health. Many patients with lung cancer—especially smokers—have existing pulmonary or cardiovascular problems that rule out surgery. Cancer that has spread to lymph nodes between the lungs was once considered inoperable, but combining surgery with pre- or postoperative chemotherapy and radiation therapy has improved cure rates.

When feasible, the preferred treatment for **nonsmall cell lung cancer** is surgery. Before the procedure, an effort is made to reduce the size of the tumor with radiation therapy or chemotherapy. During the operation, the surgeon removes the tumorous area along with surrounding lung tissue and lymph nodes; often the entire lung must be taken out. After surgery, patients stay in the hospital for several days and receive analgesics to control postoperative pain. Radiation therapy may be necessary to kill remaining cancer cells, but it is usually delayed for at least a month while the surgical wound heals. Nonsmall cell lung cancers that cannot be treated surgically are usually treated with radiation therapy.

Because of its tendency to spread extensively, **small cell lung cancer** is typically treated with combination chemotherapy—the use of more than one drug—often in conjunction with radiation therapy. For selected patients with small cell lung cancer, some doctors recommend bone-marrow transplant to allow the administration of higher doses of chemotherapy. *(See Lymphoma.)*

Patients whose cancers have metastasized, or spread to distant sites, may be treated with either chemotherapy or radiation therapy. Since metastatic lung cancer is very difficult to cure, the main goals of treatment are to provide comfort and prolong life. Current therapies can shrink tumors, which may alleviate pain and other symptoms. Patients with advanced lung cancer commonly take medication to control pain. Morphine and its various derivatives are widely used and extremely effective in the management of cancer pain.

Researchers are constantly looking for better ways to treat lung cancer, to relieve symptoms, and to improve patients' quality of life. New combinations of chemotherapy, new forms of radiation, and the use of drugs that make cancer cells more sensitive to radiation are under study. Experimental laser surgery has successfully reduced or eliminated tumors obstructing bronchi, thereby improving breathing. Trials are also under way to test various forms of immunotherapy and gene therapy against lung cancer. Immunotherapy manipulates the natural immune system in the hope of turning it aggressively against cancer, while gene therapy enlists foreign genetic material injected into tumor cells to slow or stop their spread.

### COMPLEMENTARY THERAPIES

Once conventional treatment is under way, much can be done to alleviate the pain, fear, and dis-

## ASSESSING THE RISK OF RADON

*Radon is a colorless, odorless, radioactive gas that seeps constantly from the Earth's crust. Studies of uranium miners working on the Colorado Plateau in the 1950s proved conclusively that prolonged, intense exposure to radon causes lung cancer. The U.S. Environmental Protection Agency (EPA) warns that exposure to radon in the home at a level of 4 or more picocuries may cause lung cancer. (A picocurie is one-trillionth of a curie, the standard unit for measuring radioactivity.) Smokers are believed to be particularly susceptible to radon risk, even at low levels.*

*The EPA recommends, but does not require, that all American homes be tested for and proofed against radon. Critics of the EPA's campaign contend that the costs of doing so are unwarranted, while supporters insist that the evidence—however indirect it is—justifies EPA policy. In fact, little scientific evidence supports the EPA's contention, and some studies have found that states with the highest household radon levels have a lower-than-average incidence of lung cancer. The EPA's response to the debate: "Better safe than sorry."*

comfort of cancer. Most complementary cancer therapies can be pursued safely along with standard treatment but should never be substituted for medical care. While outcomes differ among patients receiving complementary care, many have benefited from support-group therapy, improved **nutrition and diet,** and various **body work** and **mind/body** exercises. For further information on complementary cancer therapies, see Cancer.

### NUTRITION AND DIET

Some nutritional studies suggest that certain vitamins and minerals offer protection against lung cancer. Various antioxidants, including vitamins C and E as well as beta carotene (vitamin A) and some other carotenoids, are believed to protect the lungs from the harmful effects of tobacco smoke and other carcinogens. However, enthusiasm for specific nutrients must be tempered by other studies that have either contradicted or failed to support such encouraging results.

Until the full effects of specific nutrients are sorted out, most researchers are reluctant to recommend supplemental vitamins and minerals as potential lung cancer preventives. Instead they advise eating a well-balanced diet that will ensure adequate fiber and nutrients.

### AT-HOME CARE

If you've had lung surgery, your nurse or doctor can show you special exercises to improve your breathing and strengthen your chest muscles. You can relieve skin irritation associated with radiation therapy by wearing loose clothes and keeping your chest protected from the sun. Avoid using skin lotions unless approved by your doctor. For other ideas about coping with the difficulties of cancer and its treatment, see Cancer.

## PREVENTION

The best defense against lung cancer is not to smoke. Breaking the tobacco habit may be difficult, but it can be done. *(See Nicotine Withdrawal.)* While preparing yourself to quit, cut back on the number of cigarettes you smoke daily. Many people report that stopping cigarette smoking "cold turkey" is more effective than gradually tapering off. Joining a support group may help you maintain your resolve to quit. See the Appendix for a listing of substance-abuse support organizations. If you live or work with smokers, encourage them to quit and ask them not to smoke around you. If you are exposed to chemical carcinogens at work, take necessary safety measures to limit inhalation. ■

# LUPUS

## SYMPTOMS

- profound fatigue, low-grade fever, and severe muscle aches and joint pain.
- skin rash on face or body.
- extreme sun sensitivity.
- weight loss, mental confusion, and chest pain on taking a deep breath.
- nose, mouth, or throat ulcers.
- enlarged lymph nodes.
- poor circulation in fingers and toes.
- bald patches.
- discolored urine, or frequent or blocked urination.

## CALL YOUR DOCTOR IF:

- you have several of the above symptoms and suspect you have lupus. This disease is potentially fatal and requires professional medical care. Prognosis improves with early detection and rigorous treatment.
- you have a family history of lupus—especially in your mother or father or an aunt or uncle—and you have experienced several of the above symptoms.

Lupus is a chronic autoimmune disease in which the immune system mistakes the body's connective tissue for a foreign invader and attacks it. One type, **discoid lupus erythematosus (DLE)**, affects only skin that is exposed to sunlight. The other kind, **systemic lupus erythematosus (SLE)**, is more serious. It affects the skin and other vital organs, often causing a raised, scaly butterfly-shaped rash across the bridge of the nose and cheeks that can leave scars if it goes untreated. Systemic lupus may also inflame and damage the connective tissue in the joints, muscles, and skin, as well as the membranes surrounding the lungs, heart, kidneys, and brain. Inflammation of the blood vessels, especially in the fingers, can result in lesions or ulcers. Raynaud's syndrome appears in 20 percent of patients. SLE can also cause kidney disease.

Lupus is characterized by unpredictable phases of remission and exacerbation that vary in intensity and duration. The course of the disease follows no typical pattern and can range from mildly inconveniencing to debilitating.

Lupus strikes black Americans three times as often as white Americans. Most sufferers are between the ages of 20 and 35, and 90 percent are women.

## CAUSES

No single agent has been identified as causing lupus, although some research suggests that a combination of genetic, hormonal, and immunologic factors may be behind it. A predisposition to developing the disease does appear to be an inherited trait.

Environmental elements, ranging from viral and bacterial infections to severe emotional stress or overexposure to sunlight, may play roles in provoking or triggering the disease. Certain drugs such as penicillin and anticonvulsants may cause lupuslike symptoms. High estrogen levels resulting from pregnancy, estrogen replacement therapy, and oral contraceptives may aggravate lupus. There may also be a link between lupus and silicone breast implants.

#### DIAGNOSTIC AND TEST PROCEDURES

Diagnosing lupus can be difficult because symptoms often mimic other diseases and vary from patient to patient. Your doctor will first attempt to rule out chronic fatigue syndrome, mononucleosis, and autoimmune disorders other than lupus itself. Some of the tests your doctor may perform include a complete blood count, platelet count, and serum electrophoresis to indicate the levels of white blood cells and plasma proteins.

Blood testing for anti-DNA antibodies—which shows whether you have antibodies to the normal genetic material in certain cells—is the most definitive way to identify lupus.

## TREATMENT

Due to its unpredictable nature, lupus is a difficult disease to control, but close self-monitoring and proper treatment can help in most cases.

#### CONVENTIONAL MEDICINE

For milder cases, nonsteroidal anti-inflammatory drugs (NSAIDs) such as aspirin can be used to relieve joint pain. Stubborn rashes and more severe joint pain may respond to antimalarial medications such as hydroxychloroquine. A short course of corticosteroids reduces inflammation and fever and is recommended for flareups. Immunosuppressive drugs also decrease inflammation by suppressing abnormal autoimmune activity. Antidepressants and mild antianxiety drugs can help with the sleeping problems that frequently accompany the disease. Cyclophosphamides, which subdue the immune system, may be used for severe cases of lupus involving renal damage.

Mild skin rashes can be treated topically with over-the-counter corticosteroid creams; thicker lesions may require prescription fluorinated steroid creams or injections of triamcinolone.

#### ALTERNATIVE CHOICES

Although they should never be substituted for prescribed medications, a number of alternative therapies may help you control your symptoms. In addition to the remedies mentioned below, you might want to consider **acupuncture, Chinese herbs,** and various forms of **body work.** Consult a specialist for guidance in using these therapies.

#### NUTRITION AND DIET

People with lupus often have food allergies that can make symptoms worse. Identifying and avoiding problem foods can help.

A change in diet may reduce inflammation and decrease pain. Nutritionists may recommend cutting down on red meat and dairy products, and increasing consumption of fish high in omega-3 fatty acids—such as mackerel, sardines, and salmon—which have anti-inflammatory properties. Alfalfa contains a substance that has been shown in tests to aggravate symptoms, so avoiding alfalfa sprouts is strongly recommended.

The following supplements may benefit lupus patients: vitamins $B_5$, C, and E; selenium; and preparations of slippery elm *(Ulmus fulva).* Beta carotene (vitamin A) may help clear up the lesions of discoid lupus. Consult your doctor or a nutritionist for suggested dosages.

#### AT-HOME REMEDIES

- Avoid sun exposure by wearing protective clothing (hats, sunglasses, long sleeves, and long pants) along with an SPF 15 (or higher) sunscreen containing para-aminobenzoic acid (PABA).
- Pace yourself throughout the day to conserve energy, and get plenty of rest even if it means scheduling naps into your routine.

## PREVENTION

Because no one knows what causes lupus, there is no way to prevent it. Flareups can be managed, however, by avoiding known triggers such as sunlight, stress, and lack of sleep. Pay careful attention to your diet and exercise. In addition, keep a record of your symptoms—when they occur, what preceded them, and how long they last—and adjust your routine with them in mind. ■

# LYME DISEASE

## SYMPTOMS

- a circular, bull's-eye rash, often with a clear center, expanding to eight inches or more and lasting two to four weeks.
- may be accompanied by headache, fatigue, fever, chills, sore throat, and aching muscles and joints.
- if not treated, weeks later the development of a generalized and painful kind of arthritis, with swelling in one or sometimes both knees.
- paralysis (most often of the face), memory impairment; random areas of tingling or numbness.
- skin sensitivities.
- stiff neck.
- sensitivity to light.
- irregular heartbeat, chest pain, dizziness.
- psychological changes, including depression.

## CALL YOUR DOCTOR IF:

- you think you may have contracted Lyme disease, especially if you notice a bull's-eye rash or if you suddenly develop knee pain and swelling without previous injury or arthritis. Delaying treatment can result in the more serious neurological symptoms that can be difficult and sometimes impossible to cure.

Lyme disease is transmitted by tiny ticks of the Ixodidae family and afflicts about 10,000 people yearly. Initially identified in a group of children in Lyme, Connecticut, the disease has now been found in nearly all states and 18 other countries. About 90 percent of cases are reported in three areas: the northeast and mid-Atlantic states (Massachusetts to Maryland), the upper Midwest (Minnesota and Wisconsin), and the Far West (California and Oregon).

The first sign is usually an expanding bull's-eye rash that swells to several inches in diameter before disappearing after a few weeks. But in some cases, the rash may take a different form or may be absent altogether. Other early symptoms—with or without the rash—are flulike feelings of fatigue, headache, fever, sore throat, chills, or body aches.

You may also have vague pains in the joints, without swelling. In about half the patients who are not treated, this joint pain returns in about six months as painful arthritis with swelling, usually in one knee. In about 10 percent of these cases, Lyme arthritis becomes chronic. Some patients also experience a complex range of other symptoms, including stiff neck, headaches, sensitivity to light, memory loss, mood changes, chronic fatigue, recurring rashes, paralysis of one or both sides of the face, disruption of heart rhythm, and areas of tingling or numbness.

Because the symptoms are random and vague (aside from the bull's-eye rash), Lyme disease can be hard to diagnose. Unfortunately, unless Lyme disease is treated promptly, it can also be difficult to cure. This is one reason the disease has inspired considerable anxiety among residents in areas where it is common, and may be a reason it is also overdiagnosed.

The good news is that a vaccine that appears to prevent Lyme disease has been under testing. Until a vaccine is approved, however, the best protection is vigilance. Because infection does not occur until a tick has been attached for 36 to 48 hours, a thorough daily tick check can be an effective first-line defense. Be aware, however, that the ticks are very small; they are often the size of poppy seeds, although they are larger when engorged with blood.

## CAUSES

Lyme disease is spread by a spirochete bacterium usually injected by the deer tick in the East and the black-legged tick in the Far West. These tiny, hard-to-remove pests take only three meals during their lifetime, each lasting several days: at the end of the larval, nymphal, and adult stages. The nymph most often feeds on human blood, sometime between the summer months and October.

In the body the spirochete may cause flulike symptoms, invade many tissues—including the heart and the nervous system—and arouse an immune response that leads to Lyme arthritis.

### DIAGNOSTIC AND TEST PROCEDURES

The bull's-eye rash is distinctive; in its absence, Lyme disease is hard to diagnose. It mimics other diseases, such as the flu and arthritis, and there is often a long time lapse between symptoms.

Your doctor will check for flulike symptoms and take a sample of blood to check for a high antibody response to the disease. However, blood testing is neither completely reliable nor useful in the early weeks of infection, when treatment should really begin. Also, patients who have been cured often have positive blood tests for many years, raising the risk of misdiagnosis.

## TREATMENT

The treatment of choice for early-stage Lyme disease is a 10-day course of oral antibiotics, which usually kills the infectious organisms and prevents later symptoms. The sooner treatment is started, the less severe are chronic symptoms.

If the disease progresses, it may still be cured by extended treatment with antibiotics, either oral or intravenous. In some cases, however, Lyme arthritis doesn't appear to respond to antibiotics. Patients with continuing symptoms are encouraged to consult a specialized Lyme disease clinic.

There is controversy over the use of antibiotics as a preventive treatment for people who have vague symptoms or fear they may have been bitten by a tick. Because of the side effects of antibiotics, the lack of evidence that prevention is effective, and the low probability of developing symptoms after a tick bite (about 1 percent in the U.S.), this strategy is not widely recommended.

### OVERDIAGNOSIS

*Some experts warn that public concern over the dangers of Lyme disease has led to overreporting. Dr. Allen Steere of Tufts University, who first identified the disease in 1975, has reported that of 788 patients referred to his Lyme disease clinic, only 180 had the disease. Conditions often confused with Lyme disease include chronic fatigue syndrome, fibromyalgia, non-Lyme arthritis, and other disorders.*

## PREVENTION

If you spend time outdoors in areas inhabited by the deer tick, wear shoes, long pants tucked into socks, and long sleeves. Use insect repellent around your ankles. If you work or walk in brushy areas or woods, check regularly for ticks; they are easier to see against light clothing. Indoors, inspect for ticks, especially around the armpits, groin, scalp, and beltline (plus the neck and head of children). Check pets often as well.

If you do find a deer tick on your skin, remove it immediately. With tweezers or gloved fingers, grasp it as close to the skin as possible, pulling gently and steadily. Be patient; ticks secrete a special substance that "cements" them to your skin. Save the tick if possible for identification. Wash the bite with soap and water.

Even if the tick's mouthparts remain embedded in the skin, removal of the body reduces the risk of infection; the bacteria-bearing salivary glands are in the gut, far from the mouth. If redness develops around the bite, see your doctor. ■

## SYMPTOMS

**Hodgkin's disease,** one type of lymphoma, may cause no symptoms, especially in young people. When symptoms are present, they may include:
- painless lumps in the neck, armpits, or groin caused by swollen lymph nodes.
- severe itching all over the body.
- fever, chills, night sweats, loss of weight and appetite, persistent fatigue, and general weakness.
- persistent coughing, shortness of breath, and chest discomfort.

The symptoms of **non-Hodgkin's lymphoma,** in addition to those listed above, include:
- swelling or fullness in the abdomen from an enlarged spleen.
- enlarged lymph nodes in the groin.
- changes in bowel habits or bleeding from the rectum, if the disease involves the stomach or intestines.
- nasal congestion, sore throat, or difficulty swallowing, if the disease involves the throat or sinuses.

## CALL YOUR DOCTOR IF:

- you detect any symptoms associated with lymphoma. The most probable warning signs are swollen lymph nodes in the neck, armpits, or groin, although any suspicious symptom that persists for more than two weeks should be diagnosed.

Spread like a web throughout the body are thin vessels that carry a colorless fluid called lymph. Suspended in the fluid are lymphocytes, white blood cells whose purpose is to fight disease and infection. Connecting this network are small, bean-sized organs called lymph nodes; the lymph nodes, which are concentrated in the armpits, neck, groin, chest, and abdomen, filter the fluid and initiate the body's immune response. The lymphatic system—which also includes the spleen, thymus, tonsils, and bone marrow—is constantly defending the body against millions of microscopic attackers.

In some circumstances, however, lymphocytes can become cancerous and start multiplying out of control. Common types of lymphoma usually begin as a malignant tumor in a lymph node and can spread wherever healthy lymphocytes travel—through lymph and blood to other lymphatic tissue and possibly to organs outside the lymphatic system. Left unchecked, cancer cells multiply and eventually displace healthy lymphocytes, suppressing the immune system.

The term *lymphoma* refers to a varied group of diseases that range from slow-growing chronic disorders to rapidly evolving, acute conditions. **Hodgkin's disease,** named for the English physician who described it in 1832, represents one type; all others, despite their diversity, are commonly called **non-Hodgkin's lymphomas.**

Hodgkin's disease is distinguished from other lymphomas by the abnormal Reed-Sternberg cell—named for the pathologists who first detected it—which can be seen easily under a microscope. Hodgkin's disease tends to spread methodically from one cluster of lymph nodes to the next and responds predictably to treatment. It usually starts in lymph nodes in the neck or just under the collarbone; spreads into the chest, abdomen, and pelvis; and may eventually invade such organs as the spleen and the lungs, as well as bones and bone marrow.

Lymphomas represent about 5 percent of all cancers in the United States. Each year some 50,000 cases are diagnosed, about 15 percent of them Hodgkin's disease. At least 10 types of **non-Hodgkin's lymphoma** exist, each ranked as low, intermediate, or high grade according to how ag-

### THE LYMPHATIC SYSTEM

A fluid called lymph protects the body against infection by circulating lymphocytes, a type of white blood cell that attacks infectious organisms. The system's main organ is the spleen, connected by a network of tiny lymphatic vessels to clusters of lymph nodes throughout the body. Lymphocytes passing through body tissues destroy most infections before they can enter the bloodstream.

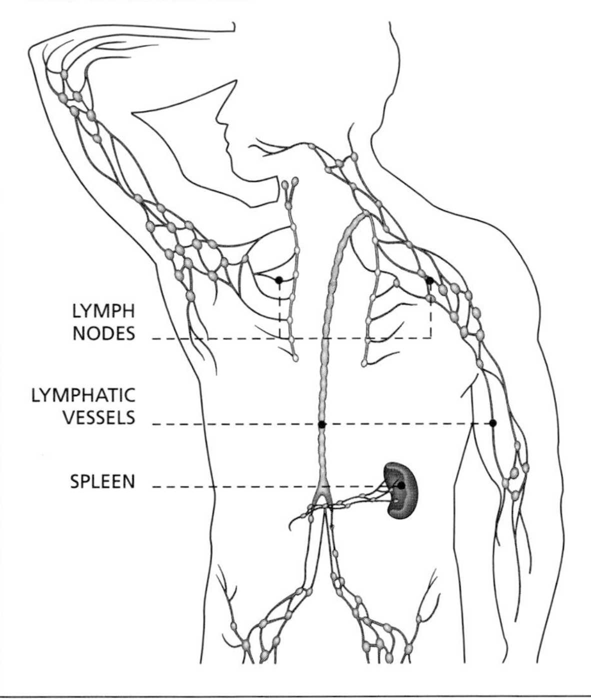


gressively it behaves. Low-grade versions usually progress slowly and tend not to spread beyond the lymphatic system. High-grade versions may spread to distant organs within a few months. Lymphoma is most commonly seen in Caucasian men. Hodgkin's disease usually appears between the ages of 15 and 30, or after 50; non-Hodgkin's lymphomas rarely strike people younger than 45.

Hodgkin's disease is now one of the most curable of all cancers, with an overall five-year survival rate of nearly 80 percent; when the disease is detected and treated early, the rate jumps to 90 percent. Although non-Hodgkin's lymphomas are typically more difficult to cure, the overall five-year survival rate has improved from 30 to more than 50 percent in recent decades. A low-grade case can be controlled for years with treatment but is difficult to eradicate completely. High-grade cases, while more immediately threatening, are potentially curable with aggressive treatment.

## CAUSES

The cause of Hodgkin's disease is unknown. Most people diagnosed with this form of lymphoma are in general good health. There may be a hereditary link, as siblings of people with Hodgkin's disease are seven times more likely than average to get the disease.

The causes of non-Hodgkin's lymphoma are also largely unknown. A form called **Burkitt's lymphoma** is strongly associated with infection by the Epstein-Barr virus, a herpesvirus most commonly found in Africa. Other lymphomas have been linked to infection by either HIV—the cause of AIDS—or HTLV, another member of the HIV family. Since the onset of AIDS in the early 1980s, the incidence of non-Hodgkin's lymphoma has increased 65 percent, while the incidence of Hodgkin's disease has decreased. Other conditions that compromise the body's immune function, such as organ transplantation, treatment with radiation or chemotherapy, or such autoimmune disorders as lupus and rheumatoid arthritis, also increase a person's risk for non-Hodgkin's lymphoma.

### DIAGNOSTIC AND TEST PROCEDURES

Doctors do not know how to detect lymphoma before it starts causing symptoms. Swollen lymph nodes in the neck, armpits, or groin usually offer the first clue. A patient may report the swelling, or it may be detected during a routine checkup. A doctor may also suspect lymphoma when swelling in lymph nodes or the spleen is accompanied by more general symptoms such as fatigue, chills, or night sweats.

Blood and urine studies coupled with imaging tests can reveal abnormalities that help early diagnosis of lymphoma, but the disease must be confirmed by a biopsy—usually of a lymph node but sometimes of affected skin or lung tissue that is removed surgically and studied by a pathologist. The size, shape, and pattern of cells under a microscope can determine whether lymphoma exists and, if so, what type.

If cancer is found, further testing can determine how widespread it is. Doctors can examine the lymphatic system using CT scans or an x-ray procedure called a lymphangiogram. For this procedure, the patient is injected with a dye that highlights the lymphatic system on x-ray. A bone-marrow biopsy is usually performed to check for the presence of cancer cells in the bone marrow. Exploratory surgery may be required to determine the full extent of the affected lymph nodes.

## TREATMENT

Lymphomas are among the cancers most responsive to radiation and chemotherapy. As these treatments have become more sophisticated, the survival rates for lymphoma have risen steadily. Most lymphoma patients now survive at least five years with conventional treatment. Success has been especially remarkable with Hodgkin's disease: At least 75 percent of newly diagnosed cases are now considered curable.

### CONVENTIONAL MEDICINE

Specifics of treatment vary from case to case, depending on the type of lymphoma involved, the presence or absence of symptoms, and the patient's age and general health. Given the complexity of decision making, lymphoma patients should be encouraged to solicit the opinion of a lymphoma specialist at a major cancer center before starting a particular treatment regimen.

When limited to one or a cluster of lymph nodes, **Hodgkin's disease** can be treated effectively with radiation therapy. To treat large tumors or Hodgkin's disease that has begun to spread, however, chemotherapy—sometimes along with radiation therapy—is the best treatment option. Such treatment pursued aggressively cures up to 40 percent of advanced cases of Hodgkin's disease.

Since success depends on high doses of toxic drugs and radiation, treatment frequently results in unpleasant side effects and can cause residual complications such as infertility. Medication along with various complementary therapies can help control some side effects. Male patients may want to consider banking their sperm before treatment begins. Premenopausal women often stop menstruating during treatment, but menstruation may resume after treatment ends.

Treatment decisions for **non-Hodgkin's lymphoma** depend largely on the grade of the disease. Low-grade disease usually progresses very slowly and—although responsive to chemotherapy—often recurs. Rather than having a patient endure unnecessary treatment, a doctor may choose to monitor a low-grade case closely and act only when it begins to accelerate. By contrast, high-grade cases merit immediate and aggressive radiation therapy, chemotherapy, or both.

Researchers continue to investigate new treatment methods in the hope of improving cure rates for advanced and recurrent lymphoma. The underlying objective is—and always has been—to kill cancer cells, but without harming healthy cells. Various ways to do so are under study. Immunotherapists are experimenting with certain biological agents, such as interferon, to stimulate immune cells into attacking cancer cells more aggressively. Other researchers are synthesizing special proteins called monoclonal antibodies that specifically target cancer cells. When fused with toxic chemicals or radioactive agents, these antibodies are intended to deliver lethal blows to cancer cells without harming the surrounding healthy cells. The anticancer arsenal includes many other techniques for making cancer cells more sensitive to radiation and drug treatment. In some cases, bone-marrow transplantation is used to allow the administration of higher-dose chemotherapy. *(See box at right.)*

Lymphoma patients who achieve remission should have regular cancer-oriented checkups, because lymphoma recurs in a significant percentage of survivors within two or three years. With successful treatment of Hodgkin's disease, relapse after five years of remission is rare.

*(See Cancer for further information on chemotherapy, radiation therapy, and other forms of cancer treatment.)*

L

### BONE-MARROW TRANSPLANTATION

*A few decades ago, oncologists (cancer specialists) faced a frustrating problem. They knew that heavy doses of chemotherapy or radiation could force some cancers "over the threshold" into remission. They also knew that such treatment could irreparably damage bone marrow, without which a person cannot live. But what if the bone marrow were sacrificed to wipe out the cancer, then resupplied? Bone-marrow transplantation emerged as a potential solution. Today, bone-marrow transplantation is accepted as a risky but appropriate therapy for some types of cancer, curing a significant number of otherwise incurable patients.*

*Transplantation for lymphoma relies on using the patient's own bone marrow. A small amount of marrow is removed, treated with chemicals to eliminate cancer cells, then placed in cold storage. Meanwhile, the patient receives chemotherapy—sometimes with radiation therapy. As the cancer cells are wiped out, so too are the remaining marrow cells. The stored, cancer-free bone marrow is then returned to the patient's body intravenously.*

*Gradually, immature blood cells in the replacement bone marrow start to multiply. Until this occurs, a patient's immune system is severely suppressed and the possibility of infection is a constant concern. To minimize this dangerous phase, doctors employ "growth factors" that speed the regrowth of healthy bone marrow. This and other refinements promise to make bone-marrow transplantation an increasingly safe and valuable cancer therapy.*

### COMPLEMENTARY THERAPIES

Lymphoma and its standard treatment of toxic drugs and radiation contribute to weakening of the immune system. Many therapies that are believed by some researchers to enhance the body's immune function can complement standard treatment safely, may sustain general health, and actually may help the body fight cancer. Rest, relaxation, and sound nutrition are the foundation for restoring good health. Joining a support group may help release emotions that contribute to stress. See Cancer for more suggestions.

### AT-HOME CARE

Chemotherapy and radiation therapy can cause unpleasant side effects, such as nausea, vomiting, diarrhea, fatigue, and vulnerability to infection. Your doctor can prescribe medication to address some of these problems, and you can do a number of things to relieve symptoms: Eat light meals. Avoid dairy products and sweet, fried, or fatty foods. Drink plenty of liquids before and after meals. If the smell of cooked food makes you feel nauseated, try eating foods cold or at room temperature. Wear loose-fitting clothing. Be careful about keeping your skin clean and scratch free, and avoid contact with obviously sick people. Rest whenever you feel the need, but otherwise keep yourself busy with activities that will help take your mind off the immediate discomfort.

## PREVENTION

With only limited knowledge of what causes lymphoma, doctors cannot provide detailed preventive guidelines. Staying as healthy as possible may reduce your risk for cancer in general. Standard advice includes eating a well-balanced diet, keeping your weight in check, exercising regularly, and getting adequate sleep. All these measures contribute to healthy immune function. Unless you are absolutely certain that your sexual partner is HIV negative, be sure to use a condom during sexual intercourse to avoid infection. ■

# MACULAR DEGENERATION

## SYMPTOMS

- dim or distorted vision, especially while reading.
- gradual, painless loss of precise central vision.
- blank spots in your central field of vision; straight lines that appear wavy.

## CALL YOUR DOCTOR IF:

- you exhibit any of the symptoms above and have never seen an ophthalmologist. Ask your doctor for a referral.
- you exhibit any of the symptoms above and have hypertension, diabetes, or heart disease. You are in the high-risk category for the advanced **wet** form of macular degeneration. Any abnormality in your vision is a sign that you may be developing the disorder.
- you have been diagnosed with **age-related macular degeneration** and then you discover blank spots in your field of vision, printed matter appears distorted, or straight lines appear wavy. You may be developing the advanced **wet** form of macular degeneration.

Macular degeneration is the leading cause of vision loss in the United States, with more than 13 million Americans showing some sign of the disorder. Because the symptoms usually do not appear in people under 55 years of age, the disorder is often referred to as **age-related macular degeneration (ARMD).** If you are over 65, macular degeneration may already affect your central vision, even though most sufferers of the disease maintain functional side, or peripheral, vision throughout life. The disorder occurs in two forms, **dry** and **wet.** The less common **wet** form of ARMD requires immediate medical attention; any delay in treatment may result in loss of your central vision.

## CAUSES

Macular degeneration is scarring of the macula, a spot about 1/16 inch in diameter at the center of the retina. The macula enables you to read, watch television, drive, sew—anything that requires focused, straight-ahead vision. Although the rest of the retina can continue to process images at the sides of your field of vision, the scarring distorts or obscures part of the central image that your eye transmits to your brain.

In the **dry** form of ARMD, tiny yellow deposits develop beneath the macula, signaling a degeneration and thinning of nerve tissue. A small number of cases develop into the **wet,** or **neovascular,** form of ARMD, in which abnormal blood vessels grow beneath the macula. As these vessels leak blood and fluid onto the retina, retinal cells die, causing blurs and blank spots in your field of vision.

You are more susceptible to ARMD as you get older, especially if there is a history of the disorder in your family. Atherosclerosis, diabetes, heart disease, high blood pressure, and nutritional deficiencies are also risk factors.

### DIAGNOSTIC AND TEST PROCEDURES

Your ophthalmologist will inspect the macula as part of a routine eye exam. A painless photographic procedure, fluorescein angiography, shows the pattern of your eye's blood vessels and can detect any abnormalities.

## TREATMENT

Macular degeneration is not reversible, so people who develop **dry** ARMD typically compensate with large-print publications and magnifying lenses for everyday activities. **Wet** ARMD may be successfully treated with laser surgery. Both forms respond positively to ophthalmology treatment as well as to alternative remedies.

### CONVENTIONAL MEDICINE

The more common **dry macular degeneration** cannot be cured, but it can be kept from getting worse under an ophthalmologist's care. For the **wet** form, a surgical procedure called laser photocoagulation destroys leaking blood vessels that have grown under the macula, halting the damaging effects to your vision. This procedure must be done before leakage from abnormal blood vessels causes irreversible damage.

### ALTERNATIVE CHOICES

Drawing on the body's natural abilities and functions, alternative treatments attempt to restore nutrient deficiencies that can damage the macula.

#### HERBAL THERAPIES

Collagen, one of the most abundant proteins in the body, plays an integral role in maintaining the strength and function of your eye tissue. The collagen structure of your retina may be strengthened and reinforced by taking 100 mg of bilberry *(Vaccinium myrtillus)* extract daily.

Dried ginkgo *(Ginkgo biloba)*—40 mg three times a day—may guard against damage to your macula by free radicals, unstable molecules found in the body that can harm cells.

#### NUTRITION AND DIET

Many older people exhibit deficiencies in zinc, which normally appears in high concentrations in the retina, particularly the macula. Ask your doctor about taking a zinc supplement to help protect the macula from damage and improve sharpness of vision. Antioxidants are said to fight the negative effects free radicals have on your retinal blood vessels. To increase your intake of antioxidants, take 1,000 mg of vitamin C three times a day, 600 IU of vitamin E a day, 200 mcg of selenium a day (avoid higher doses), or 20 mg of beta carotene (vitamin A) a day.

**AMSLER GRID**

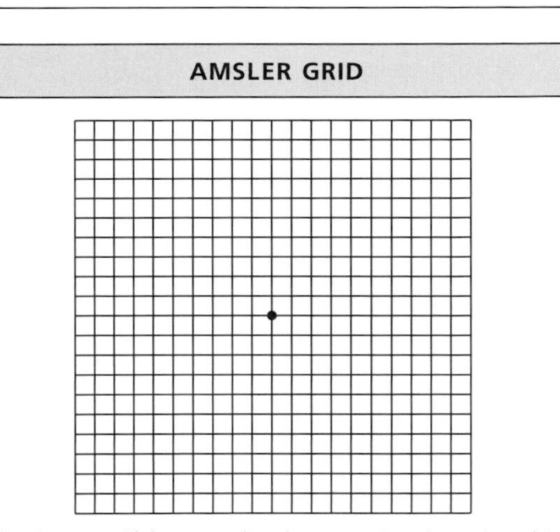

Check yourself for macular degeneration by using this Amsler grid. Place this page on a flat surface in good light. Wearing reading glasses or contact lenses, cover one eye and look at the dot at the center of the grid from a distance of 12 to 15 inches; repeat with your other eye. If any of the lines on the grid appear wavy, distorted, or missing, discuss the condition with your ophthalmologist.

### AT-HOME REMEDIES

Your ophthalmologist will suggest large-print reading material, magnifiers, and other aids to enhance your eyesight. You can monitor changes in your eyesight at home with an Amsler grid *(above)*.

Eat more fruits and vegetables rich in vitamin C, such as citrus fruits, cauliflower, and broccoli. Snack on nuts and seeds, which contain vitamin E. Yellow vegetables containing carotene, as well as cherries, blackberries, and blueberries, all of which contain antioxidant flavonoids, are also said to help stave off degeneration of the macula. Cut back on consumption of alcohol, tobacco, and coffee, all of which may aggravate eye problems.■

# MALARIA

## SYMPTOMS

- headache, fatigue, low-grade fever, and nausea.
- sudden chills and, sometimes, severe shaking.
- a fever that can be as high as 107°F, accompanied sometimes by rapid breathing.
- profuse sweating.

## CALL YOUR DOCTOR IF:

- you experience the symptoms of malaria while in an area of the world where malaria is transmitted or up to several months after returning.
- you will be traveling to an area where malaria is common; your doctor can prescribe a preventive antimalarial medication.

M

Malaria is an infectious disease transmitted by mosquitoes. Worldwide, about 300 million to 500 million people get malaria each year, including about 1,000 people in the United States—all but a handful of whom contract the disease abroad. Almost all tropical and subtropical countries have malaria-transmitting mosquitoes.

Early symptoms of malaria include headache, fatigue, low-grade fever, and nausea. Within about 24 hours, the illness frequently progresses into three distinct stages. First comes the cold stage, characterized by sudden chills and, sometimes, violent shaking, which lasts one to two hours. The second, or hot, stage is marked by a fever, which can go as high as 107°F, at times accompanied by rapid breathing; this lasts three to four hours. The wet stage follows: two to four hours of profuse sweating.

## CAUSES

Malaria is caused by a bite from the female *Anopheles* mosquito, which injects the malaria parasites into the bloodstream. Four species of a parasite known as *Plasmodium* cause malaria in humans: *P. vivax, P. ovale, P. malariae,* and *P. falciparum.* Once in the bloodstream, the plasmodia travel to the liver, where they multiply at a tremendous rate. Within a week or so, up to 40,000 of them flow back into the bloodstream, where they continue to multiply and begin to destroy red blood cells. It is this destruction that causes the characteristic symptoms of malaria.

Although all four species can be deadly, *P. falciparum* is particularly dangerous—and more likely to be fatal—because it multiplies much more quickly than the others, destroying many more blood cells. This species is also more resistant to antimalarial drugs.

Forms of both the *P. vivax* and *P. ovale* parasites can remain dormant in the liver without creating any apparent symptoms of malaria for months or, in rare cases, years. Then one day, for reasons as yet unknown to scientists, they leave the liver and return to the bloodstream, causing a malaria attack. So if you have at any time traveled to a part of the world where malaria is prevalent, be sure to report that fact to your doctor if you develop an unexplained illness with a fever.

### DIAGNOSTIC AND TEST PROCEDURES

If your doctor suspects that you have malaria, a sample of your blood will be examined for evidence of the parasites. If the first smear is negative but malaria is strongly suspected, samples may be taken and examined every 12 to 24 hours for three consecutive days.

## TREATMENT

Left untreated, *P. falciparum* malaria can be fatal. Quick and appropriate conventional treatment, however, can result in a speedy and complete recovery. Other forms of malaria rarely cause death but still require treatment to avoid complications and ease recovery.

### CONVENTIONAL MEDICINE

If you are infected with *P. vivax, P. ovale, or P. malariae,* you will receive chloroquine orally for three days. To help avoid later recurrences caused by dormant *P. vivax* or *P. ovale* parasites, you will also be given oral doses of primaquine for 14 more days. Because primaquine can destroy red blood cells and thus threaten the health of a fetus, it is not given to pregnant women; if you are pregnant, you will be kept on chloroquine.

If you became infected with *P. falciparum* in an area of the world where it has not been shown resistant to chloroquine, you will be treated with that drug. Otherwise, you will be given oral doses of either quinine and tetracycline, or quinine and a combination product of pyrimethamine and sulfadoxine for several days. If you are vomiting or have serious medical complications, you may be given intravenous quinidine until you are well enough to take the other drugs.

### ALTERNATIVE CHOICES

Alternative therapies can treat the symptoms of malaria and help your body recover from antimalarial medications, which can cause unpleasant, although temporary, side effects, such as nausea, dizziness, diarrhea, tinnitus, and skin rashes. All remedies should be taken in conjunction with conventional medications and under professional supervision.

#### HERBAL THERAPIES

Boneset *(Eupatorium perfoliatum),* sometimes called feverwort, was used by Native Americans and early American colonists to treat feverish illnesses, including malaria. Make a tea, using 1 to 2 tsp of the dried herb; drink it as hot as possible and as often as every half hour.

#### HOMEOPATHY

Remedies prescribed for malaria include Arsenicum album and Sulphur. Consult a homeopath for dosages and length of treatment.

## PREVENTION

If you are going to an area where malaria exists, tell your doctor several weeks before you leave. Your doctor will put you on a regimen of mefloquine, doxycycline hyclate, or chloroquine. If you plan to travel in an area where malaria is a problem, take the following precautions:

- Take a preventive antimalarial medication before, during, and after the trip.
- Sleep under mosquito netting treated with an insecticide, such as permethrin or deltamethrin.
- Stay in buildings with air conditioning or screened doors and windows.
- Stay indoors from dusk to dawn, the time when mosquitoes feed.
- If you go out in the evening, wear long pants and a long-sleeved shirt.
- Use a mosquito repellent: a permethrin spray for clothing and a lotion with 35 to 40 percent diethyltoluamide (DEET) for exposed skin.

### TIP FOR TRAVELERS

For current information on malaria hot spots in the world, call the Centers for Disease Control and Prevention hot line at 404-332-4555 or fax information service at 404-332-4565. ■

# MANIC-DEPRESSION

## SYMPTOMS

Dramatic and unpredictable mood swings are the primary sign of manic-depression. The illness has two strongly contrasting phases.

**In the manic phase:**

- euphoria or irritability.
- excessive talk; racing thoughts.
- inflated self-esteem.
- unusual energy; less need for sleep.
- impulsiveness, a reckless pursuit of gratification—shopping sprees, impetuous travel, more and sometimes promiscuous sex, high-risk business investments, fast driving.
- hallucinations.

**In the depressive phase:**

- depressed mood and low self-esteem.
- overwhelming inertia and apathy.
- sadness, loneliness, helplessness, guilt.
- slow speech, fatigue, and poor coordination.
- insomnia.
- suicidal thoughts and feelings.
- use of psychostimulants such as amphetamines to boost energy and spirits.

## CALL YOUR DOCTOR IF:

- you notice some of these symptoms in a family member. Note: Manic-depressives often deny anything is wrong, especially in the manic phase. If you are worried about a family member or close friend, a doctor can offer advice on how to handle the situation.
- you notice some of these symptoms in yourself.

Manic-depression, known to mental health professionals as bipolar disorder, is a serious, double-edged mental illness. In contrast to the sustained bleakness of generalized depression (technically described as unipolar disorder), manic-depression is characterized by cyclical swings between elation and despair. The pattern of the mood alternations varies widely among sufferers. In some cases, years of normal functioning can separate manic and depressive episodes. In others, the episodes cycle frequently, three or four times a year, with respites between. For some patients, depression and mania cycle continuously and sometimes rapidly. And for a rare few, an episode of manic-depression may occur only once in a lifetime. (If it occurs twice, it is usually followed by other episodes.) Generally, the depressive phase lasts longer than the manic phase, and it also tends to be more frequent; the cycle can be erratic.

Manic-depression is known to afflict about 1 percent of the U.S. population, although its incidence may be much higher because almost 75 percent of cases go untreated. Men and women are equally susceptible. Much evidence suggests that the illness has a genetic basis, but its origins are still uncertain. The symptoms apparently result from chemical imbalances in the brain, and they lie beyond voluntary control. The disorder is not only life-disrupting but can also be dangerous: About 20 percent of manic-depressives commit suicide, usually when they are passing from one phase to another and feel disoriented. Some 11 percent of sufferers take this drastic action in the first decade after diagnosis.

Fortunately, great strides have recently been made in treating this illness; in most cases, the symptoms can be controlled effectively by medication and other therapies.

The disorder occurs in two main forms, known as **bipolar I** and **bipolar II;** they may have separate genetic origins. In **bipolar I,** both phases of the illness are apt to be very pronounced. In **bipolar II,** mania is often mild (it is termed hypomania), and the depression can be either mild or severe. Bipolar II is more difficult to diagnose and is often mistaken for generalized depression. It has fewer and shorter periods of remission than bipolar I, tends to run in families, and is somewhat less responsive to treatment. It may be the more common form of manic-depression.

The illness is sometimes linked to seasonal affective disorder, with depression occurring in late fall or winter, giving way to remission in the spring, and progressing to mania or hypomania in the summer.

About 1 case of manic-depression in 5 begins in late childhood or adolescence; adolescents are more likely than adults to have physical and psychotic symptoms such as hallucinations and delusions, and they are more apt to be misdiagnosed *(see Diagnostic and Test Procedures, below).* Usually, however, the illness strikes young adults between the ages of 25 and 35. The first episode in males is likely to be manic; the first episode in females, depressive—and frequently, a woman will experience several episodes of depression before a manic episode occurs. As patients grow older, recurrences of either bipolar I or bipolar II tend to come more frequently and last longer.

## CAUSES

Manic-depression is thought to result from chemical imbalances in the brain, caused by a defective gene or genes. Among the neurotransmitters possibly involved are serotonin and norepinephrine, but the neurochemical interplay in manic-depression is complex and not yet completely understood. The likelihood that genes play a role is supported by the fact that usually there is some family history of mood swings, depressive illness, or suicide.

### DIAGNOSTIC AND TEST PROCEDURES

Because of the stigma still attached to manic-depression (and to many other mental diseases), patients are frequently reluctant to acknowledge that anything is amiss, and physicians often fail to recognize the disorder. In addition, the symptoms may sometimes seem to be merely exaggerated versions of normal moods. In any event, research suggests that almost 75 percent of all cases go untreated or are treated inappropriately.

The American Psychiatric Association has established a long list of specific criteria for recognizing the disorder. Evaluation involves investigating the patient's history and also any family history of mood swings or suicide. Other disorders must be ruled out—particularly such childhood problems as school phobia and attention deficit disorder, as well as dementia, schizophrenia, and psychotic states induced solely by alcohol or drugs. Substance abuse is common in manic-depressives and can mask the symptoms, thus complicating diagnosis and treatment *(see Drug Abuse).* Recognizing and treating any substance abuse is a priority, since it is a strong predictor of suicide, especially in men.

Before treatment begins, the patient receives a careful physical exam, and blood and urine are tested to detect conditions that could put medical constraints on the choice of treatment. A thyroid analysis is particularly important both because hyperthyroidism *(see Thyroid Problems)* can look like mania and because lithium—the principal drug treatment for manic-depression—is known to lower thyroid function. During treatment, frequent blood tests are necessary to see that adequate drug levels have been reached and to detect adverse reactions at an early stage.

IMPORTANT!

- **Be on the lookout for suicidal tendencies, especially when someone is passing from one phase to another—a time of disorientation.**
- **As a parent or spouse, make sure you understand bipolar disorder and its specific manifestations in your family member.**
- **If you find yourself or a family member consistently taking psychostimulants such as amphetamines to boost spirits and energy, consider the possibility of manic-depressive illness. Untreated bipolar disorder is very serious, and early detection can minimize its lifetime effects.**

## TREATMENT

At present, manic-depression is treated most often with a combination of the drug lithium and psychotherapy. While drug therapy is primary, ongoing psychotherapy is important to help patients understand and accept the personal and social disruptions of past episodes and better cope with future ones. In addition, since denial is often a problem, routine psychotherapy helps patients stay on their medications. (Patient compliance is particularly tricky in adolescence.) Almost all forms of psychotherapy can be used—cognitive, behavioral, or psychodynamic; individual, family, or group.

The family or spouse of a patient should be involved with any treatment. Having full information about the disease and its manifestations is important for both the patient and loved ones.

### CONVENTIONAL MEDICINE

Lithium carbonate is the principal drug used in treating manic-depression; it can be remarkably effective in reducing mania, although doctors still do not know why. Lithium may also prevent recurrence of depression, but it is often given in conjunction with varying combinations of antidepressants. The newly developed selective serotonin reuptake inhibitors (SSRIs)—specific to the neurotransmitter serotonin—are usually the antidepressants of choice because they have fewer side effects than older drugs. Among the SSRIs are fluoxetine, sertraline, and paroxetine. Other antidepressants include the tricyclics—such as desipramine, imipramine, and amitriptyline—and bupropion, a class of drug different from but similar to the SSRIs.

Haloperidol is sometimes given to patients who fail to respond to lithium, or to treat acute symptoms of mania before lithium can take effect (7 to 10 days). In severe cases, or when a patient does not respond to lithium, other drugs such as carbamazepine and valproic acid, used alone or in combination with lithium, may be prescribed.

Many of these drugs can be toxic and should be closely monitored through blood tests to see that adequate levels have been reached and to detect any adverse reactions early on. When beginning treatment, the psychiatrist will need to experiment with medications. It is almost impossible to predict which patient will react to what drug or what the dosage should be.

**Electroconvulsive therapy (ECT)** is sometimes used for severely manic or depressed patients and for those who don't respond to medication. Because it acts quickly, it can also help patients who are considered to be at high risk for committing suicide. ECT fell out of favor in the 1960s, but the procedure has been greatly refined since then. The patient is first anesthetized. Then an electric current is passed through the temporal lobe to produce a grand mal seizure of short duration—no more than a few seconds. During the course of ECT treatments—usually two to three weeks—lithium is discontinued to prevent neurotoxic complications.

**Light therapy** has proved effective when bipolar disorder has a connection to winter depression. For those people who usually become depressed in winter, sitting for 20 to 30 minutes a day in front of a special light box with a full-spectrum light of about 10,000 lux can effectively treat their depression *(see Seasonal Affective Disorder)*.

### ALTERNATIVE CHOICES

With severe manic-depression **(bipolar I),** alternative medicines and practices may not be very useful during the episodes themselves. The depressed patient is often too low to initiate any exercise or energizing techniques; the manic, too hyperactive to undertake relaxation practices. However, alternative approaches may be beneficial between episodes and for less severe manic-depression **(bipolar II).**

One research study has suggested that magnesium may be a possible replacement for lithium in cases that involve frequent shifts from one manic-depressive phase to the other. It has the advantage of being nontoxic and is available in health food stores. Further studies are needed, but researchers believe that the outlook for the use of magnesium is favorable. Talk to your doctor or psychiatrist about this option.

M

**ACUPRESSURE FOR MANIC PHASE**

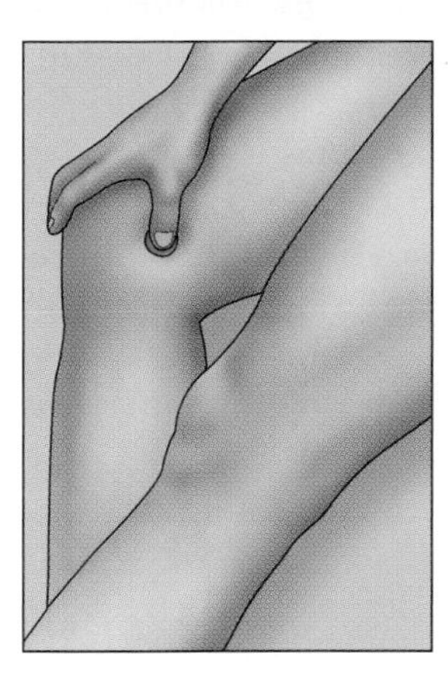

Pressing Liver 8 may help relieve the effects of manic-depression. Bending your right knee, place your thumb above the inside knee crease, just below the joint of the knee (swing your leg a few times to find it). Press for one minute, two or three times, then repeat on your left leg.

**YOGA FOR DEPRESSIVE PHASE**

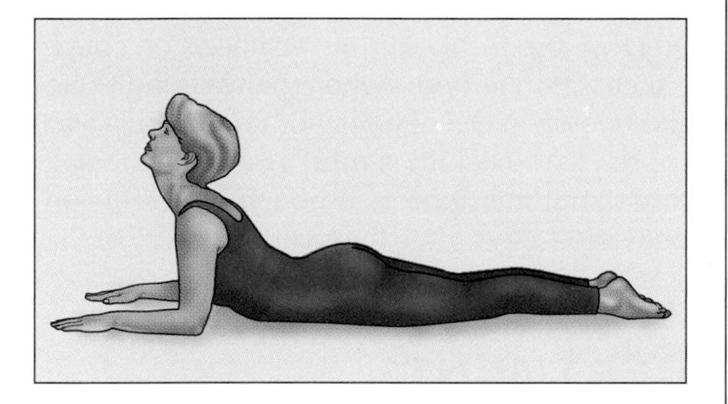

For the **Sphinx,** place both forearms on the floor, palms down and elbows directly under your shoulders. Inhale and push your chest away from the floor as far as comfortably possible. Hold for a few deep breaths, then relax and exhale.

**Chinese herbs** may soften mood swings, bringing some relaxation to the manic phase and reducing depression in the depressive phase. But be sure to seek a practitioner of Chinese medicine who is experienced in treating depression and knows how to use herbs. (Not all people who practice Chinese medicine are skilled in treating mood states or in using herbs to do so.)

A diet low in vanadium (a mineral found in meats and other foods) and high in vitamin C can be similarly helpful, but the diet should be monitored by a nutritional expert or an orthomolecular physician. A skilled **homeopath** may also ameliorate the intensity of mood swings.

Certain **acupuncture** treatments are designed to either energize or relax the body, depending on the acupuncture points used. Oil **massage** can also be relaxing or energizing.

### BIOFEEDBACK

Practitioners report that EEG biofeedback is effective in training manic-depressives to control some of the brain-wave states underlying hyperactivity, racing thoughts, irritability, lack of sleep, and poor self-control; it also seems to work for brain-wave activity associated with low energy, low self-esteem, and poor motor coordination. If the manic-depression is mild, this form of biofeedback may substitute for lithium and other drugs, although it can be used safely together with lithium. Because EEG biofeedback is new, only a thousand or so practitioners in the U.S. are trained in the technique. See Health Associations and Organizations in the Appendix for more information.

## AT-HOME REMEDIES

Maintain a calm environment, particularly when someone is in a manic phase. Keep to regular routines for daily activities—sleeping, eating, and exercise. Adequate sleep is very important in preventing the onset of episodes. Avoid excessive stimulation: Parties, animated conversation, and long periods of watching television or videos can exacerbate manic symptoms.

In the manic phase, patients may engage in risky activities, such as fast driving or certain sports; they should be monitored and prevented from taking chances, especially in a car. Drinks and foods containing caffeine—tea, coffee, cola, and chocolate—should be eliminated in the manic phase. Avoid alcohol at all times. ■

# MEASLES

## SYMPTOMS

If your child has measles, he will be very sick. Look for the following symptoms:

- Days 1-3: mild to high fever, harsh cough, runny nose, red eyes, and sneezing; tiny white spots on gums near upper molars or inside cheeks.
- Days 4-8: high fever; characteristic rash, spreading from face to trunk, then to arms and legs. Skin starts to peel in 2 to 3 days. Rash fades from the face by the time it reaches the arms and legs.

Your child may also develop inflammation of the eyes (conjunctivitis), which will make the eyes sensitive to light. *(See also the Visual Diagnostic Guide.)*

## CALL YOUR DOCTOR IF:

- you think your child has measles; your doctor may have received notice of an epidemic and may be able to confirm your diagnosis over the phone.
- your child has measles and his cough becomes harsher or more productive, which could indicate viral pneumonia.
- your child has measles and is having trouble staying fully awake; is extremely lethargic; or is suffering from irritability, disorientation, or convulsions within a week of the onset of the rash. This could indicate encephalitis.
- your child has measles and develops difficulty hearing or pain in the ears, which may indicate an ear infection *(see Otitis Media).*

Measles is one of the most contagious childhood viral infections and one of the most severe, with complications ranging from ear infections to pneumonia and encephalitis (an inflammation of the brain that occurs in 1 out of 1,000 patients). Measles can easily become an epidemic in schools. Preventive immunization is usually recommended, if not required by state law *(see page 33).*

Adults can contract measles if they have not been previously exposed or immunized. People who have once had measles develop a natural immunity and cannot contract it again.

## CAUSES

Measles is a virus that is transmitted by direct contact or by droplets from a sneeze or cough. The incubation period—when the virus multiplies in the body and the child is not contagious—is 8 to 12 days. Your child is most contagious 2 days before symptoms appear, although he is still contagious for 4 days after the rash begins.

## TREATMENT

If you suspect that your child has measles, you should always consult your child's pediatrician, who will want to notify the schools and will also want to monitor your child's progress so as to be ready to intercede if complications arise. Infected children should not return to school until a week after the rash appears.

### CAUTION!

**Never give your child aspirin—even baby aspirin—or other products containing the salt called salicylate to reduce a fever or to relieve pain. Aspirin has been linked to Reye's syndrome, a rare but very dangerous illness that causes inflammation of the liver and brain.**

### IDENTIFYING THE RASH

In the first 24 hours, small, pale red spots appear along the hairline and behind the ears, then spread across the face and down the torso *(right);* they later spread onto the arms and legs. The spots typically expand into irregular patches.

By the third day, the rash becomes more profuse and pronounced. As it wanes, it may become scaly and take on a brownish tinge. The rash usually disappears within a week.

## CONVENTIONAL MEDICINE

Your child's pediatrician will prescribe bed rest, a soft-foods diet, and increased liquid intake. The doctor may also give a gamma globulin injection to family members not previously exposed or immunized. While this won't prevent measles from spreading, it may make the course of the illness less severe for at-risk individuals.

## ALTERNATIVE CHOICES

Do not rely on home treatment alone; consult the child's primary healthcare practitioner.

### HERBAL THERAPIES

No herbs treat measles specifically. However, a number of preparations may help alleviate the symptoms. Teas of yarrow *(Achillea millefolium),* catnip *(Nepeta cataria),* and linden (*Tilia* spp.) may help reduce fever. An eyebright *(Euphrasia officinalis)* eyewash or a chamomile *(Matricaria recutita)* compress may ease sensitive eyes. You can seek help from a medical herbalist.

### HOMEOPATHY

Always consult a homeopath for appropriate dosages for children. In homeopathic medicine, Aconite is thought to help a child who suffers a sudden onset of fever; has red eyes; is restless, anxious, or fearful, and sensitive to light. Belladonna is suggested when the child has flushed red hot skin, a hot head and face but cold extremities, and high fever. Pulsatilla may help if your child has a mild fever, is weepy, is not thirsty, and has a creamy yellow discharge from the eyes or nose.

### OSTEOPATHY

Gentle, rhythmic pressure applied over the spleen, a procedure known as spleen pumping, may enhance the release of white blood cells into the blood. Seek help from an osteopath.

## AT-HOME CARE

- Children need to be isolated for most of the time they are contagious. A dimmed room may help if their eyes are sensitive to light; in such a case, limit TV viewing and reading.
- Calamine lotion, distilled witch hazel, or cornstarch or baking soda baths alleviate itching. Acetaminophen may reduce fever.
- A humidifier can ease a bad cough. Be sure to use one with a humidistat for the proper amount of mist in the air. Always clean the humidifier thoroughly before and after use.

# PREVENTION

Many alternative practitioners feel it is better for an otherwise healthy child to contract measles than to be vaccinated, because fighting the illness strengthens the immune system. However, immunization is usually required by state law, as measles can cause epidemics in schools. The MMR (measles, mumps, and rubella vaccine) is now given at 12 or 15 months, with a booster at the age of 4 to 6 or 10 to 12. The homeopathic version of immunization is not an accepted equivalent and will not provide adequate protection, but some homeopaths will prescribe remedies to ease the potential side effects of the MMR. ■

# MÉNIÈRE'S DISEASE

## SYMPTOMS

- intermittent dizziness (vertigo), sometimes accompanied by nausea and vomiting, pallor, and exhaustion.
- hearing problems, including increasing hearing loss, tinnitus (a ringing, roaring, or buzzing sound in the ears), a sensitivity to loud noises, and the sensation of not hearing the same sounds in both ears.
- a feeling of fullness in the ears, sometimes beginning before the attack of dizziness.
- headache.

## CALL YOUR DOCTOR IF:

- you suspect you have Ménière's disease, which requires a medical evaluation.
- you have recurrent episodes of dizziness; difficulty in maintaining balance may point to problems in your inner ear that need medical attention.
- you find it more and more difficult to hear; a gradual loss of hearing over time may indicate a problem in any part of your ear (inner, middle, or outer) or in your brain.
- sounds are different to each ear; this may be a sign of other types of inner ear disorder in addition to Ménière's.

Approximately 2.4 million Americans have Ménière's disease, a disorder of the inner ear that can worsen over time, often leading to poor job performance, accidents, and psychological distress. First described over a century ago by French physician Prosper Ménière, this disease is characterized by numerous symptoms, all relating to problems in the inner ear, home of the body's sensory organs for hearing and balance.

More than 96 percent of Ménière's disease patients suffer bouts of vertigo, or dizziness. These dizzy spells can last anywhere from less than an hour to two days, striking as infrequently as once a year or as often as several times a year. Following an attack, the patient often feels completely exhausted and falls asleep, waking up later feeling fine.

People with Ménière's disease can also have a variety of hearing complaints with or without vertigo. A person might, for example, experience a gradual loss of hearing, a roaring, buzzing, or ringing in the ears (tinnitus), or the sensation that tones sound different in one ear than in the other, a phenomenon known as diplacusis.

Ménière's disease usually occurs in people between the ages of 20 and 60, striking on average at the age of 40. However, the disorder has also affected children as young as 4 and seniors as old as 90. The trouble usually starts in one ear and, in many patients, progresses to the other ear. Sometimes, though, the disease simply goes away on its own for reasons that are unclear. Unfortunately, no one knows which patients will get better and which will not.

## CAUSES

Attacks of Ménière's disease can be triggered by anxiety, tension, or excessive salt intake. And while scientists are still debating the exact cause of the disorder, they do know that it involves an overabundance of endolymph, the fluid that fills the inner ear, or labyrinth *(above, right).*

The inner ear is actually a pair of sensory organs squeezed into the temporal bone, a tiny compartment in the side of the skull. One component of the inner ear, the spiral-shaped cochlea, converts sound waves into electrical impulses and sends them to the brain. Another part contains a series of rings called semicircular canals. Inside these rings is a fluid that responds to changes in your body's position (lying down, standing up, or leaning to one side, for example). Signals from the canals, together with information streaming in from the eyes and nerve endings in the skin, help the brain figure out if your body is upright or falling down. For some reason, in Ménière's disease the inner ear fills up with too much fluid, throwing off your sense of balance. Occasionally, the fluid can even seep into the cochlea and affect your hearing.

People with an abnormally shaped inner ear or temporal bone, whether by birth or as a result of an injury, are more likely to develop Ménière's disease. The shape and fluid levels of the inner ear can also be altered by certain diseases and conditions including middle ear infections (otitis media), syphilis, leukemia, otosclerosis (bone hardening in the middle ear), and immune problems.

### DIAGNOSTIC AND TEST PROCEDURES

Most of the time, an experienced otolaryngologist (ear, nose, and throat specialist) can tell if you have Ménière's disease simply by examining your medical history and performing some simple tests in the office. However, because dizziness and hearing problems can be caused by a wide variety of disorders—some inconsequential, some quite serious—arriving at a proper diagnosis can sometimes be tricky.

To rule out other problems, your doctor may conduct a thorough examination. Some of the diagnostic procedures your physician may order include audiometry, which tests hearing patterns in the ears; x-rays to determine the shape of your skull or any past injuries; and electrocochleography, in which a probe is inserted through the eardrum to test for electrical characteristics of your inner ear that may indicate the nature of your hearing problems.

**INNER EAR DISRUPTION**

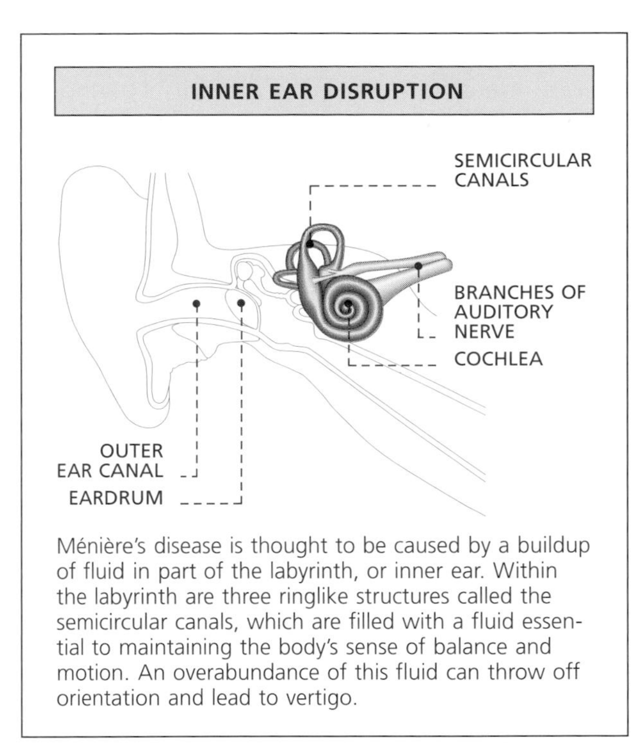


Ménière's disease is thought to be caused by a buildup of fluid in part of the labyrinth, or inner ear. Within the labyrinth are three ringlike structures called the semicircular canals, which are filled with a fluid essential to maintaining the body's sense of balance and motion. An overabundance of this fluid can throw off orientation and lead to vertigo.

## TREATMENT

Because scientists haven't yet found a cure for Ménière's disease, most treatment is directed at alleviating the symptoms and dealing with the psychological impact of the disorder. Surgery is reserved as a last resort for patients with extremely serious cases.

### CONVENTIONAL MEDICINE

Treatment for Ménière's disease often begins with medications that attempt to reduce the pressure and fluid in the inner ear. Typically prescribed drugs include diuretics (to increase fluid excretion) and sedatives (to calm the patient and reduce feelings of dizziness). Meclizine and diazepam are two drugs commonly prescribed to reduce dizziness; some physicians also use antihistamines, such as promethazine and dimenhydrinate, to reduce feelings of vertigo. Recently, physicians have also recommended skin patches of scopolamine, used to combat seasickness.

Some patients may find these medications helpful, but scientific studies don't uniformly support their use. For one thing, many of these drugs can cause unwanted side effects, and none will cure the disorder.

Some physicians also prescribe "pressure chamber" treatments in an attempt to improve the pressure in the ear by changing the pressure outside it. If a patient is experiencing severe dizziness, a doctor might prescribe a type of drug called an aminoglycoside in an attempt to destroy the balance function of the labyrinth while preserving the patient's ability to hear. This type of drug is usually prescribed when a patient has the disease in both ears.

A number of surgical procedures with a similar aim—intentionally destroying the labyrinth of the inner ear to halt the debilitating dizziness—have also been developed. Surgical techniques include vestibular neurectomy, which involves cutting the nerves going to the balance side of the inner ear, and labyrinthectomy, or removal of the labyrinth. These drastic procedures, which seriously disrupt balance and completely destroy the hearing apparatus, are generally reserved for patients with severe vertigo.

In another operation, called endolymphatic-sac surgery, the physician tries to preserve both hearing and balance by draining the inner ear or installing little valves, or shunts, in the labyrinth to relieve pressure. Results are usually good after the first year, but some people report a return of their dizziness later.

## ALTERNATIVE CHOICES

Like most conventional remedies for Ménière's disease, alternative treatments seek to relieve stress and other symptoms.

### ACUPUNCTURE

For dizziness, consult an acupuncturist for stimulation at the following ear points: neurogate, sympathetic, kidney, occiput, adrenal, and heart. For chronic cases, an acupuncturist may treat body points on the kidney, triple warmer, and spleen meridians. See pages 22–23 for point locations and page 20 for more information about meridians.

### AROMATHERAPY

To relieve stress, bathe with essential oils of lavender, geranium, and sandalwood. Or you might try a gentle massage with lavender essence and chamomile oil.

### BODY WORK

For chronic cases of Ménière's disease, consult an **osteopath** or **chiropractor** for adjustments to the head, jaw, neck, and lower back relating to movement restriction that might affect the inner ear. For acute cases of dizziness, a **reflexologist** might suggest massaging the ear area; this and

**REFLEXOLOGY**

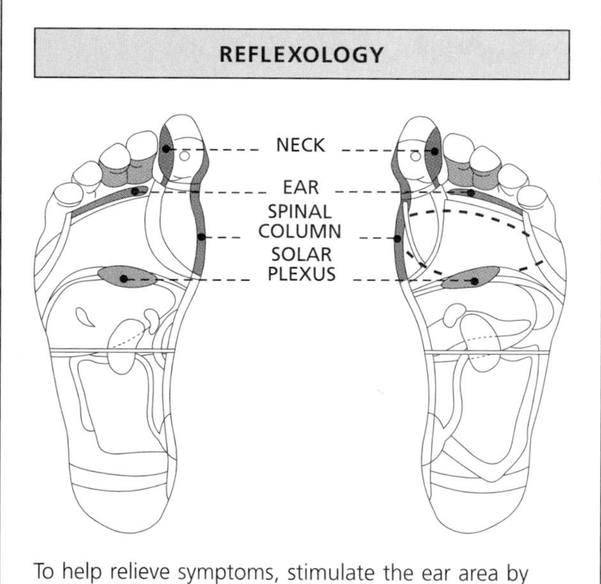


To help relieve symptoms, stimulate the ear area by walking your thumb along the base of the small toes and the shafts of the second and third toes. Walk your thumb up and down the upper portion of the spinal column area, and work the neck area on the big toe. Then stimulate the solar plexus area.

other areas that may prove beneficial are illustrated below, left.

#### CHINESE HERBS

Although some practitioners of Chinese medicine distinguish types of dizziness, a general all-purpose remedy includes xanthium *(Xanthium sibiricum)*, magnolia flower *(Magnolia liliflora)*, licorice *(Glycyrrhiza uralensis)*, honeysuckle flower *(Lonicera japonica)*, and other herbs. Visit a practitioner of Chinese medicine for a proper prescription; bear in mind that you may be allergic to some Chinese herbs.

#### HOMEOPATHY

A patient with Ménière's disease has several homeopathic options—all of which call for a dosage of 12x every four to six hours. For dizziness during an acute attack that is worse from sensitivity to motion and that is accompanied by a headache and a roaring or buzzing in the ears, try Bryonia. For dizziness and nausea in an acute attack, use Cocculus. And for dizziness that is worse when lying down or turning over and that is accompanied by sensitivity to light, try Conium. If you don't feel better in a day or two, or if you have a chronic case of Ménière's disease, you should seek the advice of a professional homeopathic practitioner.

#### MIND/BODY MEDICINE

In Ménière's disease, patients undergo a vicious cycle of attacks followed by anxiety and stress, which in turn can provoke an attack. A number of communities across the country sponsor Ménière's disease support groups where people can discuss their problems with sympathetic listeners. Various forms of **massage** therapy and **yoga** are also great ways to reduce stress.

#### NUTRITION AND DIET

Some nutritionists recommend a diet for Ménière's disease that seeks to increase calories, fat, and protein, although there is no evidence that such a regimen can cure the disease. Specialists also recommend a daily intake of the following: 2,000 mg of vitamin C; 50 mg each of vitamins $B_1$, $B_2$, and $B_6$; 20 mg of zinc; and other vitamins and minerals. If you have Ménière's disease, you may want to stay away from salt—which causes your body to retain fluid—and to restrict your intake of liquids. Some experts speculate that lowering fluid levels in your body helps relieve the buildup of pressure in your inner ear, but this has not been proved. A nutritionist or dietitian can help prescribe a diet for any specific problems you may have.

### AT-HOME REMEDIES

- During an attack of Ménière's disease, lie still and try to relax.
- Try reducing your intake of liquids and salt; some people believe that lowering fluid levels in the body can help reduce the pressure of fluid buildup in the inner ear.
- Avoid caffeine, smoking, and alcohol, which may increase stress and interfere with a proper resting state.
- Try to get a good night's sleep.
- Avoid driving, swimming, climbing on ladders, and other activities in which an attack of dizziness might lead to a serious injury.

## PREVENTION

The best way to prevent an attack of Ménière's disease is to reduce the stress in your life. Seek out enjoyment, perhaps through a hobby or a sport. Give yourself time off to pursue the things that give you pleasure: Listen to music, take a soothing bath, read a magazine, drink a relaxing tea—chamomile *(Matricaria recutita)* is a good choice—or simply take some time to sit and do nothing. If stress and anxiety continue to be problems, you may want to seek the advice of a counselor or a psychotherapist. ■

# MENINGITIS

## SYMPTOMS

- fever.
- severe headache.
- stiff neck, shoulders, or back.
- severe shooting pain down the back of the neck and sometimes along the spine when bending the neck forward.
- inability to tolerate bright light (photophobia).
- a bumpy and splotchy dark red or purplish rash anywhere on the body.
- drowsiness and mental confusion.
- vomiting.
- seizures and coma.
- in infants, a bulge of the fontanel, the soft spot on the skull.
- in infants, an eerie high-pitched cry.

## CALL YOUR DOCTOR IF:

- you develop the symptoms listed above—particularly a combination of severe headache, stiff neck, and painful aversion to light; **seek emergency medical care immediately.**
- your infant develops the symptoms listed above; **seek emergency medical care immediately.**

Meningitis is an infection of the delicate membranes, or meninges, that cover the spinal cord and brain. It is almost always a complication of another bacterial or viral infection that began elsewhere in the body, such as in the ears, sinuses, or upper respiratory tract. The bacterial form is an extremely serious illness, which requires immediate medical care. If not treated quickly, it can lead to death within hours or to permanent neurological damage. Viral meningitis tends to be less severe; most people recover from it fully, with no aftereffects.

Meningitis is relatively rare. In the United States, fewer than 3,000 cases occur each year, mostly in children under the age of two. The illness begins with simple flulike symptoms—fever, headache, and vomiting—followed by progressive drowsiness and often severe neck pain, particularly when the head is bent forward. Very young children often react to the pain by arching their backs uncontrollably. Some forms of meningitis produce a dark red or purplish rash anywhere on the body. In babies, the swelling of the meninges may also cause the fontanel—the soft spot on the top of the skull—to bulge.

Meningitis can be contagious among people living close together—in university dorms, for example. Outbreaks of meningitis, particularly the bacterial form, have been rare in the United States, although since 1991 such outbreaks have been increasing for reasons not yet understood.

## CAUSES

Bacterial meningitis is caused by any one of several bacteria. Three types—*Hemophilus influenzae* type b, *Neisseria meningitidis* (meningococcus), and *Streptococcus pneumoniae* (pneumococcus)—account for about 80 percent of bacterial meningitis cases in the United States. These bacteria are often carried harmlessly in the nasal passages or elsewhere on the bodies of a small percentage of healthy people, and are spread from person to person through coughing and sneezing. Some research indicates that people are more vulnerable to bacterial meningitis after a bout of the flu because inflamed nasal tissues offer bacteria an easy entranceway into the body.

Viral meningitis can be triggered by a variety of viruses, including several that cause diarrhea and one that can be transmitted to humans from infected hamsters and other rodents. Meningitis can also be caused by a fungus; the most common one is cryptococcus, which is found in pigeon droppings. Fungus-related meningitis is rare in healthy people, but not uncommon in people with HIV, the human immunodeficiency virus that causes AIDS.

### DIAGNOSTIC AND TEST PROCEDURES

Confirmation of meningitis requires a lumbar puncture, or spinal tap. This moderately painful procedure is done in a hospital under a local anesthetic. A needle is slipped between two of the bones of the spine to extract a small sample of spinal fluid. If the normally clear fluid appears cloudy and contains pus cells, meningitis is suspected. Further examination will determine which specific organism is involved.

Samples of your blood, urine, and secretions from your nose or ears may also be taken. Because the disease can progress so rapidly, treatment will begin immediately—even before the results of the tests are known.

## TREATMENT

The bacterial form of meningitis in particular is life-threatening. It must be treated swiftly by conventional means. Seek emergency medical care at the first sign of symptoms.

### CONVENTIONAL MEDICINE

If you have meningitis, you will be admitted to the hospital and remain there until the infection has been eradicated—possibly as long as two weeks. If you have a bacterial form of the disease, you will be given very high doses of antibiotics, perhaps intravenously. A class of antibiotics called cephalosporins is widely used to treat bacterial meningitis. Because antibiotics are not effective against viral meningitis, treatment usually involves intravenous fluids and rest.

Meningitis is contagious, so you will probably be put in an isolated room for at least 48 hours. If the meningitis has caused your eyes to be oversensitive to light, your room will be darkened. You will receive plenty of liquids and perhaps aspirin to relieve fever and headache.

Doctors may need to drain an infected sinus or mastoid (an area of the bone behind the ear) to prevent reinfection.

If you have meningococcal meningitis, your doctor may recommend that people with whom you have been in close contact undergo preventive antibiotic treatment. A vaccine for some types of meningococcal meningitis is sometimes prescribed to larger groups of people when a small epidemic of the disease has broken out, as well as to individuals traveling overseas to a meningitis risk area, such as sub-Saharan Africa. Further, vaccination against the *Hemophilus influenzae* type b bacterium is now a routine part of childhood immunizations.

### ALTERNATIVE CHOICES

Because meningitis is a quickly progressing life-threatening illness, you should use alternative treatments only after you have received emergency medical care. Alternative treatments are designed to help your body recover and to build up your resistance to a recurrence. Consult a **homeopath,** for a constitutional remedy, or a practitioner of Chinese medicine, who might advise **acupuncture, acupressure,** or a combination of **Chinese herbs** to strengthen your immune system. A **chiropractor** or **osteopath** may also prescribe treatments to help you regain strength.

#### NUTRITION AND DIET

To maintain a healthy immune system and prevent recurrences of infections that can lead to meningitis, eat a low-fat, high-fiber, nutrient-dense diet; avoid sugar and processed foods. Vitamin supplements can also be helpful. Take vitamin A (2,500 to 10,000 IU once a day), vitamin B complex (500 mg three times a day), and vitamin C (500 to 2,000 mg once a day). ■

# MENOPAUSAL PROBLEMS

## SYMPTOMS

Not all women experience symptoms with the onset of menopause. If symptoms occur, they may include:

- hot flashes—sudden reddening or heating of the face, neck, and upper back, which may produce sweating. Flashes typically last only a few minutes.
- night sweats, which may disrupt sleep and lead to insomnia.
- pain during intercourse, caused by thinning of vaginal tissues and loss of lubrication.
- increased nervousness, anxiety, or irritability.
- the need to urinate more often than before, especially during the night.

## CALL YOUR DOCTOR IF:

- you experience bleeding after menopause; among other possibilities, it may be a sign of uterine cancer, so you should be checked by your doctor.

Menopause simply means the end of menstruation, but the term is also used to refer to the months and years in a woman's life before and after her final period—a time that may or may not bring with it some physical or emotional changes.

Most women menstruate for the last time at about 50 years of age; a few do so as early as 40, and a very small percentage as late as 60. Most women notice some menstrual changes—such as irregular periods and light menstrual flow—up to a few years before menstruation ceases.

Some symptoms—including hot flashes and mood swings—are temporary and will pass as your body adjusts. But more-permanent problems can also result. Decreased levels of estrogen, for example, affect the way bones absorb calcium and can raise cholesterol levels in the blood; postmenopausal women thus face increased risk for developing both osteoporosis and cardiovascular diseases such as atherosclerosis.

## CAUSES

Typically during a woman's forties, her ovaries slow and then cease their normal functions, including the production of eggs. Even more significant, they decrease their production of estrogen and progesterone. As levels of these hormones—especially estrogen—decline, they cause changes throughout the body and particularly in the reproductive system, the most notable change being the end of menstruation. Decreased estrogen levels may also be responsible for the various symptoms associated with menopause.

## TREATMENT

In both conventional and alternative medicine, the most common approach to treating menopausal problems is to resupply the body with the estrogen it no longer produces in sufficient quantities. Known in conventional medicine as **hormone replacement therapy,** this technique is somewhat controversial because of certain side effects, so you should carefully consider the risks and the benefits in consultation with your doctor.

## CONVENTIONAL MEDICINE

**Hormone replacement therapy (HRT)** consists of estrogen and progestin supplements—usually given orally or through a skin patch. Most HRT patients take a combination of estrogen and progestin because estrogen alone has potentially serious side effects, such as endometrial cancer and uterine cancer. Progestin can cause side effects such as irregular bleeding, headaches, bloatedness, and breast swelling and pain. You may even develop an artificial monthly period, depending on the dosage regimen you're on. If you have had a hysterectomy and have no uterus, you do not need progestin.

### MENOPAUSAL MYTHS AND FACTS

***MYTH:*** *Menopause makes women emotionally unstable.*
***FACT:*** *Most women experience no emotional problems; those that occur can be treated.*

***MYTH:*** *Menopause puts an end to sexual desire.*
***FACT:*** *Vaginal dryness can make intercourse painful, reducing desire, but this is readily treated with vaginal lubricants or estrogen creams. Menopause itself can affect libido either positively or negatively; some women actually have increased libido with menopause.*

***MYTH:*** *Menopause disrupts a woman's life.*
***FACT:*** *Most women experience few or no menopausal problems; 25 percent have moderate, treatable symptoms. In countries where age is respected, women report the fewest symptoms during menopause.*

Your doctor may recommend HRT to help prevent cardiovascular disease and osteoporosis, particularly if these diseases run in your family.

Your doctor may prescribe a vaginal estrogen cream to help stop the thinning of vaginal tissues and improve lubrication.

If you have had breast cancer, endometrial cancer, liver disease, or blood clots, you should not take estrogen, because it increases your chance of a recurrence. But progestin alone may relieve hot flashes.

## ALTERNATIVE CHOICES

### CHINESE HERBS

Some Chinese herbs—including dong quai *(Angelica sinensis)* and Asian ginseng *(Panax ginseng)*—contain a form of estrogen known as phytoestrogen, or plant estrogen. Exact proportions are important, and some dosages are toxic; consult an herbalist.

### HERBAL THERAPIES

Phytoestrogen is found in a variety of herbs and foods. Extracts and teas made from black cohosh *(Cimicifuga racemosa)* may supply beneficial amounts of phytoestrogen. Estrogenic herbal creams may help relieve vaginal dryness and dry skin. Combinations of motherwort *(Leonurus cardiaca),* chaste tree *(Vitex agnus-castus),* wild yam *(Dioscorea villosa),* and other herbs may help with the rapid heartbeat that comes with hot flashes.

### NUTRITION AND DIET

Eating foods high in plant estrogens, such as soy beans and lima beans, may alleviate symptoms; other sources include nuts and seeds, fennel, celery, parsley, and flaxseed oil.

## AT-HOME REMEDIES

- Raise your calcium intake and engage in weight-bearing exercises to avoid osteoporosis and maintain general good health.
- Take 400 to 800 IU of vitamin E daily to treat hot flashes and reduce the risk of cardiovascular disease. ■

# MENSTRUAL PROBLEMS

## SYMPTOMS

- Menstruation does not occur. Called **amenorrhea,** this can come from pregnancy, overexercise, or anorexia nervosa.
- Menstruation is painful and produces clots. Called **dysmenorrhea,** this may be entirely normal, but it may also be caused by endometriosis; polyps, fibroids, or other lesions of the uterus; or an intrauterine device (IUD).
- Menstrual flow is heavy. Called **menorrhagia,** this condition can be a result of stress, endometriosis or other pelvic lesions, pelvic infection, or an IUD.

## CALL YOUR DOCTOR IF:

- you have heavy menstrual flow that fills a tampon or sanitary napkin within an hour; heavy flow can cause anemia.
- you have missed a period and think you may be pregnant; a late flow that is unusually heavy could indicate a miscarriage.
- you experience sharp abdominal pain before periods or during intercourse; you could have endometriosis.
- you get your period after menopause.

Menstruation is a normal part of a woman's reproductive cycle. When an ovary releases an egg, it also releases the hormone estrogen, which stimulates the lining of the uterus to grow and engorge with blood. If the egg is not fertilized, the ovary releases progesterone, which makes the uterus shed its lining; the resulting menstrual flow typically consists of a few tablespoonfuls of blood and tissue fragments. This series of events repeats on a cycle of approximately 28 days until interrupted by pregnancy or ended by menopause.

The degree of discomfort or pain a period causes, as well as the amount of menstrual flow, varies widely among individuals. Also, your own period may occasionally be heavier or more painful than usual. Such problems, while unpleasant, generally do not signal underlying disease. But you should be aware that the same complaints can sometimes indicate more serious conditions, such as endometriosis or an ovarian cyst.

The three main categories of menstrual irregularities are **lack of period** (amenorrhea), **painful periods** (dysmenorrhea), and **heavy periods** (menorrhagia). The following text explains these problems and what you can do about them.

## LACK OF PERIOD

Although often no cause for concern, amenorrhea can be a sign of an underlying problem. It might indicate, for example, that you have low levels of estrogen in your system and are therefore at a greater risk of developing osteoporosis. Or it may signal a lack of progesterone and that you are at a greater risk for endometrial problems, including endometrial cancer *(see Uterine Problems)*. Also, of course, if you do not menstruate, you cannot become pregnant.

### CAUSES

The lack of a period in a woman who has not yet begun to menstruate is known as primary amenorrhea; in a woman who has temporarily stopped menstruating, it is known as secondary amenorrhea. Primary amenorrhea has several causes, the most likely of which is that a girl has simply not yet reached puberty. (It is perfectly normal for puberty to occur as late as the age of 17.) But delayed puberty in a girl who is very thin or who exercises excessively is worrisome, because it could indicate anorexia nervosa; women with very low body fat do not menstruate.

Primary amenorrhea can also point to other problems. In rare cases, for example, a girl might actually lack ovaries or a uterus and therefore not be able to menstruate. Or a tumor, an injury or trauma, or a structural defect might be interfering with some aspect of the menstrual cycle, from the production of hormones to the actions of the organs and tissues that the hormones affect.

Secondary amenorrhea can also be traced to injuries or structural abnormalities; one common cause is ovarian cysts. But factors such as stress can also disrupt the balance of hormones and thereby interrupt the normal cycle. Also, as in adolescence, extreme underweight can stop menstruation; if your period stops while you are dieting or in athletic training, you may be overdoing it. And, of course, amenorrhea could signal the onset of menopause or pregnancy.

### MENSTRUAL MYTHS AND FACTS

***MYTH:*** *A bath causes or worsens menstrual cramps.*
***FACT:*** *Soaking in a warm bath can soothe and relax muscles, thereby reducing pain.*

***MYTH:*** *Menstruating women should restrict their activities, and even stay in bed and rest.*
***FACT:*** *Women can carry on normal activities during their period. Exercise may actually help lessen pain by stimulating muscles to release endorphins.*

## TREATMENT

### CONVENTIONAL MEDICINE

Treatment for primary amenorrhea may involve no more than waiting to see if nature takes its course. For a girl who exercises strenuously or who is very thin, a doctor might advise a lighter training regimen or an effort to gain weight. Treatment for anorexia nervosa might also be necessary. If the doctor suspects a hormonal irregularity, drug treatment to replace missing hormones might be prescribed. In rare circumstances, surgery to remove a cancerous or noncancerous growth—or to correct a structural problem—might be called for.

For secondary amenorrhea, if you think stress may be to blame, take steps to reduce stress in your life; this alone may restore your cycle. If you are underweight, your doctor will advise you to gain some weight and try to maintain it. If you have been diagnosed with some other condition that may be causing amenorrhea—such as endometriosis or an ovarian cyst—seek treatment for that problem, and ask your doctor whether your periods will return. If not, or if your amenorrhea is related to the onset of menopause, your doctor may prescribe estrogen or ask you to take calcium to lower your risk of osteoporosis. *(See also Menopausal Problems and Ovary Problems.)*

### ALTERNATIVE CHOICES

#### HERBAL THERAPIES

To help initiate menstrual flow, make a tincture of one part chaste tree *(Vitex agnus-castus),* two parts blue cohosh *(Caulophyllum thalictroides),* and two parts mugwort leaf *(Artemisia argyi);* take 2 ml three times daily until menstrual flow begins.

#### NUTRITION AND DIET

To address nutrient deficiencies that may be causing amenorrhea, take supplements of or eat foods rich in zinc (fish, poultry, lean meats) and vitamin B complex (brewer's yeast, wheat germ).

YOGA

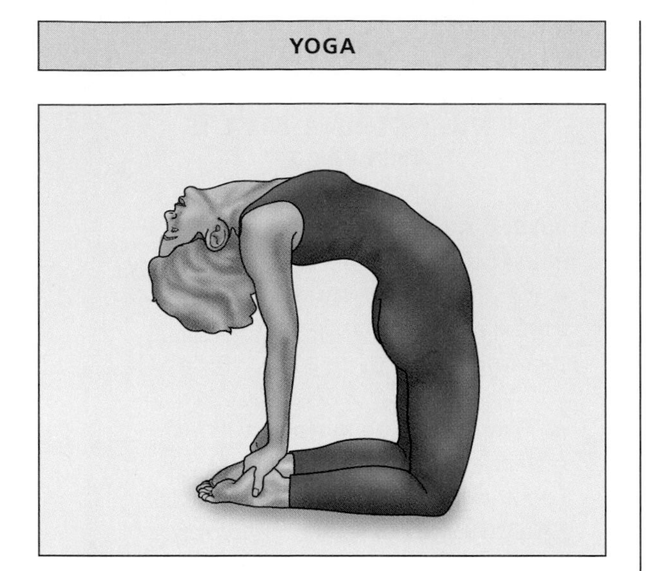

**1** Regular use of the **Camel** may help amenorrhea. First, kneel down. Lean backward as you exhale, placing your palms on the floor behind you and tilting your head back. Inhale as you squeeze your buttocks and press your pelvis forward. Then place your hands on the soles of your feet *(above)*. Breathe slowly as you hold for 20 seconds.

To release, exhale as you sit back on your heels. Then inhale as you bring your body up, raising your head last. Breathe slowly and relax for 20 seconds. Do once or twice a day.

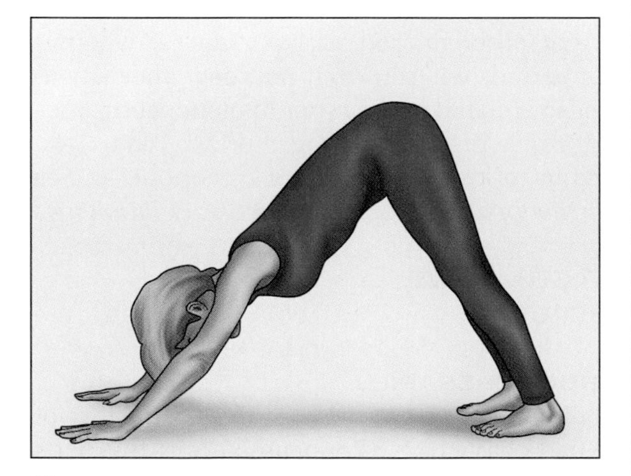

**2** The **Downward Dog** pose helps release pelvic tension. From the Table position on your hands and knees, inhale and raise your pelvis to form an inverted V with your knees slightly bent.

Press your palms and heels against the floor as you breathe deeply, keeping your arms and shoulders open and your back and legs straight *(above)*. Hold for 20 to 30 seconds.

To release, exhale as you resume the Table position. Sit back on your heels, bring your head up, and relax before attempting to stand up again.

## PAINFUL PERIODS

Menstrual pain, or dysmenorrhea, is hardly unusual and in most cases is completely normal, even if troublesome. But there are situations in which painful periods may signal a condition that requires further evaluation by your doctor. And if your pain interferes with your normal activities, you should consider some of the treatments listed here, which may help bring you relief.

## CAUSES

If you have always had painful periods, they are probably the result of hormonal changes during your menstrual cycle. The factor most likely to be causing pain is that your body is producing an excess of prostaglandins—hormonelike substances that cause contractions of the uterus during menstruation and when a woman goes into labor. During menstruation, these contractions ensure that all the menstrual blood and tissue are expelled from the body, but excess prostaglandins can cause repeated contractions—and perhaps even spasms—which are experienced as cramping. It is common for these pains to persist throughout your reproductive years, but many women find that menstrual cramps become milder after they have had a baby.

Dysmenorrhea may, however, also be caused by an underlying condition, such as endometriosis, an infection, or growths in the uterus *(see Uterine Problems and Uterine Cancer)*.

## TREATMENT

In addition to the suggestions listed below, see the appropriate entries for treatment advice related to an underlying condition.

### CONVENTIONAL MEDICINE

Analgesics such as aspirin and acetaminophen can relieve mild discomfort, but if your pain is more intense, try an analgesic such as ibuprofen, mefenamic acid, or naproxen, all of which inhibit the release of prostaglandins. Your doctor may also prescribe birth-control pills or progesterone, which may affect your balance of hormones in ways that will help relieve pain.

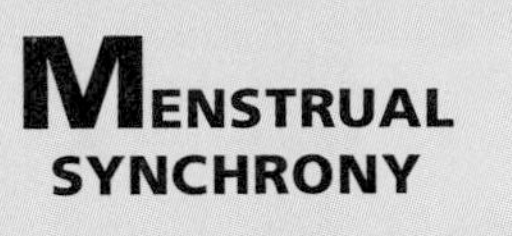

### MENSTRUAL SYNCHRONY

*Women who live or work together in close quarters may notice that they're all getting their periods at the same time. This is known as menstrual synchrony, and it often happens in closed communities such as convents, prisons, and dormitories. What causes this phenomenon is not clear, but it may be linked to pheromones—chemical messengers that are carried in the air from person to person (or from animal to animal) and that have powerful effects on body functions and behaviors, even though people are not consciously aware of them.*

## ALTERNATIVE CHOICES

Most of the alternative therapies for menstrual cramps focus on promoting the relaxation of tense muscles or on reducing tension in general.

### ACUPRESSURE

An acupressure technique that may prove effective in relieving menstrual pains is illustrated on the following page.

### AROMATHERAPY

Massage the lower abdomen, back, and legs with oil or lotion containing chamomile *(Matricaria recutita).*

### CHIROPRACTIC

Chiropractic techniques can sometimes help relieve menstrual cramps; see a chiropractor for treatment.

### HERBAL THERAPIES

To relieve cramps, drink a hot tea of 2 tsp cramp bark *(Viburnum opulus)* simmered for 15 minutes in 1 cup water; use this three times a day. Bilberry *(Vaccinium myrtillus)* and bromelain will also relax muscles. Dong quai *(Angelica sinensis)* and feverfew *(Chrysanthemum parthenium)* can relax uterine muscles; feverfew may work by inhibiting prostaglandin synthesis. Valerian *(Valeriana officinalis)* helps relax cramping muscles; however, it may be addictive and should be used only for a limited time. Consult an herbalist.

Evening primrose oil *(Oenothera biennis)* applied over painful areas can also bring relief, but don't use it if there's a chance you may get pregnant. In addition, a castor-oil pack placed over painful areas can be helpful.

Tension, anxiety, and painful spasms may be relieved with treatments of black haw *(Viburnum lentago),* skullcap *(Scutellaria baicalensis),* and black cohosh *(Cimicifuga racemosa).* Take equal parts of these herbs in 5-ml doses as needed.

### NUTRITION AND DIET

Eating a balanced diet consisting of small meals throughout the day rather than three larger meals and avoiding sugar, salt, and caffeine may help relieve or prevent cramping. You may get relief from a multivitamin, multimineral supplement containing vitamin B complex, calcium, and magnesium. You can also try taking 50 mg of vitamin $B_6$ twice a day. Because your overall goal is to keep your body relaxed, avoid caffeine and other stimulants.

### YOGA

Poses for relaxation and relief of cramps are illustrated opposite.

ACUPRESSURE

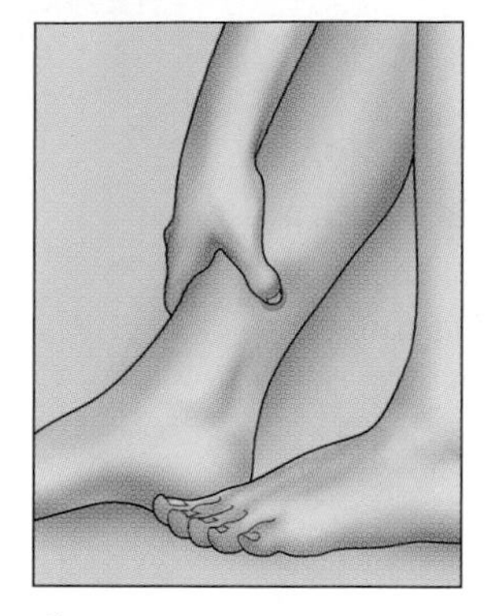

**1** Water retention during menstruation may make you uncomfortable. Find SP 6 on the inside of your leg, four finger widths above the anklebone, near the inner edge of your shinbone. Hold for one minute. Repeat on the other leg. Do not use this point if you are pregnant.

**2** To help improve your overall circulation during menstruation, apply pressure to SP 8, four finger widths below the knee on the inside of your leg. Press firmly between your calf muscle and your leg bone, and hold for one minute. Repeat on the other leg.

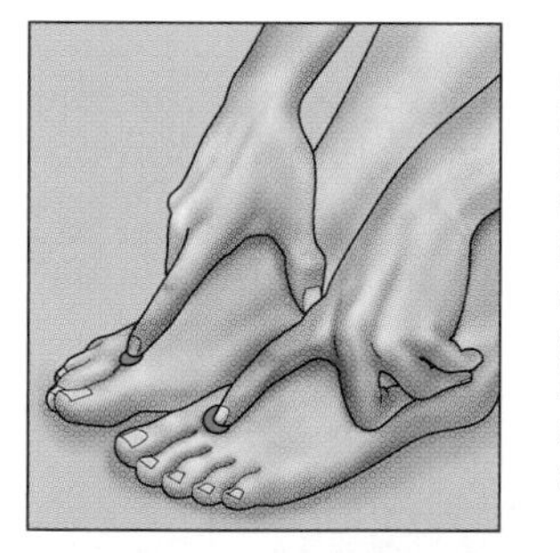

**3** Working LV 3 may help relieve cramps and spasms. Place your index fingers in the spaces between the bones of your big toes and second toes as shown. Angle the pressure toward the bones of your second toes and rub firmly. Hold for one minute.

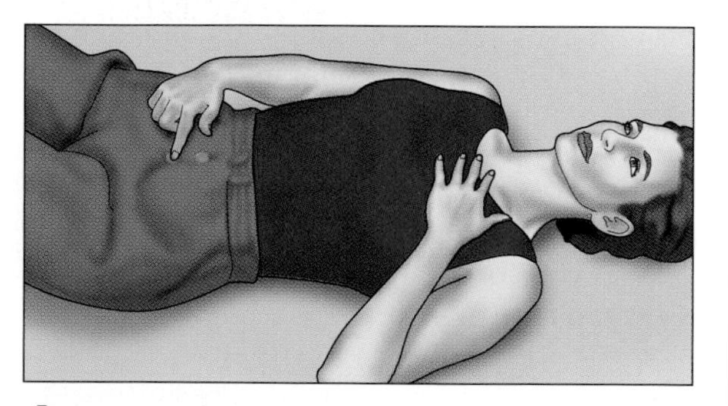

**4** You may be able to correct irregular menstrual periods by working point CV 4. Measure four finger widths down from your navel. Press your index finger firmly into your abdomen and hold for one to two minutes. Do this twice a day every day.

## HEAVY PERIODS

A heavy period (menorrhagia) is a menstrual flow that lasts longer than eight days, saturates tampons or napkins within an hour, or includes large clots of blood.

## CAUSES

Heavy periods may be caused by a hormonal imbalance, endometriosis, a pelvic infection *(see Pelvic Inflammatory Disease),* use of an IUD, or uterine growths such as fibroids *(see Uterine Problems).* Excessive bleeding may signal other irregularities in your cycle: lack of ovulation, low levels of progesterone, or an excess of prostaglandins. Heavy periods can cause iron deficiency anemia.

## TREATMENT

### CONVENTIONAL MEDICINE

Treatment for menorrhagia may include iron and folic acid supplements to treat and prevent anemia, antiprostaglandin analgesics such as ibuprofen and naproxen, and hormones to correct any imbalance in your hormone levels. Your doctor may suggest that you reduce your level of physical activity and see whether this has an effect.

Danazol, a male hormone, temporarily stops the menstrual cycle; its side effects include menopausal symptoms such as hot flashes, as well as acne, weight gain, and increased hairiness. Your doctor may prescribe other hormones, such as progesterone and birth-control pills, to balance your hormones.

The minor surgical procedure of dilation and curettage (often called a D and C) may bring relief from menorrhagia; in this operation, the doctor widens the cervical opening, then uses a spoonlike instrument or gentle suction to clean the inside of the uterus. In some cases, your doctor may suggest a hysterectomy—removal of the uterus and perhaps other reproductive organs. Seek a second opinion before deciding to undergo this surgery.

## ALTERNATIVE CHOICES

### ACUPRESSURE AND ACUPUNCTURE

Both these disciplines use techniques that rely on spleen points to help control blood flow. See a practitioner for points and techniques to relieve excessive menstrual flow.

### AROMATHERAPY

Practitioners of aromatherapy find that oils of geranium, juniper *(Juniperus communis),* and cypress, rubbed on the abdomen, may bring relief for sufferers of heavy menstrual flow.

### HERBAL THERAPIES

Tea made from yarrow *(Achillea millefolium)* may help control bleeding. You may also benefit from taking a tincture made of equal parts life root *(Senecio aureus),* shepherd's purse *(Capsella bursa-pastoris),* and wild cranesbill *(Geranium maculatum);* take it twice daily in 5-ml doses.

## AT-HOME REMEDIES

- Take extra calcium and magnesium to stop uterine muscle cramps and to lessen the flow.
- Take a warm, relaxing bath.
- Take antiprostaglandin analgesics, such as ibuprofen and naproxen.
- Drink herbal teas containing yarrow to help control bleeding.
- Apply a castor-oil pack to the abdomen to relax the muscles and lessen the flow.

**REFLEXOLOGY**

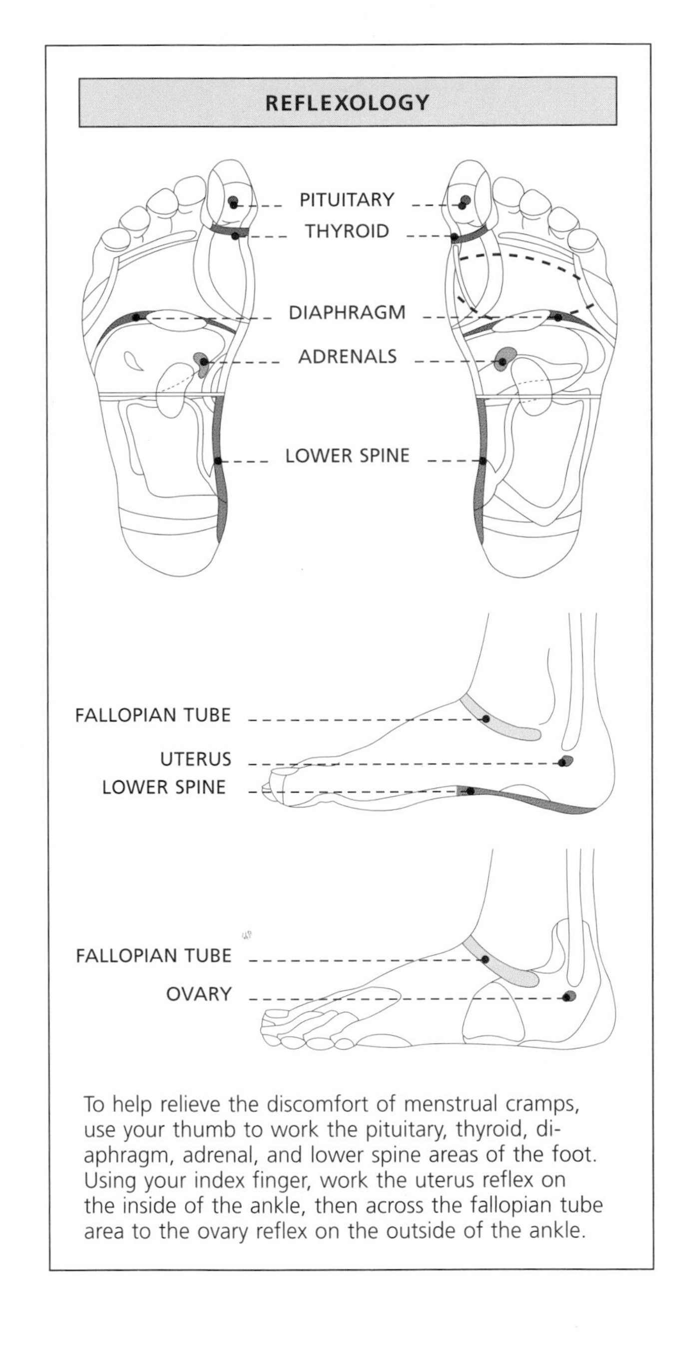


To help relieve the discomfort of menstrual cramps, use your thumb to work the pituitary, thyroid, diaphragm, adrenal, and lower spine areas of the foot. Using your index finger, work the uterus reflex on the inside of the ankle, then across the fallopian tube area to the ovary reflex on the outside of the ankle.

# PREVENTION

Maintain normal weight for your build, which helps prevent excess fat and estrogens in the body. Overweight women tend to have abnormal menstrual periods, perhaps because of an increase in estrogen-secreting cells.

Take a multivitamin, multimineral supplement including vitamins A, B complex, C, and E, as well as calcium and iron. ■

# MONONUCLEOSIS

## SYMPTOMS

The early symptoms of mononucleosis resemble those of the flu, including:

- severe fatigue.
- headache.
- sore throat, sometimes very severe.
- chills, followed by a fever.
- muscle aches.

After a day or two, the following additional symptoms may occur:

- swollen lymph nodes, especially in the neck, armpits, or groin.
- jaundice (a yellow tinge to the skin and eyes).
- a measles-like skin rash anywhere on the face or body; sometimes the rash develops suddenly after taking amoxicillin for a severe sore throat.
- bruiselike areas inside the mouth.
- soreness in the upper left abdomen (from an enlarged spleen).

## CALL YOUR DOCTOR IF:

- you have these symptoms, particularly for longer than 10 days, or if you have a severe sore throat for more than a day or two; you need to be examined by a doctor to rule out other illnesses, such as strep throat or—less likely—leukemia or infectious hepatitis.
- you develop swollen lymph nodes all over your body, which may be a sign of tuberculosis, cancer, or human immunodeficiency virus *(see AIDS)*.
- you develop abdominal pain, which may indicate a ruptured spleen. Seek emergency medical treatment immediately.

Mononucleosis, often referred to as "mono," is a very common viral illness. About 90 percent of people over age 35 have antibodies to mono in their blood, which means that they have been infected with it, probably during early childhood. When mono strikes young children, the illness is usually so mild that it passes as a common cold or the flu. When it occurs during adolescence or adulthood, however, the disease can be much more serious.

Mono comes on gradually. It begins with flu-like symptoms—fever, headache, and a general malaise and lethargy. After a few days, the lymph glands—especially those in the neck, armpits, and groin—begin to swell, although this symptom is not noticeable in everyone. Most people develop a sore throat, which can be very severe, with inflamed tonsils. A fever—usually no higher than 104°F—can also develop and may last up to three weeks. About 10 percent of people with mono develop a generalized red rash all over the body or darkened areas in the mouth that resemble bruises. In about half of all cases, the spleen may also enlarge, causing an area in the upper left abdomen to become tender to the touch.

In 95 percent of cases, the illness affects the liver. However, only about 5 percent of individuals with mono develop jaundice, a yellowing of the skin and eyes caused by an increase of bile pigment in the blood. In rare cases of mono, the liver fails. Other major complications that can develop from mono include rupturing of the spleen, meningitis, and encephalitis, an inflammation of the brain; but these, too, are extremely rare.

Most people who come down with mono feel much better within two or three weeks, although fatigue may last for two months or longer. Sometimes the disease lingers for a year or so, causing recurrent, but successively milder, attacks. In the past, some research suggested that the virus causing mono might be linked to a persistent and debilitating form of the illness known as chronic fatigue syndrome, which can last for years. Most recent research has shown no such link, however, and the cause of chronic fatigue syndrome remains unknown.

## CAUSES

Mono is caused by the Epstein-Barr virus, named after the two British researchers who first identified it in 1964, although the disease itself had been recognized many years earlier. A common member of the herpes family of viruses, Epstein-Barr is spread primarily through the exchange of saliva, which is why mono is sometimes known as the "kissing disease." However, coughing or other contact with infected saliva can also pass it from one person to another.

The mono virus can stay active in a person weeks or months after all overt symptoms are gone, so close contact with someone who shows no sign of the disease can still put a person at risk. On the other hand, not everyone who lives in proximity to an individual infected with mono comes down with the illness. Scientists believe that a healthy immune system may make it possible to fight off the infection successfully.

### DIAGNOSTIC AND TEST PROCEDURES

The wide range of symptoms associated with mono can make diagnosis difficult. Your doctor will begin by giving you a complete physical exam. A throat culture may be taken to rule out strep throat. The doctor may take a blood sample to look for the presence of abnormal white blood cells. A monospot test, in which your blood is examined for special antibodies to mono, will probably be done also. The results of these tests are not always clear, however, and additional ones may be needed.

## TREATMENT

Mononucleosis is usually a self-limiting illness. Most people recover on their own without any treatment within two weeks. Thus, the primary prescription for mono by both conventional and alternative practitioners is complete bed rest with a gradual return to normal activity.

### CONVENTIONAL MEDICINE

In addition to bed rest, your doctor may prescribe aspirin or acetaminophen for the fever, sore throat, and other discomforts of the illness. If your sore throat is so severe that you have trouble breathing or eating, your doctor may give you prednisone, a steroid drug.

### ALTERNATIVE CHOICES

Like their conventional counterparts, practitioners of alternative medicine recommend rest and various medications and treatments to help relieve the symptoms of mono. They also offer treatments to help strengthen your body's immune system and thus ensure a quick and complete recovery.

#### AROMATHERAPY

Lavender *(Lavandula officinalis),* peppermint *(Mentha piperita),* bergamot *(Citrus bergamia),* and eucalyptus *(Eucalyptus globulus)* are sometimes recommended to relieve fatigue and other symptoms of mono. Add a few drops of the essential oils of one or more of these herbs to a warm bath.

#### CHINESE HERBS

Teas made from ginseng—either the Asian *(Panax ginseng)* or the American *(Panax quinquefolius)* form—are sometimes recommended to help relieve the tiredness associated with mono. Drink three times a day.

#### HERBAL THERAPIES

To help fight the infection, drink teas made from echinacea (*Echinacea* spp.) or calendula *(Calendula officinalis),* more commonly known as marigold. Drink either tea three times daily.

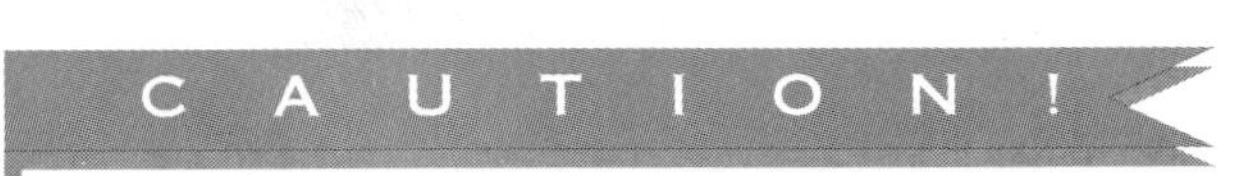


**To protect your spleen from rupturing, do not participate in any strenuous exercise until you have fully recovered.**

To reduce the fever associated with mono, try drinking a tea made from elder *(Sambucus nigra)* flowers or yarrow *(Achillea millefolium).* Drink either tea three times a day. Or, if you prefer, take 2 to 4 ml of the tincture of either herb three times a day.

To help cleanse the lymphatic system, try teas made from cleavers (*Galium* spp.) or wild indigo *(Baptisia tinctoria).* Drink either tea three times a day. Alternatively, take 2 to 4 ml of tincture of cleavers or 1 ml of tincture of wild indigo three times daily.

To help with the anxiety and depression that sometimes accompany long-term bouts with mono, try St.-John's-wort *(Hypericum perforatum)* or vervain *(Verbena officinalis).* Both herbs, when taken internally, appear to act as mild sedatives. Vervain is also recommended for jaundice, one of the symptoms of mono. Make a tea out of either herb and drink three times daily. Or take in tincture form: 1 to 4 ml of St.-John's-wort or 2 to 4 ml of vervain three times a day.

### HOMEOPATHY

Mononucleosis calls for a constitutional treatment—a set of remedies prescribed specifically for you, based on your symptoms and medical history. You will need to consult an experienced homeopath for such a treatment.

### MIND/BODY MEDICINE

Stress can exacerbate the fatigue associated with mononucleosis. It can also weaken the immune system, thus making it more difficult for your body to recover from the illness. Various relaxation techniques, such as **meditation, biofeedback,** and **guided imagery,** can be helpful in reducing the stress.

### NUTRITION AND DIET

To strengthen your immune system and help speed your recovery, eat plenty of whole (not processed) foods, especially fresh fruits and vegetables. Avoid foods that are high in saturated fats, animal proteins, and sugar, as they are difficult to digest and put stress on your body.

To maintain a better balance of blood sugar, and thus a more even energy level, eat four to six

### ACUPRESSURE

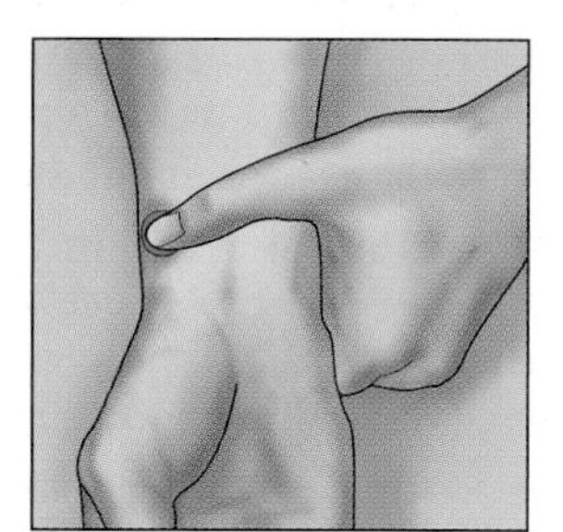

Pressing Lung 7 may bolster immunity and lung function. The point is located on the thumb side of the inner forearm, two finger widths above the crease in the wrist. Apply steady, firm pressure for one minute, then repeat on the other arm.

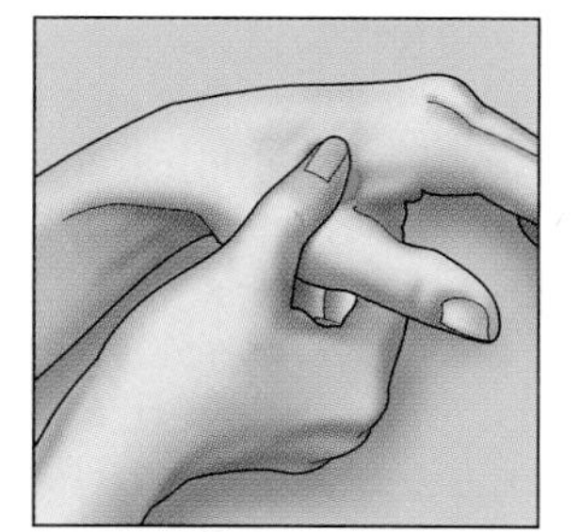

To help relieve muscle aches, use Large Intestine 4, located in the web between the thumb and index finger. Using the thumb and index finger of the right hand, press the web of the left hand for one minute; then repeat on the right hand. Do not use LI 4 if you are pregnant.

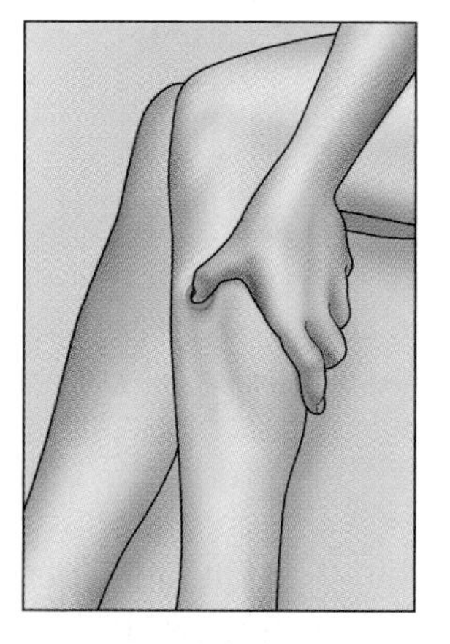

Pressing Stomach 36 may enhance immunity and increase overall vitality. The point can be found four finger widths below the kneecap, just outside the shinbone. You can verify the location by flexing your foot; a muscle should bulge at the point site. Press with your thumb for one minute.

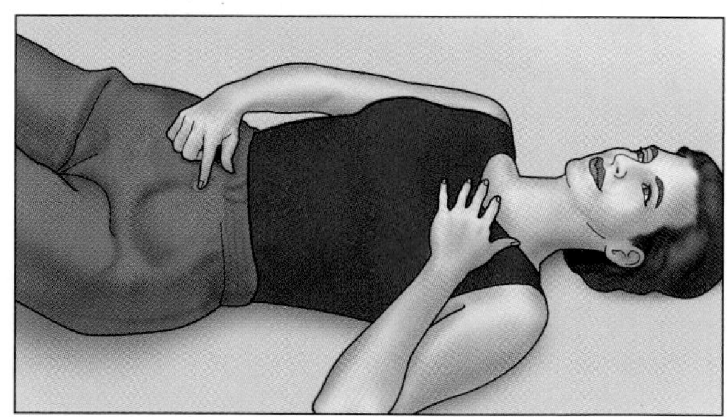

The body's energy reserve may be increased by pressing Conception Vessel 6. The point is three finger widths below the navel, midway to the pubic bone. Gradually apply deep pressure with your index finger until you feel resistance, then hold for one minute.

small meals throughout the day; try not to overeat at any one meal. Some people also find that eating a small portion of low-fat protein immediately on awakening in the morning and again in the evening before going to bed can help raise energy levels. Good choices of protein for this purpose include low-fat cheese as well as tofu, lentils, and other legumes.

Vitamin supplements may also enhance your immune system. Take vitamin A (2,500 to 10,000 IU daily), vitamin C (500 to 2,000 mg daily), and vitamin B complex (50 mg three times a day). You may also wish to try daily magnesium (200 to 700 mg) and potassium aspartate (50 to 200 mg) supplements. Research has shown that these supplements can dramatically improve energy levels after six weeks of constant use.

#### YOGA

Yoga can help reduce the fatigue associated with mononucleosis. The exercises are gentle enough to be done even by someone with the illness. One recommended pose is the **Bow** *(see page 696).*

### AT-HOME REMEDIES

- Rest your body. Do not plan to return to your normal activity level for at least a month.
- Drink plenty of liquids to prevent dehydration.
- Watch what you eat. Enrich your diet with whole foods, especially fresh fruits and vegetables. Avoid foods high in saturated fats, sugar, caffeine, and alcohol; these ingredients can diminish your energy reserves and weaken your immune system. To keep your blood sugar—and energy—level steady throughout the day, eat small but frequent meals.
- Take aspirin or an aspirin substitute to treat headache and sore throat.
- For sore throat, use a saline gargle—½ tsp salt in a glass of warm water.
- To help ease the fatigue associated with mononucleosis, massage your kidneys daily. With loose fists, rub your lower back for three to five minutes. A good occasion to do this is in the shower with warm water running down your back.

### REDUCING STRESS, STRENGTHENING IMMUNITY

Early in the 20th century, scientists began studying how humans adapt to stress. They soon discovered that humans have a biochemical reaction to danger—the fight-or-flight response. When a person experiences feelings of fear or anger, the brain releases a stream of stress hormones. One of these is epinephrine (more commonly known as adrenaline). Its release causes the heart to pump faster, blood pressure to shoot up, and blood vessels to redirect blood from the body's extremities to the muscles for greater strength. To ensure further that all the body's resources go toward either fighting or fleeing the danger, the epinephrine inhibits the digestive system and—as researchers have learned more recently—the immune system. Specifically, the stress leads to a lowering of the body's supplies of interferon and natural killer cells, which are needed to help fight disease.

The fight-or-flight response enabled our ancestors to deal with the immediate physical dangers of their frequently hazardous environment. In today's world, however, stressors tend to be more emotional than physical, and they generally occur continually over a long period of time. As a result, our immune systems often suffer from chronic suppression, making it more difficult to fight off and recover from disease.

Studies indicate that several stress-reduction techniques—including **biofeedback, hypnotherapy, meditation,** and **guided imagery**—can be effective in decreasing the fight-or-flight response and restoring the body's immune system to full strength. Practicing these techniques may therefore help you recover more quickly from mononucleosis. Research has shown that they may also protect you from other illnesses, including heart disease, diabetes, and cancer. ■

# MOTION SICKNESS

## SYMPTOMS

- sweating, dizziness, pallor, and nausea—sometimes leading to vomiting—while traveling by car, bus, train, ship, or airplane.

## CALL YOUR DOCTOR IF:

- you are planning a trip and are concerned that you will be bothered by motion sickness; your doctor may prescribe antinausea drugs.

The nausea and dizziness that afflict some people when they are traveling in a vehicle certainly cause discomfort—especially if they lead to vomiting—but they do not represent a serious illness. The symptoms of motion sickness usually subside either once your body adjusts to your mode of travel or shortly after the trip ends.

Nearly 80 percent of the population has suffered at some time from motion sickness. Fortunately, ways to prevent it abound.

## CAUSES

Motion sickness may occur because your brain is receiving conflicting information from your sensory organs: Your eyes may not detect motion to the same degree as the balance mechanism in your inner ear registers the movement of the vehicle. Your central nervous system reacts to this stress-producing phenomenon by activating the nausea center in your brain.

## TREATMENT

The surest way to cure motion sickness is to stop the activity that's causing your discomfort, but that's not always practicable. If you are prone to motion sickness, preparations for any trip should include measures to prevent the disorder or mechanisms to cope with it.

### CONVENTIONAL MEDICINE

Your doctor may recommend over-the-counter antinausea pills, such as dimenhydrinate, which counter nausea by reducing the sensitivity of the motion-detecting nerves in the ear. If you need something stronger, your doctor may prescribe the same medication in a higher potency. In order to be effective, oral antinausea medications need to be started well before your departure (up to a day ahead).

If you are going on a long trip, your doctor may prescribe scopolamine, in the form of a timed-release skin patch, to reduce the muscle spasms and contractions that trigger vomiting.

Worn behind your ear, the patch releases scopolamine into your bloodstream over a three-day period. If you are especially prone to motion sickness, your doctor may encourage you to take antinausea pills in addition to wearing the patch.

## ALTERNATIVE CHOICES

Many alternative treatments rely on similar remedies to prevent or relieve motion sickness. Ginger *(Zingiber officinale)* is a favorite motion sickness remedy of naturopaths. It causes none of the side effects of antinausea drugs and can be drunk as a tea, eaten candied, or taken in capsule form (two capsules every four hours the day before and as needed during travel); it should be taken on an empty stomach.

### ACUPRESSURE

Much scientific research exists to substantiate the use of wrist point Pericardium 6 in relieving nausea. You might want to purchase acupressure wristbands to place over this point when you travel. When worn as directed, the nodules on the bands put pressure on points acupressure proponents say reduce nausea. The bands are often recommended by conventional physicians and alternative practitioners alike, and are sold in many pharmacies and travel-goods stores.

Acupressure applied at the base of the rib cage (Spleen 16) is also said to be especially effective in relieving nausea.

See the illustrations *(below, left),* and pages 22–23 for information on point locations.

### HOMEOPATHY

Homeopathic remedies sometimes come in kits that contain motion sickness remedies, which can be taken before and during travel as directed. Your homeopathic physician may prescribe remedies such as Cocculus, Petroleum, Ipecac, or Nux vomica to take before or during travel to relieve nausea.

## PREVENTION

There are many strategies you can use to lower your vulnerability to motion sickness. In addition to the suggestions above, the following may help:

- Get plenty of fresh air. Open a car window, get on the ship's top deck, or open the overhead air vent in a plane.
- Keep your head as still as possible, close your eyes or focus on the horizon or another stationary object, and sit where motion is felt the least—in the front seat of the car, amidships or in a forward cabin of the ship, or over the wings of the plane. Avoid sitting facing backward on a bus, train, or plane. Don't read while in motion.
- Eat light meals of low-fat, starchy foods and avoid strong-smelling or -tasting foods.
- Don't drink or smoke, which can increase nausea.
- If nausea does set in, try eating olives or sucking on a lemon; these foods make your mouth dry and help diminish nausea. Soda crackers may help absorb excess saliva and acid in your stomach. If you feel too sick to eat, try a drink of ginger ale (made from real ginger) or any carbonated cola drink. ■

**ACUPRESSURE**

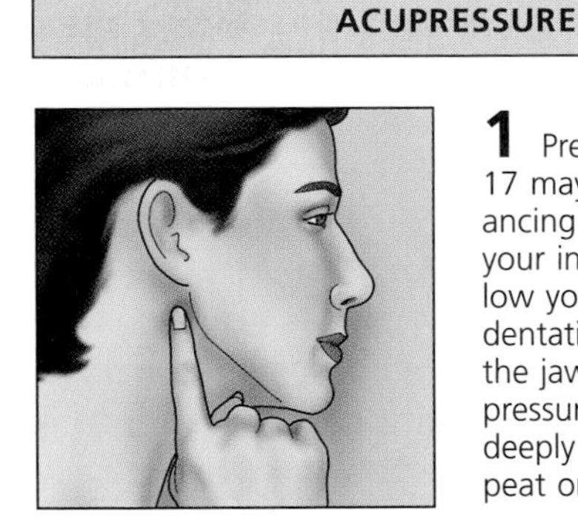

**1** Pressing Small Intestine 17 may aid the ear's balancing mechanism. Place your index fingers just below your earlobes in the indentations at the back of the jawbone. Apply light pressure while breathing deeply for one minute. Repeat one to two times.

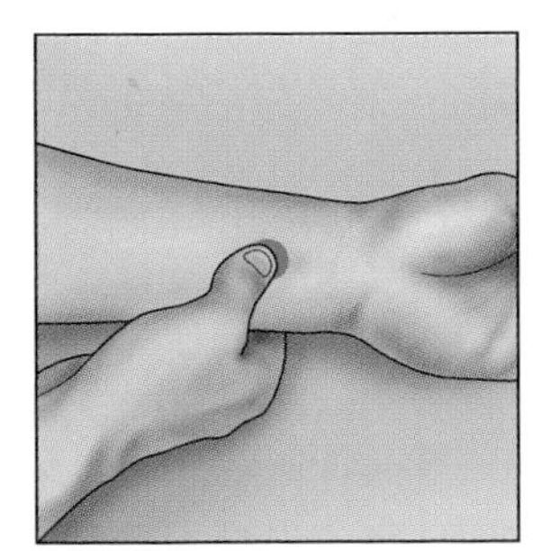

**2** To help calm nerves and reduce nausea, press Pericardium 6. Place your thumb in the center of your inner wrist between the two forearm bones, two finger widths from the wrist crease. Press firmly for one minute, three to five times; then repeat on the other arm.

# MULTIPLE SCLEROSIS

## SYMPTOMS

The first attack is generally mild, lasts only a few days, and is followed by a long period of remission—perhaps years—before the next episode. Symptoms vary considerably. They include:

- weakness, stiffness (spasticity), or numbness in one or more limbs.
- sensations of tingling, pins and needles, heaviness, a bandlike tightness around one or more limbs or the trunk of the body.
- tremors, instability, or a lack of balance or coordination.
- blurred or double vision, or rapid, involuntary eye movement.
- bladder or bowel incontinence.
- fatigue: either a feeling of general tiredness or extreme exhaustion.

## CALL YOUR DOCTOR IF:

- you or someone you know has symptoms associated with multiple sclerosis. Because other diseases share some of the same symptoms, a proper diagnosis is essential to your treatment.
- you are suffering from an acute attack; steroid injections can help relieve pain.

Multiple sclerosis is a disease of the central nervous system, typically slow and fitful in its progress, with effects that can range from relatively minor physical annoyances to major disabilities. The root problem is electrical. Normally, most nerves in the body are insulated by a fatty substance called myelin, which permits the efficient transmission of electrical impulses—the nerve signals. Multiple sclerosis, or MS, occurs when this protective sheath becomes inflamed and ultimately destroyed in places, short-circuiting the electrical flow. Among the possible consequences of the disruption are loss of muscular coordination, impaired vision, and incontinence.

The initial attack—occurring as early as the teenage years—may be brief and mild, and may not even be recognized. The symptoms temporarily abate or disappear for reasons that are not known, but recurrence is highly likely—although usually after a long latency period. Generally the first full-fledged bout, lasting weeks or months, takes place between the ages of 20 and 40, and further attacks follow at erratic intervals. The repeated inflammation of the nerves produces scarring (sclerosis), and although myelin can normally repair itself, the scarring happens too rapidly for healing to take place; the effects of the lesions become permanent. As a result of such lasting damage, 77 percent of MS sufferers are limited to some degree in their activities, and about 25 percent become wheelchair-bound.

Doctors recognize four basic categories of MS:

- **Benign.** Cases of this kind are typically limited to one attack, and there is no permanent disability. The most common symptoms are limb numbness and temporary vision problems caused by inflammation of the optic nerve. About 20 percent of MS cases are of the benign type.
- **Relapse-remitting.** This and the next category refer to on-again, off-again cycles of attacks and remissions. Cases of this type involve sudden and strong debilitating attacks followed by periods of almost total remission. About 25 percent of MS cases are of this kind.
- **Relapse-progressive.** In this type, attacks are less severe, but the recovery is less complete.

The cumulative effect of many cycles of attacks slowly leads to some degree of disability. This is the most common form of MS, accounting for about 40 percent of all cases.

- **Chronic-progressive.** This form of MS quickly becomes disabling and has no periods of remission. It accounts for about 15 percent of cases.

Multiple sclerosis not only is unpredictable in its on-again, off-again patterns and its broad spectrum of symptoms, it also strikes the population in mystifyingly uneven ways. Women are twice as susceptible as men, and the disease is twice as common among Caucasians as among African Americans. Moreover, the incidence is higher in northerly regions: The rate of MS in Canada is twice that of the United States.

**MYELIN LOSS**

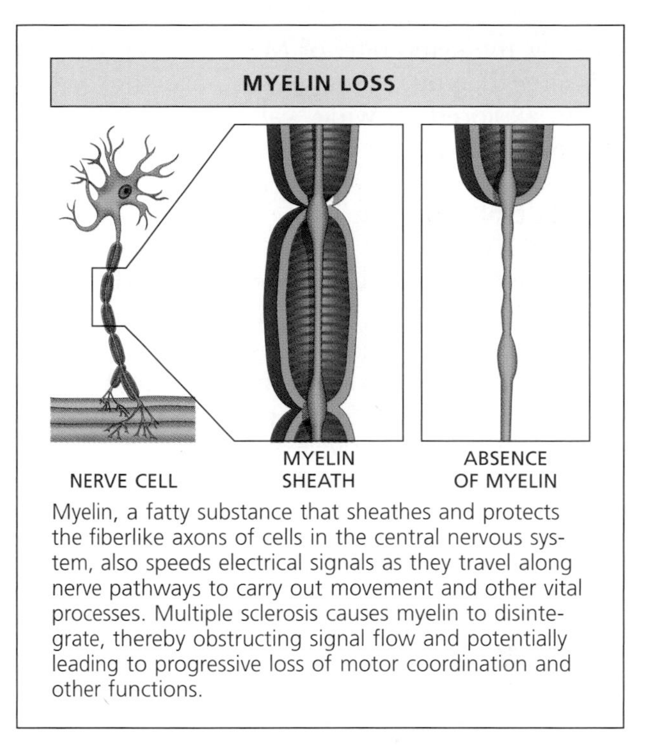


Myelin, a fatty substance that sheathes and protects the fiberlike axons of cells in the central nervous system, also speeds electrical signals as they travel along nerve pathways to carry out movement and other vital processes. Multiple sclerosis causes myelin to disintegrate, thereby obstructing signal flow and potentially leading to progressive loss of motor coordination and other functions.

## CAUSES

No one is sure what causes MS, but most researchers think the immune system plays a major role. Perhaps the disease arises from an inherited problem in the immune system. Perhaps a virus provokes an autoimmune response—a situation in which the immune system attacks the body's own tissue, mistaking it for a foreign invader. It has also been proposed that MS can be triggered by a profound emotional shock or physical trauma, which could affect the immune system.

Dietary factors have also been cited as possible causes. In attempting to explain the higher incidence of MS in northern regions, some researchers note that people there tend to eat more red meat, milk products, and other foods high in saturated fat. MS patients have a lower-than-normal ability to absorb polyunsaturated fatty acids, which are essential to the body's processing of all foods, especially saturated fat. The result is an excess of saturated fats in their systems. Many remedial diets have been devised to correct this imbalance, and some have met with sustained success—but none can be considered a cure *(see Nutrition and Diet, page 603)*.

Some researchers suspect environmental factors. The list of possible culprits includes lead, pesticides, diesel fumes, chemicals in tap water, solvents, fumes from domestic gas water heaters, and carbon monoxide pollution.

### DIAGNOSTIC AND TEST PROCEDURES

A common test for MS is the visual evoked response, in which electrodes attached to the back of the head detect electrical activity in response to visual tracking of a changing checkerboard pattern. Other tests include magnetic resonance imaging (MRI) and lumbar puncture.

## TREATMENT

Multiple sclerosis is difficult to treat—and to study, for that matter—for two reasons: Its diverse symptoms vary greatly, and the cycling of attacks and remissions makes tracking the course of the disease and determining the effectiveness of a given treatment especially problematic. (A remission, for example, could be due to medication or might have occurred on its own.)

In general, medicines are effective only in

treating the symptoms of MS, and then only to a limited degree. MS sufferers have thus vigorously explored a wide variety of alternative treatments as well.

## CONVENTIONAL MEDICINE

Although the unpredictable nature of MS makes treatments difficult to evaluate, a number of medications are regarded as effective. Among them: interferon beta, which can cut the frequency and severity of relapses; corticosteroids, which can shorten attacks and reduce inflammation; baclofen and dantrolene, which act to suppress spasticity; and muscle relaxants, which relieve stiffness and pain. A corticosteroid is frequently recommended to treat inflammation of the optic nerve, the cause of the double vision or involuntary rapid eye movement that sometimes occurs with MS. Amantadine, an antiviral drug, may promote stamina.

Some medications specifically target muscle stiffness, bladder and bowel problems, tremors, fatigue, and the pins-and-needles sensation. Others are directed at the immune system. In several trials run in 1994, cladribine, a drug used to treat leukemia, either stabilized or improved the conditions of MS patients; it apparently works by killing lymphocytes that may be attacking the central nervous system.

Researchers are exploring various other treatments. In one study, replacement myelin from cows seemed to greatly reduce the number of attacks. Physical therapy has proved effective in relaxing stiff limbs, maintaining motion in the joints, and improving circulation. A physical therapist can also help design an exercise program tailored to the individual's particular limitations.

## ALTERNATIVE CHOICES

You'll need professional guidance for some of the alternative therapies described below, but you can learn to do many yourself at home.

### ACUPUNCTURE

With MS patients, the goal of acupuncture is to reduce limb stiffness and relax muscles. Acupuncture, which stimulates nerve pathways, may enable messages to bypass damaged nerve fibers.

### APITHERAPY

The administering of stings from honeybees *(Apis mellifica)* has been used to treat arthritis for centuries—and recently, MS sufferers, too, have found relief with apitherapy, also known as bee venom therapy (BVT). The recommended treatment involves three weekly sessions of painful stings (from a live bee) for six months. Apitherapy stimulates the immune system. When an already inflamed area is stung and becomes swollen, the body's natural anti-inflammatory agents act to shrink swelling, reducing the inflammation of the original condition in the process.

Bee venom may be beneficial in other ways. It is rich in polyunsaturated fatty acids, which MS patients lack.

BVT has short-lived side effects: itching, swelling, and skin reddening. It has been known to cause fatal shock in some people and severe allergic reactions in others. Be sure to check with your doctor before embarking on a series of treatments. Some doctors will administer the stings themselves, or they may refer you to someone more experienced. You can contact the American Apitherapy Society or your state chapter of the Multiple Sclerosis Foundation for qualified practitioners, who may also help you learn how to administer treatments yourself.

### BODY WORK

Although multiple sclerosis cannot be cured through physical movement or exercise, regularly working your muscles is advised in order to keep them from atrophying.

The **Feldenkrais method** involves a series of lessons designed to retrain your neuromuscular system and expand your range of motion. More than a thousand different exercises are covered in the lessons, which you can take either in a group session or in a one-on-one meeting with a practitioner. Movements are performed lightly, slowly, and without strain.

Proprioceptive Neuromuscular Facilitation, or PNF Stretching, is another body-work technique that operates on the principle of reeducating the body. Proprioceptors are sensory receptors—concentrated in muscle tissue around the joints—that monitor physical movements and enable the brain to coordinate the body's motions. In PNF Stretching, a therapist arranges your body in a stretched position and holds you stationary while urging you to move; as you try to respond, your muscles stretch farther. With repetition, the muscles' flexibility increases and, in effect, the proprioceptors "learn" how to achieve a fuller range of motion.

### LIFESTYLE

Exercise is highly recommended for MS patients—although it should not be performed during an attack, nor too strenuously at other times, since overexertion can bring on an attack. Because muscle contractions are stimulated by nerve impulses, the exercise of muscles where nerves have been damaged can be difficult. Nonetheless, swimming, stretching, and low-impact aerobics are all within the capabilities of many people with MS, and even patients in wheelchairs can exercise to some degree.

Gentle stretching is particularly helpful for the spasticity, stiff gait, and foot and toe dragging that can accompany the disease. Performing gentle stretches in cool water, a form of **hydrotherapy,** can also help relax spastic limbs.

Studies have demonstrated that regular **yoga** exercises increase secretions of the adrenal medulla, a nervous-system stimulator, which can help to slow degeneration.

### NUTRITION AND DIET

Certain foods can bring on attacks in some MS sufferers. Among problem foods are milk and dairy products, caffeine, yeast, and gluten (found in wheat, barley, oats, and rye). Ketchup, vinegar, wine, and corn can also prove problematic. The best way to isolate sensitivity to a particular food is to stop eating it for a month, then reintroduce it into your diet to see if it provokes a reaction.

A number of special diets attempt to correct the fatty imbalance in MS sufferers. Two approaches (sometimes used together) appear to have the greatest impact in managing the disease: One is to increase the intake of fatty acids; the other, to decrease the intake of saturated fats. The latter tactic is the more common, although in many recommended diets, saturated fats are not the only targets for reduction or elimination. For example, allergen-free diets forbid foods known to produce allergic reactions such as hives, hay fever, and asthma attacks. Diets that are gluten-free eliminate wheat, rye, barley, and oats. Pectin- and fructose-free diets ban fruits and fruit juices. The **Evers Diet** consists primarily of raw food. The **MacDougal Diet** is gluten- and fructose-free and includes megadoses of vitamins. The **Cambridge Liquid Diet** is a balanced, very low-calorie diet usually used for obese MS patients.

The best-known diet for MS sufferers is the **Swank Diet**, devised by Dr. Roy Swank of the Oregon Health Sciences University. In many cases, it has apparently slowed the course of the disease and reduced attacks. Very low in saturated fats, it calls for specific amounts of polyunsaturated oils—sunflower, safflower, olive, and sesame oils, for example, as well as oils in beans, leafy green vegetables such as spinach and kale, and most fish. The diet also includes proteins, supplements of cod-liver oil, and high doses of vitamins. Butter, margarine, shortening, and hydrogenated oils (such as coconut and palm oil) are strictly forbidden. In the first year, you are advised to avoid red meat entirely, as well as peanut butter, cheese, sour cream, sauces, gravies, pastries, whole milk, and snack foods—all of which are high in saturated fats.

Supplements figure in many diets recommended for MS sufferers. Linoleic acid, found in sunflower oil and known for its role in regulating the immune system, is said to reduce the severity of MS attacks and to produce longer remissions. Evening primrose oil *(Oenothera biennis)* is beneficial because of its specialized fatty-acid content. Nerve sheaths may be strengthened with 5 daily grams of lecithin (kept refrigerated). Coenzyme Q, or CoQ10, in 30 mg doses two or three times a day, may help cells utilize more oxygen. Niacin may help with tingling and numbness. ■

# MUMPS

## SYMPTOMS

- swollen, inflamed salivary glands located above the angle of the jaw, on one or both sides of the face.
- fever and fatigue.
- in some cases, swelling of the salivary glands under the tongue.
- especially in teens and adults, secondary inflammation of the testes, which is visible, or of the ovaries or pancreas, which is felt as abdominal pain.

## CALL YOUR DOCTOR IF:

- you suspect your child has the mumps, to confirm your diagnosis.
- your child has the mumps and has a severe headache and neck pain; these could be signs of meningitis.
- your child has the mumps and has severe abdominal pain and vomiting—symptoms of an inflamed pancreas.
- any teenage or adult male family member with the mumps has swollen testes, which in extremely rare cases can lead to sterility.

M

You will have little trouble recognizing a child with the mumps, a mild viral infection that occurs most frequently between the ages of 3 and 10. The telltale sign: swelling on one or both sides of your child's face, above the angle of the jaw. Once your child has had the mumps, the child will never get it again, having developed what is known as natural immunity. Most states require a child to be immunized against mumps before starting school if not already naturally immune *(see page 33)*.

Mumps is only mildly contagious; there is little risk that other family members will get sick at the same time. Though mumps is usually a childhood illness, teens and adults can also contract it. The case is likely to be no more severe for an older individual, but swelling of the testes in a teenage or adult male should be checked out by your doctor because of a very slight risk of its causing sterility.

## CAUSES

Mumps is a virus and is transmitted through the air in droplets from a sneeze or cough, or by direct contact. The incubation period—when the virus multiplies in the body and the person is not contagious—is 16 to 18 days from exposure. A person is contagious 2 days before symptoms appear and for 9 days while symptoms are present.

## TREATMENT

Call your child's pediatrician to confirm your diagnosis of mumps, as well as to ensure that the physician can intercede if complications arise and to keep your child's health history current. Children with the mumps should stay home from school until all symptoms are gone.

### CONVENTIONAL MEDICINE

Your pediatrician will prescribe rest, a soft-foods diet, increased liquids, and heat or ice on the glands to relieve pain. The doctor may also recommend an acetaminophen-based pain reliever.

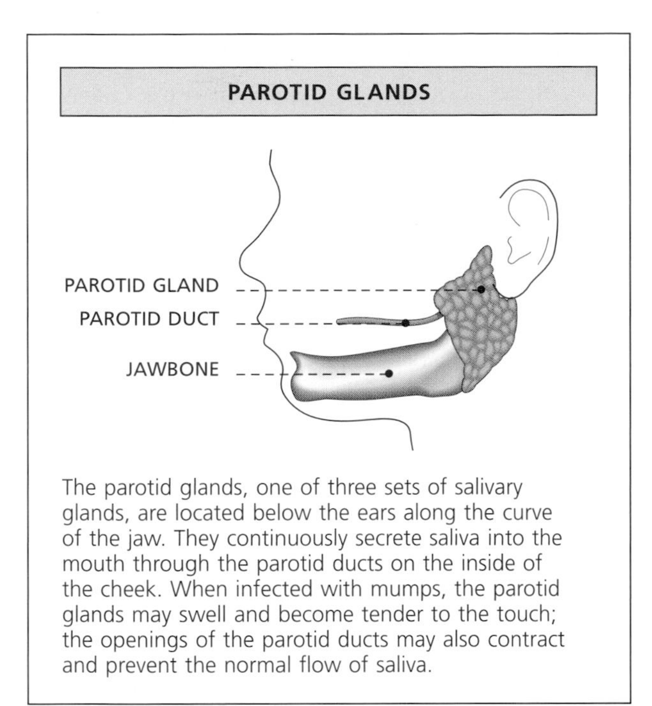

The parotid glands, one of three sets of salivary glands, are located below the ears along the curve of the jaw. They continuously secrete saliva into the mouth through the parotid ducts on the inside of the cheek. When infected with mumps, the parotid glands may swell and become tender to the touch; the openings of the parotid ducts may also contract and prevent the normal flow of saliva.

#### ACUPRESSURE

To relieve pain caused by swollen glands, place your middle fingers in the hollows just behind your child's earlobes, and hold lightly for two minutes. Encourage your child to breathe deeply. (Older children can do this by themselves.)

#### HERBAL THERAPIES

No herbs specifically treat mumps, but to reduce swelling, try cleavers *(Galium aparine)* or echinacea (*Echinacea* spp.). Echinacea may help clear the infection. Consult a medical herbalist for dosages.

#### HOMEOPATHY

Always consult a homeopathic physician for appropriate dosages for children. The homeopath may recommend Belladonna when a child is flushed, red, and has swelling on the right side; Bryonia when a child is irritable, thirsty, and doesn't want to move; or Phytolacca for extremely swollen glands. Stop treatments that don't help within 24 hours; you need to try another remedy.

#### NUTRITION AND DIET

Offer your child light foods such as soups, vegetables, and fruits. Avoid dairy products, which are hard to digest, and citrus fruits or juices, which can aggravate the swollen salivary glands.

#### OSTEOPATHY

Gentle, rhythmic pressure applied over the spleen, a procedure known as spleen pumping, may enhance the release of white blood cells into the blood. Consult an osteopath.

### AT-HOME CARE

- Keep your child quiet, especially if he's feverish; confinement to bed is not required.
- An ice pack or a heating pad applied to the swelling may relieve pain. An acetaminophen-based pain reliever may also help.
- A tea made from apple juice and cloves can help relieve painful swallowing. Gently boil eight whole cloves in 1 qt apple juice. Strain and stir, and cool to room temperature.

## PREVENTION

Because fighting the illness strengthens the immune system, many practitioners of alternative medicine believe it is better for an otherwise healthy child to contract mumps than to be vaccinated. You should discuss immunization with your child's doctor. The MMR (measles, mumps, and rubella vaccine) is now given at 12 or 15 months, with a booster between the ages of 4 and 6 or 10 and 12. The homeopathic version of immunization is not an accepted equivalent and will not provide the same protection, but some homeopaths will prescribe remedies to decrease the potential side effects of the MMR.

### CAUTION!

**Never give a child aspirin—even baby aspirin—or other products containing the salt called salicylate to reduce a fever or to relieve pain. Aspirin has been linked to Reye's syndrome, a rare but very dangerous illness that causes inflammation of the liver and brain.** ■

# MUSCLE CRAMPS

## SYMPTOMS

Once you've experienced a muscle cramp, you'll probably recognize any future ones by the nature of the pain they inflict. Common symptoms include:

- a sharp, sudden, painful spasm—or tightening—of a muscle, especially in the legs.
- the affected muscle's hardness to the touch.
- in some cases, visible distortion or twitching of the muscle beneath the skin.
- in other cases, extremely severe cramps in the arms and legs, beginning without warning, and sometimes affecting the abdominal muscles as well. These symptoms are typical of heat cramps.
- persistent cramping pains in lower abdominal muscles, which may occur with back problems or during menstruation.

M

## CALL YOUR DOCTOR IF:

- you experience frequent muscle cramps.
- your muscle cramp lasts more than an hour.
- your cramp is in your chest or arms; this may indicate a serious heart or abdominal problem. **Seek immediate medical help.** *(See also Heart Attack.)*

From a stitch that grabs your side while you're running to a charley horse in your calf awakening you in the dead of night, muscle cramps can be an all-too-common source of discomfort. Normally, a muscle at work contracts—tightening to exert a pulling force—then stretches out when the movement is finished or when another muscle exerts force in the opposite direction. But sometimes a muscle contracts with great intensity and stays contracted, refusing to stretch out again; this is a muscle cramp.

## CAUSES

Muscles contract or lengthen in response to electrical signals from nerves; minerals such as sodium, calcium, and magnesium, which surround and permeate muscle cells, play a key role in the transmission of these signals. Imbalances in those minerals—as well as in certain hormones, body fluids, and chemicals—or malfunctions in the nervous system itself can foul up the flow of electrical signals and cause a muscle to cramp.

Physical overexertion depletes fluids and minerals and can lead to cramping, particularly in people who work or exercise in conditions that overheat their bodies. Activities like working in the garden on a hot summer day, if you are not careful to drink plenty of fluids, may cause heat cramps. And if you do not take steps to alleviate them, heat cramps can progress to much more serious **heatstroke** and **heat exhaustion** *(see Emergencies/First Aid, page 68).*

## CAUTION!

**Cramping pain in your chest and arm muscles may indicate a heart problem. Call your doctor or get medical help immediately. If you suffer from circulatory problems, diabetes, heart disease, or varicose veins, or if you have had a stroke or been warned that you might be susceptible to one, avoid massage until you talk to your doctor.**

Hormone imbalances caused by diabetes and thyroid problems can also cause cramps, as can a reduced supply of blood-borne oxygen to muscles. Blood oxygen levels often fall in smokers, for instance, causing muscles to cramp—especially when smokers engage in hard physical labor. If you move in your sleep, you may pinch a nerve, signaling a muscle to contract and perhaps leading to a cramp. If you're prone to night cramps, do stretching exercises before you go to bed.

## TREATMENT

There are simple techniques for easing common, occasional muscle cramps *(see At-Home Remedies, right),* but if you suffer from frequent or severe cramps, see your doctor. Frequent cramps might indicate a more serious illness. And severe cramps in your chest, shoulders, or arms can be symptoms of a heart attack; call immediately for medical help.

### CONVENTIONAL MEDICINE

No medicinal treatment of common muscle cramps is required. Massaging a cramping muscle or drinking water to relieve heat cramps is usually sufficient remedy. For frequent or severe cramps, your doctor will diagnose and treat the underlying cause.

### ALTERNATIVE CHOICES

#### ACUPRESSURE

If the cramp is in your calf, acupressurists recommend applying pressure for two to three minutes at the lower end of the calf muscle bulge.

#### HERBAL THERAPIES

An infusion of ginkgo *(Ginkgo biloba)* may help improve circulation and relieve leg spasms. Pour a cup of boiling water onto 2 tsp of the dried herb and steep for 15 to 20 minutes; drink three times a day. An herbalist might prescribe Japanese quince *(Chaenomeles speciosa)* as an antispasmodic for cramps in the calves.

#### HOMEOPATHY

Over-the-counter homeopathic preparations (in tablet form) of Cuprum metallicum (6c), sucked slowly, are said to relieve the spasm and ache.

#### NUTRITION AND DIET

Nutritionists recommend taking vitamin E supplements (300 IU daily) to prevent night cramps. You may also find relief by increasing your intake of calcium. Good sources include milk, cheese, yogurt, dark green leafy vegetables, and canned fish.

### AT-HOME REMEDIES

To relieve a typical cramp, you need to make the muscle stop contracting—by physically either stretching it or massaging it, or both. You can stretch a calf muscle simply by standing on your toes and then slowly lowering your heels. For a greater stretch, put your hands or forearms against a wall, and keeping your feet flat on the floor, slide backward until you are leaning against the wall from several feet away. For even more stretch, keep edging your feet backward.

To massage away a cramp, from a sitting position stretch your heel down, pointing your toes up—toward your head—and firmly squeeze your calf with your hand. Begin at the edges of the cramp and move in toward the center with gentle pressure. For an obstinate cramp, immerse the muscle in a hot bath, perhaps while stretching and massaging it. To treat heat cramps, drink plenty of cool water. This is also the best way to prevent heat cramps: Drink a cup of cool water before and after exercise, and every 15 minutes during exercise. If you use a sports beverage instead, drink one low in sugar; sugar in an overheated body can bring on stomach cramps. Dilute juices with 3 parts water.

## PREVENTION

Drink 6 to 8 cups of water every day. Be sure to acclimate yourself to exercise routines and sports, especially in early summer. Do stretching exercises regularly, particularly before bed. If you smoke, enroll in a program to help you quit. ■

# MUSCLE PAIN

*Read down this column to find your symptoms. Then read across.*

| SYMPTOMS | AILMENT/PROBLEM |
| --- | --- |
| ◆ muscle and joint pain after excessive or strenuous activity. | ◆ Overexertion |
| ◆ cramping muscle pain, often in your calf; may awake you from sleep. | ◆ Muscle cramp |
| ◆ muscle pain following vigorous activity or an injury; possibly, swelling. | ◆ Strained muscle or muscles |
| ◆ pain in your neck muscles after a jolt. | ◆ Whiplash |
| ◆ muscle and joint aches; fever, chills, headache, weakness, runny nose, cough, sore throat; possibly, vomiting or diarrhea. | ◆ Flu |
| ◆ muscle pain after taking medication. | ◆ Drug reaction |
| ◆ chronic burning or radiating muscle pain, especially in your shoulders, neck, and hips; fatigue; often, a sleep disorder such as insomnia; typically affecting people in their late forties or older. | ◆ Fibromyalgia |
| ◆ pain and stiffness in the muscles of your neck, shoulders, and arms, or your lower back, thighs, and hips. | ◆ Polymyalgia rheumatica |

| WHAT TO DO | OTHER INFO |
|---|---|
| ◆ Use ice packs for swelling. Consider heat rubs, warm baths, a heating pad, or massage when swelling is gone. Take an anti-inflammatory painkiller such as ibuprofen. | ◆ A cream containing aspirin or the homeopathic remedy Arnica may help relieve pain. Because muscles require 48 hours to recover from exertion, try exercising only every other day. |
| ◆ Massage the muscle, rubbing upward and toward the heart. For recurrent cramps avoid heavy blankets and tight pajamas when sleeping. | ◆ Extra calcium, magnesium, or vitamin E, or a 12-oz glass of tonic water (which contains quinine) taken at night, may reduce the frequency of cramps. |
| ◆ Try RICE: rest, ice (wrapped in a thin cloth), compression (with an elastic wrap), and elevation of the affected area. Take an anti-inflammatory painkiller such as ibuprofen. *(See Sprains and Strains.)* | |
| ◆ Rest on a firm bed without a pillow. Take an anti-inflammatory painkiller such as ibuprofen. Call your doctor if you are no better in 24 hours. | ◆ Your doctor may recommend that you wear a supportive collar. |
| ◆ Rest, drink plenty of fluids, and if needed, take an anti-inflammatory painkiller such as ibuprofen. | ◆ Flu shots are often recommended for prevention in people over the age of 65 and in those with chronic diseases. |
| ◆ If the drug is by prescription, call your doctor. If the drug is over-the-counter, stop taking it and seek your doctor's advice. | ◆ Clofibrate, a lipid-lowering drug, often causes muscle pain. Corticosteroids may cause such pain indirectly by depleting potassium. |
| ◆ Call your doctor. Take pain relievers recommended by your doctor; a muscle relaxant or a low dose of an antidepressant may be recommended for pain relief or sleep improvement. | ◆ Women are affected by this illness 10 times more frequently than men. Physical therapy, aerobic exercise, biofeedback, acupuncture, and improved sleeping habits may be helpful. |
| ◆ Call your doctor. The usual treatment is with corticosteroids and, possibly, anti-inflammatories. | ◆ Patients with this disease typically are over 50 years old, and it occurs more often in women than in men. |

# MUSCLE WEAKNESS

*Read down this column to find your symptoms. Then read across.*

| SYMPTOMS | AILMENT/PROBLEM |
|---|---|
| ◆ muscle weakness (inability to exert or sustain much pressure, weight, or strain, or to grasp objects or resist force; lacking vigor; weakness may be actual or perceived) after excessive or strenuous activity or exercise. | ◆ Overexertion |
| ◆ muscle weakness and aching; fever, chills, headache, malaise, runny nose, cough, sore throat; possibly, vomiting or diarrhea. | ◆ Flu or other infection |
| ◆ muscle weakness after sweating, vomiting, or diarrhea; possibly, muscle cramps. | ◆ Dehydration and/or electrolyte abnormality |
| ◆ muscle weakness with fatigue; bluish lips, pasty skin, slick-feeling tongue; shortness of breath, faintness, dizziness. | ◆ Anemia |
| ◆ muscle weakness, trembling hands, nervousness; weight loss despite increased appetite; increased heart rate and blood pressure; excessive perspiration. | ◆ Hyperthyroidism |
| ◆ muscle weakness and aching; joint pain; fatigue; low-grade fever; skin rash; sun sensitivity; weight loss; mental confusion; chest pain on taking deep breaths; poor circulation in fingers and toes. | ◆ Lupus |
| ◆ unexplained muscle weakness that spreads throughout the body; possibly, tingling, numbness, paralysis. | ◆ Neurological disease such as Guillain-Barré syndrome, Lou Gehrig's disease, multiple sclerosis, or myasthenia gravis |
| ◆ weakness in hip or shoulder muscles; pain, swelling, warmth, and redness in small joints. | ◆ Polymyositis or dermatomyositis (inflammation of muscles caused by immune system dysfunction) |
| ◆ muscle weakness that progresses in severity; coordination and gait difficulties; patient always male and usually younger than five years at onset. | ◆ Muscular dystrophy |

| WHAT TO DO | OTHER INFO |
|---|---|
| ◆ Slow down for a few days, but continue light activity. | ◆ Overexertion may cause weakness from fatigue or fluid losses. |
| ◆ Rest, drink plenty of fluids, and if needed, take an anti-inflammatory painkiller such as ibuprofen. | ◆ The flu virus can cause inflammation of the muscle fibers, interfering with their contraction. It is best to return to exercise slowly. |
| ◆ Drink fluids, especially a carbohydrate-electrolyte drink (sports drink). Call your doctor if symptoms persist. | ◆ An imbalance of the group of minerals called electrolytes, which give signals to the muscles to contract, may be caused by loss of fluid or other factors, such as medications, alcohol abuse, or various diseases. |
| ◆ If the cause is a deficiency of iron, folic acid, or vitamin $B_{12}$, you may need a dietary change or supplement. | ◆ Weakness may occur because tissues are deprived of oxygen from blood loss or from a lack of red blood cells. |
| ◆ See Thyroid Problems. Your doctor may suggest antithyroid medication, surgery, or other treatment. | ◆ Muscle weakness can also be caused by an underactive thyroid gland (hypothyroidism) or by a deficiency of another endocrine gland, the adrenal gland. |
| ◆ Call your doctor. Treatment may involve anti-inflammatory painkillers, corticosteroids, immunosuppressive drugs, and/or antidepressants or mild antianxiety drugs. | ◆ In this autoimmune disease the immune system attacks the body's connective tissue as if it were foreign matter. |
| ◆ Call your doctor. You may be referred to a neurologist for testing and treatment; treatment depends on the specific disease. | ◆ Physical therapy is commonly used to increase function in these disabling disorders. |
| ◆ Call your doctor. The usual treatment is with the corticosteroid prednisone. | ◆ Although these disorders may disappear within a few months, they can be serious if lung problems develop. |
| ◆ Call your doctor. The only treatment is to lessen deformities through physical therapy. | ◆ The muscles in people with this rare, inherited disease lack a protein needed for proper functioning. |

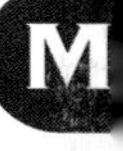


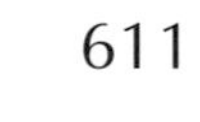

# NAIL PROBLEMS

*Read down this column to find your symptoms. Then read across.*

| SYMPTOMS | AILMENT/PROBLEM |
|---|---|
| ◆ split, brittle, and/or bent nails following extensive hand washing or a visit to a manicurist. | ◆ Possibly, an allergic reaction to a soap, nail polish, or other substance |
| ◆ nails that become pale and spoon-shaped or develop a temporary groove. | ◆ Anemia; damaged nail matrix (the nail-forming region underlying the cuticle) |
| ◆ cracked, thickened, and discolored nails accompanied by an itchy, scaly rash that usually starts between the fourth and fifth toes. | ◆ Athlete's foot |
| ◆ greenish black spots under the nail. | ◆ Potentially serious bacterial infection |
| ◆ black specks, especially on fingernails; bluish gray spots on the nail bed, and nails that curve over the ends of fingers or toes (also called clubbed nails). | ◆ Possibly, heart valve or other heart problems |
| ◆ a nail that grows into the side of the nail bed, causing inflammation; most common in the big toe, especially in women who wear narrow, tight shoes. | ◆ Ingrown nail |
| ◆ swollen, red, painful cuticle or nail fold (at the side of the nail); the cuticle may lift away from the base and ooze pus when pressed. | ◆ Paronychia (infection of tissue near a nail) |
| ◆ white spots on a nail, usually following a slight blow; similar patches on one or more nails. | ◆ Minor physical trauma; vitamin or mineral deficiency |
| ◆ thickened nails, which may be difficult to cut. | ◆ Circulatory problems, possibly related to atherosclerosis or diabetes |

| WHAT TO DO | OTHER INFO |
|---|---|
| ◆ See Allergies. Stop using nail lacquers, polishes, or adhesives (for false nails) and see if the problem clears up. | ◆ Acetate-based nail polish removers are less irritating to the skin than acetone-based nail polish removers. |
| ◆ Consult with your doctor. You may only need to increase your iron intake, but you may need other medical treatment. | ◆ Be sure your doctor tests for a vitamin $B_{12}$ deficiency as well as an iron deficiency. |
| ◆ Use over-the-counter antifungal medications. Dry your feet thoroughly after washing, and change your socks and shoes regularly. | ◆ A persistent or recurring case may require a trip to the doctor for more aggressive treatment. |
| ◆ **Call your doctor now.** See also Staph Infections. | |
| ◆ See Heart Disease. Call your doctor without delay if you suspect a heart condition. | ◆ Clubbed nails are a late—not an early—sign of heart problems. |
| ◆ Trim the excess nail and put a thin strand of sterile cotton under the corner of the nail to lift it away from the skin until it grows out. | ◆ Soak the affected foot in warm salt water or a calendula *(Calendula officinalis)* solution to soften the nail and help in easing it out from the nail fold. |
| ◆ See your doctor for antibiotic or antifungal treatment. | ◆ Occasionally a case of paronychia is caused by *Candida albicans,* so women should get checked for vaginitis or yeast infections. |
| ◆ No treatment is necessary for minor nail bruising. Take vitamin and mineral supplements if there was no trauma to the affected nail or nails. | ◆ The most likely deficiency is of zinc or vitamin $B_6$. |
| ◆ See the entries listed at left. | |

N

# NASAL POLYPS

## SYMPTOMS

- chronic blockage of nasal passages.
- difficulty breathing through nose.
- difficulty smelling.
- headaches.
- nosebleeds.

## CALL YOUR DOCTOR IF:

- you suspect you have nasal polyps. (You may be able to see them by looking in a mirror while shining a light up your nostrils; they look like pearly gray lumps.)
- you have a stuffy nose for more than two weeks; this may be a sign of an allergy or a sinus infection *(see Sinusitis),* which may require medical care.
- you have a fever along with your stuffy nose; this could be a sign of an infection, which may require medical care.
- the drainage from your nose is thick and colored; this could indicate a nasal infection, which may require medical care.

When the mucous membrane lining the inside of the nose becomes swollen, it can sometimes distend into the nasal cavity, creating protuberances known as nasal polyps. The polyps look something like small, pearly grapes and can appear singly or in clusters. Although harmless, they often obstruct the nasal passages, making breathing difficult and sometimes affecting the sense of smell. If the polyps block the opening between the nasal cavity and one of the sinuses, headaches can occur.

## CAUSES

Nasal polyps are caused by an overproduction of fluid in the mucous membrane lining the nose. People with chronic allergies and sinus infections are at greatest risk of developing them. Children with cystic fibrosis also tend to develop nasal polyps. In addition, the overuse of aspirin or other salicylate medications can cause polyps to form in some susceptible people.

### DIAGNOSTIC AND TEST PROCEDURES

If you think you have polyps, your doctor will examine the inside of your nose with a special medical instrument called a nasal speculum. If polyps are diagnosed in a child, further tests to rule out cystic fibrosis may be performed.

## TREATMENT

The only way to completely rid yourself of nasal polyps is to have them surgically removed. The polyps often recur, however, so it is important that you take preventive steps to manage or control the chronic allergies or sinus infections that usually cause them to form.

### CONVENTIONAL MEDICINE

To temporarily reduce the polyps, your doctor may treat them with a corticosteroid, either by directly injecting the medication into the polyps or by spraying it into your nostrils. You may also be given medications to treat the underlying cause of the polyps: an antihistamine for allergies or an antibiotic for a sinus infection.

If the polyps are causing serious discomfort or breathing problems, your doctor may recommend that you have them surgically removed. The operation, which uses a wire snare to clip off the polyps, is considered minor surgery and is usually performed under local anesthesia. Because the polyps often reappear, the surgery may need to be repeated. In very persistent cases, the lining of the sinuses where the polyps originate must be removed as well. This operation requires general anesthesia.

### ALTERNATIVE CHOICES

Many of the alternative treatments for nasal polyps are aimed at managing or controlling their underlying causes—the allergies and infections that make the nasal membranes swell with fluid.

#### AROMATHERAPY

Tea tree oil (*Melaleuca* spp.), eucalyptus *(Eucalyptus globulus)*, and peppermint *(Mentha piperita)* are often recommended for clearing stuffy noses. Add 2 drops of each to a warm bath, and soak for 15 minutes or so. Or you can place a drop of each on a tissue and inhale deeply whenever necessary.

#### HOMEOPATHY

Homeopaths believe that an appropriately chosen medication may help decrease some of the discomfort and problems caused by polyps. Consult a homeopath for a prescription, which might include the following remedies:

- ◆ If the polyps are accompanied by loss of smell, swelling around the bridge of the nose, and yellow mucus, Calcarea carbonica.
- ◆ If the polyps bleed easily, Phosphorus.
- ◆ If mucus drips down the back of the throat and you feel weak and chilled, Psorinum or Thuja.
- ◆ If the polyps are accompanied by sneezing and a crawling sensation in the nose, and mucus forms into large dry pieces, Teucrium.

Treatments can be lengthy—up to six months—and require many follow-up visits.

### AT-HOME REMEDIES

- ◆ To help decongest a stuffy nose and keep the mucous membranes from swelling and forming polyps, try hot baths or showers. Or try steam inhalations: Run very hot water in a sink until steam builds up. With the water running, lean over the sink, and drape a towel over your head to trap the steam. Breathe deeply through your mouth and nose for 5 to 10 minutes. Repeat several times a day.
- ◆ You can also decongest your nose with a homemade saline nasal spray: Mix 1 tsp table salt and 1 tsp baking soda in 1 qt boiled water that has been cooled. Fill a sprayer from the drugstore with the solution and use as many times during the day as necessary.

## PREVENTION

- ◆ If you have allergies, limit your exposure to whatever is causing them and take an antihistamine at the first sign of an allergic reaction.
- ◆ Avoid aspirin, which can stimulate the formation of nasal polyps.
- ◆ Drink plenty of fluids to keep your nasal membranes moist and healthy.
- ◆ Avoid beer, wine, and cordials, which contain tyramine and tannin, ingredients that can cause the nasal membrane to swell.

### CAUTION!

**Follow directions carefully when using over-the-counter nose drops or spray to clear up a stuffy nose. Overuse of these products can cause your mucous membranes to produce more fluid, making the congestion even worse than it was before. Never use one of these products more frequently or longer than directed on the label.** ■

# NAUSEA

*Read down this column to find your symptoms. Then read across.*

| SYMPTOMS | AILMENT/PROBLEM |
|---|---|
| For other conditions that may involve nausea, see also Vomiting. | |
| ◆ You feel nauseated (sick to your stomach) after a specific event or stimulus, such as a ride on a roller coaster, an unpleasant odor, or a stressful encounter. | ◆ Anxiety, motion sickness, stress, or merely a natural reaction to an unpleasant stimulus |
| ◆ frequent, burning pain in your upper middle abdomen, usually relieved by eating; possibly, nausea. | ◆ Gastritis; stomach ulcer |
| ◆ nausea; severe headache, possibly with vomiting; symptoms may worsen with exposure to bright light. | ◆ Migraine headache; possibly, meningitis |
| ◆ nausea while you are undergoing chemotherapy to treat cancer. | ◆ Common side effect of cancer treatment |
| ◆ sudden attacks of nausea accompanied by bouts of vomiting, extreme dizziness, and severe earache, sometimes with ringing or buzzing in your ears. | ◆ Ménière's disease |
| ◆ nausea, diarrhea, vomiting, and fever lasting 48 hours or less; may occur after eating rich, spicy, or possibly spoiled foods, drinking an excessive amount of alcohol, or ingesting a drug you have never taken before. | ◆ Gastroenteritis (also called stomach or intestinal flu) |
| ◆ nausea lasting one to two weeks, headache, malaise, and fatigue; sometimes sore throat, fever, and rash. | ◆ Mononucleosis; scarlet fever, which may follow strep throat |
| ◆ severe nausea with pain starting in the upper abdomen and moving to the right shoulder blade. | ◆ Gallstones; gallbladder infection |

| WHAT TO DO | OTHER INFO |
|---|---|
| ◆ If you have become nauseated at a sight, sound, or smell, close your eyes or plug your ears or nose, and focus on something pleasurable. | ◆ Mind/body medicine, including meditation and biofeedback, can help you lower your stress levels. Ginger *(Zingiber officinale)* capsules often alleviate motion sickness, as do acupressure wristbands. |
| ◆ If symptoms are constant or recurrent, see a doctor. Avoid irritating substances such as alcohol, tobacco, and caffeine; antacids may help alleviate symptoms. | ◆ Herbal teas of chamomile *(Matricaria recutita)* or lemon balm *(Melissa officinalis)* may reduce symptoms. |
| ◆ If you suspect meningitis, **call 911 or your emergency number now.** Migraines may respond to various analgesics (over-the-counter and prescription varieties). | ◆ Migraines often have specific triggers, such as red wine or chocolate. Identifying and avoiding your triggers is the best way to control the headaches. |
| ◆ Ask your doctor about specific ways to counteract this effect of your treatment. | ◆ Discuss any alternative therapies with your doctor before trying them. See Cancer for suggestions. |
| ◆ See your doctor. The regimen for minimizing symptoms may include keeping your sodium intake low and taking daily prescription medications to counteract fluid retention and dizziness. | ◆ Mind/body medicine, yoga, and massage therapy can help you learn to deal effectively with stress, which can trigger attacks. When Ménière's flares, avoid reading and bright lights to reduce dizziness. |
| ◆ Rest, drink plenty of fluids, and eat bland foods. You may need an antibiotic if your stomach bug is the result of a bacterial infection. | ◆ Gastroenteritis can be caused by a bacterial or viral infection, food poisoning, overindulgence in alcohol or rich foods, or some medications (including antibiotics). If you suspect that a prescription drug is causing the problem, see your doctor. |
| ◆ See your doctor. For mononucleosis, complete bed rest is essential, with a gradual return to normal activity; scarlet fever requires treatment with antibiotics. | ◆ Scarlet fever, though once a common childhood disease, is now quite rare. |
| ◆ Call your doctor today for an evaluation; gallstone attacks may require prompt treatment. | ◆ A doctor's care is required, but some alternative therapies, including Chinese herbs (which may help dissolve gallstones), can augment conventional treatment. |

| SYMPTOMS | AILMENT/PROBLEM |
|---|---|
| ◆ recurrent attacks of nausea, heartburn, and indigestion, particularly after meals; possibly, reduced appetite and weight loss. | ◆ Stomach ulcer; possibly, colorectal cancer |
| ◆ You are addicted to alcohol, have recently quit "cold turkey," and experience nausea, anxiety, insomnia, or delirium tremens (DT). | ◆ Common effect of recovering from alcohol abuse |
| ◆ nausea accompanied by increased thirst and urination; dehydration; drowsiness; confusion; possibly, a fruity odor on your breath. | ◆ Diabetes; possibly, diabetic shock |
| ◆ nausea coming in attacks once or twice every several months, accompanied by intense, steady abdominal pain and, in some cases, fever, diarrhea, and vomiting. | ◆ Crohn's disease; pancreatic problems |
| ◆ nausea and vomiting that persist after a viral infection; alternating periods of hyperactivity and fatigue. | ◆ Reye's syndrome (a neurological disorder typically in children, which may follow an upper respiratory tract infection or chickenpox, especially if aspirin has been given during treatment) |
| ◆ nausea with shortness of breath, chest pain, and sweating. | ◆ Heart attack |
| ◆ You are allergic to a specific food, drug, or insect sting, and experience nausea, vomiting, and difficulty breathing after encountering the allergen. | ◆ Allergies; possibly, anaphylactic shock (a severe allergic reaction that causes tissues to swell, preventing blood from traveling properly; tissues then become starved for oxygen) |
| ◆ You are or could be pregnant; you have nausea, a bloated feeling in the pelvic area and breasts, and possibly, vomiting. | ◆ Normal effects (sometimes called morning sickness, though it can occur any time of day) often felt during the first three months of pregnancy |

| WHAT TO DO | OTHER INFO |
|---|---|
| ◆ Call your doctor today for diagnosis. | ◆ Early detection is crucial for successfully treating colorectal cancer. |
| ◆ Consult with your doctor; some withdrawal symptoms may require immediate medical treatment. | ◆ Prescription medications are available that make alcohol withdrawal a much easier process. |
| ◆ Call your doctor. If you suspect diabetic shock, **call 911 or your emergency number now.** | ◆ Ketoacidosis, a potentially fatal condition of extremely high blood sugar levels, requires an immediate insulin injection. |
| ◆ Call your doctor today; a combination of medications may be necessary to control Crohn's disease. | ◆ Conventional medical treatment is essential, but discomfort can be lessened with acupuncture, herbal therapies, homeopathy, and mind/body medicine. |
| ◆ **Call 911 or your emergency number now.** Reye's syndrome progresses quickly, and immediate treatment is essential. | ◆ Never give aspirin to a child with a fever or an infection; use acetaminophen or other nonaspirin pain relievers when needed. |
| ◆ **Call 911 or your emergency number now.** | |
| ◆ If you suspect anaphylactic shock, **get emergency medical treatment.** See Emergencies/First Aid: Shock. While waiting for emergency care, monitor the patient's breathing and pulse, and give nothing to eat or drink. | ◆ Particularly if you have allergies, ask your doctor about preparing an anti-anaphylactic shock kit. |
| ◆ Avoid extremely salty foods, get plenty of rest, and eat small meals several times a day instead of three large meals. See Pregnancy Problems. | ◆ Ginger *(Zingiber officinale)* tea is helpful in relieving nausea due to morning sickness, but check with your doctor before trying any remedy. |

# NECK PAIN

*Read down this column to find your symptoms. Then read across.*

| SYMPTOMS | AILMENT/PROBLEM |
| --- | --- |
| ◆ neck stiffness or pain upon awakening that wasn't there when you went to bed. | ◆ A stiff neck, from sleeping in a position that strained your neck muscles or joints |
| ◆ swelling or a lump on the side or back of your neck; possibly accompanied by neck pain. | ◆ Swollen lymph nodes, in response to an infection somewhere in your body |
| ◆ neck stiffness that progressively worsens. | ◆ Osteoarthritis |
| ◆ intense neck pain that shoots into your arms or shoulders, especially when you move your head. | ◆ A ruptured or slipped vertebral disk, which is pressing against a nerve |
| ◆ severe neck pain that started in the last 24 hours after some sort of jolt (as when a car stops suddenly); may be accompanied by dizziness, difficulty walking, vomiting, difficulty controlling arms or legs, or loss of bladder or bowel control. | ◆ Whiplash |
| ◆ dull, throbbing pain on one side of your neck that may radiate into your cheek, eye, or ear; pain is worse when you chew, yawn, or move your head; symptoms may follow another illness (such as sore throat), or may be associated with migraine headache. | ◆ Carotidynia (dilation of the carotid artery, which carries blood to the brain; possibly caused by a virus or bacteria) |
| ◆ pain at the front of your neck when you swallow; possibly, pain along the jaw and below the ear; mild fever; neck may be red and tender. | ◆ Thyroiditis (inflammation of the thyroid, possibly the result of infection or an autoimmune disorder) |
| ◆ severe headache followed by neck pain that is worse when the head is bent forward; any one of the following: nausea, vomiting, confusion, drowsiness, sensitivity to bright light. | ◆ Meningitis |

| WHAT TO DO | OTHER INFO |
|---|---|
| ◆ If the stiffness or pain does not go away within 24 hours, call your doctor. | |
| ◆ See your doctor to identify the infection; you may need an antibiotic. | |
| ◆ See Arthritis. Pain is often relieved by a daily regimen of over-the-counter nonsteroidal anti-inflammatory drugs (NSAIDs). | ◆ Osteoarthritis most commonly affects people over the age of 50. |
| ◆ See Disk Problems. Take aspirin or nonsteroidal anti-inflammatory drugs (NSAIDs) to relieve pain. Your doctor may suggest wearing a soft collar to limit movement until the disk returns to position, and possibly stronger pain relievers as well. | ◆ Chiropractors, massage therapists, and yoga instructors often have success treating these problems. |
| ◆ **Call your doctor now,** and apply ice to your neck until you can get medical care. If the pain is mild and unaccompanied by other symptoms, you may only need to take aspirin or nonsteroidal anti-inflammatory drugs (NSAIDs), but call your doctor if you feel no better after 24 hours. | ◆ Wearing a soft padded collar will immobilize and stabilize your neck, but don't use it for more than a week or so or your healing will actually take longer. For more comfortable sleeping, lie on a firm bed and don't use a pillow. |
| ◆ Call your doctor. Pain may be relieved with rest, nonsteroidal anti-inflammatory drugs (NSAIDs), and a cold or hot compress; prescription antimigraine drugs sometimes help. | ◆ Differentiating between carotidynia and sore throat, sinus infection, an abscessed tooth, or oral cancer can be difficult. |
| ◆ Call your doctor to differentiate between thyroiditis and sore throat. See Thyroid Problems; Immune Problems. | ◆ After a bout of thyroiditis, expect frequent checks by your doctor to ensure your thyroid is working properly. |
| ◆ **Get medical care immediately.** You will need two weeks of aggressive antibiotic therapy, and you may need to stay in the hospital. | ◆ Without treatment, bacterial meningitis can be fatal; viral meningitis is rarely fatal. |

# NEURALGIA

## SYMPTOMS

Neuralgia, or nerve pain, comes in many different forms: It may be sudden, shooting, sharp, burning, or stabbing, and is sometimes accompanied by a background sensation of burning, itching, or aching, or by hypersensitivity to touch. It occurs in one part of your body, typically on one side. The pain may be intermittent or continuous; it can last for a few seconds or a few minutes, and may recur, on and off, for days or weeks.

## CALL YOUR DOCTOR IF:

- you suspect that the pain is caused by a spinal problem, a herniated disk, or a pinched nerve.
- the symptoms include impaired bladder or bowel control or a dragging foot—signs of nerve damage; **call your doctor immediately.**
- facial neuralgia spreads to an eye after a herpes attack; this could lead to blindness if untreated.
- the pain becomes too great to bear; nerve damage could result.

Neuralgia, as the name suggests, is nerve pain, occurring when a nerve is irritated or inflamed. The pain, spreading along neural pathways, may be fleeting or chronic and can range from mild to outright unbearable.

Only a few types of neuralgia are common. One, characterized by flashes of facial pain, is called trigeminal neuralgia, after the multi-branched cranial nerve that is affected; the condition occurs mostly in people over 50 and afflicts three times as many women as men. Nerves of the buttocks and legs are also vulnerable; irritation of the large sciatic nerve, for example, produces the neuralgia called sciatica. Another relatively common type is postherpetic neuralgia, which strikes after the type of herpes infection known as shingles and typically manifests itself as a continuous burning sensation.

## CAUSES

Generally, the likeliest source of neuralgias is irritation or inflammation of a nerve or pressure on a nerve from bones or connective tissue. Such pressure may be due to a muscle or spinal injury, a prolapsed disk, or years of poor posture. Trigeminal neuralgia may stem from the pressure of a blood vessel. In postherpetic neuralgia, the nerve inflammation is caused by a viral infection. In many cases of neuralgia, however, the reason for the nerve's irritated state cannot be discovered.

## TREATMENT

### CONVENTIONAL MEDICINE

Physicians often prescribe analgesics for mild neuralgia and opioid analgesics for severe cases. Trigeminal neuralgia pain can be relieved with the anticonvulsants carbamazepine and phenytoin. Capsaicin (the active ingredient in cayenne pepper) in ointment form can be an effective over-the-counter remedy for postherpetic neuralgia. Corticosteroids reduce nerve inflammation, and sedatives help with pain indirectly.

## ALTERNATIVE CHOICES

In addition to the therapies listed below, consider seeing a **chiropractor** or an **osteopath;** manipulations of the spine and of soft tissue have proved helpful in relieving several types of neuralgia.

### ACUPUNCTURE

Acupuncture has been shown to be extremely effective in treating neuralgia. If the pain is severe, 5 to 10 acupuncture sessions may be required.

### BODY WORK

In a series of lessons, an **Alexander technique** instructor can train you to adjust your body posture and movements to prevent future attacks. Deep-tissue **massage** reduces pain by probing into successively deeper layers of muscle and connective tissue, and concentrates on "clearing out" a particular area of the body. When inflammation causes the connective tissue, or fascia, that covers muscles to have an abnormally tight grip on a muscle, myofascial release therapy loosens that grip through gentle stretching, reducing pain.

### HERBAL THERAPIES

A cup of boiling water poured over 2 tsp St.-John's-wort *(Hypericum perforatum)* and steeped for 10 minutes has painkilling properties when drunk three times daily. Recent experiments on extracts from black cohosh *(Cimicifuga racemosa)* suggest it may have anti-inflammatory qualities.

### HOMEOPATHY

For sharp, shooting pain with tingling and burning, try Hypericum (6x) once an hour for three to four doses. Consult a homeopath for other remedies specific to your symptoms.

### NUTRITION AND DIET

When an attack begins, a maximum dose of 50 mg vitamin $B_6$ three times a day and vitamin B complex once a day may help; continue for one week only. For postherpetic neuralgia, add 400 IU vitamin E twice a day.

Making oats *(Avena sativa)* a regular part of your diet can improve the overall condition of nerves. A drink made from minced oat straw or oat grass steeped for two minutes in warm water and strained is thought to be a valuable tonic; drink 1 to 4 grams daily. To soothe itching skin, bathe in water that has been run over oatmeal in a muslin bag hung under the bathtub tap.

**AREAS OF PAIN**

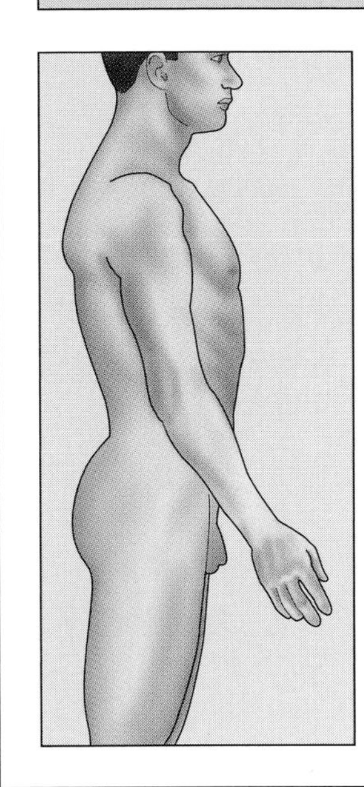

Neuralgia, or pain that results from an irritated or damaged nerve, occurs in various forms in different parts of the body. Trigeminal neuralgia, for example, affects the face. Intercostal neuralgia causes pain between the ribs, and sciatica strikes the lower back and legs. These locations are not exclusive, however; neuralgia can develop in any part of the body where a nerve has been damaged.

## AT-HOME REMEDIES

- ◆ A man suffering from trigeminal neuralgia can grow a beard to shield his face from the cold, which sometimes leads to an attack.
- ◆ An old folk remedy calls for cutting a baked potato in half and applying the cooled halves to an afflicted area to draw out the pain.

# PREVENTION

Learning how to sit, stand, and lift for proper back support is the best way to forestall some types of neuralgia. Several different **body work** therapies *(above, left)* can teach you how to move properly to avoid attacks. Consult a trained therapist. ■

# NICOTINE WITHDRAWAL

## SYMPTOMS

In active tobacco users, a lack of nicotine produces a wide range of withdrawal symptoms, including any or all of the following:

- headache.
- nausea.
- constipation or diarrhea.
- falling heart rate and blood pressure.
- fatigue, drowsiness, and insomnia.
- irritability.
- difficulty concentrating.
- anxiety.
- depression.
- increased hunger and caloric intake.
- increased pleasantness of the taste of sweets.
- tobacco cravings.

## CALL YOUR DOCTOR IF:

- you are a tobacco user concerned about your health for any reason; tobacco users are more susceptible to respiratory problems; circulatory problems such as stroke, heart attack, and occlusive vascular disorder; and many forms of cancer.
- you want to stop using tobacco; your doctor can prescribe nicotine-based aids and refer you to counseling or to other cessation programs to get you through the withdrawal stage.

Withdrawal from nicotine, an addictive drug found in tobacco, is characterized by symptoms that include headache, anxiety, nausea, and a craving for more tobacco. Nicotine creates a chemical dependency, so that the body develops a need for a certain level of nicotine at all times. Unless that level is maintained, the body will begin to go through withdrawal.

For tobacco users trying to quit, symptoms of withdrawal from nicotine are unpleasant and stressful but temporary. Most withdrawal symptoms peak 48 hours after you quit and are completely gone in six months. But even after that you may still have to deal with the fact that you are probably eating more than you did as a smoker and may need to lose some weight.

## CAUSES

The symptoms of nicotine withdrawal are physiological responses to the removal of a substance on which the body has become dependent.

## TREATMENT

### CONVENTIONAL MEDICINE

A combination of smoking cessation drugs and behavior modification appears to be the most effective treatment in helping tobacco users, especially smokers, quit.

Your doctor may recommend a smoking (or other tobacco-use) cessation program and may also prescribe nicotine-based chewing gum or a skin patch to help you through withdrawal. Most doctors recommend that patients stop using the gum or patch after a month or two. These aids are meant to help you modify your behavior, not to allow you to maintain your nicotine habit.

### ALTERNATIVE CHOICES

Alternative therapies can offer support to tobacco users trying to quit their habit. Behavior modification techniques that may help include **meditation, guided imagery, biofeedback,** and **hypnotherapy.**

### ACUPRESSURE

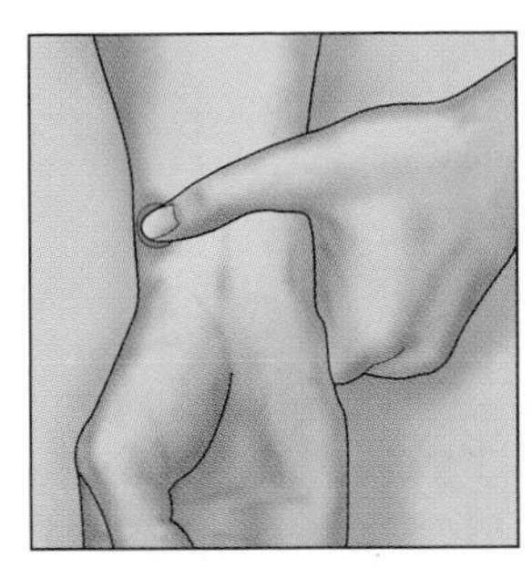

**1** To improve lung function after you quit smoking, press Lung 7. Place your left thumb two finger widths above the right wrist crease, along the radius bone, in line with the index finger. Press firmly for one minute, then repeat on the other arm. Do three times.

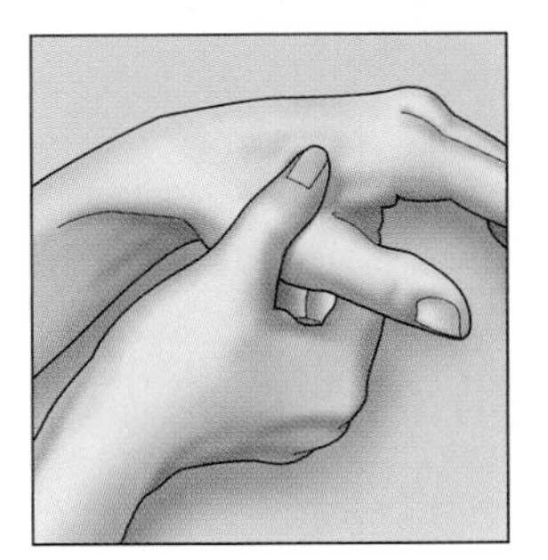

**2** Pressing Large Intestine 4, in the web between your thumb and index finger, may ease withdrawal symptoms. Use the thumb and index finger of your right hand to squeeze the web of your left hand for one minute. Repeat on the right hand. Do not use this point if you are pregnant.

### ACUPUNCTURE

Acupuncture has been shown to help relieve withdrawal symptoms. Treatment usually involves one to three sessions using points on the ear or the body. Acupuncture may be combined with herbal medicine or other nutritional support but is not appropriate when using the nicotine gum or patch.

Consult a Chinese herbalist or an acupuncturist trained in Chinese herbs for an appropriate course of therapeutic treatment.

### HERBAL THERAPIES

Lobelia *(Lobelia inflata)* has actions similar to nicotine but is gentler and longer lasting. It is often used by medical herbalists in conjunction with ephedra *(Ephedra sinica),* a stimulant, to help tobacco users quit. See a professional; too much of these herbs can cause serious side effects. Herbalists also often recommend herbs to calm the nervous system during withdrawal, including oat *(Avena sativa)* straw, chamomile *(Matricaria recutita),* hops *(Humulus lupulus),* and valerian *(Valeriana officinalis).*

### AT-HOME REMEDIES

Most tobacco-use cessation programs offer the following steps to help you quit:

- Analyze your habit for a few weeks; keep a log of when, where, and why you use tobacco.
- List the reasons you want to quit.
- Set a "quit" date and stick to it.
- Find substitutes—sugarless gum to chew or a pen or pencil to hold—and change your routines to avoid triggering a desire for tobacco.
- Reward your resolve. Treat yourself with the money you would have spent on your habit.
- Enjoy your food and eat as much low-calorie food as you want during withdrawal.
- Never let a relapse deter you from continuing your efforts to quit. Former smokers try an average of six times before they quit for good.

## PREVENTION

The best preventive step is not to start using tobacco and to educate your children to its dangers. Most tobacco users start in their teens because of peer pressure, a need to rebel, or a desire to appear more mature. Children of tobacco users are more likely to be users because they view tobacco use as acceptable. If you use tobacco and you're serious about preventing your children from doing so, you can provide the best example by quitting.

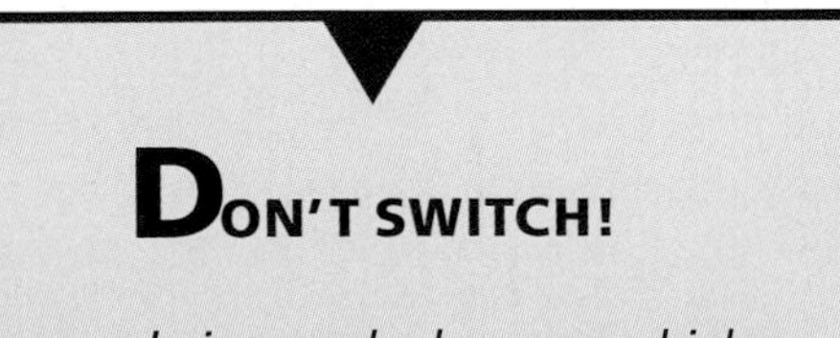

### DON'T SWITCH!

*Cigar and pipe smoke have even higher levels of nicotine and carcinogens than cigarette smoke. While most pipe or cigar smokers don't inhale this smoke, research shows that cigarette smokers who switch to cigars and pipes retain their smoking habits, so they inhale even more harmful smoke than before.* ■

# NUMBNESS AND TINGLING

*Read down this column to find your symptoms. Then read across.*

| SYMPTOMS | AILMENT/PROBLEM |
|---|---|
| ◆ numbness or tingling on one side of your body, and one or more of the following: weakness in hands or feet, dizziness, confusion, blurred vision, difficulty speaking. | ◆ Stroke or transient ischemic attack |
| ◆ numbness, tingling, or pain in one arm or one leg, with weakness on that side. | ◆ Possible herniated or prolapsed disk |
| ◆ numbness, tingling, or pain in the fingers, hand, or wrist; pain may shoot into the fingers from the wrist. | ◆ Carpal tunnel syndrome |
| ◆ tingling in any part of the body; may be accompanied by vision problems, loss of coordination and trembling of one hand, difficulty walking, or loss of bladder control. | ◆ Multiple sclerosis or other neurological ailment |
| ◆ tingling or numbness of the hands or feet, perhaps accompanied by nausea, headache, or dizziness, without underlying disease. | ◆ Environmental poisoning/illness |
| ◆ numbness or tingling that you experience in any part of your body while you are taking certain medications or vitamins. | ◆ Adverse side effect of a drug |
| ◆ numbness and a bluish color in one or more fingers or toes, quite often triggered by cold. | ◆ Raynaud's syndrome |
| ◆ numbness or tingling in your hands and face, especially around your lips, accompanied by shaking, fear, or heart palpitations. | ◆ Panic attack |
| ◆ numbness or tingling in a hand, foot, arm, or leg after sitting or sleeping in one position. | ◆ Stretching or pressing on a nerve, or decreasing the blood supply to a nerve |

| WHAT TO DO | OTHER INFO |
|---|---|
| ◆ **Call your doctor now.** Prompt treatment may prevent a full-blown stroke and damage to brain tissue. See also Angina; Heart Attack. | ◆ You may be able to prevent a full-blown stroke by lowering your blood pressure, using aspirin or other drugs to prevent the formation of clots, or having surgery. |
| ◆ See your doctor. Pain may subside when you lie down. See Disk Problems. | ◆ Many herniated, or ruptured, disks can be treated with bed rest; sometimes surgery is necessary. |
| ◆ See your doctor. For mild symptoms, a wrist splint may help. The condition can also be corrected surgically, with good long-term results. | ◆ This syndrome can be caused by repetitive manual tasks. Taking regular breaks and gently rotating the hands help prevent it. |
| ◆ See your doctor. Symptoms may be intermittent in early stages of the disease and hard to diagnose. | ◆ Multiple sclerosis destroys the thick myelin sheath that surrounds nerve fibers. Because almost any part of the nervous system may be affected, symptoms may be diverse. |
| ◆ See your doctor, who may suggest tests to check for neurological damage. See Environmental Poisoning. | ◆ People most at risk include farmers, environmental and chemical workers, pest exterminators, and people living near industrial plants. |
| ◆ Discuss any medications you are taking with your doctor, who may suggest alternatives. | ◆ Such symptoms may be caused by fluoride, anesthetics, niacin, nitrous oxide, the cancer drug taxol, and vitamin $B_6$. |
| ◆ Numbness can usually be relieved by warming or rubbing, and normally resolves itself without serious consequences. | ◆ Raynaud's may afflict people who work with their hands or are exposed to the cold, or it may have no known cause. |
| ◆ Practice relaxation techniques; consult your doctor or a psychotherapist for persistent attacks. | ◆ The physical effects of panic attacks may be triggered by rapid breathing. Attacks usually subside in a quarter of an hour or less. |
| ◆ Move your limbs around or stand up. Feeling should return to normal in a few moments. | ◆ This temporary pins-and-needles feeling is normal and does not indicate an underlying disorder. |

# OBESITY

## SYMPTOMS

- a body-fat percentage greater than 30 percent for women and 25 percent for men. (Your doctor can measure this percentage for you.)
- weighing 20 percent more than your ideal body weight. Your ideal weight is based on your gender, age, and typical activity level (whether you tend to be sedentary or active). Consult your doctor or a nutritionist for an accurate determination of your ideal weight.

## CALL YOUR DOCTOR IF:

- you suspect you weigh 20 percent more than your ideal body weight; obesity places you at much greater risk for high blood pressure, heart disease, diabetes, gallbladder problems, respiratory problems, and various cancers, including breast cancer and colorectal cancer.
- you've lost weight many times but always gain it back; you may need professional guidance to develop a long-term, permanent weight-loss program.
- you are overweight and experience a drop in your sex drive, have problems menstruating, or become noticeably hairier; you may suffer from a hormone problem or a tumor on a hormone-secreting gland.

If you consume more calories than you burn, you will gain weight. The tricky part of the equation is that some people metabolize food differently from others. Why this happens is complex and not entirely clear to researchers, who continue to be surprised by each new finding. For example, one recent study concluded that heavy people actually burn calories faster than underweight people because their metabolism speeds up as they put on pounds, and slows if they try to take them off. For obese people—generally defined as those weighing 20 percent more than their ideal weight, or "set point"—the average-sized meal really isn't very filling. Not only do these people have more fat cells sending out signals for food, but their faster metabolism burns more calories as well.

Despite such obstacles, if you are obese, you should make every effort to lose weight. If left unchecked, obesity places you at much greater risk for developing a variety of extremely serious, often life-threatening conditions, from cancer to heart disease. Be particularly concerned if your body tends to store fat around your waist (most common in men). Unlike fat around the thighs, which is more common in women and is more likely to serve as an energy reservoir, abdominal deposits deliver fatty acids directly into the bloodstream for immediate short-term energy; doctors remain uncertain why this can prove to be detrimental to your health.

Unfortunately, many people never take off—and keep off—the extra pounds. According to charts developed by the Metropolitan Life Insurance Company more than 50 years ago *(see page 37)*, which many of today's doctors consider too forgiving, anywhere from a quarter to a third of the adults in the United States are overweight.

A more reliable measuring system, the body mass index (BMI), determines obesity based on body-fat content rather than weight. Determining your body-fat level (something your healthcare practitioner can do for you) is the best way to assess your weight status. For example, you may be the same height and weight as someone considered to be obese, but if you have relatively thick bones and a lot of muscle—and therefore less body fat—you will not merit the same diagnosis.

If you are overweight, you need to realize that you have a lifelong condition that requires not only a special diet and exercise but possibly some counseling and medications to bring under control. Keeping obesity in check requires constant vigilance—no easy task in the high-fat, high-sugar, high-volume nutritional landscape of the United States.

## CAUSES

There are many reasons for a person's being obese, including diabetes, thyroid problems, poor diet, insufficient exercise, and heredity. People with a predisposition to gain weight often aggravate their condition by smoking, drinking alcohol, and leading a sedentary lifestyle. Indeed, watching TV is one of the strongest predictors of obesity. If you are obese, the key is to recognize that you have a disease and to avoid habits that aggravate it.

While most cases of obesity are related to family history, social environment, diet, and other lifestyle habits, there are rare instances in which something specific, such as a thyroid condition, is the cause. Certain drugs, in particular estrogens and progestins, insulin, and steroids, can also cause weight gain.

In addition to all these factors, a recent study showed that muscles as well as fat cells play a role in obesity. Doctors have long recognized that fat cells in your body increase in size and mass when you put on weight. What they have just learned is that your muscles become more efficient and burn fewer calories when you try to lose that weight, which helps account for your slowed metabolism.

## TREATMENT

Weight-loss programs are a billion-dollar business in the U.S., with more overweight people signing up to drop pounds (only to regain them later) every day. Unfortunately, many of these commercial enterprises follow the cultural view that obesity results from some moral inadequacy, that fat people could lose weight if they would just exercise a little will power; but research shows that the answer is nowhere near that simple. Strong biochemical and genetic forces come into play every time any of us approaches a plate of food. Lack of will power has little to do with how your body will eventually process what you eat or how it will respond when you are full.

As knowledge of obesity's causes changes, so do the treatments. For now, most conventional and alternative therapies focus on diet, exercise, and possible psychological complications.

**THE DANGERS OF HIGH BODY FAT**

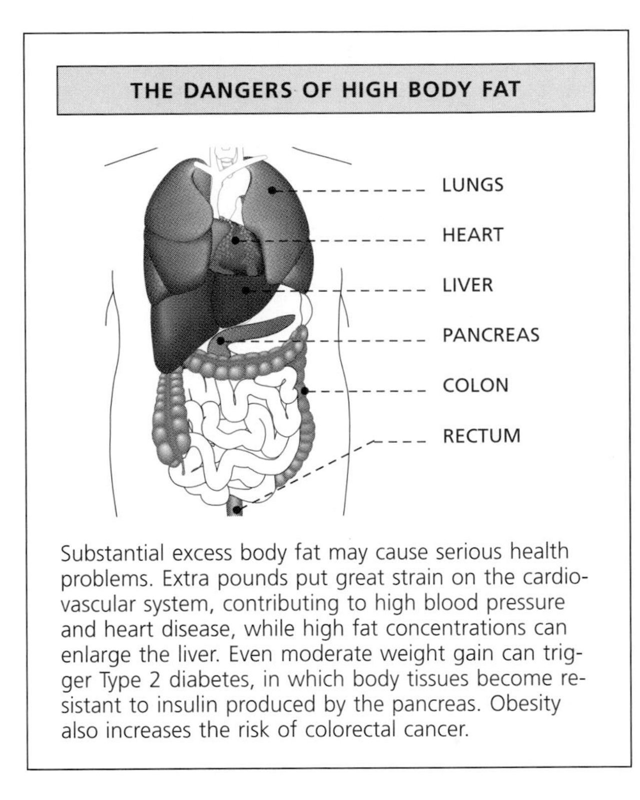


Substantial excess body fat may cause serious health problems. Extra pounds put great strain on the cardiovascular system, contributing to high blood pressure and heart disease, while high fat concentrations can enlarge the liver. Even moderate weight gain can trigger Type 2 diabetes, in which body tissues become resistant to insulin produced by the pancreas. Obesity also increases the risk of colorectal cancer.

### CONVENTIONAL MEDICINE

When it comes to obesity, the only thing everyone agrees on is that exercise is crucial to any weight-loss program. One study found that 95 percent of patients on a weight-loss diet regained the pounds they had lost if they did not include exercise as part of their overall program. Other factors, such as the fat and fiber content of your diet, also play a major role, but nothing is as important as exercise.

Indeed, you can conscientiously shun calories but never lose the fat. A key reason for the uphill battle: As you reduce the number of calories you consume, your body reacts in ways that evolved hundreds of thousands of years ago as defense mechanisms. It assumes that you are starving and as a result raises all sorts of barriers to protect against weight loss, including slowing down metabolism and storing energy more efficiently. As you try to lose weight, then, your body does all it can to keep the weight on.

If you are obese, you must think in terms of permanent change rather than short-term dieting, because you have a permanent problem. Consult your doctor about determining a good general target for your caloric intake and then maintain that level; a low-fat, low-sugar, high-fiber diet will help you achieve your goal. Add an exercise program to your weekly routine; something as simple as a 30-minute walk at lunch can be very effective. There is some evidence that a long-term, strict regimen of regular exercise and a moderate, low-fat diet can permanently lower your set point, making it easier for you to sustain a lower weight.

In some instances your doctor may recommend that you supplement your lifestyle and dietary changes with a drug that suppresses appetite. The most popular options include ephedrine, which affects metabolism by stimulating the nervous system; fenfluramine, which inhibits the uptake of calories and promotes a feeling of satiety; and fluoxetine, an antidepressant that has also been found to suppress appetite.

People desperate to lose weight are easy targets for hucksters who plug a whole host of useless remedies, from amphetamines and thyroid supplements to topical creams that purport to melt away fat. To be on the safe side, always consult with your doctor before you try any over-the-counter or mail-order weight-loss medication.

On rare occasions a doctor may suggest a surgical procedure that essentially shrinks the stomach. Only motivated, healthy patients benefit from this therapy, which has many critics. It does remove the need for appetite suppressants, but research has yet to show whether patients manage to keep weight off for the long term.

Two much simpler techniques, liposuction and jaw wiring, also have many drawbacks and should rarely if ever be considered. To perform liposuction, the surgeon makes a small incision near fatty deposits and then suctions the fat out. Very little fat can be removed, however, because of potential risks to blood vessels and nerves.

Jaw wiring can damage gums and teeth and cause muscle spasms in the jaw joint. The liquid diet that such patients must eat does result in weight loss, but as soon as the wires are removed patients almost always put back on what they lost.

The best treatment skirts these more extreme approaches and attacks obesity on several levels, including a psychological one. Learning to control what you eat, how you react to food in general, and what you do in your free time (watching television versus taking a walk) will do more for you than any surgeon's knife. Consider seeing a professional nutritionist, an exercise therapist, and possibly, a counselor if you believe you have an unhealthy attitude toward food.

## ALTERNATIVE CHOICES

Most alternative therapies work well when used to complement an existing program of proper diet and exercise.

### ACUPRESSURE

Some food addicts have found that use of a press needle or a plastic device placed over certain acupressure points on the ear helps alleviate cravings. Consult a practitioner familiar with treating eating disorders.

### CHINESE MEDICINE

The Chinese herb ephedra *(Ephedra sinica)* contains ephedrine, which increases the metabolic rate in fat tissue. Be aware that this treatment can have potent side effects, including insomnia, anxiety, heart arrhythmias, and hypertension. Do not use it if you have diabetes, thyroid problems, or heart disease. For best results see a practitioner of Chinese medicine, who will work on regulating all of your organs, especially the spleen.

### HERBAL THERAPIES

To stimulate your metabolic rate, try kelp (*Fucus*

spp.) in tablet form three to four times a day; it is thought to be especially good for thyroid-related obesity. Dandelion *(Taraxacum officinale)* may flush out the kidneys, boost metabolism, and offset a craving for sweets. Eat the leaves raw in a salad or make a tea by boiling 2 to 3 tsp of the root in a cup of water for 10 to 15 minutes. Drink three times a day.

#### HOMEOPATHY

Homeopathy offers treatments for various aspects of obesity. For example, many over-the-counter mixtures contain Argentum nitricum, which may cure intense sugar cravings. If your weight does not improve in one to two months after beginning at-home homeopathic treatment, see a professional.

#### LIFESTYLE

Smoking provides an excellent example of how a predisposition toward obesity can lure a person into an unhealthy lifestyle. Studies show that overweight teenage girls are more apt to smoke and are less responsive to programs designed to help them quit because they think cigarettes keep their weight down. While smoking does suppress appetite, it also adversely affects fat storage, leading to more deposits in the waist area. Overweight people also tend to drink alcohol more, adding to their caloric intake; alcohol is processed in the body much like fatty foods.

#### MIND/BODY MEDICINE

**Hypnotherapy, guided imagery,** and **yoga** may help with weight loss by altering the way you relate to food. Check with a specialist in these techniques.

#### NUTRITION AND DIET

A diet of complex carbohydrates, such as potatoes and pasta, as well as chicken, fish, and plenty of vegetables, should fill you up without filling you out.

Consider eating your main meal in the middle of the day, when you will burn off more of the calories you take in; a large meal eaten at night, when you are more sedentary, is less easily digested and absorbed.

Replace daily consumption of soft drinks, fruit juices, and milk with six to eight glasses of water.

Avoid diets that count calories. The grueling routine of such a diet increases your risk for developing eating disorders such as anorexia nervosa and bulimia.

Always keep in mind that you cannot shed pounds unless your energy output exceeds your energy input.

### AT-HOME REMEDIES

Certain at-home remedies can help with some side effects associated with obesity, such as constipation.

- 1 to 2 tsp a day of brewer's yeast or some dandelion will reduce a craving for sweets. Bee pollen or a dash of cayenne *(Capsicum frutescens)* may increase your metabolism.
- A tea made from rhubarb root may alleviate constipation.

## PREVENTION

If you stick to a moderate, low-fat diet and an exercise routine for several years, you may actually lower your set point. Once your body accepts the lower weight as your natural state, it will be much easier for you to sustain it without dieting. Some helpful tips to avoid obesity:

- Eat three or four moderate meals a day, with your main meal in the middle of the day.
- Eat a high-fiber, low-fat diet.
- Avoid sedentary activities, such as watching television, and get into a regular exercise routine.
- Don't turn to calorie-counting diets or diets that require you to fast or deprive yourself of normal helpings of food for extended periods of time.
- Avoid using food as a reward for yourself. ■

# OBSESSIVE-COMPULSIVE DISORDER

## SYMPTOMS

You may have obsessive thoughts or compulsive behavior or both.

**For obsession:**

- involuntary and persistent thoughts that appear to be senseless, such as an overwhelming fear of dirt; persistent worry about a past event.
- attempts to suppress such thoughts.
- recognition that these thoughts come from one's own imagination, not from outside factors (not true for children).

**For compulsions:**

- repetitive acts such as hand washing, checking and rechecking locks, tidying, repeating words.
- recognition that the repetitive behavior is excessive or unreasonable (may not be true for children).
- feverish levels of thought or activity.
- depression and distress as attempts to deal with compulsions fail.

**For children:**

- mute behavior with agitated depression.
- withdrawal and social isolation accompanied by delusional thinking.
- mood swings from anxiety to despair.
- exemplary functioning in sports or schoolwork accompanied by compulsive behavior.

## CALL YOUR DOCTOR IF:

- you or your child is experiencing some of the symptoms listed above.
- your child is anxious or depressed and has fears of aggression, sexual behavior, contamination, or disorderliness.

Obsessive-compulsive disorder (OCD) is not the ordinary "double-checking" that all of us do from time to time—making sure the doors are locked or the oven is off. For OCD patients these thoughts are so magnified that they interfere with everyday routines, jobs, and relationships. Sufferers have been known to wash their hands for eight hours or to reorganize their entire household daily. Obsessive-compulsive disorder is chronic and cannot be controlled voluntarily. Even after long periods of relative normality, sufferers may have another attack without apparent cause.

Because obsession takes hold gradually—moving slowly from simple interest to brooding to complete preoccupation—people often fail to recognize that they are suffering from a disorder. When OCD eventually produces symptoms that interfere with daily life, patients may try to hide their compulsions from others and attempt to deal with them by using will power.

Although OCD can appear in childhood, onset most often occurs in adolescence; half of adult sufferers show some symptoms by the age of 15. In the United States, between 2 percent and 3 percent of the population experiences some form of OCD during their lives. Obsessive-compulsive features are also found in Tourette's syndrome *(see Tics and Twitches)*, depression, and schizophrenia.

## CAUSES

At one time, obsessive or compulsive behavior was thought to indicate demonic possession, with exorcism one of the earliest forms of treatment. Currently, some 20 different theories exist on what might cause obsessive-compulsive disorder. The traditional hypothesis from Freudian thought holds that obsessions reflect unconscious desires from an earlier stage of development (anal stage). Although some experts in psychology still support the Freudian hypothesis, the most widely held theory today suggests that there is a genetic predisposition to OCD and that it is triggered by low levels of one of the brain's neurotransmitters, serotonin.

### DIAGNOSTIC AND TEST PROCEDURES

Often, the patients' own descriptions of their behavior offer the best clues. A family history is also important, to evaluate whether there is any genetic predisposition. Your doctor will also want to rule out other psychological disorders, such as schizophrenia, that can produce similar patterns of behavior.

## TREATMENT

The goal of treatment is to reduce anxiety, resolve inner conflicts, and help you learn more effective ways of dealing with anxiety. Conventional treatment may include psychotherapy or behavior therapy, antidepressants, and stress-reduction techniques. Drugs combined with behavior therapy seem to bring the best results.

### CONVENTIONAL MEDICINE

Currently, the most effective antiobsessional drug appears to be the tricyclic antidepressant clomipramine. Studies have shown that clomipramine, which increases serotonin levels in the brain, produces a 30 to 60 percent reduction in symptoms in adults and a 70 to 80 percent reduction in children. Other antidepressants that have demonstrated good results are the selective serotonin reuptake inhibitors (SSRIs), such as fluoxetine, paroxetine, and sertraline. For proper drug choices and dosages, consult a psychiatrist trained in anxiety disorders.

Behavior therapy emphasizes changing a specific behavior—such as compulsive cleaning—by stopping what has been triggering it or by replacing it with a more desirable response. According to some anecdotal evidence, 60 to 70 percent of OCD patients are "much improved" after brief treatment with behavior therapy. For children, family therapy is important.

### ALTERNATIVE CHOICES

Alternative therapies are helpful both for relieving the anxiety of OCD and for diminishing the compulsions themselves. **Massage** is useful for reducing the physical rigidity in the neck, shoulders, and back that many OCD patients suffer. By loosening the musculature, massage relieves anxiety and reduces the urgency of compulsions. Exercises of all kinds, particularly those such as **yoga** that stretch and flex many of the body's muscles, do much the same thing.

#### BIOFEEDBACK

Because obsession and compulsion are often the mind's way of controlling such feelings as anxiety, anger, or sadness, helping the brain reduce the intensity of these feelings reduces the OCD itself. Studies have shown that EEG (brain-wave) biofeedback (also known as neurotherapy) is a good tool for reducing the intensity of unwanted feelings. Between 30 and 60 EEG-biofeedback training sessions are needed to treat OCD effectively, but the sessions may bring about permanent change, and this technique has the advantage of giving patients control over their treatment. *(See Health Associations and Organizations in the Appendix for more information.)*

#### HOMEOPATHY

Homeopathic practitioners have specific prescriptions for OCD, which can be tailored to the individual. Among the remedies that may be used by an experienced homeopath are Arsenicum album, Hyoscyamus, Medorrhinum, Nux vomica, and Pulsatilla.

#### MIND/BODY MEDICINE

Many mind/body practices may help relieve the anxiety associated with OCD. **Meditation** and other **relaxation** techniques such as progressive muscle relaxation, **yoga, t'ai chi,** and **qigong** all may be helpful. Find one or two you prefer and use them daily.

Since anxiety is almost always accompanied by shallow breathing, deep-breathing exercises are very helpful. *(See Anxiety for yoga breathing.)* Alternate nostril breathing, which specifically is thought to stimulate different areas of the brain, is also good for relieving anxiety. ■

O

## SYMPTOMS

A whitish or velvety red patch of tissue instead of normal pink membrane in the oral cavity may signal a potential precancerous condition. If left untreated, the discolored patch may grow and begin to feel like a canker sore. The symptoms of oral cancer may include:

- a persistent lump, sore, or thickening along the side or bottom of the tongue, on the floor of the mouth, inside the cheeks, or on the gums, palate, or roof of the mouth; the lump may eventually bleed or become ulcerated.
- discomfort while eating, drinking, or swallowing.
- loose teeth, or toothache or earache that does not respond to conventional treatment.
- a swollen lymph node in the neck.

Symptoms associated with advanced oral cancer include pain in the ear or roof of the mouth, unexplained spasms in facial or neck muscles, or persistent bad breath.



## CALL YOUR DOCTOR IF:

- you have persistent hoarseness, soreness, or a sensation of something lodged in your throat. You may have throat cancer.
- you feel persistent and inexplicable discomfort in your mouth or ear. The pain may very well stem from something other than cancer, but the cause should be determined in any event.

Oral cancer refers to all cancers of the oral cavity—the lips, tongue, cheeks, mouth, gums, and oropharynx, or upper part of the throat. These tumors almost always arise in the flat, squamous cells that line the pink membrane of the oral cavity and throat. Although oral cancer may spread through the head and neck, it seldom spreads farther.

Oral cancer sometimes evolves from other oral conditions: **Erythroplakia,** which is signaled by a velvety red patch of tissue inside the mouth, is always considered precancerous. **Leukoplakia,** characterized by whitish tissue, is sometimes precancerous. Both erythroplakia and leukoplakia are strongly associated with alcohol and tobacco use—as are the overwhelming majority of oral cancers.

Like any cancer, oral cancer is most treatable if detected early. Fortunately, you can often feel suspicious tissue changes that may signal oral cancer. The overall five-year survival rate for oral cancer is more than 50 percent; when treated early, 9 out of 10 patients survive more than five years, and most are cured permanently.

## CAUSES

The role of alcohol and tobacco—including chewing tobacco—in causing oral cancer cannot be overemphasized. People who use both substances regularly are 35 times more likely to get oral cancer than people who use neither. The disease usually affects tissue that is already irritated by jagged teeth, ill-fitting dentures, or habitual chewing on the inside of the cheek. Iron deficiency has been linked to tongue cancer in women, while excessive exposure to sunlight causes some types of lip cancer. People treated for oral cancer who continue to smoke and drink are very likely to develop the disease again.

### DIAGNOSTIC AND TEST PROCEDURES

Routine examination of the mouth by you, your dentist, or your doctor will improve the chance of detecting oral cancer early. In the event of a suspicious abnormality, a doctor will do a biopsy

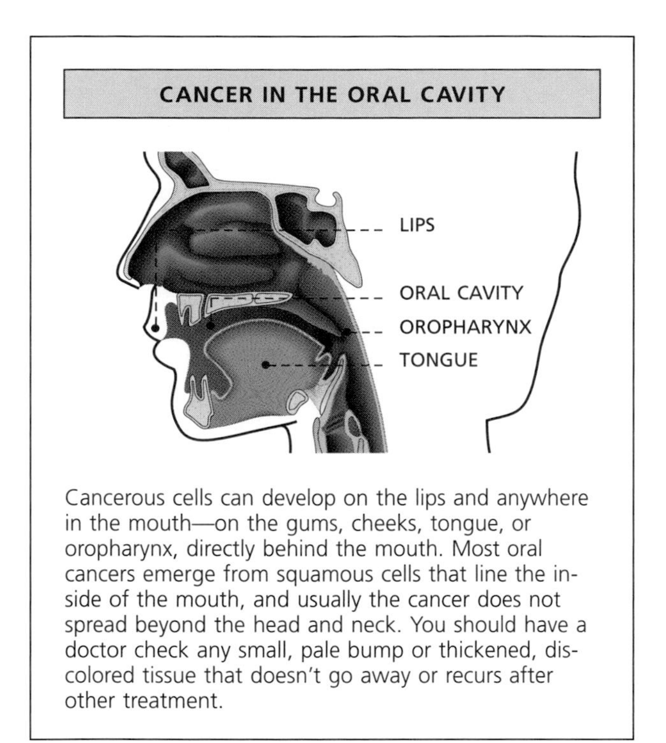

Cancerous cells can develop on the lips and anywhere in the mouth—on the gums, cheeks, tongue, or oropharynx, directly behind the mouth. Most oral cancers emerge from squamous cells that line the inside of the mouth, and usually the cancer does not spread beyond the head and neck. You should have a doctor check any small, pale bump or thickened, discolored tissue that doesn't go away or recurs after other treatment.

by taking a small tissue sample from your mouth, or fluid from swollen lymph nodes in your neck, to examine under a microscope. X-rays or other imaging tests may be needed to identify a primary tumor that is not readily apparent or to establish the extent of spread in an existing cancer.

# TREATMENT

## CONVENTIONAL MEDICINE

Small oral cancers respond equally well to either surgery or radiation therapy; advanced cancers are treated with both and sometimes with chemotherapy to relieve symptoms. For recurrent cancer, radiation therapy is the primary treatment. Laser surgery or cryosurgery—freezing cells with liquid nitrogen—can kill small tumors without affecting mouth function or the patient's looks. If significant amounts of tissue or bone are removed, reconstructive surgery may be needed. In such cases, patients must adjust to their new appearance and relearn basic chewing, swallowing, and speaking skills. Since postoperative radiation and chemotherapy typically suppress normal saliva production and may injure healthy mouth tissue, most patients must take extra measures to deter gum and tooth decay during and after treatment. *(See Cancer for more information about therapies.)*

## COMPLEMENTARY THERAPIES

For cancer, there is no acceptable alternative to conventional medical care. Other approaches can complement, but not replace, standard treatment.

### NUTRITION AND DIET

High doses of vitamin A may protect against onset and recurrence of oral cancer. Vitamin A is toxic in high doses, so take supplements only under a doctor's supervision. You can also eat plenty of fresh fruits and vegetables as healthy sources of carotenoids—dietary precursors of vitamin A—and vitamin E, which also may be protective.

## AT-HOME CARE

During radiation therapy, you may have difficulty opening your mouth, keeping your mouth moist with saliva, and brushing your teeth. Try gentle stretching exercises, drinking iced beverages, rinsing frequently, and using a soft toothbrush. For a gentle, effective mouthwash, try aloe *(Aloe barbadensis)* juice or cool chamomile *(Matricaria recutita)* tea. To combat dry mouth and restore natural saliva, rinse your mouth with an acidophilus solution, available at most health food stores. Swish the solution in your mouth, then swallow it, several times a day.

# PREVENTION

Don't smoke or chew tobacco. Drink alcohol only moderately. If you wear dentures, be sure they fit properly. Use sunscreen to protect your lips. Eat fresh fruits and vegetables daily. If you are diagnosed with a potentially precancerous oral condition, have your doctor monitor it carefully. ■

# OSTEOPOROSIS

## SYMPTOMS

Osteoporosis is usually asymptomatic until a fracture occurs.

- backache.
- a gradual loss of height and an accompanying stooped posture.
- fractures of the spine, wrists, or hips.
- loss of bone in the jaw *(see below)*.

## CALL YOUR DOCTOR IF:

- you develop a backache or a sudden severe back pain, which can indicate a spinal compression fracture caused by osteoporosis.
- dental x-rays reveal a loss of bone in the jaw, which can be an early sign of osteoporosis.

Osteoporosis, which means "porous bones," is a condition that causes formerly strong bones to gradually thin and weaken, leaving them susceptible to fractures. In the United States about 1.3 million fractures are attributed to osteoporosis each year. Although all bones are affected by the disease, those of the spine, hip, and wrist are most likely to break. In elderly people hip fractures can be particularly dangerous, because the prolonged immobility required during the healing process often leads to blood clots or pneumonia. About a third of elderly women with hip fractures die within six months.

Of the estimated 24 million Americans afflicted with osteoporosis, at least 80 percent are women. Experts believe women are more susceptible because their bones tend to be lighter and thinner, and because their bodies experience hormonal changes after menopause that appear to accelerate the loss of bone mass. In men osteoporosis is uncommon until after the age of 70.

## CAUSES

Although the exact cause of osteoporosis is unknown, the process by which the bone becomes porous is well understood. Normally, 6 to 12 percent of an adult's total skeleton is replaced each year, a process known as bone remodeling. After skeletal mass peaks—usually around the age of 35—bones begin to lose calcium, the mineral that makes them hard, faster than they can replace it. Less remodeling takes place and the bones begin to thin. For women the loss of bone density speeds up during the first three to seven years after menopause and then slows down again. Scientists believe that this rapid postmenopausal increase in bone loss is caused by a sharp decline in the body's production of estrogen, which appears to help keep calcium in the bones.

Although some loss of bone density is a natural part of aging, certain women are at higher risk than others for developing the very porous bones and the fractures associated with osteoporosis. Women who are small boned, thin, and fair haired, for example, are at higher risk, as are those who smoke, drink more than moderately, or

**AT-HOME CALCIUM ABSORPTION TEST**

*To determine whether the calcium in your supplement tablets is easily absorbed by your body, try this test: Drop a tablet into 6 ounces of vinegar at room temperature. Stir every 2 to 3 minutes. The tablet should disintegrate within 30 minutes. If it does not, try another supplement.*

live a sedentary lifestyle. Women with a family history of osteoporosis and those who have had their ovaries removed, especially before age 40, are also more prone to the condition. White and Asian women are more frequently affected than black women. Research has also indicated that women whose hair turns more than 50 percent gray before age 40 are four times as likely to develop osteoporosis as those whose hair doesn't.

Certain conditions that impair the body's ability to absorb calcium, such as kidney disease, Cushing's syndrome, and hyperthyroidism *(see Thyroid Problems)*, can also lead to osteoporosis, as can surgical removal of part of the stomach or intestine and excessive use of glucocorticoids, other steroids, or anticonvulsant drugs. Prolonged immobility because of paralysis or illness can cause calcium loss and thus, eventually, bone loss.

### DIAGNOSTIC AND TEST PROCEDURES

If your doctor suspects you have osteoporosis, he may measure you to check for a loss of height. The vertebrae are often the first bones affected, causing a loss in height of half an inch or more.

Your doctor may also recommend that your bone density be measured. Although osteoporosis is sometimes diagnosed incidentally after an x-ray has been taken for a fracture or an illness, an ordinary x-ray does not reveal bone loss until at least 20 to 30 percent of the bone mass has disappeared, limiting its usefulness for early screening of the condition. Diagnostic tools more likely to catch osteoporosis at an early stage include various forms of a technique called absorptiometry, which is specifically designed to measure bone density. A relatively new diagnostic tool known as quantitative computerized tomography is also an accurate method of measuring bone density anywhere in the body, but it uses higher levels of radiation than the other methods.

In addition to these bone measurement tests, you may be asked to supply blood or urine samples for analysis so that disease-related causes for the bone loss can be ruled out.

## TREATMENT

Because osteoporosis is difficult to reverse, prevention is the key to treatment. Both conventional and alternative medicine offer effective preventive measures for the condition.

### CONVENTIONAL MEDICINE

To prevent osteoporosis or to slow its progression, many doctors recommend hormone replacement therapy (HRT)—either estrogen alone or a combination of estrogen and progesterone—to postmenopausal women. Studies have shown that women who take long-term HRT within a few years of menopause keep their bone density and have fewer hip and wrist fractures while they are taking it than women who do not. HRT does not build new bone; it only slows the loss of existing bone, and this effect disappears after age 75, when most dangerous fractures occur. Once the hormone treatment is discontinued, the bone begins to thin again—at the same pace as at menopause. Women who take HRT for osteoporosis, therefore, must continue it indefinitely to help keep their bones from thinning. Because HRT has been associated with an increased risk of serious health problems, most notably uterine and breast cancers, many doctors recommend the treatment only for women at high risk of osteoporosis.

Calcitonin, a naturally occurring hormone that inhibits bone loss, is also sometimes prescribed for osteoporosis. It is very expensive, however, and must be given by injection. (A nasal spray available in other countries has not yet been approved by the Food and Drug Administration for use in the United States.) Because it is difficult to administer and can cause undesirable side effects, such as nausea and skin rashes, calcitonin is not widely prescribed.

As a preventive measure your doctor may suggest that you increase the amount of calcium in your diet or perhaps take calcium supplements. To help with the absorption of the calcium, vitamin D supplements may also be recommended unless you live in a sunny climate. Your doctor may also encourage you to begin a regular exercise program to keep your bones strong and free of fractures. *(For more information, see Nutrition and Diet, right, and Exercise, below.)*

## ALTERNATIVE CHOICES

Like conventional techniques, alternative therapies focus on building and retaining strong bones.

### CHINESE HERBS

Chinese practitioners recommend several herbs for preventing bone loss, most notably dong quai *(Angelica sinensis)* and Asian ginseng *(Panax ginseng),* which appear to have estrogen-like effects in the body. Consult a practitioner experienced in Chinese herbal medicine for appropriate dosages.

### EXERCISE

Studies have shown that weight-bearing exercises—those that put stress on bones, such as running, walking, tennis, ballet, stair climbing, aerobics, and weightlifting—reduce bone loss and help prevent osteoporosis. To benefit from the exercise, you must do it at least three times per week for 30 to 45 minutes. Swimming and bicycle riding, although good cardiovascular exercises, do not appear to prevent osteoporosis because they do not put enough stress on bones.

### HERBAL THERAPIES

Although acknowledging that herbal therapies cannot cure osteoporosis, herbalists believe that the use of some herbs can help slow the progression of the condition. Herbs traditionally used for the prevention of osteoporosis include horsetail *(Equisetum arvense),* alfalfa *(Medicago sativa),* licorice *(Glycyrrhiza glabra),* marsh mallow *(Althaea officinalis),* and sourdock *(Rumex crispus).* Take daily in tea or tincture form. Ask an herbalist about progesterone creams made from the wild Mexican yam; they may stimulate bone formation.

### HOMEOPATHY

In addition to a calcium-rich diet and exercise, homeopaths recommend treatments they believe help the body absorb calcium. Remedies are likely to include Calcarea carbonica, Calcarea phosphorica, Calcarea fluorica, and Silica. Consult a homeopath for remedies and dosages.

### NUTRITION AND DIET

To ensure that women get enough calcium to build and maintain strong bones, both alternative and conventional practitioners recommend eating plenty of calcium-rich foods, such as nonfat milk, low-fat yogurt, broccoli, cauliflower, salmon, tofu, and leafy green vegetables. According to a panel convened by the National Institutes of Health, women who are still menstruating or who are postmenopausal but taking hormone replacement therapy should consume 1,000 mg of calcium each day. Postmenopausal women who are not being treated with estrogen should get 1,500 mg daily. (One glass of nonfat milk provides only 300 mg of calcium.)

Because most women take in through their diet only half or a third as much calcium as they need, some practitioners recommend calcium supplements to make up the difference. Calcium supplements are available in many forms, but chelated forms, such as calcium citrate and calcium gluconate, appear to be more effective at reducing bone loss. *(See At-Home Calcium Absorption Test on page 637.)* Avoid using dolomite or bone meal as calcium supplements or calcium carbonate supplements labeled "oyster shell," as they may contain lead and other toxic metals.

To help the body absorb calcium, some practitioners suggest taking vitamin D (400 to 800 IU) and magnesium (250 to 350 mg) supplements. A veal bone supplement that provides calcium and trace minerals is sometimes prescribed as well.

CAUTION: Calcium supplements can inhibit the absorption of salicylates, tetracycline, and other medications. Check with your practitioner before beginning a supplementation program.

In addition to eating calcium-rich foods you should also avoid phosphorus-rich ones, which can promote bone loss. High-phosphorus foods include red meats, soft drinks, and those with phosphate food additives. Indeed, several studies have indicated that vegetarians tend to have denser bones later in life than meat eaters, although other studies have shown no such difference. Excessive amounts of alcohol and caffeine are also thought to reduce the amount of calcium absorbed by the body and should be avoided.

To help keep estrogen levels from dropping precipitously after menopause and thus help prevent osteoporosis, some alternative practitioners advise postmenopausal women to consume more foods containing plant estrogens, especially tofu, soybean milk, and other soy products.

### AT-HOME REMEDIES

Here are two easy ways of increasing the amount of calcium in your diet:

- Add nonfat dry milk to everyday foods and beverages, including soups, stews, and casseroles. Each teaspoon of dry milk adds about 20 mg of calcium to your diet.
- Add a little vinegar to the water you use to make soup stock from bones. The vinegar will dissolve some of the calcium out of the bones, for a calcium-fortified soup. A pint can contain as much as 1,000 mg of calcium.

## PREVENTION

- Eat foods rich in calcium, such as nonfat milk, low-fat yogurt, broccoli, cauliflower, salmon, tofu, sesame seeds, almonds, and leafy green vegetables.
- Eat foods that contain plant estrogens, especially tofu and other soy products.
- Avoid foods that can interfere with your body's absorption of calcium, such as red meats, soft drinks, and excessive amounts of alcohol and caffeine.
- Do weight-bearing exercises for 30 to 45 minutes at least three times a week.
- Do not smoke. Some studies have shown that women who smoke increase their risk of developing osteoporosis by 50 percent.
- Avoid antacids containing aluminum, as they can prevent calcium absorption by binding with phosphorus in the intestines.

### ASSESS YOUR RISK

*To help determine whether you are at risk for osteoporosis, ask yourself the following questions. The more "yes" answers, the greater your risk.*

- *Is there a history in your family of osteoporosis and hip fractures?*
- *Have you had both of your ovaries removed, especially before age 40?*
- *Are you small boned or slender?*
- *Are you light complexioned?*
- *Did your hair turn 50 percent or more gray before you turned 40?*
- *Do you lead a sedentary lifestyle?*
- *Do you smoke?*
- *Has your diet been low in calcium-rich foods?*
- *Do you drink two or more alcoholic beverages a day?*
- *Do you drink more than 24 ounces of carbonated soft drinks a day?*
- *Do you drink more than two cups of caffeinated coffee a day?*
- *Do you eat red meat and other high-protein foods frequently?*
- *Are you taking corticosteroids?*
- *Have you been on long-term thyroid medications?* ■

# OTITIS MEDIA

## SYMPTOMS

**In adults:**
- earache (either a sharp, sudden pain or a dull, continuous pain).
- fever and chills.
- nasal congestion.
- feeling of fullness in the ear.
- nausea and diarrhea accompanying earache.
- muffled hearing.

**In children:**
- tugging at the ear.
- fever.
- irritability, restlessness.
- nasal discharge.
- diminished appetite.
- crying at night when lying down.

## CALL YOUR DOCTOR IF:

- body temperature rises above 101°F or 102°F; a fever signals the possibility of a more serious infection.
- you or your child frequently develops otitis media; repeated bouts with the disorder can lead to hearing loss or more serious infections.
- you or your child has hearing problems; the infection may be affecting the ability to hear.
- you suspect that your young child has otitis media; it's often difficult for a parent to tell if a child has trouble hearing.

Otitis media, sometimes referred to simply as an ear infection or inflammation, is the most common cause of earaches. Although this condition is a frequent cause of infant distress and is often associated with children, it can also affect adults. Otitis media is an infection of the middle ear, whose tiny bones pick up vibrations from the eardrum and pass them along to the inner ear. But very often, otitis media accompanies a common cold, the flu, or another type of respiratory infection. This is because the middle ear is connected to the upper respiratory tract by a pair of tiny conduits known as Eustachian tubes.

Most parents are frustratingly familiar with otitis media. Except for wellness baby visits, ear infections are the most common reason for trips to the pediatrician, accounting for 30 million doctor visits a year in the United States. Today, almost half of all antibiotic prescriptions written for children are for otitis media, and the cost of treating middle ear infections in the U.S. is estimated at $2 billion a year. Untreated, otitis media can lead to more serious complications, including mastoiditis (a rare inflammation of a bone adjacent to the ear), hearing loss, perforation of the eardrum, meningitis, facial nerve paralysis, and possibly Ménière's disease.

## CAUSES

Cells in the middle ear manufacture a fluid that, among other things, helps keep out invading organisms. Normally, the fluid drains out through the Eustachian tube and into the throat. But if the Eustachian tube becomes swollen, the fluid can become trapped in the middle ear, causing the area to become inflamed and infected. This tube lies in a more horizontal position and is shorter in children, which may put them at even greater risk of infection. To the physician, the eardrum of an infected patient appears red and bulging.

The most common cause of otitis media is an upper respiratory viral infection, such as a cold or the flu. These disorders can make the Eustachian tube so swollen that middle ear fluid cannot escape. Allergies—to pollen, dust, animal dander, or food—can produce the same effect, as can smoke, fumes, as well as other environmental toxins.

Bacteria can cause otitis media directly, but usually these organisms come on the heels of a viral infection or an allergic reaction, quickly finding their way into the warm, moist environment of the middle ear. Invading bacteria can wreak major havoc, turning inflammation into infection and provoking fevers. Among the bacteria most often found in infected middle ears are the same varieties responsible for sinusitis, pneumonia, and other upper respiratory infections. (Note: Flu shots do not offer protection from otitis media.)

Otitis media occurs in various degrees of severity. A single, isolated case that is easily cured is called acute otitis media. If the condition clears up but comes back as many as three times in a six-month period (or four times in a single year), it is known as recurrent otitis media. If it continues for weeks without clearing up, it is called chronic otitis media. A fluid buildup in the ear without infection is termed serous otitis media.

In recent years, scientists have identified the characteristics of people most likely to suffer recurrent middle ear infections: males, individuals with a family history of ear infections, babies who are bottle-fed (breast-fed babies get fewer ear infections), children in day-care centers; Native Americans and Australian Aborigines, people living in households with tobacco smokers, and people with poor or damaged immune systems.

### DIAGNOSTIC AND TEST PROCEDURES

If you or your child has an earache accompanied by a stuffy or runny nose, sore throat, and fever, chances are good that the problem is otitis media. Your doctor will most likely examine the eardrum with an instrument called an otoscope for signs of infection—not an easy task if the patient is a fussy infant.

To check for a bacterial infection, the doctor may make an opening in the eardrum, draw out a sample of fluid from the affected middle ear, then culture the sample in a laboratory dish. This more extreme measure is usually used only for serious or particularly stubborn infections.

## TREATMENT

The goal of most doctors and therapists is to rid the middle ear of infection before more serious complications set in. Treatment usually involves eliminating the causes of otitis media, killing any invading bacteria, boosting the immune system, and reducing swelling in the Eustachian tubes.

### CONVENTIONAL MEDICINE

Otitis media is typically caused by a viral infection, in which case the only relief doctors can offer is treatment of the symptoms. This may involve trying to reduce swelling in the Eustachian tubes with a decongestant, such as pseudoephedrine, and an antihistamine, possibly diphenhydramine. (Note: Antihistamines will not cure otitis media, and they may cause minor side effects, including drowsiness and nervousness.) To ease the pain, your doctor may recommend an analgesic, typically acetaminophen, which also helps reduce a fever. (Aspirin should be avoided in children because of the threat of Reye's syndrome.)

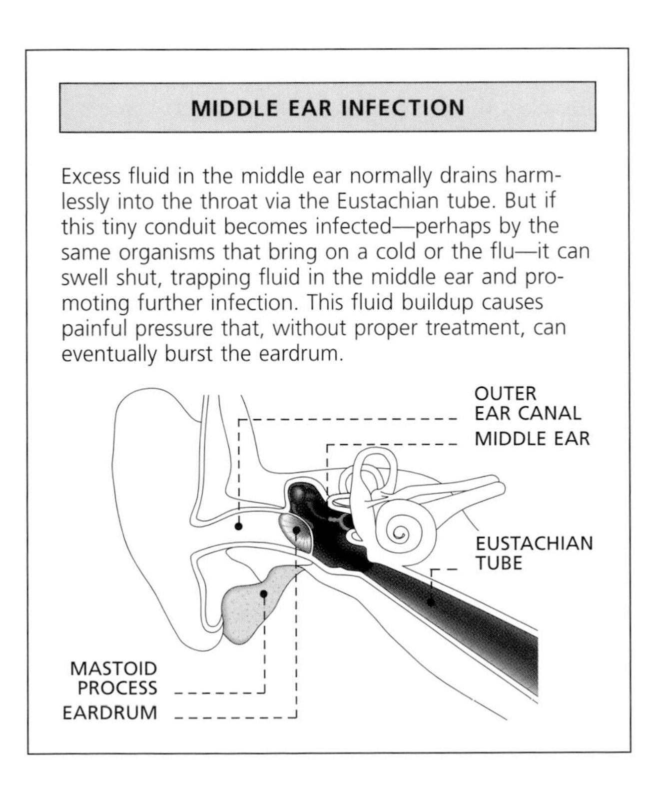


**MIDDLE EAR INFECTION**

Excess fluid in the middle ear normally drains harmlessly into the throat via the Eustachian tube. But if this tiny conduit becomes infected—perhaps by the same organisms that bring on a cold or the flu—it can swell shut, trapping fluid in the middle ear and promoting further infection. This fluid buildup causes painful pressure that, without proper treatment, can eventually burst the eardrum.

A controversy surrounds the use of antibiotics in treating bacterial middle ear infections. In England, most physicians treat only the symptoms of otitis media, without the help of bacteria-killing drugs. Studies have shown that up to 88 percent of otitis media cases got better when treated this way. Other research, in fact, suggests that 80 percent of otitis media cases are viral in origin and therefore will not respond to antibiotics.

But many doctors, particularly in the U.S., are concerned that without antibiotics, bacteria lurking inside the middle ear can grow out of control, possibly causing a serious complication such as hearing loss or mastoiditis. After all, they point out, these complications have become rare, largely as a result of antibiotic therapy. To be on the safe side, many American physicians treat all otitis media cases as if bacteria were present.

Amoxicillin is the antibiotic of choice for treating bacterial otitis media. The drug is generally considered safe because it is less likely to cause allergic reactions than penicillin, from which it is derived. The drug is highly effective: A single course of amoxicillin can knock out an ear infection in 7 to 10 days, at little cost.

Lately, however, doctors have noticed trouble with this wonder drug. As it turns out, some types of bacteria have learned to make a defensive protein that renders amoxicillin useless. Critics of routine antibiotic use in the U.S. charge that the millions of prescriptions of amoxicillin written for otitis media that had no bacterial element helped to create these resistant strains.

Whatever their origin, amoxicillin-resistant bacteria have shown up in a number of communities, prompting many doctors to prescribe other antibiotics for otitis media. Some of these substitutes, which tend to be more expensive than amoxicillin, are taken from a class of medications called cephalosporins. Others are combination drugs—amoxicillin and clavulanate, for instance. For those allergic to amoxicillin, doctors may prescribe sulfamethoxazole and trimethoprim, or erythromycin mixed with a sulfa drug like sulfisoxazole. For patients at least two years of age with severe, recurrent otitis media, doctors can stimulate the immune system by using a special vaccine that causes the body's immune system to recognize and attack certain bacteria.

If a case of otitis media develops serious complications, physicians may suggest surgery to eliminate infection or drain the middle ear. One technique, called myringotomy, involves piercing the eardrum to release fluid from the middle ear. If the Eustachian tubes become completely closed off due to swelling, a surgeon may insert a ventilation tube inside to keep them open. However, this procedure—called tympanostomy—is often expensive and may lead to infection and scarring. If recurring infections in the adenoids or tonsils cause repeated episodes of otitis media, a physician may suggest having the glands removed. *(See Adenoid Problems and Tonsillitis.)*

## ALTERNATIVE CHOICES

Some alternative treatments for otitis media attempt to fight the viruses or bacteria responsible for the infection, while others try to relieve the symptoms or boost the immune system.

### AROMATHERAPY

Lavender *(Lavandula officinalis)* essence may sometimes help to reduce the inflammation and pain of ear infections. Other oils used include chamomile *(Matricaria recutita),* cajuput, evening primrose oil *(Oenothera biennis),* fatty acid, flax oil, and borage.

### AYURVEDIC MEDICINE

To open and drain the Eustachian tubes, Ayurvedic physicians massage the lymph nodes outside the ears. The massage is complemented with a drink made with the herb amala, a source of vitamin C that also has antiviral and antibacterial properties. Amala is often given with raw honey. (CAUTION: Raw honey may contain the organism responsible for botulism and should not be given to infants or people with weak immune systems.)

### CHINESE HERBS

Practitioners use certain herbs to help fight infection and open up ear passages. Mixtures might include skullcap *(Scutellaria baicalensis),* alisma *(Alisma plantago-aquatica),* plantain *(Plantago major),* bupleurum *(Bupleurum chinense),* and licorice *(Glycyrrhiza uralensis)*. Contact a practitioner for exact recipes.

### HERBAL THERAPIES

A number of herbs that help fortify the immune system—including echinacea (*Echinacea* spp.), chamomile *(Matricaria recutita)*, and goldenseal *(Hydrastis canadensis)*—are available in oral tablets. Ear-drop solutions cannot penetrate the middle ear and should be reserved for outer ear infections. *(See Swimmer's Ear.)*

### HOMEOPATHY

In the early stages of an ear infection with sudden onset and feverish restlessness, use Aconite (30c every four to six hours). For throbbing and sharp pain accompanied by fever, intense heat, and flushing in the outer ear and along the side of the face, use Belladonna (30c every four to six hours). WARNING: Use extreme caution when treating with Belladonna, an extract from a poisonous plant of the nightshade family. Check dosages with your practitioner and follow label directions carefully. For children with otitis media who are very irritable, in great pain, and can't be consoled, try Chamomilla (30c every four to six hours). When a child is weepy, clingy, feels better in the open air, and has a yellowish green discharge coming from the nose, use Pulsatilla (30c every four to six hours). For ear congestion without infection, try Kali muriaticum (30c every four to six hours). If there is no improvement after two days, try a different remedy or consult a homeopathic practitioner.

### NUTRITION AND DIET

Although diet alone won't cure an ear infection, nutritionists suggest using the following vitamins and supplements to fight a viral infection:

- Beta carotene (vitamin A). Multiply your child's age times 20,000 IU for the daily dosage, with 200,000 as the maximum.
- Vitamin C. Daily dosage: Your child's age times 500 mg. (WARNING: High doses of vitamin C can cause diarrhea; it is important to spread the dose out evenly over the course of a day. Although for adults and adolescents there is no strict daily maximum, many people cannot tolerate more than 1,000 mg every two hours.)
- Zinc. Daily dosage: Your age times 2.5 mg. Do not take more than 50 mg per day without consulting a nutritionist.
- Bioflavonoids. Daily dosage: Your child's age times 50 mg, with 250 mg as the maximum.

### OSTEOPATHY

Consult an osteopathic practitioner for therapies that may help drainage of the Eustachian tubes.

## AT-HOME REMEDIES

- You can provide a great deal of symptomatic relief for an infected ear at home. Many find that warmth, perhaps from a warm compress, brings comfort. Steam inhalations and hot footbaths may also help.
- If you take antihistamines, which may rob your body of moisture and dry out your throat and respiratory passages, try to replace lost fluids by drinking lots of water.
- Gargling with salt water helps soothe an aggravated throat and clear the Eustachian tubes.
- Holding your head erect also helps drain your middle ear.
- Some people find relief with over-the-counter nasal sprays, which act as decongestants. Used for more than three days, however, sprays can become habit-forming and lead to rebound congestion, or a worsening of your condition.

## PREVENTION

Because bottle-fed babies are more likely to get otitis media, it is better to breast-feed your infant, if possible, to prevent ear infections. (If you must bottle-feed, never lay your baby down and prop the bottle up.) Also, remove as many environmental pollutants from your home as you can, including dust, cleaning fluid and solvents, and tobacco smoke. Food allergies may play a role in otitis media, so if you or your child is susceptible to the disease, try cutting back on wheat products, corn products, and food additives, as these tend to be more allergenic than other foods. ■

# OVARIAN CANCER

## SYMPTOMS

Although ovarian cancer rarely produces symptoms in its earliest stages, eventual warning signs may include:

- vague digestive disturbances, such as mild indigestion, bloating, feeling of fullness, or loss of appetite.
- diarrhea, constipation, or a frequent need to urinate.
- pain or swelling in the abdomen, or pain in the lower back.
- vaginal bleeding between menstrual periods or after menopause.

Symptoms associated with advanced ovarian cancer include severe nausea, vomiting, pain, and weight loss.

## CALL YOUR DOCTOR IF:

- you have otherwise unexplained abdominal pain or vaginal bleeding, particularly if these conditions accompany the more general symptoms listed above. Do not allow such symptoms to continue undiagnosed for more than two weeks.

Flanking the uterus are the two ovaries, each about the size of an almond, which produce eggs and female hormones. Over a lifetime, the ovaries may develop abnormal but noncancerous growths; for example, fluid-filled ovarian cysts are always benign—or noncancerous—as are 3 out of 4 ovarian tumors. Yet despite those odds, about 1 in 70 women in the United States will develop ovarian cancer. It can occur at any age, even in childhood, but is most common after menopause. The disease accounts for about 20,000 new cases and 12,500 deaths in the United States annually.

If ovarian cancer could be readily detected in its earliest stages, more women would be cured. But like many cancers, it usually has spread by the time it is diagnosed. The importance of early detection is clear: The five-year survival rate for ovarian cancer detected early is 88 percent; the rate for all cases is only about 40 percent.

## CAUSES

Most women with ovarian cancer have no family history of the disease, yet a woman is more likely to get the disease if her mother or sister has had ovarian, breast, or uterine cancer; the more relatives affected, the greater the risk. Women who have had few or no children, who delay childbearing until their thirties, or who have trouble conceiving are also at greater risk for ovarian cancer. Those who have several children, who breast-feed their infants, or who use birth-control pills are at reduced risk. The difference may be linked to less-frequent ovulation. Evidence suggests that the more saturated fat a woman consumes, the greater her ovarian cancer risk. Many high-fat foods contain estrogen, and all stimulate natural estrogen production. Because most ovarian cancers grow more rapidly in the presence of estrogen, some experts believe that abnormally elevated estrogen in a woman's body promotes the onset of ovarian cancer. Exposure to asbestos is also believed to be a factor in some cases.

### DIAGNOSTIC AND TEST PROCEDURES

Annual pelvic examinations help detect ovarian

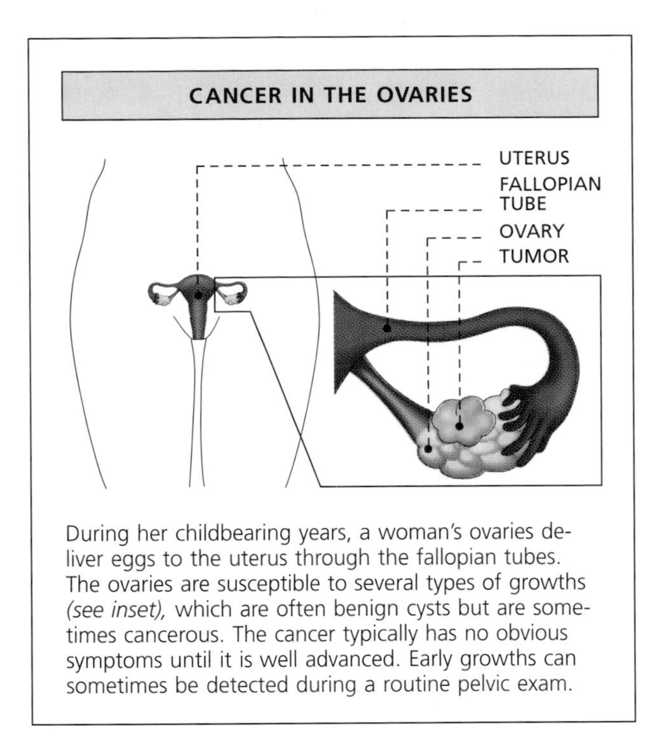


During her childbearing years, a woman's ovaries deliver eggs to the uterus through the fallopian tubes. The ovaries are susceptible to several types of growths *(see inset),* which are often benign cysts but are sometimes cancerous. The cancer typically has no obvious symptoms until it is well advanced. Early growths can sometimes be detected during a routine pelvic exam.

cancer early. Researchers are developing special blood tests that may help early diagnosis, but the tests are not yet reliable enough for general screening. If an ovarian growth is suspected, a sonogram of the ovaries is made; any visible abnormality justifies further testing in a hospital. Blood studies and other imaging tests may be done, and ultimately a tissue biopsy is necessary to confirm or rule out the diagnosis.

## TREATMENT

See Cancer for further information about some of the conventional treatment options below.

### CONVENTIONAL MEDICINE

Surgery is standard treatment for ovarian cancer. Ordinarily, the two ovaries and the other reproductive organs are removed. Young women who have only a small tumor in one ovary and who still want to have children may have just the diseased ovary removed; the second can be removed later to prevent cancer recurrence. In most patients, some cancer remains after surgery. A patient's prognosis depends on how much cancer remains and how well it responds to follow-up treatment. Most patients receive chemotherapy, which can prolong survival and may result in cure. Radiation therapy may be used after surgery to prevent recurrence or to help treat advanced or recurrent cases. Once remission occurs, follow-up examinations are essential; women who have had the disease may be at greater risk for breast and colorectal cancer.

New chemotherapeutic agents, new biological agents designed to stimulate the immune system, and new methods of delivering treatment with fewer adverse effects are under study. One of the more promising new drugs for treating advanced and recurrent ovarian cancer is taxol, originally extracted from the Pacific yew tree but now manufactured in the laboratory.

### COMPLEMENTARY THERAPIES

Maintaining a healthy immune system is important for people with cancer. Get regular exercise, adequate sleep, and essential vitamins and minerals by eating fresh fruits and vegetables. Cut down on dairy products, meats, and other high-fat foods. Various herbs with demonstrated immune-enhancing properties may complement standard treatment, but check with your doctor before using them.

## PREVENTION

Depending on your stage of life, you should discuss with your doctor the pros and cons of using birth-control pills or hormone replacement pills. Low-dose birth-control pills are considered protective, but hormone replacement therapy may heighten the risk of ovarian cancer; neither practice may be appropriate for women with a family history of the disease. If you are considered high-risk for ovarian cancer, ask your doctor about current recommendations for routine blood screening. For women at extremely high risk, a doctor may recommend having the ovaries removed as a preventive measure. ■

# OVARY PROBLEMS

## SYMPTOMS

- feeling of fullness or pressure on one side of the abdomen.
- abdominal pain during intercourse.
- sharp abdominal pain.
- irregular vaginal bleeding or absent menstrual periods.
- increase in facial or body hair.
- irregularities in bowel movements or urination.

Many small benign ovarian cysts and tumors produce no symptoms.

## CALL YOUR DOCTOR IF:

- you experience sudden sharp or severe abdominal pain, with or without fever; it may be a ruptured or twisted **ovarian cyst** or another problem, such as appendicitis, that requires immediate medical attention.
- you notice any significant increase in facial or body hair; you may have an ovarian problem that is altering your body's hormonal balance. See your doctor as soon as possible for treatment.
- your menstrual periods become irregular or stop altogether; you may have an ovarian problem that has altered your body's production of hormones or another disease or condition that requires medical treatment, such as diabetes. See your doctor as soon as possible.

The ovaries are a pair of almond-shaped organs located deep within the pelvis, on each side of the uterus. Each ovary contains thousands of eggs. Once a month during the years a woman is menstruating, one egg (or sometimes more) begins to grow in a small cystlike structure known as a follicle. When the egg is mature, the follicle ruptures and releases the egg, a process called ovulation. The egg then floats down to the uterus through the fallopian tube, propelled by hairlike cilia within the tube. The journey from the ovary to the uterus takes about three days.

The ovaries also produce the hormones estrogen and progesterone. While the egg is maturing, the follicle releases estrogen to help thicken the lining of the uterus in case the egg is fertilized and grows into an embryo. After the follicle ruptures it develops into a structure known as the corpus luteum, which produces progesterone to help the uterus prepare for a fertilized egg. If no pregnancy occurs, the level of progesterone decreases, menstruation occurs, and the cycle repeats itself.

Several problems can develop in the ovary. It can become infected, sometimes alone but more often as part of an infection that involves other pelvic organs *(see Pelvic Inflammatory Disease).* Cysts and tumors can also form on the ovaries. Most often these are benign—or noncancerous—and produce no symptoms. They are discovered only through a routine pelvic examination. Sometimes many small cysts form on the ovaries, a

### STEPPING ON A NEW OLD WIVES' TALE

***MYTH:*** *Wearing high-heeled shoes contributes to ovarian cysts by blocking circulation to the pelvic area.*

***FACT:*** *Absolutely no evidence supports the notion that footwear has any effect on circulation to the pelvic area, including the ovaries.*

condition known as polycystic ovary syndrome.

Although most benign **ovarian cysts** and tumors disappear after a few menstrual cycles, some grow large enough to cause discomfort. Sometimes the growths disrupt the production of ovarian hormones, causing irregular bleeding or an increase in body hair, or they press on the bladder, leading to more frequent urination. A cyst or tumor that has ruptured or become twisted on its attachment to the ovary can cause significant abdominal pain and may lead to an infection.

## CAUSES

Ovarian infections are most frequently caused by sexually transmitted diseases. Some **ovarian cysts** are the result of a follicle or corpus luteum that continues to grow and fill with fluid long after the egg has been released. **Polycystic ovary syndrome** occurs when egg follicles get trapped just under the surface of the ovary, unable to release their eggs, and form into multiple small cysts.

### DIAGNOSTIC AND TEST PROCEDURES

Your doctor will give you a complete physical and pelvic exam. If he or she suspects you have an ovarian cyst or tumor, you may need to undergo an ultrasound scan, which uses sound waves to produce a detailed image of the pelvic organs. The organs can be visualized directly by means of laparoscopy, a surgical procedure in which a special viewing instrument is inserted into the abdominal cavity under general anesthesia.

## TREATMENT

Treatment for an ovarian problem depends on the nature of the disorder. Treating **ovarian cysts** is often unnecessary; they tend to disappear on their own. Because of the possibility that a growth on an ovary may be cancerous, you should always seek out a conventional practitioner for the diagnosis of an ovary problem. Alternative treatments should be used only to help ease any discomfort associated with the condition.

### CONVENTIONAL MEDICINE

If diagnostic tests reveal an ovarian infection, your doctor will prescribe an antibiotic. If an **ovarian cyst** or tumor is diagnosed, he or she may recommend prompt surgery to rule out the possibility of cancer. If you are under age 40 and your cyst is soft and smaller than two inches in diameter, your doctor may suggest that you delay surgery for one or two menstrual cycles to see whether the cyst will disappear spontaneously.

Some doctors prescribe birth-control pills to women with a suspected ovarian cyst in the belief that hormones in the pills will help the cyst regress, thus eliminating the need for surgery.

For **polycystic ovary syndrome** doctors prescribe hormonal treatment to reestablish regular menstrual cycles. Either progesterone or birth-control pills, which contain both progesterone and estrogen, are used. Fertility drugs are also sometimes prescribed for women with polycystic ovaries to induce ovulation.

### ALTERNATIVE CHOICES

Alternative treatments for ovary problems should be used only as supplements to conventional treatment methods.

#### HERBAL THERAPIES

Herbalists recommend blue cohosh *(Caulophyllum thalictroides)* and false unicorn root *(Chamaelirium luteum)* as general tonics for the female reproductive organs. You may take these herbs in either tea or tincture form.

#### NUTRITION AND DIET

To help prevent and treat **ovarian cysts,** some alternative practitioners recommend a vegetarian diet rich in foods believed to nourish the liver, especially beets, carrots, dark-green leafy vegetables, and lemons. Others prescribe supplements of zinc and vitamins A, E, and C. Supplements of black currant oil, borage oil, and evening primrose oil *(Oenothera biennis)* may also be recommended because they are believed to help regulate the body's hormone levels. Consult your alternative practitioner for specific dosages. ■

# PAIN, CHRONIC

## SYMPTOMS

Any pain that lasts longer than six months is defined as chronic. The condition may include weakness, numbness, tingling, or other sensations, along with sleeping difficulties, a lack of energy, and depression. Some common forms of chronic pain are:

- continuing muscle pain, accompanied by cramping, soreness, swelling, and muscle spasms or stiffness.
- lingering back pain, which may be sharp or aching, constant or intermittent, localized, radiating, or diffuse.
- enduring joint pain, with tenderness and a sensation of heat in the affected area as well as radiating pain and a restricted range of motion.

## CALL YOUR DOCTOR IF:

- your pain continues for several weeks and doesn't respond to over-the-counter analgesics and rest; early care may keep acute pain from becoming chronic.
- your pain is unrelenting and unresponsive to prescription medications; your doctor may administer tests to rule out cancer or other possible causes.
- the symptoms of your chronic pain change abruptly. You may be at risk of complications, or you may have developed a different, unrelated problem.

Tens of millions of Americans suffer from chronic pain, the medical term used to describe any pain that, despite treatment, persists for longer than six months. Chronic pain can be mild or excruciating, episodic or continuous, merely inconvenient or totally incapacitating. The most common versions are headaches, arthritis, joint pain, pain from injury, and backaches. Other kinds of chronic pain include Achilles tendonitis, sinusitis, other forms of degenerative joint disease besides arthritis, carpal tunnel syndrome, and pain affecting specific parts of the body, such as the shoulders, pelvis, and neck. Generalized muscle or nerve pain can also develop into a chronic condition. *(See separate entries for more specific information about these ailments.)*

In some cases, chronic pain is self-perpetuating. For example, although rubbing a tender area may offer temporary relief, it can also inhibit healing; similarly, favoring an injured limb may set up musculoskeletal stresses that create new problems. The emotional toll of chronic pain also can become part of a vicious cycle. Anxiety, stress, depression, anger, and fatigue interact in complex ways with chronic pain and may decrease the body's production of natural painkillers; moreover, such negative feelings may increase the level of substances that amplify sensations of pain, worsening the spiral. Even the body's most basic defenses may be compromised: There is considerable evidence that unrelenting pain can suppress the immune system.

Because of the mind/body links associated with chronic pain, effective treatment may require addressing psychological as well as physical aspects of the condition.

## CAUSES

The causes of chronic pain are exceedingly diverse. One frequent factor is the development of any of a number of conditions that can accompany aging and may affect bones and joints in ways that cause chronic pain. Other common reasons for persistent pain are nerve damage and injuries that fail to heal properly. Some kinds of chronic pain have numerous possible causes: Back pain, for example, may be traceable to years of poor posture; to improper lifting and carrying of heavy objects; to being overweight, which puts excess strain on the back and knees; to a congenital condition such as curvature of the spine; to a traumatic injury; to wearing high heels; to sleeping on a poor mattress; or to no obvious physical cause.

Disease can also be the underlying cause of chronic pain. Rheumatoid arthritis and osteoarthritis are well-known culprits, but persistent pain may also be due to such ailments as cancer, multiple sclerosis, stomach ulcers, AIDS, and gallbladder disease.

In many cases, however, just what the source of chronic pain is can be a very complex and even mysterious issue to untangle. Although it may begin with an injury or illness, continuing pain can develop a psychological dimension after the physical problem has healed. This fact alone makes pinning down a single course of treatment tricky, and it is why doctors and other healers often find they have to try a number of different types of curative steps.

## TREATMENT

Many people suffering from chronic pain are able to gain some measure of control over it by practicing mind/body techniques on their own *(see Mind/Body Medicine, page 652).* But others may need professional help. For them, pain clinics—special care centers devoted exclusively to dealing with intractable pain—are often the answer. Some pain clinics are associated with hospitals and others are private; in either case, both inpatient and outpatient treatment are usually available. The length of a full treatment program can vary from several weeks to several months.

Pain clinics generally employ a multidisciplinary approach, involving physicians, psychologists, physical therapists, and alternative healthcare practitioners; the patient as well will take an active role in his or her own treatment. The aim in many cases is not only to alleviate pain but also to teach the chronic sufferer how to come to terms with pain and function in spite of it. The first step in many cases is to wean the patient from a dependence on painkilling medications. Other methods used by pain specialists include **biofeedback** and **relaxation** techniques to control brain-wave activity, behavior-modification therapy to revise the way pain is perceived, **acupuncture, hypnotherapy, meditation,** and other forms of alternative therapy. One high-tech method involves a miniature device controlled by the patient or an implanted electronic nerve stimulator that transmits tiny pulses of electric current to block pain signals.

Various studies have shown as much as 50 percent improvement in pain reduction for chronic pain sufferers after visiting a pain clinic, and most people learn to cope better and can resume normal activities.

### CONVENTIONAL MEDICINE

Over-the-counter painkillers such as aspirin and ibuprofen can control milder cases of musculoskeletal pain and reduce inflammation. Your doctor may prescribe stronger drugs, such as muscle relaxants, antianxiety drugs (such as diazepam), antidepressants, prescription nonsteroidal anti-inflammatory drugs (NSAIDs), or a short course of stronger painkillers (such as opioid analgesics). A limited number of corticosteroid injections at the site of an injury can reduce swelling and inflammation. Oral doses of the amino acid D-phenylalanine appear to release endorphins, the brain's natural painkillers, which can relieve all types of pain. For injuries that require immobilization to heal, a doctor may also advise wearing a brace, collar, splint, or surgical corset that binds your torso for short periods of time only. Extreme cases of injuries requiring immobilization might call for traction or surgery.

### ALTERNATIVE CHOICES

A broad array of alternative options exists to address chronic pain. Some focus on physical aspects of the condition, others on psychological factors, and still others on where physiological and psychological factors overlap.

## UPPER-BODY ACUPRESSURE

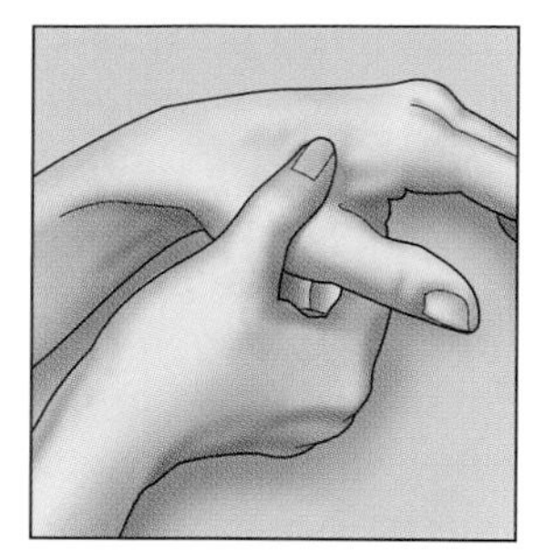

**1** Pressing Large Intestine 4, in the web between your thumb and index finger, may help relieve facial pain. Use the thumb and index finger of your right hand to squeeze the web of your left hand for one minute. Repeat on the right hand. Do not use this point if you are pregnant.

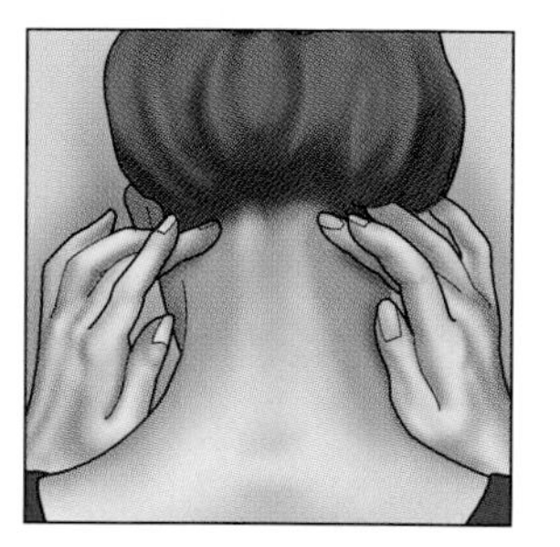

**2** To reduce neck muscle stress that may cause head or back pain, try pressing Gall Bladder 20. Place the tips of both middle fingers in the hollows at the base of your skull, about two inches apart, on either side of the spine. Press firmly for one minute.

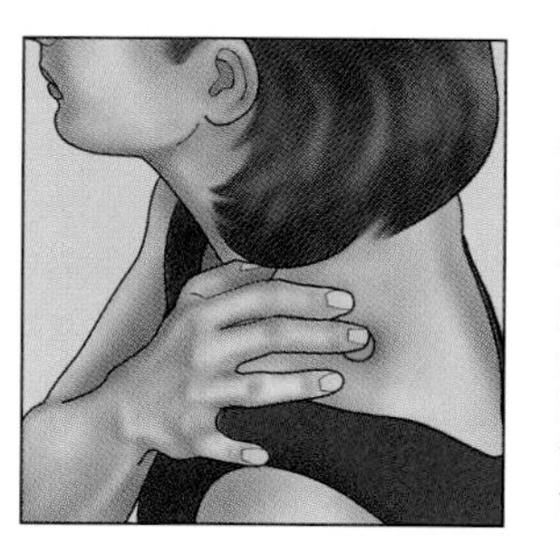

**3** Pressing Gall Bladder 21 may help release tension in the shoulders. Place your right middle finger on the highest point of your left shoulder muscle, one or two inches from your lower neck. Press two or three times, then repeat on the other side.

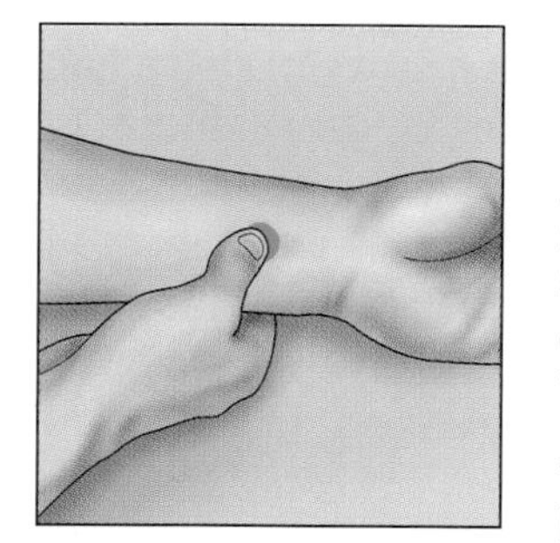

**4** To help ease pain in the chest and upper abdomen, press Pericardium 6. Place your thumb in the center of your inner wrist, two finger widths from the wrist crease and between the two bones of the forearm. Press firmly for one minute, three to five times, then repeat on the other arm.

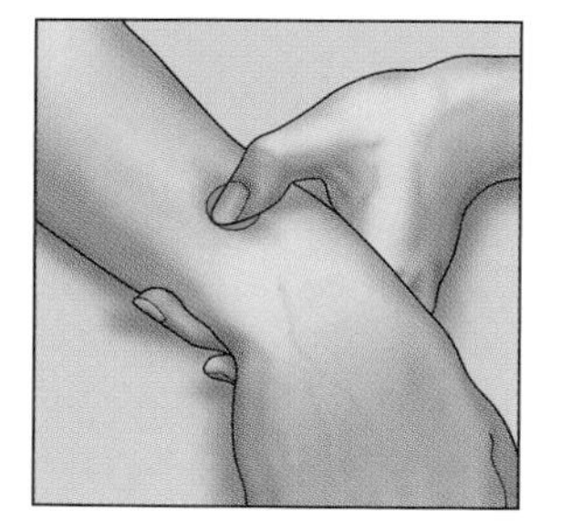

**5** Pressing Triple Warmer 5 may help soothe areas of pain in the upper body. Center your thumb on the top of your forearm, two thumb widths from the wrist joint. Press firmly for one minute, then repeat on the other arm. Do two or three times.

## LOWER-BODY ACUPRESSURE

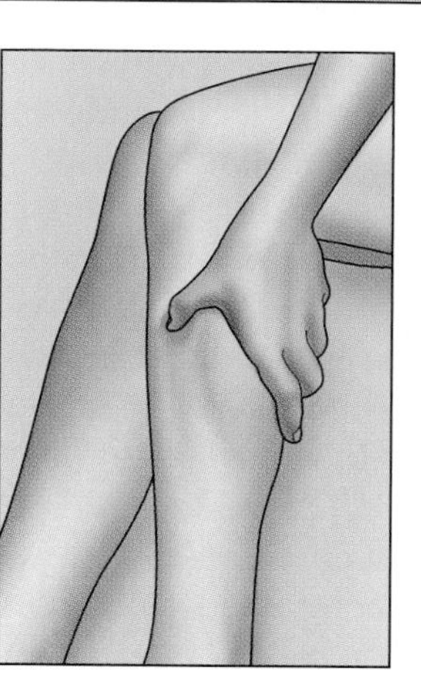

**1** Abdominal pain may be eased by steady finger pressure on Stomach 36, four finger widths below the kneecap just outside the shinbone. Maintain pressure for one minute, then switch legs. To verify the location, flex your foot; you should feel a muscle bulge at the point site.

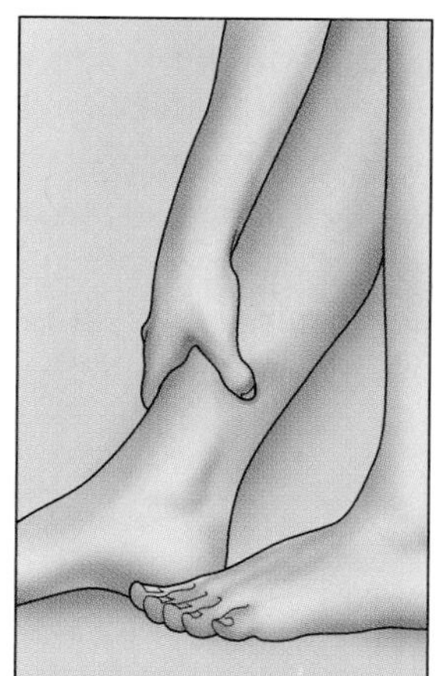

**2** Abdominal cramping may be relieved by pressing Spleen 6. Place your thumb four finger widths from your right inside anklebone, near the edge of the shinbone. Press for one minute, then switch legs. Do two or three times. Do not use this point if you are pregnant.

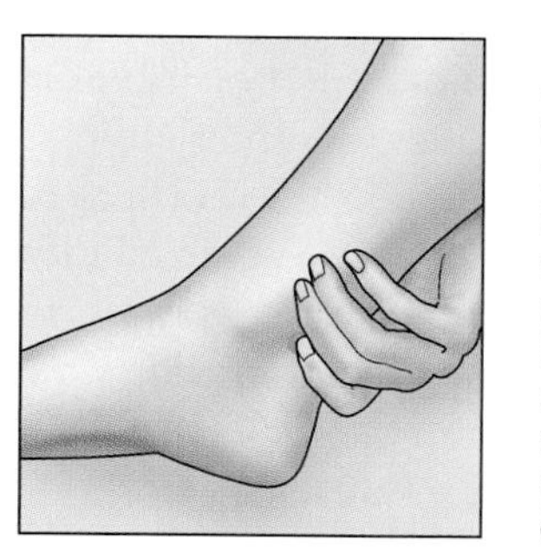

**3** Kidney 3, located on the inside of the ankle between the anklebone and the Achilles tendon, may ease back pain. Press firmly with your index finger and hold for one to two minutes, then repeat on the other foot. Do not use this point after the third month of pregnancy.

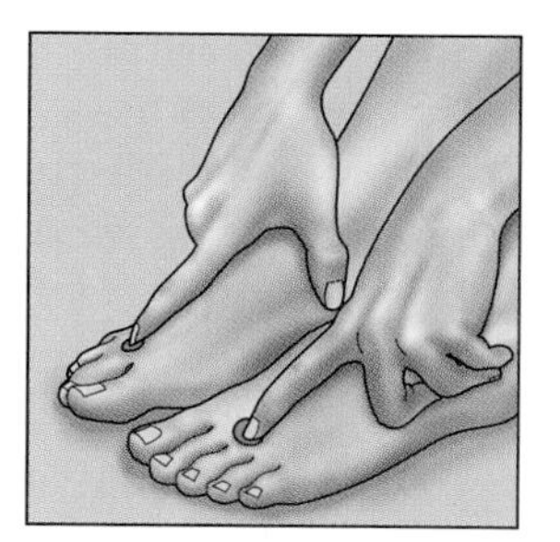

**4** Ankle and foot pain may be relieved by pressure on Stomach 44, located on the top of the foot in the web between the second and third toes. Press lightly on both feet with your index fingers for one minute, two or three times.

### ACUPRESSURE
Acupressure therapy is based on the belief that specific points on your hands, feet, and limbs correspond to various parts of your body where you may be feeling chronic pain. Self-administered, it generally involves pushing straight down with a bent thumb or finger (but not your fingernails) on the indicated point for about a minute, removing the pressure, then pressing deeply again. For techniques targeting specific instances of chronic pain, see the illustrations at left.

### ACUPUNCTURE
Acupuncture may be used to reduce swelling and inflammation associated with chronic pain. The treatment may include placing needles along the large-intestine meridian, considered the most effective of pain-relieving channels. One theory holds that acupuncture works by stimulating the release of endorphins, the body's natural painkillers. Because this therapy is thought to have a cumulative effect, it is most beneficial if done on a regular basis. For the best results, consult an acupuncturist who has experience treating a wide range of types of chronic pain.

### AROMATHERAPY
Mix together the following essential oils with a carrier oil such as sweet almond, apricot kernel, or jojoba oil, and massage the blend into your skin at the site of the pain: lavender *(Lavandula officinalis)* to reduce inflammation and relax muscles; eucalyptus *(Eucalyptus globulus)* to bring down swelling and accelerate healing; ginger *(Zingiber officinale)* to relieve pain and stiffness associated with arthritis and other types of degenerative joint disease.

### BODY WORK
The **Alexander technique** reeducates you in the way you move to avoid adding unnecessary tension to skeleton-supporting muscles, thus preventing neck and back problems. This therapy has been shown to be especially helpful for correcting poor posture that can cause backaches.

**Massage** therapy may provide temporary relief of muscle tension, stiffness, and spasms. Its muscular manipulation may break the pain-spasm-pain cycle of many types of chronic pain by reducing muscle tension, which can produce sudden, involuntary contractions and lead to more pain.

Massage with ice packs may interrupt pain messages sent along nerve pathways, replacing those messages with signals about temperature and, in this way, providing relief.

### CHIROPRACTIC
Chiropractic manipulation seeks to restore joint mobility in cases of bursitis and tennis elbow. It is also used as a means of reducing back or neck pain or muscle spasms.

### HERBAL THERAPIES
Capsicum, the active ingredient in cayenne *(Capsicum frutescens),* is believed to increase blood flow to joint tissues, thereby reducing inflammation. An over-the-counter ointment made with cayenne may bring temporary relief of osteoarthritis and rheumatoid arthritis, although it is very hot and should be used for only short periods. Infusions of black cohosh *(Cimicifuga racemosa)* or six 500-mg capsules of evening primrose oil *(Oenothera biennis)* taken daily may also lessen inflammation. Rubbing a dilution of peppermint *(Mentha piperita)* oil on the affected area may have a temporary numbing effect.

Topically applied dilutions of wintergreen *(Gaultheria procumbens)* oil—which contains methyl salicylate, an ingredient similar to those found in aspirin—may have an analgesic effect. Geranium *(Pelargonium odoratissimum)* and white willow *(Salix alba)* bark are natural painkillers. Chamomile *(Matricaria recutita)* is an antispasmodic and anti-inflammatory agent. Consult an herbalist to determine the best treatment for your specific condition. You must also take special precautions if you are pregnant.

### HOMEOPATHY
Try Rhus toxicodendron for joint, back, and arthritic problems that feel worse when first rising in the morning and become better with warmth. Persistent pain may be relieved by Kali bichromicum. If you eat a lot of salt and have severe low-back pain that abates when firm pres-

sure is applied, try Natrum muriaticum. For burning lower-back pain that improves with movement and grows worse after rest, take Calcarea fluorica. Sepia may be good for lower-back pain that is worsened by sitting. Consult a homeopathic practitioner for the appropriate remedies and dosages.

Topical homeopathic creams that have Arnica as a main ingredient can help with muscle pain and other kinds of pain that are not associated with your joints.

#### LIFESTYLE

Although resting for short periods can alleviate pain, too much rest can make muscles shorter, tighter, and weaker, actually increasing pain and putting you at greater risk of injury when you again attempt movement. If chronic pain has sidelined you for a long period, try a technique called "shaping" to get moving again: Determine the length of time you can painlessly perform an activity and establish a regular schedule for doing it; if your pain threshold is 10 minutes of stretching or walking, cut that time in half, but instead of stretching for only five minutes per day, stretch twice a day for five minutes each. You'll achieve the same benefits without feeling the pain. Gradually, you'll be able to increase your exercise time while increasing your pain threshold.

Research has shown that regular exercise can diminish pain in the long run by improving muscle tone, strength, and flexibility. Exercise may also release endorphins, the body's natural painkillers. Some exercises are easier for certain chronic pain sufferers to perform than others; try swimming, biking, walking, or rowing.

#### MIND/BODY MEDICINE

Some healthcare practitioners propose that, instead of resisting chronic pain, you should find ways to accept it and adjust to it. They suggest that this attitude, far from being defeatist, can enable you to escape a victim mentality. The pain may dissipate as a result, since psychological factors can play a major role in its perception.

The psychotherapeutic method called cognitive restructuring teaches you to replace negative, self-destructive beliefs with positive affirmations to "solve" pain problems. Your internal monologue is changed from "I can't do this; I'll never be better" to "I don't know what the future holds, but this is what I can do now."

**REFLEXOLOGY**

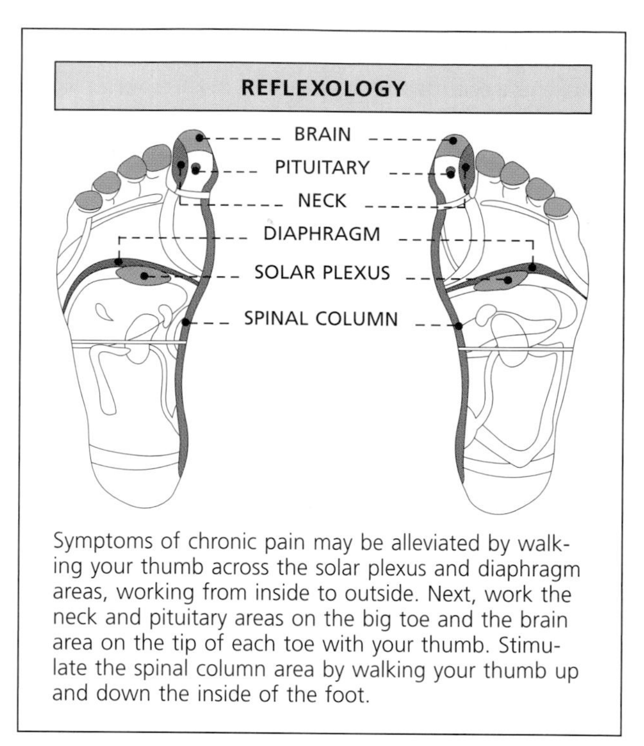


Symptoms of chronic pain may be alleviated by walking your thumb across the solar plexus and diaphragm areas, working from inside to outside. Next, work the neck and pituitary areas on the big toe and the brain area on the tip of each toe with your thumb. Stimulate the spinal column area by walking your thumb up and down the inside of the foot.

Visualization may be another worthwhile pain-controlling technique. Try the following exercise: Close your eyes and try to call up a visual image of the pain, giving it shape, color, size, motion. Now try slowly altering this image, replacing it with a more harmonious, pleasing—and smaller—image. Don't expect this imaging technique to work right away; it takes practice.

Another approach is to keep a diary of your pain episodes and the causative and corrective factors surrounding them. Review your diary regularly to explore avenues of possible change. Strive to view pain as part of life, not all of it.

Electromyographic (EMG) **biofeedback** may alert you to the ways in which muscle tension is contributing to your pain and help you learn to control it.

**Hypnotherapy** and self-hypnosis may help you block or transform pain through refocusing techniques. One self-hypnosis strategy, known as glove anesthesia, involves putting yourself in a trance, placing a hand over the painful area, imagining that the hand is relaxed, heavy, and numb, and envisioning these sensations as replacing other, painful feelings in the affected area.

**Relaxation** techniques such as **meditation** or **yoga** have been shown to reduce stress-related pain when they are practiced regularly. The gentle stretching of yoga is particularly good for strengthening muscles without putting additional strain on the body. Try the following so-called Corpse pose for 10 minutes of relaxation: Find a quiet place where you won't be disturbed and lie on your back with small pillows under your neck and the small of your back; consciously attempt to relax every part of your body, beginning with your toes and working upward to your face; let your breathing slow, and pay attention to how your body feels.

If you can't get your mind off your concerns, visualize two lists; in one column, list the concerns in order of priority, and in the other, visualize potential solutions to them. Place an imaginary check mark by each one after you've found a solution for it, then put both lists out of your mind and try the relaxation exercise again.

#### NUTRITION AND DIET

To reduce inflammation, try the following supplements (taken in increments throughout the day): 2,000 mg daily of calcium pantothenate, or pantothenic acid (vitamin $B_5$); 800 to1,000 mg daily of calcium citrate-malate; and 600 mg daily of the enzyme bromelain. For chronic back pain, a beneficial regimen may be 500 mg of vitamin C three times a day with meals, 1,200 mg daily of calcium, and 400 IU daily of vitamin E. CAUTION: Be sure to check with your doctor or a nutritionist before taking large doses of vitamin supplements. Foods high in calcium and magnesium relax muscles and may help reduce muscle-related pain.

For rheumatoid arthritis and other musculoskeletal pain, you may want to avoid dairy products, meat, and other foods that are high in saturated fats; they boost the body's production of prostaglandins, hormonelike fatty acids in the body that may contribute to inflammation.

Food has occasionally been implicated as a cause in some diseases that result in chronic pain. This type of food intolerance is then manifested as symptoms of the disease. Allergies to wheat, corn, citrus fruits, tomatoes, or potatoes, for example, can be expressed as rheumatoid arthritis. Consult your doctor or a recommended specialist to address this type of problem. You will probably be advised to try eliminating certain types of food from your diet to see if they are the source of your trouble.

#### OTHER THERAPIES

A transcutaneous electrical nerve stimulator, or TENS, is a small battery-powered device that is attached to painful areas by electrodes; the device stimulates nerves, which may block transmission of pain impulses to the brain. With training, this technique can be self-administered.

Hot and cold **hydrotherapy** treatments can relieve aches. Pour hot water into one container and ice water into another. Dip a rolled-up towel in the hot water, wring it out, and place it on the affected area for three minutes; then dip another rolled-up towel in the cold water and apply it for one minute. Repeat these alternating applications for 20 minutes three times a day.

### AT-HOME REMEDIES

- Treat the acute pain of an injury to a muscle, ligament, or cartilage with immediate rest, ice, compression, and elevation—acronymically known as RICE. Rest the injured body part, apply ice (a pack of frozen vegetables or ice pack) alternately for 20 minutes on, 20 off, compress the area with an elastic bandage, and keep the injury elevated to reduce swelling. Once swelling has subsided, apply heat (a hot-water bottle or heating pad). Finally, aspirin-based creams can help reduce pain and inflammation. It's important to treat acute pain before it has the chance to become chronic.
- Take capsules or drink infusions of one of the herbal remedies suggested above on a regular basis or as directed by an herbalist.
- A **yoga** class or bicycle-riding club has the benefit of stimulating endorphins—your body's natural painkillers. ■

# PANCREATIC CANCER

## SYMPTOMS

Pancreatic cancer usually produces no symptoms until it reaches an advanced stage. Symptoms that may arise, in typical order of occurrence, include:

- significant weight loss accompanied by abdominal pain—the most likely warning signs.
- vague but gradually worsening abdominal pain, often severe at night, which may radiate to the lower back.
- digestive or bowel complaints such as diarrhea, constipation, gas pains, bloating, or belching.
- nausea, vomiting, loss of appetite, and weight loss.
- jaundice, indicated by yellowish discoloration of the skin or eye whites.
- sudden onset of diabetes.
- black or bloody stool, indicating bleeding from the digestive tract.

A few rare types of pancreatic cancer cause hormonal imbalances that produce their own symptoms, which might include:

- episodes of weakness, sweating, rapid heartbeat, irritability, or skin flushing related to low blood sugar.
- severe ulcer symptoms, such as stomach pain and watery diarrhea, which do not respond to ulcer medication.

## CALL YOUR DOCTOR IF:

- any symptoms listed above endure longer than two weeks. You should have a full physical examination.

The pancreas, a small gland located deep in the abdomen, has two vital functions: It supplies the intestines with digestive juices, and it secretes hormones—including insulin—that regulate the body's use of sugars and starches. Endocrine cells in the pancreas are devoted to hormone regulation; they form clusters called islets and are found mostly in the tail and body sections of the gland. Exocrine cells, which outnumber endocrine cells 99 to 1, are spread throughout the gland and perform the digestive functions.

At least 90 percent of pancreatic cancers are **exocrine cell cancers,** usually originating in the head of the gland. **Endocrine cell cancers**—or **islet cell carcinomas**—are slower growing, generally more treatable, and quite rare. Because early pancreatic cancers cause few symptoms, and because indicators of most pancreatic cancer may be misattributed to more benign digestive disorders, the disease is rarely detected before it has spread to nearby tissues or distant organs through the bloodstream or lymphatic system. A few rare types of endocrine cell cancer are likely to be detected early, because they produce abnormal quantities of hormones that cause telltale hormonal imbalances.

Like many other cancers, pancreatic cancer is characteristically a disease of the elderly, usually striking after age 60. It is more commonly diagnosed in men than in women, and most cases are incurable. The incidence of pancreatic cancer has risen with an increase in the average life span, causing some 27,000 new cases and about the same number of deaths annually in the U.S., making it one of the leading cancer killers.

## CAUSES

Aside from advanced age, smoking is the main risk factor for pancreatic cancer; a smoker is three times more likely than a nonsmoker to acquire the disease. People frequently exposed to certain petroleum products may also be at increased risk. Excessive dietary fat and protein may promote the disease. Diabetes is also linked to pancreatic cancer: 10 to 20 percent of patients diagnosed with pancreatic cancer also have dia-

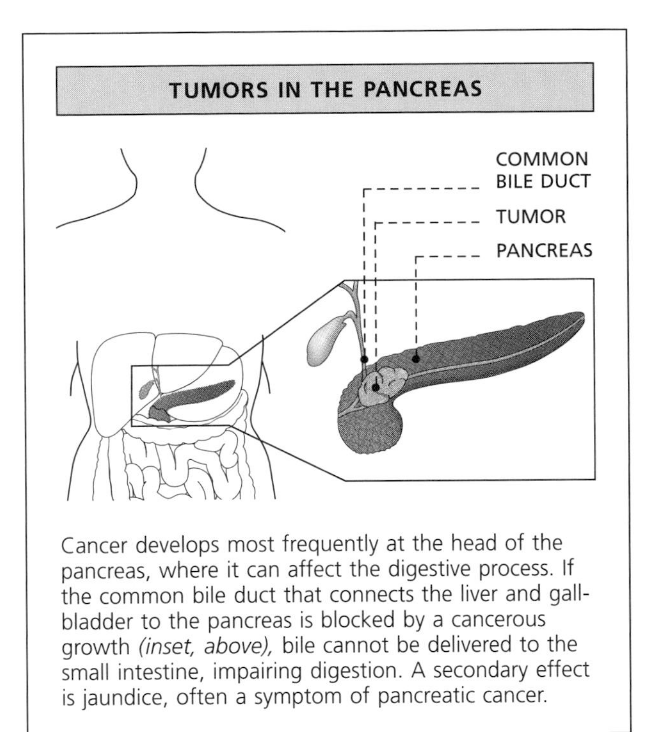


Cancer develops most frequently at the head of the pancreas, where it can affect the digestive process. If the common bile duct that connects the liver and gallbladder to the pancreas is blocked by a cancerous growth *(inset, above)*, bile cannot be delivered to the small intestine, impairing digestion. A secondary effect is jaundice, often a symptom of pancreatic cancer.

betes. Other diseases associated with pancreatic cancer include hereditary pancreatitis, an inflammatory pancreatic problem; Gardner's syndrome, characterized by growths within and outside the colon; neurofibromatosis, or elephant man's disease; and multiple endocrine neoplasia, a condition that promotes growth of benign islet cell tumors; all these conditions are hereditary.

### DIAGNOSTIC AND TEST PROCEDURES

To check for tumors in the pancreas, a doctor relies on imaging studies of the gland. The most common tests are sonograms and CT scans of the abdomen. If necessary, detailed images are obtained by inserting an endoscope through the mouth to the pancreas, injecting dye, then taking x-rays. A tissue sample for biopsy can also be extracted through the scope. If a biopsy confirms cancer, further tests are done to determine how far the disease has advanced. Sometimes exploratory surgery is necessary so the surgeon can study the tumor directly, determine if nearby lymph nodes are cancerous, and take tissue samples for microscopic examination.

## TREATMENT

See Cancer for more information about the conventional treatments described below.

### CONVENTIONAL MEDICINE

Because most cases of pancreatic cancer are advanced when diagnosed, cure is rarely a realistic goal. Instead, treatment usually aims to extend survival and relieve uncomfortable symptoms. Surgery may cure the cancer, but only if it has not spread beyond the pancreas. If possible the surgeon removes the malignant tumor, leaving as much of the pancreas as possible to allow continued function. More often, however, the entire pancreas must be removed. Then the patient must have a lifelong regimen of replacement enzymes and hormones, including insulin.

Depending on the type of cancer, patients may also be administered radiation or chemotherapy treatments, either after surgery in an effort to extend survival time, or as a means of relieving symptoms. **Exocrine cell cancer** responds best to radiation, sometimes in combination with chemotherapy, while **endocrine cell cancer** responds best to chemotherapy. Prescription medication, usually including narcotics, is given to help manage the pain that is common with advanced pancreatic cancer.

### COMPLEMENTARY THERAPIES

For many advanced pancreatic cancer sufferers, pain is significant. Besides taking prescription medication, patients can try pain control through **massage, acupuncture,** and **biofeedback** training, as well as such **relaxation** techniques as **guided imagery** and self-hypnosis.

## PREVENTION

Pancreatic cancer is not easily prevented, but you can take measures to reduce your risk. If you work around petroleum products, take precautions to avoid unnecessary exposure to both materials and fumes. And if you smoke, quit now. ■

# PANCREATIC PROBLEMS

## SYMPTOMS

For **acute pancreatitis:**

- sudden, intense pains in the middle of the abdomen, often beginning 12 to 24 hours after a large meal or a bout of heavy drinking. The pain may radiate to your back.
- fever.
- nausea or vomiting.
- clammy skin.
- abdominal distention and tenderness.
- rapid pulse.

For **chronic pancreatitis:**

- intense, long-lasting abdominal pain that may radiate to the back and chest; the pain may be persistent or intermittent.
- excessively foul, bulky stools.
- nausea or vomiting.
- weight loss.
- abdominal distention.

## CALL YOUR DOCTOR IF:

- you think you may have pancreatitis. Patients with acute pancreatitis must have professional care to avoid serious, possibly life-threatening complications. Chronic pancreatitis also requires professional evaluation and treatment.
- you continue to lose weight after treatment for pancreatitis; you may have a complication that prevents the body from digesting food properly.
- you are pale, cold, clammy, have a rapid heartbeat, or are breathing rapidly; you may be in **shock** and need emergency care. *(See page 75 in Emergencies/First Aid.)*

**Chronic pancreatitis** and **acute pancreatitis** are inflammations of the pancreas, a gland that produces both digestive enzymes and the hormone insulin, which your body uses to metabolize carbohydrates and fats. The symptoms of acute pancreatitis are typically severe and need to be treated. If they aren't, you may develop pancreatic cysts, abscesses, and leaks of pancreatic fluid into the abdomen, which can lead to other long-term problems. Shock is a possibly fatal complication of acute pancreatitis.

Chronic pancreatitis develops over a number of years, usually after a history of recurrent attacks of acute pancreatitis. Chronic pancreatitis may cause you to lose the ability to secrete the enzymes your body needs to digest foods. The resulting condition, known as exocrine insufficiency, is a principal characteristic of chronic pancreatitis and is signaled by weight loss—either gradual or sudden—and foul-smelling stools. Chronic pancreatitis can also lead to diabetes mellitus and pancreatic calcification, in which small, hard deposits develop in the pancreas.

## CAUSES

**Acute pancreatitis** is associated with excessive alcohol drinking, gallstones, viral and bacterial infections, drugs, and blockage of the pancreatic duct. These factors appear to encourage pancreatic digestive enzymes to act on the pancreas itself, causing swelling, hemorrhage, and damage to blood vessels in the pancreas. More than half the people who develop **chronic pancreatitis** are heavy drinkers; heavy consumption of alcohol is the most frequent cause of exocrine insufficiency in adults. (The leading cause of exocrine insufficiency in children is cystic fibrosis.)

### DIAGNOSTIC AND TEST PROCEDURES

Your doctor will probably press on your abdominal area to see if it is tender, and check you for low blood pressure, low-grade fever, and rapid pulse. Your blood will be tested for abnormal levels of pancreatic enzymes, white blood cells, blood sugar, and calcium. Abdominal x-rays will show if your pancreas is calcified. Ultrasound tests or CT scans will show bile duct problems.

To diagnose **chronic pancreatitis,** your doctor will take blood samples and check your stool for excess fat, a sign that the pancreas is no longer producing enough enzymes to process fat. You may be given a stimulation test to see how well your pancreas releases its digestive enzymes into the duodenum. You may also be screened for diabetes mellitus.

## TREATMENT

Conventional medicine treats pancreatitis with drugs, diet, and surgery. Alternative choices focus on alleviating symptoms of pancreatitis and bolstering your overall health.

### CONVENTIONAL MEDICINE

If you have an attack of **acute pancreatitis,** your doctor will try to stem the flow of pancreatic enzymes by feeding you intravenously. You may receive meperidine—a strong analgesic—for pain. You may have to have your stomach drained with a tube placed through your nose. If your pancreatitis is caused by gallstones or an obstructed pancreatic duct, you may need surgery once your symptoms have subsided.

If you have **chronic pancreatitis,** your doctor will focus on treating you for pain—guarding against your possible addiction to prescription analgesics—and for complications that affect your digestive abilities. You may be placed on an enzyme replacement therapy to restore your digestive tract's ability to digest nutrients; this will also likely reduce the frequency of new attacks. You may have to avoid fatty foods, and will have to abstain from drinking alcohol. If your pain does not respond to medication, the damaged pancreatic tissue may be surgically removed, but only as a last resort.

### ALTERNATIVE CHOICES

Alternative treatments can be used in conjunction with conventional treatment to help improve your overall responsiveness to medical therapy. Because both acute and chronic pancreatitis require conventional treatment, you should discuss any other approaches with your doctor before proceeding with them.

#### CHINESE MEDICINE

A practitioner will treat pancreatitis in the context of a complete body system imbalance.

#### HERBAL THERAPIES

A combination of equal parts of glycerates of fringe-tree bark *(Chionanthus virginicus),* balmony *(Chelone glabra),* and milk thistle *(Silybum marianum)* may help promote fat digestion; take 1 tsp of the mixture three times daily.

#### NUTRITION AND DIET

Take chromium supplements, 300 mcg daily, to help maintain normal blood sugar levels. Supplements of buffered vitamin C as well as vitamin B complex with extra niacin ($B_3$) and pantothenic acid ($B_5$) may help reduce stress and fight infection. Do not drink alcohol.

#### REFLEXOLOGY

Press the adrenal gland areas to help your body fight infection, the stomach and pancreas areas to improve digestion, and the solar plexus areas to relieve stress. *(See page 25 for area locations.)*

## PREVENTION

- Limiting yourself to one or two alcoholic drinks per day may significantly lessen your chances of developing pancreatitis. Once you have had pancreatitis, though, you should not drink at all; any drinking carries the risk of new attacks.
- Controlling your weight and maintaining a healthful diet and lifestyle may prevent gallstones. ■

# PANIC ATTACK

## SYMPTOMS

If you have four or more of the following, you are having a panic attack:

- heart palpitations.
- sweating.
- shaking.
- a "smothering" sensation.
- a feeling of choking.
- chest pain or discomfort.
- nausea.
- dizziness or faintness.
- a sense of unreality.
- a fear of going crazy.
- a fear of dying.
- numbness or tingling.
- chills or hot flashes.

If you have recurrent panic attacks and persistent fear of subsequent attacks or change your behavior significantly because of such attacks, you have **panic disorder.**

## CALL YOUR DOCTOR IF:

- you think you have **panic disorder.** An isolated panic attack, while extremely unpleasant, is not uncommon or life-threatening.
- you think you may be having an actual heart attack, whose symptoms can be similar. However, most people having a panic attack have had one before, triggered by a similar event or situation. Also, the chest pain of a panic attack usually stays in the mid-chest area (the pain of a heart attack commonly moves toward the left arm) and is accompanied by rapid breathing, palpitations, and fear.

P

You are engaged in some ordinary aspect of life when suddenly your heart begins to pound, and you hyperventilate, sweat, and tremble. You fear you are having a heart attack, going crazy, or even dying. Then, 10 or so minutes later, it's gone. Where did that feeling come from?

Unfortunately, there is no clear answer. You have had a panic attack, and for a small minority of sufferers, they recur again and again in a pattern known as **panic disorder.** Between attacks, sufferers live in dread of the next one.

Many people with panic disorder relate an attack to what they were doing when it occurred. They may assume that the restaurant, elevator, or classroom caused the attack, and decide to avoid that situation. In this case, panic disorder may lead to **agoraphobia**—the fear of leaving home or being in public places—though the relationship between the two conditions is unclear. *(See Phobias.)*

Panic attacks are fairly common, afflicting about 35 percent of the population each year. About 1 to 2 percent will develop panic disorder. Attacks usually begin between ages 15 and 25.

## CAUSES

The underlying cause of panic disorder is not clear. There is evidence of both a genetic and a biochemical basis. There is also an association with phobias, such as school phobia or agoraphobia, and with depression, alcohol abuse, suicide risk, and seasonal affective disorder. The sudden feeling of terror or doom often brings on hyperventilation—uncontrollable, rapid, shallow breathing. This in itself can cause many of the other physical symptoms by upsetting the balance of oxygen and carbon dioxide in the bloodstream.

Panic disorder may begin after a serious illness or accident, the death of a close friend, separation from the family, or the birth of a baby. Attacks may also accompany the use of mind-altering drugs. Most often, however, a panic attack comes "out of the blue"; it may even begin during sleep.

Some medical problems and medications can cause panic attacks, including antidepressants at high dosage. Panic disorder that begins after age 40 suggests depression or another underlying medical disorder.

## TREATMENT

Because the cause of most panic attacks is not clear, treatment must be based on particular cases and may involve psychotherapy, cognitive-behavioral therapy, or medication. Alternative treatments fight anxiety and relax the body.

### CONVENTIONAL MEDICINE

Psychotherapy offers support and helps to minimize the fearfulness of symptoms; sometimes this is sufficient to clear up the disorder. Recurrent attacks, however, require additional measures.

Cognitive-behavioral therapy, which exposes patients to the bodily sensations of panic in a safe setting, is often helpful. These sensations may be induced by rapid breathing, head rolling, or running up stairs. Patients are taught coping skills such as muscle relaxation and breathing techniques. This therapy also helps them learn that panic does not lead to the catastrophic events they fear, such as having a heart attack.

Antidepressants, such as imipramine, often help reduce anxiety and the frequency and severity of panic attacks. Antianxiety drugs (such as alprazolam) work faster than antidepressants but carry the risk of dependence. Halting the medicine, however, often leads to relapse. Medication is most successful when used with cognitive-behavioral therapy.

### ALTERNATIVE CHOICES

A number of alternative techniques may help reduce the anxiety that underlies panic disorder.

#### AROMATHERAPY

Studies have shown that essential oil of lavender *(Lavandula officinalis)* can relieve anxiety and stress. Try carrying a small bottle with you and sprinkling a few drops on a handkerchief to inhale at stressful moments.

#### BODY WORK

Both **qigong** and **yoga** can relax the body and help with the anxiety that patients experience between panic attacks. Either can be learned from a teacher and then practiced at home.

#### HERBAL THERAPIES

A number of herbs function as relaxants and tranquilizers and may soothe anxiety. Try a tea made from skullcap *(Scutellaria lateriflora),* valerian *(Valeriana officinalis),* vervain, or lemon balm.

#### HYPNOTHERAPY

Hypnosis is effective for many patients with anxiety or phobias, partly because the therapy itself brings deep relaxation. This may be combined with other therapies to enable patients to discover and overcome the cause of the panic.

#### MIND/BODY MEDICINE

Because hyperventilation is a central feature of panic attacks, the practice of slow and deep breathing can help reduce the severity and perhaps even the frequency of attacks. **Meditation** and other relaxation exercises, such as taking two minutes each hour to breathe slowly, are helpful in both calming the rhythm of breathing and reducing anxiety.

#### NUTRITION AND DIET

Magnesium has a tranquilizing action; try a 250-mg tablet twice a day. Avoid caffeine and other stimulants, alcohol, and sugar.

## PREVENTION

You can take steps to lessen the chance of attacks and learn to manage them better.

- Learn to recognize a panic attack. When you sense the first symptoms, know that others may come. You have survived them before and can do so again. Try slow, deep breaths.
- Take your time. It's important not to hope for a quick cure. Therapy takes time, and improvement comes in small steps.
- Go easy on yourself. People who feel panic tend to be overly critical of themselves. ■

# PARKINSON'S DISEASE

## SYMPTOMS

The disease takes hold slowly, beginning with a sense of weakness and a slight tremor of the head or hands, then gradually progressing to more generalized symptoms. These can include:

- slow, jerky movements; a shuffling gait; and stooped posture.
- unsteady balance; difficulty rising from a sitting position.
- continuous "pill-rolling" motion of the thumb and forefinger.
- indistinct speech; voice weakened to a monotone.
- swallowing problems in later stages.
- in severe cases, rigid trunk and limbs; fixed facial expression and unblinking, staring eyes.

## CALL YOUR DOCTOR IF:

- you suspect Parkinson's disease might be at the root of any of the above symptoms. In the disease's early stages, drugs can be very beneficial.

Parkinson's disease, which mostly afflicts older people, results from gradual degeneration of nerve cells in the portion of the midbrain that controls body movements. The first signs are likely to be barely noticeable—a feeling of weakness or stiffness in one limb, perhaps, or a fine trembling of one hand when it is at rest (activity causes the tremor to disappear). Eventually, the shaking will worsen and spread, muscles will tend to stiffen, and balance and coordination will deteriorate. Depression and other mental or emotional problems are common.

Usually the disorder begins between the ages of 50 and 65, striking about 1 percent of the population in that age group; it is slightly more common in men than in women. Medication can treat its symptoms, and the disorder is not directly life-threatening. About half of all patients treated with drugs have no major disabilities 10 years after the onset of the disease.

## CAUSES

Bodily movements are regulated by a portion of the brain called the basal ganglia, whose cells require a proper balance of two substances called dopamine and acetylcholine, both involved in the transmission of nerve impulses. In Parkinson's, cells that produce dopamine begin to degenerate, throwing off the balance of these two neurotransmitters. Researchers believe that genetics sometimes plays a role in the cellular breakdown, and in rare instances, Parkinson's may be caused by a viral infection or by exposure to environmental toxins such as pesticides, carbon monoxide, or the metal manganese. But in the great majority of Parkinson's cases, the cause is unknown.

### DIAGNOSTIC AND TEST PROCEDURES

Usually, the outward symptoms of Parkinson's are distinctive enough for a diagnosis to be made. The metabolic changes in the brain can be traced with imaging tests such as PET—positron emission tomography.

## TREATMENT

Most treatments aim at restoring the proper balance of the neurotransmitters acetylcholine and dopamine by increasing dopamine levels. Drugs are the standard way of doing this, but neurosurgeons have had some success with experiments involving operative procedures.

### CONVENTIONAL MEDICINE

Symptoms can be effectively controlled for years with medication. The drug most often prescribed is levodopa—also called L-dopa—which the body metabolizes to produce dopamine. (Direct administration of dopamine is ineffective; the brain's natural protections block its uptake.) To suppress nausea and other possible side effects, levodopa is often used in conjunction with a related drug called carbidopa.

But some patients cannot tolerate carbidopa and so take levodopa alone. If you take only levodopa, it's important not to take it at the same time as food or vitamins containing vitamin $B_6$, which interferes with its effectiveness.

Most doctors try to postpone starting patients on levodopa as long as possible, because the medication tends to lose effectiveness over time. However, there is some controversy about waiting to begin treatment with levodopa because it can be so beneficial. Researchers have thus investigated ways to offset the loss of effectiveness. Some studies have found that, when used in conjunction with levodopa and carbidopa, the antioxidant selegiline hydrochloride reduces many of the adverse effects associated with long-term drug use.

A new class of dopamine-like drugs imitates dopamine's activity rather than adding to the amount of it in the brain. Two of them, bromocriptine and pergolide, appear promising. Other medications prescribed for Parkinson's disease include apomorphine, benztropine, amantadine, and anticholinergic drugs; all can help control various symptoms—in some cases by releasing dopamine from nerve cells, in others by reducing the effects of acetylcholine rather than increasing the amount of dopamine.

Neurosurgeons have explored various ways of grafting dopamine-producing cells in the brain rather than trying to correct the neurotransmitter imbalance with drugs. One promising approach uses fetal-tissue implants. Some improvements have been observed, but because of the source of the cells, the technique is highly controversial.

Another experimental technique, stereotactic surgery, creates lesions in the thalamus, the brain's inner chamber. In some studies, this procedure appears to eliminate tremor in 80 percent of patients and to relieve rigidity in almost all. A similar form of surgery—using electrical stimulation instead of lesions—also shows promise.

Scientists are also investigating the use of glial cell-derived nerve growth factor to treat Parkinson's and other neurodegenerative diseases. This substance is produced naturally by tissues throughout the body; some experiments indicate that injections of this nerve growth factor may help preserve and even restore nerve cells in the brain and spinal cord—specifically those that produce dopamine and that help initiate muscle movement.

Some treatments focus on the effects of the disorder rather than the causes. Your doctor might refer you to a physical therapist to restore normal body alignment, enhance your balance and motor responses, and improve your ability to initiate motion. A physical therapist may also give you muscle-strengthening exercises to help with speaking or swallowing.

In many Parkinson's patients, a weakening of social ties because of physical difficulties can lead to depression. Antidepressants can help. In addition, the American Parkinson Disease Association *(see the Appendix)* can provide information about support groups and exercise classes in your area—valuable sources of companionship.

### ALTERNATIVE CHOICES

Conventional medicines such as levodopa are widely acknowledged as the best treatments for Parkinson's disease. However, many of the alternative therapies mentioned below can be very helpful for relieving symptoms or easing tight muscles. Some of the herbal and dietary therapies can be applied in conjunction with conventional medicines, but be sure to consult your doctor about possible adverse interactions.

#### ACUPUNCTURE

According to some studies by acupuncturists, Parkinson's disease may be accompanied by an imbalance of energy along one or more meridians *(see page 20)*. The muscle stiffness, soreness, and imbalance of Parkinson's may be alleviated by a series of treatments.

#### BODY WORK

Deep-muscle **massage** stretches the connective tissue around tight muscles, ridding them of cramping and allowing greater freedom of movement. Massage can also improve motion in your joints, soften hardened muscle tissue, and stimulate your lymphatic system.

**Reflexology** practitioners say that the brain, head, and spine all respond to indirect massage. See the illustration below for reflexology techniques that may help relieve some Parkinson's symptoms.

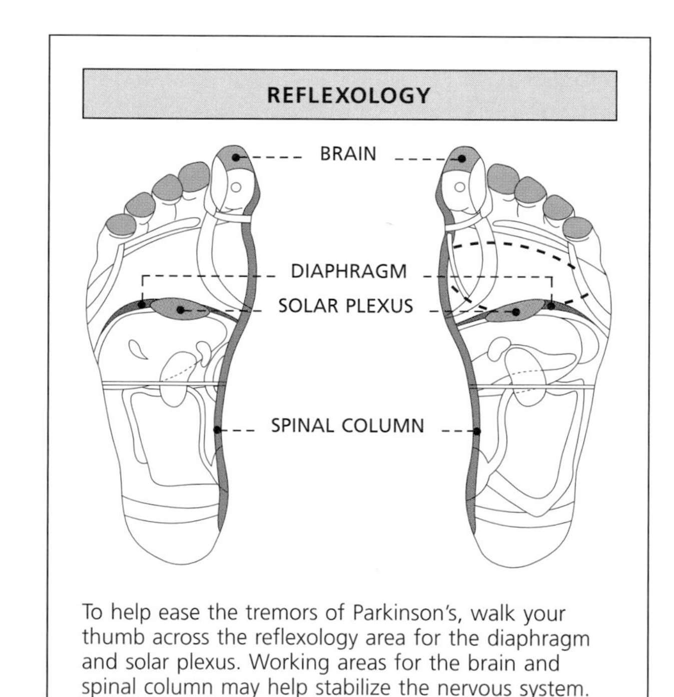


To help ease the tremors of Parkinson's, walk your thumb across the reflexology area for the diaphragm and solar plexus. Working areas for the brain and spinal column may help stabilize the nervous system.

Chi yi, a Chinese deep-breathing exercise, increases the oxygen supply in the blood and may thereby help alleviate depression. Sit with your back against the back of a chair and your feet flat on the floor. Reach toward the ceiling with both arms, inhaling deeply through your nose as you do so. Hold your breath as you ball your hands into fists, squeezing your arm muscles. Exhale slowly through your nose to a count of six as you bring your tensed arms down, crossing them on your chest over your heart. Lower your chin to your chest. Take four short breaths, completely filling your lungs, and feel your chest expand. Hold for a few seconds, then exhale slowly. Repeat this exercise several times each day, concentrating on the rhythm and depth of each breath. If tremor prohibits arm or head movements, concentrate on the breathing, working toward a rate of only four or five breaths per minute. Limit practice to five minutes per day.

**Yoga** is an ideal form of exercise for Parkinson's patients because of its slow movements. Regular exercise is important to avoid the atrophying of muscles and shrinking of tissues from disuse. See the illustration opposite for one useful type of yoga exercise.

#### CHINESE HERBS

Taken several times a day, combinations that include rhubarb *(Rheum palmatum)*, peony *(Paeonia officinalis)*, licorice *(Glycyrrhiza uralensis)*, and magnolia bark *(Magnolia officinalis)* are said to stop tremors and relax stiff muscles. Because using Chinese herbs is complicated, consult an expert in the field for correct dosages.

#### HERBAL THERAPIES

Passionflower *(Passiflora incarnata)* acts as an antispasmodic when ½ tsp of tincture is taken three times a day. Or take it twice daily as a tea: Pour one cup boiling water over 2 tsp dried leaves; steep for 15 minutes. Passionflower has been shown to reduce passive tremor when taken in combination with levodopa better than when either remedy is taken alone. But be sure to check with your doctor first if you are already taking levodopa.

Daily doses of 500 mg of evening primrose oil *(Oenothera biennis)* may reduce tremors.

YOGA

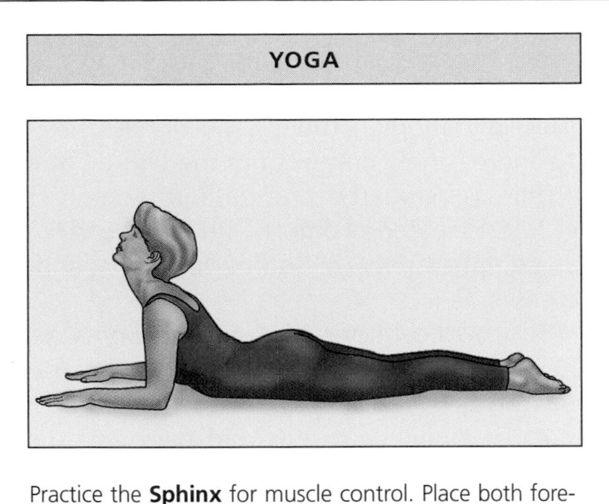

Practice the **Sphinx** for muscle control. Place both forearms on the floor with your palms down and elbows under your shoulders. Inhale and push your chest away from the floor as far as comfortably possible. Hold for a few deep breaths, then relax and exhale.

#### HOMEOPATHY

A trained homeopath might prescribe a single remedy, a series, or a combination of remedies for the many different symptoms of Parkinson's.

#### MIND/BODY MEDICINE

The **Feldenkrais method,** which consists of a large number of exercises performed either in group classes or solo with a practitioner, aims at improving autonomic motor responses. While lying down, you are guided through a series of light, slow movements designed to support your neuromuscular system and alter habitual patterns of movement.

#### NUTRITION AND DIET

Parkinson's patients should pay close attention to diet; weight loss—possibly caused by persistent involuntary movements—is a common problem.

A diet called the 7:1 plan—for the ratio of carbohydrates to proteins—is designed for patients taking levodopa (proteins reduce the drug's effectiveness). Researchers disagree as to whether the proteins should be eaten throughout the day or restricted to the evening meal, when interference with levodopa might be less of a problem. Consult your doctor to determine which method works best for you. Either way, a low-protein diet can lead to deficiencies in calcium, iron, and B vitamins; supplements are therefore advised. (If you are taking levodopa without carbidopa, however, avoid vitamin $B_6$; the vitamin will interfere with the levodopa.)

Fava beans, also called broad beans, are a natural source of levodopa. One-half cup contains 250 mg, or the same amount as one pill. But don't substitute beans for pills without first consulting your doctor.

Patients attempt to relieve the constipation that often accompanies Parkinson's by eating bran. But recent research shows that bran is high in vitamin $B_6$, which interferes with the effectiveness of levodopa when the drug is taken alone. Prune juice, grains, and fiber laxatives should be substituted instead.

Foods seasoned with hot spices have been known to cause uncontrollable physical movement in some people with Parkinson's. Avoid such foods.

### AT-HOME CARE

- Adding banisters in hallways and along walls can make it easier for a Parkinson's patient to get around.
- Chairs and sofas that are equipped with higher arms make sitting down and rising more manageable.
- Thick carpeting offers protection in falls, common with Parkinson's patients. ■

P

# PELVIC INFLAMMATORY DISEASE

## SYMPTOMS

**With acute pelvic inflammatory disease (PID):**

- severe pain and tenderness in the lower abdomen with vaginal discharge, often accompanied by fever.

**With chronic PID:**

- mild, recurrent pain in the lower abdomen, sometimes accompanied by backache or irregular menstrual periods.
- pain during intercourse.
- infertility.
- irregular menstrual periods.
- heavy, unpleasant-smelling vaginal discharge.

## CALL YOUR DOCTOR IF:

- you experience sudden abdominal pain with or without fever; it may indicate acute pelvic inflammatory disease or another serious condition that requires immediate medical attention, such as appendicitis, endometriosis, a ruptured ovarian cyst *(see Ovary Problems)*, or an ectopic pregnancy.
- you experience any abnormal menstrual bleeding; you may have pelvic inflammatory disease or another serious condition, such as endometriosis or cervical cancer.
- you experience a vaginal discharge that is foul-smelling or unusually heavy; you may have pelvic inflammatory disease or another condition that requires medical treatment, such as vaginal, uterine, or cervical problems, or a sexually transmitted disease.

Pelvic inflammatory disease (PID) is the term used to describe an infection of any of a woman's pelvic organs, including the uterus, ovaries, or fallopian tubes. The disease has become increasingly common in the United States, affecting an estimated one million women each year. If not treated promptly, PID can lead to serious complications, including infertility and, in rare cases, death.

PID can be either acute or chronic. Acute PID comes on suddenly and is apt to be more severe. Chronic PID is a low-grade infection that may cause only recurrent mild pain and sometimes backache. Some women with PID have no discernible symptoms and discover they have had the infection only when they later attempt to get pregnant and discover that they are infertile.

## CAUSES

PID is caused by bacteria from contaminated semen that ascend from the vagina into the normally sterile uterus. Most cases of PID used to be caused by gonococcus, the organism responsible for the sexually transmitted disease gonorrhea, or by chlamydia. Recently, researchers have linked other organisms to PID, including some commonly found in the vagina and elsewhere in the body.

The risk of PID increases after childbirth, miscarriage, abortion, the insertion of an intrauterine device (IUD) for contraception, or certain operations, such as a dilation and curettage (D and C), all of which cause the cervix, or opening to the uterus, to widen temporarily. Douching also increases the risk of PID.

### DIAGNOSTIC AND TEST PROCEDURES

Your doctor will give you a pelvic examination. If there is evidence of an infection, he or she will use a cotton swab to obtain a sample of pus from inside your vagina. The sample will be analyzed to determine which organism is causing the infection. Sometimes a laparoscopic exam—a surgical procedure in which a special viewing instrument is inserted into the abdominal cavity—is necessary for an accurate diagnosis. Your doctor may also use ultrasound to help with the diagnosis.

## TREATMENT

Because PID can lead to serious complications, such as infertility, it must be treated with conventional antibiotics. Alternative therapies may be used, however, to complement the antibiotics and to help with recovery and prevention.

### CONVENTIONAL MEDICINE

Your doctor will prescribe one or more oral antibiotics, such as tetracycline, erythromycin, or doxycycline, to clear up the infection. You may be treated on an outpatient basis, but if you are pregnant or have severe symptoms or if your case presents other complicating factors, you may be hospitalized and given the antibiotics intravenously.

If you have an IUD, your doctor will remove it. Until the PID is eradicated, you should avoid intercourse, which can cause the pelvic organs to move, spreading infected pus.

If your infection is chronic or recurrent and does not respond to oral antibiotics, your doctor may order intravenous antibiotics. When pelvic abscesses have developed, even intravenous antibiotics may not work; it may then be necessary to operate and drain the abscesses. If your pain is persistent and does not respond to other treatments, your doctor may recommend pelvic surgery to remove or repair infected tissue. Sometimes it is possible to spare one ovary, thus preventing premature menopause, and still get relief from the pain. Discuss this possibility with your doctor.

### ALTERNATIVE CHOICES

Use alternative methods during or after conventional antibiotic treatment to speed recovery and help prevent recurrences. To relieve the pain of a PID infection, for example, use castor-oil packs or get **acupressure** or **acupuncture** treatments from an experienced practitioner.

#### HERBAL THERAPIES

To help fight PID infection, herbalists recommend echinacea (*Echinacea* spp.) or calendula *(Calendula officinalis)*. Both these herbs are believed to have antimicrobial properties. Blue cohosh *(Caulophyllum thalictroides)* and false unicorn root *(Chamaelirium luteum)*, which are prescribed as general tonics for the female reproductive organs, are also recommended. You may take these herbs in either tea or tincture form.

#### NUTRITION AND DIET

To strengthen your immune system and help speed your recovery, eat plenty of whole (unprocessed) foods, especially fresh fruits and vegetables.

Vitamin supplements may also enhance your immune system. Take vitamin A (10,000 IU daily), vitamin C (500 to 2,000 mg daily), and vitamin B complex (50 mg three times a day).

## PREVENTION

- Use barrier contraception (condoms, diaphragm, or a cervical cap with spermicides).
- Avoid putting anything in your vagina for two to three weeks after an abortion, a miscarriage, or a D and C and for six weeks after childbirth. This means no intercourse, no douching, and no tampons. You should also avoid bathing and swimming during this period; take showers or sponge baths instead.
- Do not use an IUD. Women wearing an IUD are three to five times more likely to get PID than those not wearing one, especially if they have more than one partner.
- If you have a history of pelvic infections or have several sexual partners, use barrier methods of contraception and avoid intercourse during your menstrual period. The cervix—the opening to the uterus—widens during menstruation to allow blood and uterine tissue to flow out.
- Get prompt treatment for any sexually transmitted disease. ■

# PENILE PAIN

*Read down this column to find your symptoms. Then read across.*

| SYMPTOMS | AILMENT/PROBLEM |
|---|---|
| ◆ a bend in the penis that may be painful during erection. | ◆ Peyronie's disease—a fibrous thickening along the shaft of the penis. |
| ◆ persistent, painful erection unrelated to sexual desire. | ◆ Priapism—a state of continuous erection, usually traceable to a disease or other disorder. |
| ◆ painful urination and a clear, thin discharge from the penis. | ◆ Chlamydia—a sexually transmitted infection caused by a microscopic organism. |
| ◆ painful urination and a cloudy, thick, puslike discharge from the penis. | ◆ Gonorrhea—a sexually transmitted bacterial infection. |
| ◆ painful blisters along the penis that break and expose raw skin. | ◆ Genital herpes—a sexually transmitted viral infection. |
| ◆ itchy, hard, flesh-colored warts along the penis, which may bleed and be mildly painful. | ◆ Genital warts—a sexually transmitted viral infection. |
| ◆ pain, redness, and swelling on the foreskin or head (glans) of the penis. | ◆ Balanitis—an infection or inflammation of the penis. |
| ◆ pain occurring after injections for erectile dysfunction, or impotence. | ◆ Drug-induced pain. |
| ◆ pain and difficulty retracting the foreskin. | ◆ Phimosis—an overly tight foreskin. |
| ◆ a lump, swelling, or open sore on the penis. | ◆ Possibly a sign of cancer of the penis. |

| WHAT TO DO | OTHER INFO |
|---|---|
| ◆ See your doctor. Although many cases need no treatment, others require surgery. Taking 200 IU of vitamin E with each meal may help. | ◆ Most common in middle-aged men. Scar tissue from repeated vascular injuries prevents penile skin from sliding normally during intercourse. |
| ◆ See your doctor. Untreated priapism can cause impotence; you need to be evaluated for the existence of another health problem. For temporary relief, take acetaminophen and apply an ice pack to the penis. | ◆ Priapism has various causes—including sickle cell anemia. Treating the condition promptly should restore normal erections. |
| ◆ See your doctor or a clinic for a blood test. Chlamydia can be successfully treated with antibiotics. | ◆ Sexual partners must also be treated for the infection. |
| ◆ See your doctor. Discontinue sexual relations until you are analyzed and treated. | ◆ This infection may be transmitted by vaginal, anal, or oral sex, and may spread to other parts of the body. |
| ◆ See your doctor. Wash and dry the area regularly. Avoid sexual intercourse for two weeks after an outbreak. | ◆ Herpes usually spreads only during the active phase of the disease. Acyclovir lotion may relieve pain and reduce the length of the active phase. |
| ◆ See your doctor. Avoid sexual contact until warts disappear. Never treat genital warts with over-the-counter wart preparations. | ◆ Genital warts may disappear on their own but often recur, though less often and less severely over time. |
| ◆ Wash beneath the foreskin when bathing. If infection is chronic, circumcision—surgical removal of the foreskin—may be necessary. | ◆ May be caused by irritating clothing or by secretions that collect under an uncircumcised foreskin. |
| ◆ See your doctor, who may add sodium bicarbonate or the painkiller procaine to the medication. | ◆ Sodium bicarbonate neutralizes the acidity of injected medications used to treat erectile dysfunction. |
| ◆ See your doctor. If you have persistent pain, circumcision may be necessary. | ◆ The cause may be inflammation or a genetic condition. Contrary to myth, circumcision has no noticeable effect on sexual function or satisfaction. |
| ◆ See your doctor immediately, even if there is no pain. Prompt diagnosis increases the chance of successful treatment. | ◆ Cancer may begin as small growths beneath the foreskin. Circumcised men rarely develop this cancer. |

# PHLEBITIS

## SYMPTOMS

For **superficial phlebitis:**
- a red, cordlike vein visible in your leg; the vein will feel hard, warm, and tender, and surrounding tissue may become itchy and swollen.
- a throbbing or burning sensation beneath the skin's surface.
- pain and heaviness when lowering your leg.

For **deep phlebitis:**
- potentially no symptoms.
- pain and swelling throughout the entire affected limb.
- fever, skin ulcers, or swellings in your leg that stay indented when pressed.

## CALL YOUR DOCTOR IF:

- you suspect you have phlebitis; you need proper diagnosis and treatment.
- symptoms of **superficial phlebitis** do not dissipate within 7 to 10 days; you may have developed a more serious condition.
- you experience unusual bleeding when taking anticoagulant drugs; your doctor may have to adjust the dosage.
- you notice lumps, high fever, or pervasive pain or swelling throughout a limb. All are signs of **deep phlebitis,** possibly accompanied by infection, that requires immediate medical care.
- you have phlebitis and develop an associated infection (which may occur after childbirth or a wound or trauma to a vein, or if you have a heart valve infection). Even in mild cases, infection introduces a risk of blood poisoning.

Doctors often use the general term "phlebitis" (meaning inflammation of a vein) to refer to a more specific condition known as thrombophlebitis, which involves the formation of blood clots, or thrombi, where inflammation occurs. These clots cause pain and irritation, and may also partially or fully block blood flow in affected veins.

The most common form of phlebitis, called **superficial phlebitis,** occurs in veins near the skin's surface, typically in the legs. Though annoying, it is relatively harmless, usually resolving itself in a matter of days. **Deep phlebitis,** which affects interior veins of the legs, is less common and more dangerous: Because interior veins are larger, blood clots tend to be bigger and are more likely to break free and travel to the lungs. Also, people with deep phlebitis often are not aware that they have it and don't seek proper care.

## CAUSES

People with varicose veins are prone to phlebitis. Anyone immobilized for any length of time, such as after surgery, is also vulnerable because blood is not flowing as strongly and clots form more easily. The elderly are also susceptible, because circulatory problems and vascular diseases that can trigger phlebitis tend to worsen with age.

Phlebitis can also develop in response to infection or trauma of some kind. It may occur at the site of an intravenous injection, particularly when that site has been prodded repeatedly.

Researchers have identified several other risk factors. About 70 percent of phlebitis sufferers are women. Pregnant women and those on birth-control pills are more likely to develop the condition. People whose blood tends to clot too readily are at higher risk. Obesity, a sedentary lifestyle, and smoking have also been linked to phlebitis.

## TREATMENT

Treatment depends on the type of phlebitis. **Superficial phlebitis** usually responds to simple at-home measures. **Deep phlebitis,** however, often requires a short stay in the hospital. In either

## RISK IN DIFFERENT VEINS

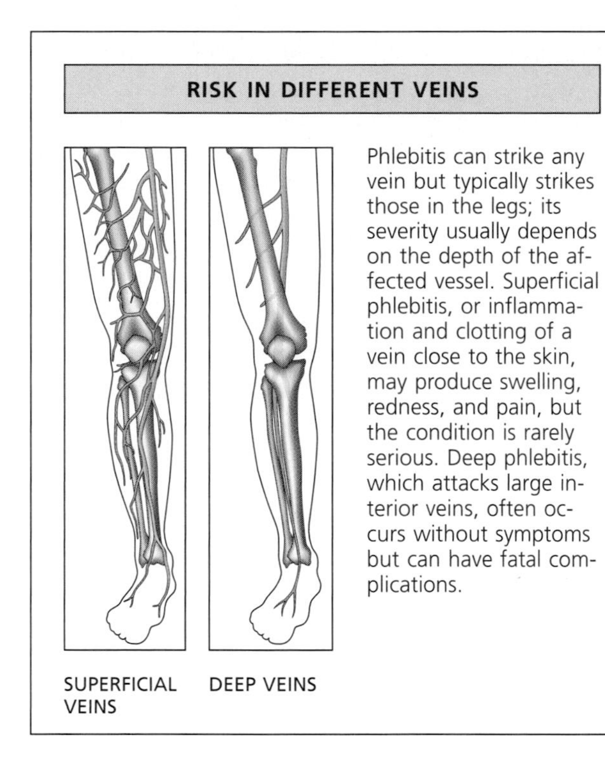


Phlebitis can strike any vein but typically strikes those in the legs; its severity usually depends on the depth of the affected vessel. Superficial phlebitis, or inflammation and clotting of a vein close to the skin, may produce swelling, redness, and pain, but the condition is rarely serious. Deep phlebitis, which attacks large interior veins, often occurs without symptoms but can have fatal complications.

case, if you smoke, stop; smoking greatly aggravates all circulatory problems. Also, switching from birth-control pills to another form of contraception may help prevent a recurrence.

### CONVENTIONAL MEDICINE

If you think you have phlebitis, your doctor may order x-rays to confirm the diagnosis and to determine whether deep veins are involved.

To help relieve the symptoms of **superficial phlebitis,** your doctor may recommend aspirin to reduce inflammation. You may be given an antibiotic if your doctor thinks there is an infection. If you're bothered by pain and swelling, inquire about elastic support stockings. Although pantyhose often constrict circulation, specially prescribed compression stockings can greatly improve blood flow; for many, they bring immediate and lasting relief. See also At-Home Remedies.

If you're diagnosed with **deep phlebitis,** you will be hospitalized. Doctors routinely prescribe a one-week treatment of heparin, an anticoagulant usually given intravenously. You will rest in bed with your legs elevated and be evaluated for signs of lung clots. Your doctor will probably also start you on a 90-day course of another anticoagulant known as warfarin, taken orally. Warfarin is a powerful drug, so you'll need to watch for side effects your doctor will tell you about.

### ALTERNATIVE CHOICES

Some alternative therapies may help with **superficial phlebitis.** Consult a **homeopath,** or a practitioner of Chinese medicine, who might advise **acupressure, acupuncture,** or a combination of **Chinese herbs** designed to reduce inflammation. You might also try increasing your intake of vitamin E, a natural blood thinner, and vitamin C; both help keep blood vessels in good shape.

### AT-HOME REMEDIES

For **superficial phlebitis,** there are several things you can do at home to ease discomfort and speed your recovery:

- Get plenty of rest.
- When you lie down, prop up your legs so they are 6 to 12 inches above your heart level. This encourages blood to drain from your legs, easing the burden on veins affected by phlebitis.
- Use a heating pad or apply a moist, warm pack to swollen areas for relief. If surrounding skin itches, try a dab of zinc oxide.

### C A U T I O N !

**It's quite natural to rub an aching muscle to relieve pain, but be careful if you have phlebitis. Though the risk is slight, massage—particularly vigorous massage—might dislodge a blood clot, which could potentially travel to your lungs and cause a life-threatening pulmonary embolism. Don't worry if you forget and find yourself rubbing a sore area without thinking, but try to resist the urge.** ■

# PHOBIAS

## SYMPTOMS

Phobias are anxiety disorders. Three main types of phobias exist:

- If you have a persistent, irrational fear of particular objects or situations, such as snakes, spiders, heights, blood, flying, or elevators, you have a **specific phobia.**
- If you have a persistent, irrational fear of situations where you may be scrutinized or criticized or embarrassed by other people, you have **social phobia.**
- If you fear leaving home, being alone, or being away from home in a situation where you feel trapped or helpless, you have **agoraphobia.**

## CALL YOUR DOCTOR IF:

- you have a phobia that interferes with a normal social or working life. Treatment can often lessen your anxiety and may diminish or even remove the phobia.

Phobias (from the Greek *phobos,* meaning fear or flight) are irrational and disabling fears that produce a compelling desire to avoid the dreaded object or situation. A phobic person understands that the fear is excessive or groundless, but the effort to resist it only brings more anxiety. Phobias affect about 7 percent of the population, often beginning in childhood.

**Specific phobias** are the most common; they involve things such as school, dentists, driving, water, balloons, snakes, fat, age, high places (acrophobia), and enclosed spaces (claustrophobia). The fear is usually not of the object itself but of some dire outcome, such as falling from an airplane. Even though phobics acknowledge that their fear is excessive, this knowledge does not diminish their fear.

A victim of **agoraphobia** suffers multiple fears that center around three main themes: fear of leaving home, of being alone, and of being in a situation where one cannot suddenly leave or obtain help. If agoraphobia progresses, a person may go to almost any lengths to avoid leaving home.

In **social phobia,** which often affects adolescents, a person's central fear is of being humiliated in public. People with this kind of phobia may even balk at eating in a restaurant. They avoid public speaking, parties, and public lavatories; such situations and places may bring blushing, palpitations, sweating, tremors, stuttering, or faintness. As many as 25 percent of professional performers struggle with severe, lifelong performance anxiety—a form of social phobia. A person whose phobia is left untreated may become withdrawn, depressed, and socially incapacitated.

## CAUSES

Some **specific phobias** can be explained by early traumatic events, such as the bite of a dog, but the majority have no obvious cause. Most are thought to be produced when an underlying fear or conflict is displaced onto an unrelated object. **Agoraphobia** may develop in response to repeated panic attacks. Precursors of **social phobia** may be observable early in childhood, but the true cause is unknown.

## TREATMENT

The effectiveness of treatment depends partly on the phobia's severity. While some phobias are never completely cured, many people can learn to function effectively, especially after attending phobia clinics and support groups including people who have recovered from phobias.

### CONVENTIONAL MEDICINE

For **specific phobias,** treatment by systematic desensitization therapy is highly successful. For example, someone who is afraid of flying may be led through a series of steps, beginning with looking at pictures of airplanes in the relaxed environment of a therapist's office. This is followed by an imaginary trip in an airplane, then a visit to an airport, and finally an actual flight. Each stage should be accompanied by **relaxation** techniques. The support of a trusted person is very important.

Treating **social phobia** usually involves gradual exposure to social situations, along with role playing and rehearsal. Individuals are taught to reduce anxiety and encouraged to be less self-critical and learn appropriate behavior. Medications may also be used. Many musicians, actors, and lecturers reduce their symptoms with beta-adrenergic blockers (such as propranolol).

The best treatment for **agoraphobia** is to gradually move out into the places and situations that trigger anxiety. Taking small steps each day, in the company of a trusted person, a sufferer eventually learns to cope with situations that once inspired terror. This may be assisted by antidepressants (such as imipramine), which reduce the fear of panic. Antianxiety drugs may also be used, but with caution because of the risk of dependence. **Relaxation** techniques should be used to facilitate treatment.

### ALTERNATIVE CHOICES

Phobias are difficult to treat by yourself. A number of self-help therapies may help to ease the way, but they should be followed only with professional guidance.

#### AROMATHERAPY

Studies have shown that essential oil of lavender *(Lavandula officinalis)* can bring relief from anxiety. Carry a small bottle with you; sprinkle on a handkerchief to inhale at stressful moments.

#### HERBAL THERAPIES

Valerian *(Valeriana officinalis)* tea may ease anxiety. Pour a cup of boiling water over 1 to 2 tsp of the root and steep for 15 minutes.

#### HYPNOTHERAPY

Hypnosis, in the hands of a skilled professional, may help reduce symptoms, diminish fear, and sometimes uncover the cause of a phobia.

#### MIND/BODY MEDICINE

Numerous relaxation techniques, including **yoga, meditation,** and **biofeedback** exercises, can help reduce the anxiety that surrounds phobias.

### AT-HOME REMEDIES

By taking one small step at a time, most phobic people can reduce their terrors and, in many cases, move beyond them. Work with a trusted friend or therapist. Here are some guidelines:

- Feel free to ask for feedback or a reality check on a feared object or situation: Is it safe? Will it hurt me?
- Practice shifting your thoughts in a positive direction—from "That dog will bite me" to "That dog is tied up and can't hurt me."

## PREVENTION

- Do regular deep breathing and relaxation exercises, especially when anxiety starts to rise.
- Regular exercise helps burn up adrenaline, which accompanies panic attacks.
- Avoid alcohol, barbiturates, and antianxiety medicine whenever possible; drugs simply mask the symptoms. Also avoid caffeine, which can mimic some of the symptoms of panic attacks. ■

# PINCHED NERVE

## SYMPTOMS

- tenderness, tingling, or numbness in one part of your body, often a limb.
- prickly, burning, or lacerating pain where a nerve is being irritated, with a dull ache farther along the nerve's length.
- weakness in the affected area; atrophy of muscles because of disuse, so that one arm or leg may look thinner than the other.

See also Carpal Tunnel Syndrome, Disk Problems, and Sciatica.

## CALL YOUR DOCTOR IF:

- the pain persists for several days and does not respond to over-the-counter analgesics; your doctor may prescribe anti-inflammatory drugs or physical therapy.
- the pain is so great that you are unable to move without severe discomfort; your doctor may want to perform tests in order to rule out other ailments.

Any pressure applied to a nerve by the surrounding tissue will produce irritation and will disrupt the nerve's functioning, with consequences that can range from aches and pains to a loss of feeling or weakening of muscles. The pinching can occur for many reasons—pregnancy, an injury, repetitive motions, or joint disease, to name just a few. It may also occur anywhere in the peripheral nervous system (that is, nerves outside the brain and spine). Nerves passing over a rigid prominence, such as a bone, are particularly vulnerable.

The most typical pinched nerves are the median, ulnar, and radial nerves, which extend down the arms from the shoulders to the hands. Other commonly compressed nerves include the femoral, which extends from the pelvis to the knee; the plantar nerves in your feet; nerves between disks in your spinal column; the peroneal nerve running along the side of your leg; and the sciatic nerve, a large nerve that runs the length of each leg from the base of your spine to your foot *(see Sciatica).*

With treatment, a pinched nerve generally heals in a few days to a few weeks. Chronic cases can result from persistent irritation of the affected nerve. In some cases, damage to the nerve can become permanent.

## CAUSES

Pressure on a peripheral nerve from the surrounding tissue causes inflammation of the nerve. Such pressure can be the result of injury, disease, and even genetic inheritance. Sometimes the source of the problem is constant repetition of arm or leg movements, common with keyboard operations and assembly-line jobs. *(See Carpal Tunnel Syndrome.)*

Another common cause of nerve irritation is a damaged spinal disk—the cushioning between vertebrae. If a disk becomes injured or degenerates, it can tear, allowing the soft jellylike center to bulge out and press on an adjacent nerve. This condition—popularly known as a slipped disk *(see Disk Problems)*—tends to occur in the parts of the spine that are the most mobile: the lower

HERNIATED DISKS AND PINCHED NERVES

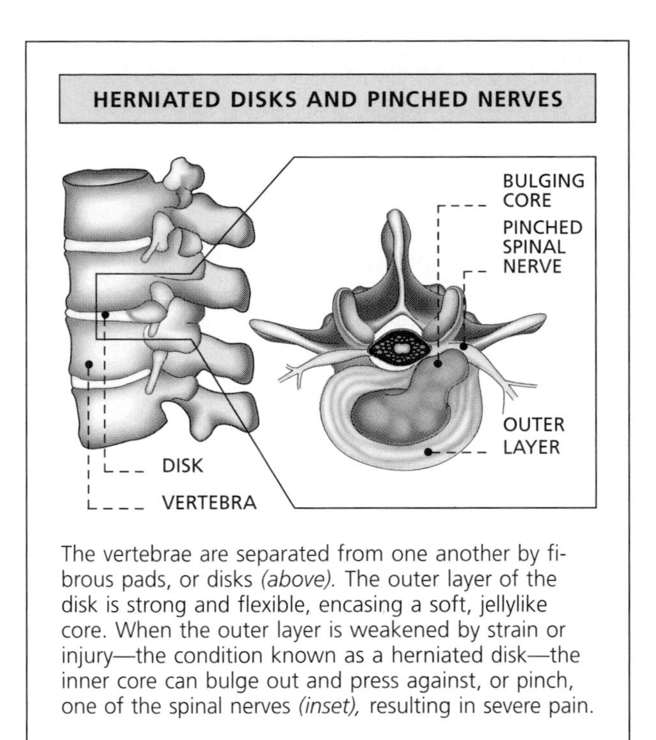


The vertebrae are separated from one another by fibrous pads, or disks *(above)*. The outer layer of the disk is strong and flexible, encasing a soft, jellylike core. When the outer layer is weakened by strain or injury—the condition known as a herniated disk—the inner core can bulge out and press against, or pinch, one of the spinal nerves *(inset)*, resulting in severe pain.

back (lumbar spine) and neck (cervical spine). Heavy lifting, obesity, and contact sports can contribute to the problem.

### DIAGNOSTIC AND TEST PROCEDURES

Your doctor may test your reflexes and look for problems of restricted movement. An EMG test may be performed to determine the motor conduction speed in your arms and legs.

## TREATMENT

### CONVENTIONAL MEDICINE

Your doctor may advise adjustment or cessation of an activity that is causing pressure on a nerve and may suggest wearing a splint, brace, or some other support. Physical therapy can strengthen surrounding muscles. Anti-inflammatory drugs or a short course of corticosteroids can promote healing. Small doses of amitriptyline or another tricyclic antidepressant, sometimes prescribed for pain, may help if your case is chronic.

### ALTERNATIVE CHOICES

#### CHIROPRACTIC

A chiropractor may x-ray your back to measure any abnormalities in your posture. Dislocated vertebrae are manipulated to relieve pressure on nerves and ease pain. Acute cases of pinched nerves might be helped by intramuscular injections of vitamin $B_{12}$.

#### HERBAL THERAPIES

Try a tea combining equal parts of St.-John's-wort *(Hypericum perforatum),* skullcap *(Scutellaria lateriflora),* and Siberian ginseng *(Eleutherococcus senticosus).*

#### HOMEOPATHY

For low-back pain that feels better when warmth is applied, try Rhus toxicodendron. Taking Arnica when your back pain follows an injury may lessen symptoms. Consult a homeopathic practitioner for proper dosages.

#### NUTRITION AND DIET

Taking 1,000 mg of lecithin with meals may help regenerate nerves. Nerve impulse conduction may benefit from 2,000 mg daily of calcium chelate.

### AT-HOME REMEDIES

Try the herbs discussed above or tinctures of all three combined with the tincture of oats *(Avena sativa);* mix them together in equal portions and take 1 tsp in a glass of water three times a day. If made into a tea, drink 3 cups daily.

## PREVENTION

Try to avoid tasks that involve repetitive hand, wrist, arm, or shoulder motions. When avoidance is impossible, perform the motions for short periods of time with breaks in between. *(See Carpal Tunnel Syndrome for specific guidelines.)* If symptoms begin to appear, consult a physical therapist to learn about possible modifications in the task or the equipment. ■

# PLANTAR WARTS

## SYMPTOMS

- small, bumpy growths on the soles of the feet, one-quarter inch to two inches in diameter, sometimes with tiny black dots on the surface.
- pinpoint bleeding from warts when they are scratched.
- pain in the soles of the feet when standing or walking.

*(See also the Visual Diagnostic Guide.)*

## CALL YOUR DOCTOR IF:

- the area becomes red, hot, painful, and tender after treatment; an infection may have set in.
- you are unsure whether you have a plantar wart or another condition, such as a corn, callus, mole, or skin lesion. Most such growths are harmless, but some can become cancerous.

Plantar warts are tough, horny growths that develop on plantar surfaces—that is, the soles of the feet. Normal standing and walking tends to force them into the skin, and the pressure makes the feet very painful. Like all warts, they are benign and will eventually go away even without treatment, but in most cases they are too painful to ignore. Plantar warts that grow together in a cluster are known as **mosaic warts.**

## CAUSES

Plantar warts are caused by a virus that invades the skin through tiny cuts or abrasions. The warts may not appear for weeks or months after the initial exposure. Like other viral infections, plantar warts are contagious, commonly spread in public swimming pools or communal showers. Virtual epidemics of plantar warts sometimes break out among people who share gym or athletic facilities or who engage in group activities where bare feet are the rule. Because most people build immunity to the virus with age, plantar warts are more common in children than in adults.

## TREATMENT

Deciding how to treat your plantar wart may depend on your ability to tolerate the pain that the various treatments can inflict. Folk remedies for treating warts abound, and there is no single treatment that works every time. Conventional treatment focuses on removal, while alternative approaches emphasize gradual remission. Whatever you do, do not try to cut off a plantar wart yourself; let nature or a doctor do the work.

### CONVENTIONAL MEDICINE

Your doctor may first try applying salicylic-acid plasters to eliminate the warts. Such treatment may take several weeks to be effective. Burning, freezing with liquid nitrogen dioxide, and surgical removal are more aggressive options for more severe conditions.

## ALTERNATIVE CHOICES

In general, alternative treatments emphasize proper nutrition, since a healthy diet will not only enhance your immunity to the virus but help your body combat it. Various substances can be applied directly to the wart as aids to removal.

### AROMATHERAPY

Two drops of essential lemon oil in 10 drops of cider vinegar may help remove plantar warts: Apply daily and cover during the day with an adhesive bandage, but leave the wart exposed at night. Or you can put a drop of tea tree oil (*Melaleuca* spp.) on the center of the wart daily and bandage it. Continue treatment until the wart goes away, which may take several weeks.

You can try strengthening your immune system by massaging your legs with the essential oils of rosemary *(Rosmarinus officinalis),* geranium *(Pelargonium odoratissimum),* or juniper *(Juniperus communis)*—or a blend of any two—using long strokes from ankles to thighs.

### HERBAL THERAPIES

Various herbal remedies are recommended for removing warts. Whichever herbal remedy you try, first protect the surrounding skin with petroleum jelly and cover the treated wart with a clean bandage. Repeat daily until the warts are gone.

- Apply the juice from dandelion *(Taraxacum officinale)* stems morning and evening.
- Put a clove of raw garlic *(Allium sativum) or a* drop or two of garlic oil on the wart twice daily.
- Apply a few drops of yellow cedar *(Thuja occidentalis),* available in either oil or tincture form, to the wart twice daily.

### NUTRITION AND DIET

Poor diet can be a factor in persistent or recurring warts. Foods high in vitamin A—eggs, coldwater fish, onions, garlic, and dark green and yellow vegetables such as broccoli, cabbage, Brussels sprouts, squash, and carrots—will help sustain your immune system, as will yogurt and other fermented milk products. You can also consult a nutritional therapist about the potential benefits of supplemental vitamins A, B complex, C, and E; L-cysteine; and zinc.

## AT-HOME REMEDIES

- Try an over-the-counter topical medication that contains salicylic acid, which is best absorbed by the skin after a bath, a shower, or a soak in warm water. Protect the healthy skin around your warts with petroleum jelly.
- Mix castor oil and baking powder into a paste and apply to the wart nightly. Cover with a bandage until the wart disappears.
- Cut or scrape off some of the white material from the inside of a banana peel—preferably from a green banana, since it is said to have more of the enzymes that help fight the wart-causing virus. Apply a piece of the material to the wart before going to bed, and cover with first-aid tape. Repeat nightly until the condition improves.
- Apply vitamin E twice daily or vitamin A nightly; open a capsule of the vitamin, apply the oil to the wart, and cover with a bandage. Continue applications until the wart goes away.
- To ease the pain until the wart is gone, wear a foam pad in your shoe. Cut a hole in the pad at the location of the wart to take pressure off the wart while you are standing or walking.



# PREVENTION

Protect yourself against exposure to the virus that causes plantar warts by wearing shower shoes, thongs, or rubber swimming shoes whenever you visit a public pool or use a communal shower. Be sure to wash your feet thoroughly with a disinfectant soap after being in an area where the virus can spread. ■

# PLEURISY

## SYMPTOMS

**Pleurisy:**
- severe, fleeting, sharp pain in your chest, possibly on one side only, when breathing deeply, coughing, moving, or sneezing.
- severe chest pain that goes away when you hold your breath.

**Pleural Effusion:**
- shortness of breath.
- a dry cough.

## CALL YOUR DOCTOR IF:

- you are experiencing any of the symptoms above, particularly if you have not been diagnosed for the underlying disease; pleurisy and pleural effusion can be symptoms of such serious diseases as pneumonia and lung cancer.
- the symptoms above are accompanied by fever, no matter how slight. You may have a type of infection called empyema that requires treatment with antibiotics.

P

Pleurisy, also called pleuritis, is an inflammation of the pleura—the moist, double-layered membrane that surrounds the lungs and lines the rib cage. The condition can make breathing extremely painful and, if not treated promptly, can lead to the development of pleural effusion, in which the area between the membrane's layers, called the pleural space, fills with excess fluid.

Strictly speaking, pleurisy and pleural effusion are not diseases; rather, they are complications of an underlying lung infection or disease, such as pneumonia, tuberculosis, or systemic lupus erythematosus. A number of other conditions—most commonly congestive heart failure but including chest injuries, viral infections, rheumatoid arthritis, and cancer—can also irritate the pleura.

Pleurisy and pleural effusion are generally only as serious as the underlying disease. If you have either of these conditions, you may already be undergoing treatment for the underlying disease; if not, seek medical attention immediately.

## CAUSES

The double-layered pleura protects and lubricates the surface of the lungs as they inflate and deflate within the rib cage. Normally, a thin, fluid-filled gap—the pleural space—allows the two layers of the pleural membrane to slide gently past each other. But when these layers become inflamed by an infection in the chest, their roughened surfaces rub painfully together with every breath, sneeze, and cough. This condition is known as pleurisy.

In some cases of pleurisy, excess fluid seeps into the pleural space, resulting in pleural effusion. This fluid buildup usually has a lubricating effect, relieving the pain associated with pleurisy as it reduces friction between the membrane's layers. But at the same time, the added fluid puts tremendous pressure on the lungs, reducing their ability to move freely and causing shortness of breath. In some cases of pleural effusion, this excess liquid becomes infected, causing a condition known as empyema.

### DIAGNOSTIC AND TEST PROCEDURES

To diagnose pleurisy, a physician will listen to your chest through a stethoscope as you breathe. If this examination reveals pleural friction rub—the abrasive sound of the pleura's two layers sliding against each other—the diagnosis is clear. Pleural friction rub produces a scraping, raspy sound that occurs at the end of your inhalation and the beginning of your exhalation, and it comes from the area directly over the pleural inflammation. By gently tapping that area on your chest, your doctor might be able to hear a rattling vibration, another indication of pleurisy.

Your doctor may also take x-rays of the area or draw a sample of pleural fluid for analysis. After injecting your back or chest with a local anesthetic, the physician will use a syringe to extract the fluid. The doctor may run tests on the sample to determine, for example, if the underlying cause of the fluid buildup is cancer.

**PLEURISY**

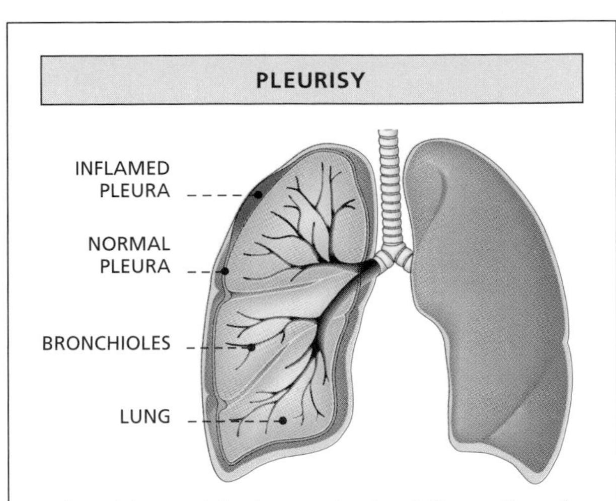


A lung injury or infection can lead to inflammation of the pleura, a thin, two-ply membrane that encases the lungs and lines the inside of the rib cage. Between the pleural layers is a fluid-filled space that normally cushions the contact between them during respiration. When inflamed, however, the surfaces can become roughened and tender; breathing forces them to rub together, intensifying the pain.

## TREATMENT

Conventional medicine usually treats the underlying disease that causes pleurisy or pleural effusion. In some cases of pleural effusion, however, excess fluid must be drained. Alternative treatments may help relieve some of the discomfort associated with these conditions.

### CONVENTIONAL MEDICINE

In addition to antibiotics and other appropriate medications aimed at treating the underlying disease, your physician will probably prescribe anti-inflammatory drugs or analgesics, such as aspirin, to remedy the inflammation. Sometimes, a codeine-based cough syrup will be prescribed to control a painful cough.

In the case of pleural effusion, your physician may recommend a diuretic to help drain excess fluid. As a preventive measure, antibiotics may also be prescribed to combat empyema. If the amount of pleural fluid is excessive, the doctor may drain it through a tube inserted in your chest, a procedure that requires hospitalization.

### ALTERNATIVE CHOICES

The cure for pleurisy and pleural effusion lies with conventional treatment of the underlying disease. Even so, a number of alternative remedies, including **acupuncture,** may alleviate some of the discomfort associated with these conditions.

#### CHINESE HERBS

The Chinese herb ephedra *(Ephedra sinica)* is a potent bronchodilator, which can help ease breathing. CAUTION: Large quantities of ephedra have the same effect as large quantities of epinephrine; do not use the herb if you have high blood pressure or heart disease. Prepare an infusion by combining 5 grams ephedra, 4 grams cinnamon *(Cinnamomum cassia)* sticks, 1.5 grams licorice *(Glycyrrhiza uralensis),* and 5 grams apricot seed *(Prunus armeniaca).* Let the mixture steep in cold water for several minutes, then bring it to a boil. Drink it hot. ■

# PNEUMONIA

## SYMPTOMS

- A combination of low fever and chills, muscle aches, fatigue, enlarged lymph nodes in the neck, chest pain, sore throat, and coughing are typical symptoms of **viral pneumonia.**
- A combination of high fever, cough with thick yellow-green sputum that may contain blood, shortness of breath, rapid breathing, sharp chest pain that is worse when you breathe deeply, abdominal pain, and severe fatigue are symptoms of **bacterial pneumonia.**
- Loss of appetite and weight, fever, coughing with sputum, perhaps following a period of unconsciousness, may indicate **aspiration pneumonia**.
- In children, labored and rapid breathing (more than 45 breaths a minute), sudden onset of fever, cough, wheezing, and bluish skin are general signs of pneumonia.

## CALL YOUR DOCTOR IF:

- your symptoms indicate you have any form of pneumonia. You need immediate treatment to recover and avoid complications.
- your sharp chest pain does not respond to prescribed treatment; you have increased shortness of breath; or your fingernails, toenails, or skin becomes dark or develops a bluish tinge after diagnosis. Your lungs are not getting enough oxygen and you need medical assistance.
- you cough up blood; you may need additional treatment for a worsening infection.

Pneumonia is the relatively common inflammation caused by various viral, bacterial, and fungal infections, or chemical exposure of the lungs. In response, the lungs become congested with fluids and cells that leak from the affected tissue. If the inflammation is limited to one lobe of one lung, it is classified as **lobar pneumonia;** inflammation spreading from the bronchi to other parts of one or both lungs is **bronchopneumonia.** If both lungs are inflamed, the condition is called **double pneumonia.** Depending on your overall health, pneumonia usually lasts about two weeks, although you may feel exhausted a month or more after it has cleared up.

**Viral pneumonia** is generally mild; you can usually treat it at home once the doctor has made a diagnosis. **Bacterial pneumonias** are more complex and more serious. Until the development of antibiotics, cases were frequently fatal, and they remain one of the leading causes of death in the U.S. As recently as 1976, **legionnaire's disease** killed 29 people before it was identified and treated as a bacterial pneumonia. Of the many other types of pneumonia, **walking pneumonia** is

**EVIDENCE OF INFECTION**

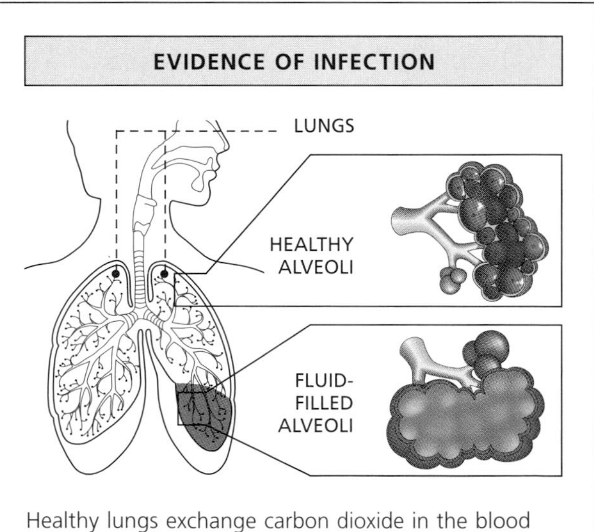


Healthy lungs exchange carbon dioxide in the blood for oxygen through tiny air sacs called alveoli *(inset, top).* A pneumonic infection—whether it is caused by bacterial, viral, or chemical agents—makes tissue in the alveoli swell and fill with fluid *(inset, bottom).* Shallow, labored breathing brought on by an insufficient oxygen supply is often a symptom of pneumonia.

most common in children and in young adults.

Pneumonia is a common complication of many illnesses, and like the common cold and flu, any type can be transmitted from one person to another. Patients hospitalized for other ailments may become infected with bacterial pneumonia that is resistant to the usual course of antibiotic treatment. The strains of bacterial pneumonia outside hospitals are usually much less severe and respond readily to antibiotics.

## CAUSES

Various common viral organisms are responsible for **viral pneumonia. Bacterial pneumonia** is most commonly caused by *Streptococcus pneumoniae,* sometimes called pneumococcus. The bacterium *Hemophilus influenzae* is often responsible for pneumonia that develops as a complication of flu. Pneumonia is also on the rise as a result of infection by tuberculosis bacteria. The Legionella bacterium responsible for **legionnaire's disease** and similar pneumonias can be transmitted through contaminated water from many sources, including hot tubs and air-conditioning units.

**Aspiration pneumonia** develops when bacteria from the mouth or stomach enter the lungs, generally during sleep, unconsciousness, or a seizure. Such bacteria normally inhabit the digestive tracts of healthy people. A small amount of inhaled mucus won't harm most people, but it can cause lung inflammation in alcoholics or other people with weakened immune systems. Bacteria can also be carried into the lungs by inadvertently inhaling vomit, usually when unconscious.

**Pneumocystis pneumonia (PCP)** develops when the body's immune defenses are exhausted by AIDS, Hodgkin's disease, or other diseases that suppress the immune system. It develops as a secondary infection in over half of all AIDS patients, but treatment is readily available.

### DIAGNOSTIC AND TEST PROCEDURES

Pneumonia's forms range from a mild condition treatable at home to a potentially fatal infection requiring hospitalization, so you must have a professional diagnosis to guarantee appropriate treatment and a successful recovery. Your doctor will first listen to your chest for crackling noises and tap your chest to check for dull thuds indicating fluid-filled lungs. If necessary, an x-ray can confirm the diagnosis, showing where air sacs in the lungs are filled with fluid and debris. Blood and sputum samples, sometimes obtained by inserting a tube into the lungs, may be tested for microorganisms, but the results are not always conclusive.

ATTENTION!

**POSTURAL DRAINAGE**

**To help clear phlegm out of your lungs, try postural drainage for 5 to 15 minutes three times a day. This technique is physically demanding, so make sure that your doctor approves, and have a support person with you at all times.**

**Lie on a bed with the top half of your body off the mattress, using your forearms on the floor as support. Cough up phlegm from deep in your lungs and spit it into a container on the floor. At the end of the session, flush the phlegm down the toilet.**

**If this technique is too strenuous for you, have a friend or family member pound gently with cupped hands on your upper back for several minutes to help loosen chest secretions.**

## TREATMENT

The goal of treatment for any form of pneumonia is speedy recovery, since complications can set in if the disease is allowed to linger. All treatments include bed rest. Conventional medicine focuses on curing the infection, while alternative treatments may help to ease uncomfortable symptoms.

### CONVENTIONAL MEDICINE

For most types of pneumonia, the two essential keys to recovery are bed rest and "productive coughing"—bringing up phlegm and other fluid from your lungs.

If you have a mild case of **viral pneumonia,** you can probably recover at home, taking aspirin or acetaminophen to lower your fever and reduce pain, drinking lots of fluids, and eating lightly. If you have **bacterial pneumonia,** your doctor will probably prescribe an antibiotic such as penicillin or erythromycin. You will need to stay in bed until your fever drops and your breathing becomes normal. If your lungs are severely congested, you may need oxygen or to be put on a respirator temporarily, which will require a hospital stay. **Aspiration pneumonia** almost always requires intravenous antibiotics and a lengthy hospital stay. **Pneumocystis pneumonia** is usually treated with bed rest, antibiotics such as pentamidine or sulfamethoxazole and trimethoprim, and decongestants to reduce congestion.

A vaccine is available for many identifiable types of bacterial pneumonia, and more are being developed. Vaccination against pneumonia is recommended for everyone over the age of 65, and for people with chronic lung disease, sickle cell anemia, heart disease, alcoholism, and immune deficiency diseases such as AIDS, as well as for people whose spleen has been damaged or removed. Vaccines are also available for some forms of influenza and are recommended for older people; a flu shot may protect you from either catching the disease or developing such a serious case that complications like pneumonia set in.

**ATTENTION!**

**BEWARE OF THE BIRDCAGE**

**Parakeets and lovebirds can transmit psittacosis—a rare form of pneumonia commonly known as parrot fever—to their unsuspecting human owners. Sick birds can spread the infectious microorganism in dust from their feathers, in droppings, or even by biting a finger. Psittacosis symptoms include fever, chills, headaches, muscle aches, loss of appetite, nausea, vomiting, and enlargement of the spleen.**

## ALTERNATIVE CHOICES

If you are diagnosed as having pneumonia, various alternative therapies may help ease your symptoms and hasten your recovery.

### ACUPUNCTURE

Acupuncture on the lung meridian may help your recovery from pneumonia by reducing cough and congestion, making you more comfortable, and improving your energy level. Key points are LU 7 to expel matter from the lungs, LU 5 to stop cough, and LU 1 to relieve chest congestion. Depending on the condition, an acupuncturist may also work on enhancing the immune system. *(See pages 22–23 for information on point locations.)*

### AROMATHERAPY

Recovery from pneumonia may be helped if you add the essential oils of eucalyptus *(Eucalyptus globulus),* lavender *(Lavandula officinalis),* tea tree (*Melaleuca* spp.), or pine to a warm bath or a vaporizer for steam inhalation. Do not use steam inhalations if you are asthmatic, because the vapor may irritate your lungs.

### BODY WORK

After the fever is gone, **massage** the upper-back muscles to ease chest congestion. Adding a few drops of essential oil of eucalyptus *(Eucalyptus globulus)* to the massage lotion may help to loosen and release phlegm.

### HERBAL THERAPIES

Since clearing the lungs of phlegm is an important part of the healing process, using traditional herbal expectorants to promote coughing can aid recovery. To make your own expectorant, combine 2 oz licorice *(Glycyrrhiza glabra),* 1 oz wild black cherry *(Prunus serotina)* bark, 1 oz coltsfoot *(Tussilago farfara),* ⅛ oz lobelia *(Lobelia inflata),* and 1 oz horehound *(Marrubium vulgare).* Simmer 1 tbsp of the mixture in 1 cup of water for 5 minutes; let the mixture steep for 10 minutes and strain it into a clean container. Adults should

### THE ONION OPTION

*Try this homemade cough syrup that combines the soothing qualities of honey with the pungent bite of raw onion. Pour honey over slices of raw white onion and let them sit overnight in a covered container. In the morning, strain the mixture into a clean container and discard the onion slices. Take a tablespoonful of the mixture, preferably after warming it slightly, every five or six hours.*

drink one cupful every 2 hours. Lobelia can be poisonous, so never use more than the recommended amount. Stop using this mixture if you become nauseated, and never give it to children or pregnant women.

A decoction of pleurisy root *(Asclepias tuberosa)* is recommended to help fight pneumonia. Simmer 1 tbsp of the herb in a cup of water for 10 minutes, steep 5 minutes, and strain; drink four to five times daily.

Eating raw garlic *(Allium sativum)* or three garlic capsules three times a day is said to help your body fight infection. Echinacea (*Echinacea* spp.) may help you recover from infection: It can be brewed as tea—1 tsp in a cup of water—taken three times a day. It can also be taken as a tincture, 30 drops four times a day, or in over-the-counter capsules according to label directions.

#### HOMEOPATHY

Some recommended over-the-counter homeopathic remedies are Bryonia, Phosphorus, and Arsenicum album; follow label directions.

#### NUTRITION AND DIET

- Up to 1,000 mg of vitamin C an hour may offer substantial benefits in fighting pneumonia if started within two days of onset. Reduce dosage if you develop diarrhea.
- From 25,000 to 50,000 IU of vitamin A daily, for not more than two weeks, may help support your respiratory and immune systems.
- Zinc supplements, up to 60 mg daily, may also help your immune system fight infection.
- 600 IU of vitamin E daily may help support damaged lung tissue.
- If you are taking antibiotics to fight bacterial pneumonia, try *Lactobacillus acidophilus* supplements, either in capsule form or in live yogurt cultures, to help replace your beneficial intestinal bacteria.

#### AT-HOME REMEDIES

- A heating pad or hot-water bottle on the chest or back for 10-minute periods several times a day can help relieve chest pain. Wrap the pad or bottle in a towel to prevent burning the skin.
- Try a traditional mustard poultice to loosen phlegm. Mix dry mustard with enough warm water to make a thick paste. Spread the paste on thin cotton or cheesecloth, fold, and place on your chest for several minutes, but don't overdo it: Mustard may cause blistering if it is left on bare skin too long.
- Drink plenty of fluids and fresh fruit and vegetable juices to thin lung secretions and make them easier to cough up.

## PREVENTION

- Avoid smoking and exposure to tobacco smoke, which significantly damage the hairlike cilia in your respiratory tract that filter irritants from the lungs. Smoking weakens your ability to fight viral and bacterial agents that cause pneumonia.
- Don't drink large amounts of alcohol; alcohol impairs your immune system's ability to fight all sorts of infection, including pneumonia.
- If you are over 60 or suffer from a chronic condition that taxes your immune system, ask your doctor about the advisability of vaccination against pneumonia and seasonal influenza viruses that often lead to pneumonia. ■

# POISON IVY

## SYMPTOMS

- patches of red, itchy skin, usually followed by small blisters, which fill with a clear fluid and eventually break open.
- Severe cases can develop into swollen, extremely painful areas filled with fluid.
- The rash rarely appears on the soles of the feet or palms of the hand.

## CALL YOUR DOCTOR IF:

- your rash stays red and itchy for more than two weeks; you may have another type of contact dermatitis, eczema, or lupus.
- you have the rash near your eyes or the rash covers a large part of your body. You may need medical intervention.
- you have severe allergic complications, such as generalized swelling, headache, fever, or a secondary infection.
- you have been exposed to or inhale the smoke from burning poison ivy, poison oak, or poison sumac. The toxin is not killed by fire and can cause severe allergic reactions internally as well as externally.

Poison ivy, poison oak, and poison sumac cause a short-lived but extremely irritating allergic form of contact dermatitis. The rash generally develops within 2 days, peaks after 5 days, and starts to decline after about a week or 10 days. While some people survive exposure without ill effects, complete immunity is unlikely; people who seem immune at one time and place may find themselves vulnerable in other situations.

## CAUSES

The leaves, stems, and roots of poison ivy, oak, and sumac plants contain the resin urushiol, minute amounts of which on exposed skin can trigger an inflammatory allergic reaction. Urushiol can be transferred by fingers or animal fur and can remain on clothing, shoes, and tools for a number of months. Scratching the rash does not spread the poison to other parts of the body, but it can prolong the discomfort and cause a secondary infection.

## TREATMENT

You can treat most cases of the rash yourself with the application of calamine lotion or over-the-counter topical remedies containing antihistamines, benzocaine, or hydrocortisone. A cortisone shot may relieve the itching, particularly within 24 hours of exposure. Oral corticosteroids or antihistamines may also relieve the symptoms, but both drugs can have unwanted side effects. Don't take oral antihistamines if you are using an antihistamine lotion; the combination may actually make the condition worse. If you have complications from a severe case, you may need to see a doctor. If your case is so severe that general illness develops, your doctor may recommend injections of prednisone or another corticosteroid drug. *(See Dermatitis.)*

### ALTERNATIVE CHOICES

Like conventional medicine, various alternative therapies help relieve itching and swelling. In ad-

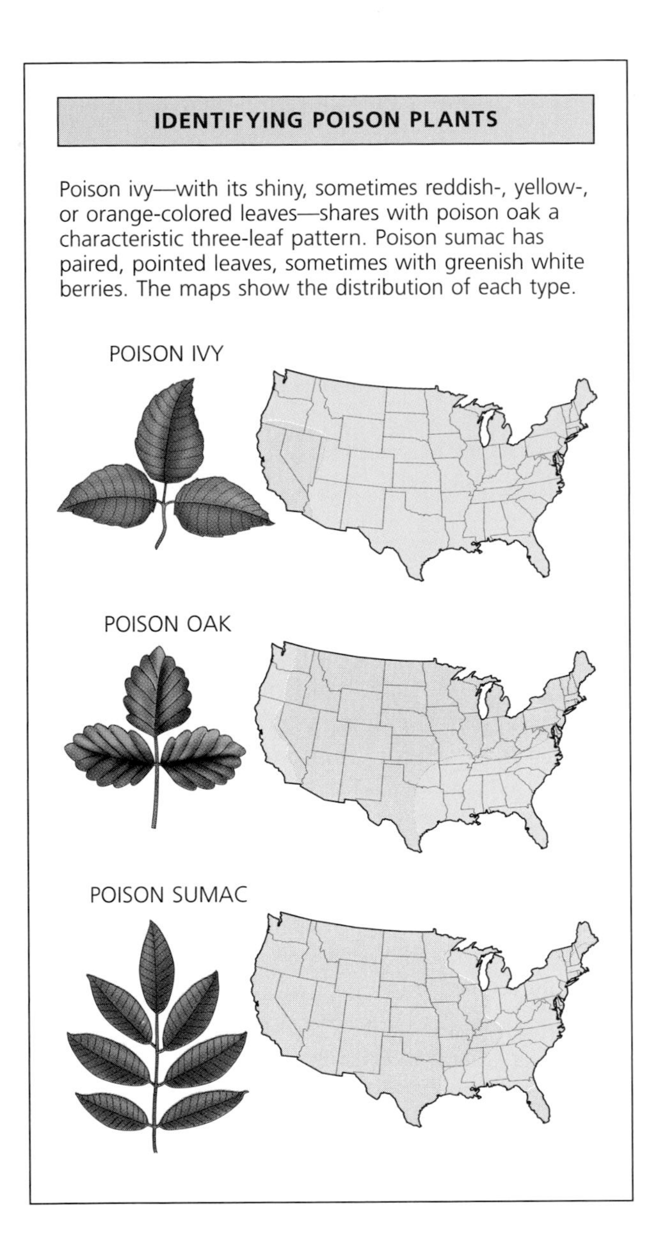


**IDENTIFYING POISON PLANTS**

Poison ivy—with its shiny, sometimes reddish-, yellow-, or orange-colored leaves—shares with poison oak a characteristic three-leaf pattern. Poison sumac has paired, pointed leaves, sometimes with greenish white berries. The maps show the distribution of each type.

dition to topical remedies, vitamin C injections are also said to provide relief.

#### HERBAL THERAPIES

The leaves of jewelweed *(Impatiens),* which often grows near poison ivy, may neutralize urushiol if wiped over the skin right after contact. For relief from itching, try the following topical remedies:

- a few drops of juice squeezed from the leaves of the common plantain *(Plantago major).*
- 1 tbsp salt in ½ cup water with enough cosmetic clay to make a paste; add 1 or 2 drops of oil of peppermint *(Mentha piperita).*
- equal parts goldenseal *(Hydrastis canadensis)* root powder and green clay, available in health food stores.

#### HOMEOPATHY

Of all the over-the-counter homeopathic remedies available, Rhus toxicodendron—derived from the poison ivy plant itself—may be the most effective. Follow directions on the label.

### AT-HOME REMEDIES

- Wash exposed skin with soap and water within 15 minutes of contact.
- Soothe the itch with calamine lotion or other over-the-counter medication.
- Cover open blisters with sterile gauze to prevent infection.
- Make a paste with water and either cornstarch, oatmeal, baking soda, or Epsom salt, and apply it to the rash. You can also use a paste made with baking soda and a few drops of witch hazel.
- Run hot water over the rash—as hot as you can stand it. The itching will intensify briefly, then abate, giving you several itch-free hours.

## PREVENTION

The best way to deal with this poisonous threesome is to learn to recognize the plants, then stay out of reach. If you suspect contact with a poison plant, wash immediately and thoroughly with soap and water—-your skin, clothes, shoes, tools—anything that might have picked up the plant's toxic resin. If you're going into poison-plant country, try one of the barrier lotions available from outdoor suppliers. The old folk tale about eating poison ivy leaves to make yourself immune is just that—a myth: Never eat the leaves or berries of wild plants, many of which can cause dangerous reactions in humans. ■

# POSTNASAL DRIP

## SYMPTOMS

- a flow of mucus that runs down the back of your throat, ranging in consistency from watery to thick, and often associated with a sore throat, a cough, hoarseness, or the feeling that something is lodged in your throat.
- inadvertent sniffing, snorting, or swallowing of nasal mucus.

## CALL YOUR DOCTOR IF:

- you have treated the condition with an over-the-counter decongestant for more than a week without success; or if the condition is accompanied by continued sneezing, wheezing, watery eyes, or persistent shortness of breath. You may be suffering from an allergy or a form of environmental poisoning.
- the condition is accompanied by a congested nose, fever, pain or abnormal pressure in the nose and face, and thick nasal discharge. You probably have sinusitis.

Postnasal drip is an annoying complication of various respiratory ailments and generally disappears after the primary ailment clears up. Mucus is a normal product of the nasal passages, but when too much is produced it finds its way into the throat instead of leaving by way of the nostrils. When the condition becomes chronic—for example, from an allergy or prolonged sinusitis—mucus can drip into the bronchial tubes, especially at night, inducing coughing and heavy phlegm. Since postnasal drip is most often a symptom of another ailment, the best approach is to identify and treat the underlying condition.

## CAUSES

Watery postnasal drip along with itching eyes, nose, palate, and throat (or sneezing, congestion, and watery eyes) is usually **allergic rhinitis** triggered by plant pollen, dust, animal hair, or other allergens. Some people develop postnasal drip when exposed to environmental irritants such as tobacco smoke or airborne contaminants.

If postnasal drip involves thick mucus, a sore throat, runny and congested nose, headache, achiness, and reduced sense of taste and smell, you probably have **viral rhinitis**—a common cold. Intermittent or continual postnasal drip that becomes very pronounced with humidity and temperature changes or periods of emotional stress may be **vasomotor rhinitis.** This condition can also be a side effect of some prescription drugs.

Thick yellow or greenish mucus can indicate a bacterial or viral respiratory infection. Whenever thick nasal discharge and postnasal drip are accompanied by fever and congestive pain or pressure in the face, it is probably from sinusitis.

Women who use hormone replacement therapy or estrogen-based birth-control drugs can develop postnasal drip as a side effect, and it can be a minor complication of pregnancy.

### DIAGNOSTIC AND TEST PROCEDURES

Laboratory tests of the mucus itself can determine if your postnasal drip is due to an allergy, some form of rhinitis, or another condition. Your

## HOMEMADE SALINE

*You can buy commercially prepared saline solution, but it's easy to make your own. Mix a teaspoon of table salt and a teaspoon of baking soda in a quart of water. Whenever you need to flush away excess mucus, tilt your head back and spray a small amount of the solution into each nostril. You'll have to buy a small spray bottle—try a well-stocked pharmacy.*

doctor will use an illuminating instrument to examine your nasal passages, and if complications from sinus problems are indicated, you may need an x-ray or other imaging procedure.

## TREATMENT

Both conventional and alternative treatment will vary depending on whether your symptoms stem from an allergy, a cold, or another condition.

### CONVENTIONAL MEDICINE

Over-the-counter decongestant drops or sprays can help alleviate postnasal drip by opening nasal passages, but prolonged use may make the problem worse. Your system can become temporarily dependent on them and must adjust after you stop their use. If you suffer from high blood pressure, you should not take oral decongestants without a doctor's approval. Some antihistamines can make you drowsy; if that happens, look for products with formulas that do not induce sleep.

### ALTERNATIVE CHOICES

Alternative treatments to clear postnasal drip rely primarily on ways to thin the offending mucus and allay the underlying causes.

#### AROMATHERAPY

Inhaling steam can help clear nasal passages. Add essential oils of eucalyptus *(Eucalyptus globulus)*, tea tree (*Melaleuca* spp.), rosemary (*Rosmarinus officinalis)*, or peppermint *(Mentha piperita)* to the water in a humidifier during the day, and use the essential oil of lavender *(Lavandula officinalis)* in the evening for a better night's sleep.

#### CHINESE HERBS

Chinese medicine relies on mixtures of traditional herbs brewed in water and drunk at prescribed intervals. The Minor Blue Dragon Combination is recommended to reduce nasal drainage; consult an experienced practitioner for the correct amounts of each herb to use for your condition.

#### HERBAL THERAPIES

Eyebright *(Euphrasia officinalis)* may help dry up postnasal drip; make an infusion or tincture with the leaves and stems, or take two 200 mg capsules of the prepared herb three times daily.

#### HOMEOPATHY

For postnasal drip with thick yellow-green mucus, try Pulsatilla (12c) three or four times a day for two days. For postnasal drip associated with symptoms of a common cold, try Nux vomica (12c) three or four times a day for two days. For other kinds of postnasal drip, a homeopath will prescribe a remedy for your particular symptoms.

### AT-HOME REMEDIES

- Use an over-the-counter cough medicine or a simple saline solution *(above, left)* as a nasal spray to help thin postnasal drip mucus.
- Drink lots of water (at least six glasses a day) to help keep the mucus as thin as possible.
- Humidify the air around you, especially in winter. If your heating system does not have a built-in humidifier, you can buy a self-contained unit at most home-supply centers. (Read the directions carefully for cleaning and maintaining a humidifier; improperly cleaned humidifiers can spread germs.) ■

# POSTTRAUMATIC STRESS DISORDER

## SYMPTOMS

Someone who has experienced severe trauma—war, combat, natural disaster, physical or sexual abuse—or witnessed violence, such as murder or physical abuse, may display one or more of these symptoms:

- repeated flashbacks or recurrent dreams of the event. Children may not remember the event directly but may recall a single image or express their fear by repeatedly playacting an event or action. Their dreams may simply be frightening with no specific content.
- hypervigilance—a preoccupation with possible unknown threats.
- traumatic dreams, sleeping problems.
- outbursts of anger.
- intense distress if exposed to anything resembling the event.
- psychological numbing; inability to relate to others.
- chronic physical symptoms—pain, headaches, irritable bowels.
- in young children, agitated behavior, difficulty concentrating, or developmental regression in such things as toilet training or speech.
- no sense of a future; no expectation of having a family, career, living to old age.

## CALL YOUR DOCTOR IF:

- you or your child or other loved one has experienced trauma and shows any of the symptoms.

A few people live through horrible events without experiencing much fear, but most of us react with feelings of horror and helplessness. The degree of a person's reaction—both physical and psychological—to such events determines whether the person will actually develop the condition known as posttraumatic stress disorder (PTSD), whose effects can be long-lasting and disabling. Once known as battle fatigue or shell shock, PTSD is now considered a mental disorder resulting from any sort of deeply shocking experience.

PTSD may begin immediately following the event or may not surface until weeks or months later. Treatment and the passage of time may diminish its duration and its severity. For a few, the symptoms disappear entirely.

Some 31 percent of Vietnam veterans have suffered from it and 15 percent continue to be affected. For battered women, 84 percent reported symptoms soon after the event and 45 percent still suffered a year later. Children are more likely to suffer from PTSD if the trauma is personal—caused by a family member or friend, rather than by a natural disaster. Also, witnessing family violence can be as harsh a trauma for a child as being attacked personally.

As might be expected, people with PTSD also often suffer from various physical ailments, depression, drug abuse, phobias, or panic attacks.

## CAUSES

PTSD is caused by a severely traumatic event that triggers feelings of intense fear, horror, and helplessness. Both its onset and its severity are directly related to the length and severity of exposure; the greater the horror and the longer it lasts, the more likely a person will suffer PTSD and the more severe it is apt to be. This is particularly true of children who experience repeated abuse or witness repetitive family violence.

Some researchers theorize that intense fear may physically damage the part of the brain that processes fear and that this damage may contribute to the symptoms of PTSD—including anger flashes, extreme vigilance, and sleep disturbance.

Risk factors that may contribute to PTSD include a family history of anxiety, early separation from parents, earlier childhood abuse, or prior exposure to traumas.

### DIAGNOSTIC AND TEST PROCEDURES

Diagnosis is based almost exclusively on a report of the patient's full history. This will include recent symptoms; a description of the event; childhood, educational, and work experiences; and relationships with others. Other disorders that often accompany PTSD are depression, anxiety, and drug abuse.

## TREATMENT

The usual treatment for PTSD is a combination of antidepressant drugs and psychotherapy. Support groups—with or without family members—allow sufferers to work through feelings with others who have had similar experiences.

Alternative treatments include a wide variety of antianxiety techniques, **biofeedback,** and a newly developed therapy called **Eye Movement Desensitization and Reprocessing** *(see Eye Movement Therapy, right).*

### CONVENTIONAL MEDICINE

To reduce PTSD stress, the antidepressant drug group called selective serotonin reuptake inhibitors (SSRIs) seems to be the most effective. When psychotherapy is prescribed—whether individual or group—the goal is to encourage the patient to recall all details of the event, express grief, complete the mourning process, and get on with life. For children, this may involve play therapy.

### ALTERNATIVE CHOICES

Because PTSD is an anxiety disorder in which the victim is left tense and jittery, the practice of any exercise or relaxation technique is extremely valuable. Choose one or two techniques that you like and practice them daily. (For various options, see Anxiety.)

#### ACUPUNCTURE

Acupuncture has been shown to ease excessive fear reactions and can reduce traumatic dreams. It works best when combined with psychotherapy. Consult an acupuncturist experienced in treating emotional disorders.

#### BIOFEEDBACK

In EEG biofeedback (a form of biofeedback also known as neurotherapy), the sufferer retrains his brain's neurological functioning. In controlled studies, some veterans who have suffered for decades have shown great improvement, sometimes total recovery. The patient is attached to an EEG machine and, by listening to the kind and amount of brain waves produced, learns to change them in ways that ultimately affect both behavior and feelings. At least 30 sessions are required to accomplish this, but the technique can result in permanent change.

#### EYE MOVEMENT THERAPY

A rather astonishing new treatment—known as **Eye Movement Desensitization and Reprocessing (EMDR)**—seems to bring remarkable results. In some clinical studies, EMDR has reportedly brought dramatic improvement in 90 percent of those tested, and it has become standard treatment in some veterans' hospitals.

The technique is relatively simple. The patient visualizes a distressing image from the traumatic event while tracking with his eyes two fingers the therapist moves quickly back and forth across his line of vision. After each set of movements, the client reports any new feelings or forgotten memories he may have. The therapist then repeats the procedure. Each session lasts about 90 minutes and is repeated as often as needed. One Vietnam veteran reported that EMDR accomplished more in one session than conventional counseling had managed in years.

#### MASSAGE

Massage has proved effective in lowering anxiety and stress for some natural-disaster victims, but it should not be used with anyone who has been physically abused. Massage should be gentle and is best performed by an experienced therapist. ■

# PREGNANCY PROBLEMS

## SYMPTOMS

Women can expect some or all of these conditions in a normal pregnancy:

- in the first trimester—absence of menstrual flow; minor weight gain; increased urination; enlarged and perhaps sore breasts; **morning sickness** or nausea.
- in the second trimester—significant weight gain (about a pound a week); stretching of the abdominal wall and pelvis; possibly backache, constipation, heartburn, and fetal movement.
- in the third trimester—swollen limbs from fluid retention; leaking breasts; constipation; hemorrhoids; insomnia; discomfort below the rib cage a few weeks before the baby drops at about 36 weeks.

## CALL YOUR DOCTOR IF:

- you have severe nausea and vomiting; dehydration; rapid heartbeat; or pale, dry skin. You may have hyperemesis gravidarum, a severe form of **morning sickness.**
- you have vaginal spotting or bleeding. You may be having a **miscarriage** or serious placental complication.
- you have sudden weight gain over a few days, severe headache, and blurred vision. You may have developed **preeclampsia,** a form of high blood pressure.
- you have a fever over 100°F and chills, backache, or blood in your urine. You may have **pyelonephritis,** a kidney infection.
- after the fetus begins to move, you feel decreased movement for more than a day or no movement; you may be experiencing **fetal distress.**

Most pregnancies are medically uneventful and end happily in the successful birth of a healthy baby. But you still have nine months to wonder whether certain physical and emotional discomforts are serious enough for medical intervention or are minor problems that you can deal with on your own.

Your first—and most important—step is signing up for a comprehensive program of prenatal care with a doctor who specializes in pregnancy and childbirth. You and your developing baby will get routine monitoring to make sure everything is going well—and if it isn't, appropriate care for any problems. You and your husband or partner will get confidence-building information about each stage of your pregnancy, including labor, childbirth, and the care and feeding of a newborn.

A pregnant woman is as likely as anyone to get minor illnesses, but when you're pregnant you should always keep your doctor informed so you get proper treatment. Your main responsibility is keeping yourself and your baby well nourished and cared for. That means you need a balanced diet, appropriate exercise, plenty of rest, and a stress-free environment. Above all, don't smoke or use alcohol while you're pregnant, and avoid all drugs except those prescribed by your doctor.

The following text describes what you can do for some of the common health problems you may face during your pregnancy; alternative therapies are included in some cases. Remember, though: You should never hesitate to call your doctor about any discomfort or illness you experience while you're pregnant.

### ABDOMINAL PAIN

To relieve sharp pains or cramps from stretched abdominal muscles and ligaments, particularly when sitting or lying down, use a warm heating pad. Regular exercise *(see the box opposite)* will strengthen and tone your abdominal muscles.

### BACKACHE

Keep your weight gain under control with proper diet and exercise. Avoid taking analgesics; instead, use a heating pad to relieve pain. Special

P

exercises to strengthen abdominal muscles can also help reduce backache. *(See Back Problems.)* Try a pregnancy girdle or elastic sling to support your abdomen. Wear shoes or shoe inserts designed for pregnant women, and avoid high heels.

Don't stand for long periods and don't stretch to reach high places. Sit straight without slouching, and whenever possible, sit with your legs elevated. Sleep on a firm mattress.

Be careful when lifting heavy loads—especially children. Bend at the knees, keep your back as straight as possible, hold the object or child close to your body, and raise yourself slowly.

**Acupressure.** Stimulate the Bladder 23 and 47 points, along your lower back, by rubbing vigorously enough with the back of your hand to create heat. Also try pressing the Bladder 48 point. *(See pages 22–23 for information about point locations.)*

**Chiropractic.** See a licensed chiropractor for treatment of possible spinal misalignment brought about by the stress of the pregnancy.

**Massage.** Sit backward on a straight chair. Lean over the back with your head resting on your crossed arms. Have the massager use long strokes, working upward and outward from the lower back, avoiding pressure on the spine.

## BREAST DISCOMFORT

Wear a bra that gives your enlarged breasts proper support. If your breasts leak small amounts of fluid, use nursing pads in your bra.

## BREATHLESSNESS

Keep your weight gain within the recommended limits and maintain good posture, especially when you are sitting. Sleep on your side, not on your back.

## CONSTIPATION

To keep stools soft and bowel movements regular, get plenty of dietary fiber from fresh fruit, vegetables, whole-grain cereals and breads, and dried fruit. Avoid using over-the-counter laxatives, but try psyllium *(Plantago psyllium),* an herbal bulk-forming agent. Drink lots of fluids and exercise regularly.

### USEFUL EXERCISES

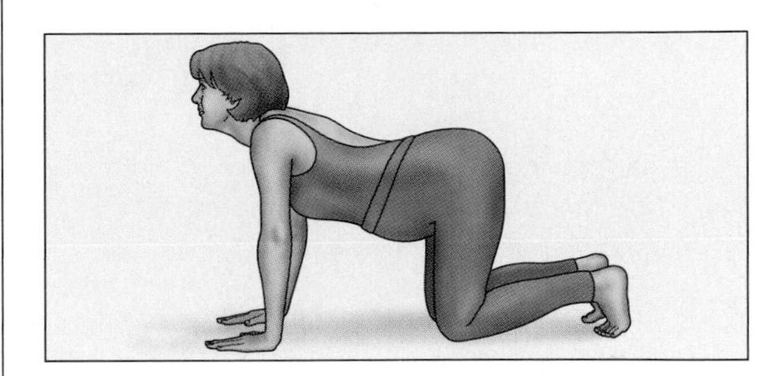

**1** To strengthen your uterus, get on your hands and knees, keeping your back flat. Inhale as you arch your back downward, keeping your head and buttocks raised. Hold this position for 10 seconds, then relax and breathe normally.

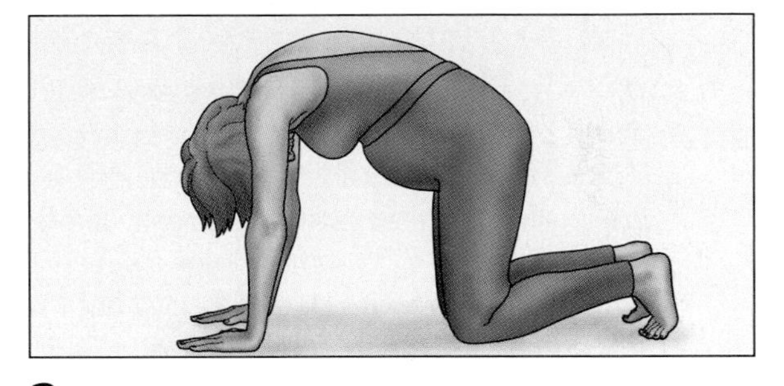

**2** Next, exhale as you arch your back upward, rounding your shoulders and upper spine. Hold this position for 10 seconds, then relax and breathe normally. Slowly repeat this up-and-down sequence 10 times.

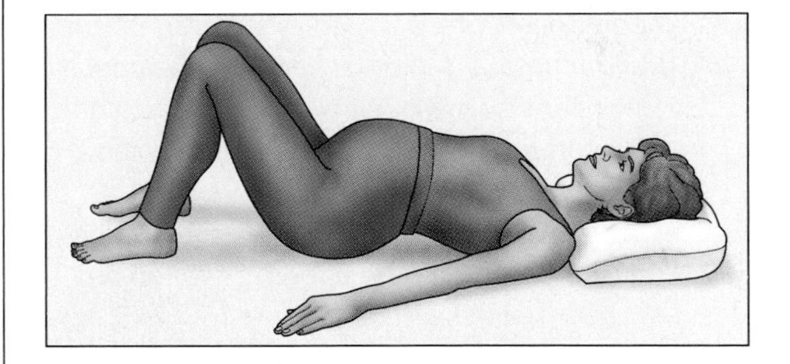

**3** Lie on your back with your knees up. Tighten your buttocks and lower abdominal muscles, pressing the small of your back to the floor. Hold the position for 20 seconds, then relax and rest for one minute. Repeat five times.

## Pregnancy Warnings

- *A growing baby can throw you off balance, so be careful walking and getting out of the shower or tub.*
- *Check with your doctor before you start exercising. Some otherwise normal activities should not be undertaken during pregnancy, and others need to be modified.*
- *Avoid inhalation of or skin contact with chemical household cleaners, paints, and insecticides.*
- *The most dangerous time to take any medication is during the first trimester, when the fetus is developing rapidly and is more vulnerable to injury. Always check with your doctor before taking any over-the-counter or prescription drugs, including those that may have been prescribed before you became pregnant.*
- *Smoking during pregnancy increases the risks of vaginal bleeding, miscarriage, stillbirth, premature birth, low birthweight, and many other potential problems that you and your baby don't need. Smoke-filled rooms, car exhaust, and industrial fumes can also be hazardous to pregnant women: Avoid prolonged exposure to environmental pollutants as best you can.*
- *Several diseases pose special hazards to pregnant women and the unborn child, among them German measles, chickenpox, fifth disease (erythema infectiosum), mumps, cytomegalovirus, chlamydia, gonorrhea, genital herpes, genital warts, syphilis, and AIDS. Check with your doctor immediately if you think you have been exposed to any of them. If possible, get vaccinated against German measles and mumps before pregnancy unless you've had them.*
- *Most couples are able to have sexual intercourse until near the time of birth. Check with your doctor about the advisability of intercourse if you have a history of miscarriages or preterm birth, any infection or bleeding, if the placenta is in an abnormal position (known as placenta previa), or during the last trimester if you are carrying multiple fetuses. Avoid sex after the amniotic sac has broken or fluids leak. If you develop pain or abdominal cramps that continue or worsen more than an hour after having intercourse, call your doctor, your cervix could be dilating.*
- *Avoid having unnecessary x-rays. If you must get an x-ray, be sure to tell the doctor or the technician you are pregnant.*
- *Don't get overheated, avoid exercising in hot and humid weather, and stay out of hot tubs, saunas, and whirlpool baths.*

**Acupressure.** Pressing the Bladder 48 point may relieve constipation. *(See pages 22–23 for information on point location.)*

### CONTRACTIONS

Mild, painless uterine contractions usually start sometime after the 20th week of pregnancy. If they cause discomfort, try changing positions. If contractions start coming at regular intervals, notify your doctor.

### CYSTITIS

If you develop a bladder infection or any type of urinary tract infection, ask your doctor about appropriate treatment. A heating pad on your lower abdomen will help relieve the discomfort. *(See also Urinary Problems.)*

**Nutrition and Diet.** Several glasses of cranberry juice a day are said to be helpful in preventing urinary tract infections.

### DIZZINESS AND FAINTNESS

Slow down when you stand up or get out of bed. Dizziness when you rise too quickly from a sitting or prone position is called **postural hypotension.** If you're in a crowd and start feeling dizzy, step away and get some fresh air; if possible, lie down with your feet elevated or sit with your head between your knees.

### EDEMA

Monitor your weight gain throughout your pregnancy. To control swelling in your legs and ankles, wear support hose and avoid standing for long periods. Wear shoes that fit well and give good support, or buy shoe inserts designed especially for pregnant women.

### FATIGUE

Get a full night's sleep and rest with your feet up for at least 15 minutes several times a day.

**Acupressure.** Stimulate Bladder 23 and 47 points by rubbing your lower back vigorously. Also try pressing the Bladder 10 point. *(See pages 22–23 for information on point locations.)*

### HEADACHES

Make sure you get enough rest, eat regularly, and drink six or more glasses of water daily. Avoid aspirin or other over-the-counter painkillers except for acetaminophen; instead, try such stress-reduction techniques as **yoga** or **meditation.** Or try taking a hot bath with a cold pack on your forehead. *(See also Headache.)*

**Acupressure.** To relieve a headache, press the Governing Vessel 24.5 point. *(See pages 22–23 for information on point location.)*

**Aromatherapy.** Soak a handkerchief or washcloth in cool water with a few drops of lavender *(Lavandula officinalis)* and place on your forehead.

### HEARTBURN

Avoid heavy meals and spicy, greasy, sugary, and acidic foods. Stick to a bland, high-fiber diet, drink lots of fluids, and exercise daily. Don't lie down right after a meal. Raise the head of your bed two to four inches with a stable support such as wooden blocks. *(See also Heartburn.)*

**Acupressure.** Pressing Stomach 45 and Spleen 16 may ease the discomfort of heartburn. *(See pages 22–23 for point locations.)*

**Herbal Therapies.** After meals, drink tea made from chamomile *(Matricaria recutita),* ginger *(Zingiber officinale),* or fennel *(Foeniculum vulgare).*

### HEMORRHOIDS

Hemorrhoids may develop as your pelvis stretches, but they usually disappear after the birth. Eat a high-fiber diet to keep your stool soft, drink lots of fluids, and don't strain during bowel movements. To relieve hemorrhoidal itching or pain, try a warm sitz bath or apply an ice pack or a cloth soaked in witch hazel. Kegel exercises, designed to strengthen the pelvic muscles, can improve circulation in the area. *(See also Hemorrhoids and Incontinence.)*

### LEG PAINS AND CRAMPS

Wear support hose during the day, and elevate your feet when resting, if possible. Use a heating pad or gentle massage on the back of your thigh to ease sciatica. When a leg cramp hits, straighten your leg and slowly flex your ankle and toes, massage your calf, or soak your leg in hot water. You may be able to prevent night cramps by wearing socks to bed or by pressing your foot against the bed board. If painful cramps persist, ask your doctor about calcium or magnesium supplements.

### MORNING SICKNESS

You may feel nauseated at any time of the day, typically in the first trimester. Try eating frequent light meals rather than three full meals. Keep your diet high in protein and complex carbohydrates, and low in sweet and fatty foods. Drink plenty of fluids, and eat fresh fruits and vegetables, which are high in water content. Do not take antacids, but try 50 mg of vitamin $B_6$ three times a day. In general, try to minimize stress in your everyday activities.

**Acupressure.** Locate the Pericardium 6 point on the inside of your left wrist, breathe deeply, and massage with your right thumb using a deep circular motion for one minute. Repeat on the other wrist. Seasickness straps, available in health stores, press the same point on the wrist. *(See pages 22–23 for information on point locations.)*

**Aromatherapy.** Add the essential oils of lavender *(Lavandula officinalis)* and mandarin to your bath, or put 2 drops each of peppermint *(Mentha piperita)* and sandalwood on a handkerchief and inhale the scent. Massage your abdomen with 2 drops each of peppermint and sandalwood mixed in 2 tsp of a carrier oil such as almond, olive, or sunflower oil.

**Herbal Therapies.** Try tea made from anise, caraway, catnip *(Nepeta cataria),* fennel *(Foeniculum vulgare),* or freshly grated ginger *(Zingiber officinale).* An infusion of dried peppermint *(Mentha piperita)* and chamomile *(Matricaria recutita)* may help your symptoms. Almonds and papaya juice are also said to ease morning sickness.

**Homeopathy.** Try Nux vomica (12c) or Tabacum (12c) for morning sickness, following label directions.

### MOUTH AND GUM DISCOMFORT

Pregnancy can be demanding on your teeth, so see your dentist early in your pregnancy for a checkup and cleaning. Brush your teeth and tongue at least twice a day, and floss regularly. Sugarless gum can be substituted for an after-meal cleaning if it isn't feasible to brush your teeth. Supplemental vitamin C, calcium, and coenzyme Q10 will strengthen your own teeth and ultimately your baby's. Or try a folic acid rinse, but do not swallow it.

### NASAL CONGESTION OR NOSEBLEEDS

Use a vaporizer to humidify your bedroom at night, and lubricate each nostril with a dab of petroleum jelly during the day to prevent nosebleeds. Avoid nasal sprays, which can constrict blood vessels.

**Acupressure.** To control nasal congestion, try finger pressure on Bladder 10. *(See pages 22–23 for information on point location.)*

### NUMBNESS

Avoid lying on your hands while sleeping. If your hand feels numb when you wake up, shake it over the side of the bed. Soaking the hand in warm water or using a heating pad twice daily may help ease numbness, or try wearing a wrist splint *(see Carpal Tunnel Syndrome).* If numbness persists try 50-mg vitamin $B_6$ supplements three times a day.

### SKIN CHANGES

Rashes from hormone changes during pregnancy generally go away after the baby is born. To prevent freckles or a dark pregnancy mask called **chloasma** on your face, wear a wide-brimmed hat or use sunblock on sunny days. Lubricate dry skin around your abdomen with a moisturizing cream; stretch marks usually fade and decrease after the birth. For heat rash, try to stay as cool as possible and use cornstarch powder under your breasts, on your thighs, or wherever your skin tends to chafe.

## TASTE CHANGES

You may find some foods unpalatable and develop a craving for others, especially sweets. Use mouthwash often; chewing gum, mints, or hard candies may also chase away unpleasant tastes. Iron supplements may leave a bad taste in your mouth; talk to your practitioner if this is a problem.

## URINATION PROBLEMS

Kegel exercises *(see Incontinence)* can help you to control stress incontinence—losing a small amount of urine when you sneeze, cough, or laugh. You can also use a sanitary napkin. Leaning forward while urinating helps to empty your bladder completely.

## VAGINAL DISORDERS

A thin, mild-smelling discharge is normal in pregnancy. Use sanitary napkins, but do not douche without your doctor's approval. Any red or brown discharge is a signal to call your doctor immediately. Vaginal itching and soreness may indicate an infection, which requires treatment by your doctor. Vaginal yeast infections may be common in pregnancy and may disappear without treatment after the baby is born. *(See also Vaginal Problems.)*

**Homeopathy.** Check with a homeopath about using Sepia (9c) to treat mild vaginal disorders.

## VARICOSE VEINS

Pregnancy puts extra strain on the blood vessels in your legs. You can get the most benefit from wearing support pantyhose or elastic stockings if you put them on while you are lying down so that body fluids are not gravitating to your legs. Exercise regularly, but don't stand for long periods. Raise your legs above hip level when sitting, if possible. Lie on your side in bed, or put a pillow under your feet. *(See also Varicose Veins.)*

**Nutrition and Diet.** Ask your doctor or a nutritional specialist about taking vitamin C supplements to strengthen blood vessels.

## VISION CHANGES

If your eyes swell from fluid retention and hard contact lenses become uncomfortable, switch to soft lenses or glasses.

C A U T I O N !

**BABY ON THE WAY**

**You can confidently treat many secondary disorders of pregnancy yourself, but only after you discuss the problem and potential treatments with your doctor. Some prescription drugs and over-the-counter medications can be dangerous to unborn babies and pregnant women. This is equally true of herbal preparations, essential oils, or anything you eat or drink. The same cautions apply to acupressure, massage, yoga, and other body work techniques; in fact, most acupuncturists will not treat pregnant women. For your comfort and safety—to say nothing of your baby's—always discuss alternative treatments with trained therapists sensitive to the special aspects of pregnancy. And make sure you have 24-hour access to your doctor to discuss any health questions or concerns.** ■

# PREMENSTRUAL SYNDROME

## SYMPTOMS

The symptoms of premenstrual syndrome recur during the same phase of the menstrual cycle, usually 7 to 10 days before your period begins. They may include any of the following:

- bloating and fluid retention.
- breast swelling and pain.
- acne, cold sores, or susceptibility to herpes outbreaks.
- weight gain of up to five pounds (from retention of fluids).
- headaches, backaches, and joint or muscle aches.
- moodiness, anxiety, depression, or irritability.
- food cravings, especially for sugary or salty foods.
- insomnia.
- drowsiness and fatigue, or conversely, extra energy.
- hot flashes or nausea.
- constipation, diarrhea, or urinary disorders.

A very small number of women with premenstrual syndrome may experience more intense symptoms:

- fits of crying.
- panic attacks.
- suicidal thoughts.
- aggressive or violent behavior.

## CALL YOUR DOCTOR IF:

- your symptoms are severe enough to interfere with your normal functions; your doctor may be able to offer treatments that will alleviate your symptoms.

Premenstrual syndrome—commonly known as PMS—is a physical condition characterized by a variety of symptoms that typically recur during a particular phase of the menstrual cycle, usually a week to 10 days before your period begins. Practically every woman experiences at least one PMS symptom sometime in her life, and between 10 and 50 percent of women in the United States suffer from PMS regularly. Specific symptoms vary from woman to woman. Some 5 to 10 percent of women experience symptoms severe enough for them to seek medical help.

PMS is uncommon in adolescents. Although some adolescents do indeed suffer from the syndrome, for most women the symptoms first develop while they are in their twenties.

Women most often affected by premenstrual syndrome are those who have experienced a major hormonal change, as may happen after childbirth, miscarriage, abortion, or tubal ligation. Women who discontinue birth-control pills may also notice an increase in PMS symptoms until their hormone balance returns.

Although PMS has been reported in the medical literature since the 1930s, its validity as a medical condition is a hotly debated subject. Many worry that it will be used to prove women too emotionally and physically unpredictable for certain jobs or responsibilities. Experts point out, however, that the syndrome—although sometimes discomforting—is rarely debilitating.

## CAUSES

Numerous theories have been proposed to explain some or all of the symptoms of PMS. Many researchers believe that PMS is the result of a hormonal imbalance, although the precise nature of that imbalance is not certain. An overproduction of the hormone estrogen is sometimes cited; however, most women do not experience PMS at the middle of their menstrual cycle, when estrogen levels are at their peak.

It has also been suggested that a deficiency in a particular hormone—such as estrogen, progesterone, testosterone, or prolactin—may be responsible for PMS, but controlled studies have ruled out these single-hormone theories. Recent research has focused on the monthly fluctuations in brain chemicals known as neurotransmitters, including mood-altering endorphins and monoamines, as a possible cause of the syndrome, but studies have been inconclusive.

Dietary deficiencies, including a lack of vitamin $B_6$ and essential fatty acids, are also considered a possible cause. One type of PMS, characterized by headache, dizziness, heart pounding, increased appetite, and a craving for chocolate, is thought by some researchers to be the result of a magnesium deficiency brought on by stress. According to this theory, the craving for chocolate, a food rich in magnesium, helps balance the deficiency; unfortunately, however, the sugar in chocolate also raises blood insulin levels, which can exacerbate the other symptoms.

The fact that identical twins are more likely to share PMS symptoms than are fraternal twins suggests that premenstrual syndrome may have a genetic component.

### DIAGNOSTIC AND TEST PROCEDURES

Before making a diagnosis of PMS, your doctor will want to rule out other possible causes of the symptoms by giving you a general physical and pelvic examination. Some doctors take blood samples to check hormone levels in the body, but many PMS experts consider these tests to be of dubious value. Instead, they suggest that the best way of accurately diagnosing PMS is for you to keep a written daily diary of your symptoms for at least two months. Keep a calendar record of when your menstrual period begins and ends, and each evening write down on the calendar any PMS symptoms you had that day. Your doctor can then use this written record not only to confirm a diagnosis but also to help decide on a possible treatment plan.

## TREATMENT

You may decide not to treat your PMS symptoms at all. But if they are severe and you seek help, be aware that some treatment approaches are controversial. Remedies for PMS basically fall into two categories: hormonal treatments, prescribed by some conventional doctors, and nutritional and lifestyle changes, prescribed by both conventional and alternative practitioners. Because of the health risks associated with hormonal treatments, many women prefer to try alternative methods first.

### CONVENTIONAL MEDICINE

Some doctors prescribe various hormones, most notably estrogen or progesterone, to relieve symptoms. The hormones are given in a variety of forms, including injection and vaginal or rectal suppositories. But hormonal treatments may produce side effects, some of which can be serious, and no controlled studies have definitively shown that these treatments work.

Some doctors prescribe hormone-containing birth-control pills to women with PMS symptoms. Although some women report that the pills alleviate their symptoms, studies have shown that they are not useful for most women with PMS and may in certain cases even worsen symptoms.

Because of the risks associated with hormonal treatments, many conventional doctors prefer approaches that emphasize good nutrition, regular exercise, and other lifestyle changes such as those described below.

### ALTERNATIVE CHOICES

A wide variety of alternative treatments may help relieve PMS symptoms. Because PMS is different from one woman to the next, you may have to try several treatments, or a combination of them, before you find the right approach for you.

#### AROMATHERAPY

To relieve anxiety and irritability, try lavender *(Lavandula officinalis)* or chamomile *(Matricaria recutita)* oil; parsley *(Petroselinum crispum)* or juniper *(Juniperus communis)* oil may also be helpful. Add several drops to a warm bath.

To relieve breast tenderness, try adding 6 to 8 drops of geranium *(Pelargonium odoratissimum)* oil to a warm bath.

### CHINESE HERBS

For relief from PMS symptoms, Chinese herbalists sometimes recommend dong quai *(Angelica sinensis),* which is believed to help balance the body's hormones and have a tonic effect on the uterus and other female organs. Take as a tea or in tincture form (4 to 6 ml) three times a day.

### NUTRITION AND DIET

Dietary changes have been shown to effectively reduce PMS symptoms in some women. Try reducing your intake of caffeine, sugar, salt, dairy products, and white flour, which studies have shown can sometimes aggravate PMS symptoms. Many women also find that eating six or more small meals throughout the day rather than three large ones reduces their symptoms, perhaps by keeping insulin levels more constant.

Some PMS symptoms, such as mood swings, fluid retention, bloatedness, breast tenderness, food cravings, and fatigue, have been linked to a deficiency of vitamin $B_6$ or magnesium. Nutritionists recommend supplements of these nutrients: 50 to 100 mg of vitamin $B_6$ daily, and 250 mg of magnesium daily, with a gradual increase if necessary. Supplements of calcium, zinc, copper, vitamins A and E, as well as various amino acids and enzymes, are also sometimes prescribed. Consult an experienced nutritionist.

Some research has indicated that a dietary deficiency in fatty acids may contribute to PMS. Many women report that taking evening primrose oil *(Oenothera biennis),* a substance that contains essential fatty acids, is effective. Your healthcare practitioner may recommend that you take one capsule (500 mg) daily throughout the month. If this amount does not bring relief, the dosage may be increased to four capsules a day. Other dosage regimens are also recommended. Consult your healthcare practitioner.

### HERBAL THERAPIES

Herbalists recommend a wide variety of herbs to help alleviate the many symptoms of PMS. Chaste tree *(Vitex agnus-castus),* for example, is sometimes prescribed because it is believed to help balance the body's hormones and relieve the anxiety and depression associated with PMS. Dan-

### YOGA

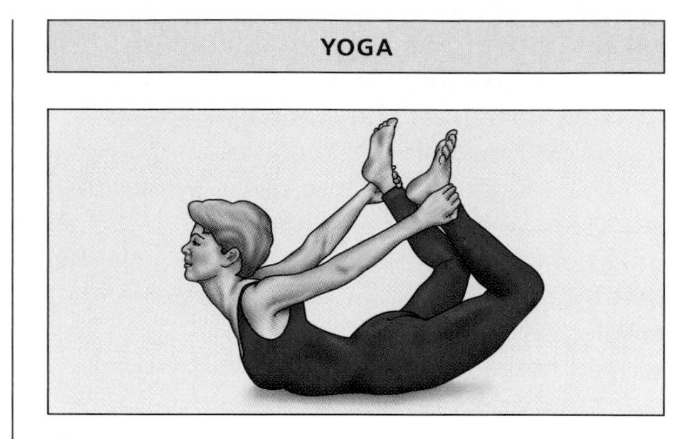

**1** To help restore hormonal balance, try the **Bow.** Lie on your stomach, legs bent, and grasp both ankles. While inhaling, squeeze your buttocks and slowly raise your head, chest, and thighs off the floor. Hold for 15 seconds, breathing slowly, and release. Do one time.

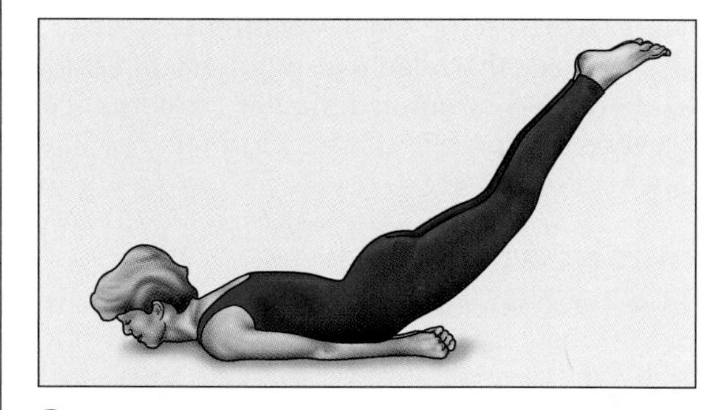

**2** The **Locust** tones muscles in the pelvic area. Lie on your stomach, arms at your sides. Squeeze your buttocks as you press down with your arms. Raise your legs, keeping them straight as you press out through the toes and heels. Hold for 15 seconds, then exhale and release. Do once or twice a day.

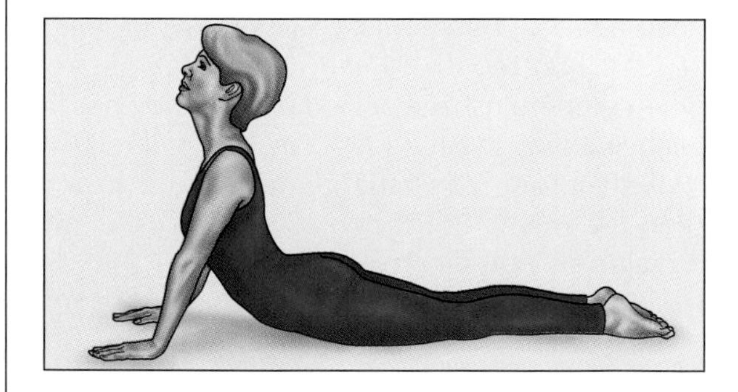

**3** You can also try the **Cobra.** Place both forearms on the floor, elbows directly under your shoulders. Inhale and push your chest up while pressing your pelvis and palms against the floor. Hold for 15 seconds, breathing deeply, then slowly relax. Do one or two times.

delion *(Taraxacum officinale),* whose leaves are thought to act as a powerful diuretic, is sometimes used to reduce the bloating and breast swelling caused by premenstrual fluid retention. Skullcap *(Scutellaria lateriflora),* believed to have a calming effect on the nerves, is also sometimes suggested. For an herbal preparation designed to relieve your particular symptoms, see an experienced practitioner.

#### HOMEOPATHY

For relief from your specific PMS symptoms, consult an experienced homeopath for individualized remedies and dosages.

#### LIFESTYLE

Studies have shown that regular exercise lessens PMS symptoms, perhaps by stimulating the release of endorphins and other brain chemicals that help relieve stress and lighten mood. Getting enough sleep is also important for the successful treatment of PMS. Lack of sleep can exacerbate fatigue, irritability, and other emotional symptoms. Experts recommend that people who have trouble getting enough rest stick to a regular sleep schedule. By going to bed and awakening at the same time each day, even on weekends, you may find it easier to get the sleep you need.

#### MIND/BODY MEDICINE

Various relaxation techniques, such as **yoga** and **meditation,** can be helpful in reducing the anxiety, irritability, and other emotional symptoms that sometimes occur premenstrually. The Cobra and Bow yoga positions *(left)* are particularly recommended for PMS.

### ACUPRESSURE

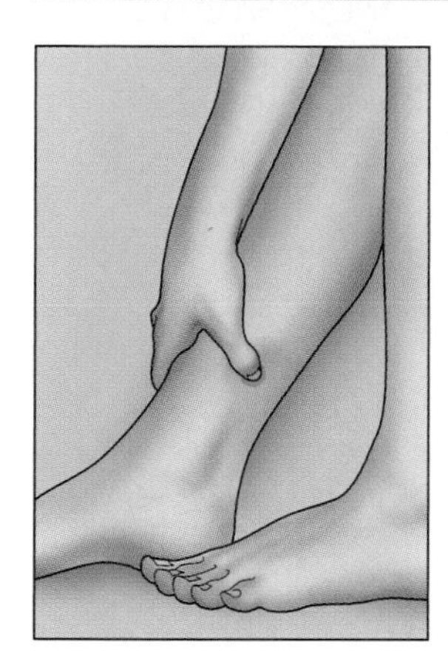

Symptoms of PMS may be relieved by pressing Spleen 6. Place your thumb four finger widths up from your right inside anklebone, near the edge of the shinbone. Press for one minute, then do the same on the other leg. Do two to three times. Do not use SP 6 if you are pregnant.

## AT-HOME REMEDIES

- Try to eat a low-fat, high-fiber diet. Avoid salt, sugar, caffeine, and dairy products right before your menstrual period.
- Exercise regularly.
- Try to reduce stress and increase sleep during the week before your period.
- Take recommended vitamin supplements.
- Try to manage your food cravings—particularly for chocolate; giving in to them may actually make your symptoms worse. Reach for fruit instead of sugary treats.
- As your period approaches, take long, warm baths to ease tension and stress.
- Use a hot-water bottle, a heating pad, or castor-oil packs to ease backaches and muscle aches associated with PMS.
- Abstain from alcohol before your period. It can aggravate PMS depression, headaches, and fatigue, and can trigger food cravings.
- Join a PMS support group. Some communities have PMS self-help organizations that meet regularly to provide support and exchange information. Check your phone book or call a local hospital for the name of a group in your area. ■

# PROSTATE CANCER

## SYMPTOMS

Early prostate cancer rarely causes symptoms. Once a malignant tumor causes the prostate gland to swell significantly, or once cancer spreads beyond the prostate, the following symptoms may be present:

- a frequent need to urinate, especially at night.
- difficulty starting or stopping the urinary stream.
- a weak or interrupted urinary stream.
- a painful or burning sensation during urination or ejaculation.
- blood in urine or semen.

Symptoms of advanced prostate cancer include:

- dull, incessant pain or stiffness in the pelvis, lower back, or upper thighs; arthritic pain in the bones of those areas.
- loss of weight and appetite, fatigue, nausea, or vomiting.

## CALL YOUR DOCTOR IF:

- you have difficulty urinating or find that urination is painful or otherwise abnormal. Your doctor will examine your prostate gland to determine whether it is swollen and, if so, whether the problem is caused by a malignant tumor or another kind of ailment.
- you have chronic pain in your lower back, pelvis or upper thighbones, or other bones. Ongoing pain without explanation always merits medical attention. Pain in these areas can have various causes but may be from the spread of advanced prostate cancer.

The prostate is a gland in the male reproductive system that helps produce semen, the thick fluid that carries sperm cells. The walnut-sized gland is located beneath a man's bladder and surrounds the upper part of the urethra, the tube that carries urine from the bladder. Prostate function is regulated by testosterone, a male sex hormone produced mainly in the testicles.

Prostate cancer is a major health concern for American men. Although the disease is rare before age 50, experts speculate that most elderly men have at least traces of it. Some 200,000 new cases and 38,000 deaths are attributed to prostate cancer each year in the U.S. For reasons not fully understood, African American men have the greatest incidence of prostate cancer in the world and the highest death rate from the disease. In other parts of the world—notably Asia, Africa, and Latin America—prostate cancer is rare.

Compared with most other cancers, prostate cancer behaves rather strangely. It often lies dormant for years, causing no symptoms and posing no threat to general health. Most men with prostate cancer die of other causes—many without ever realizing that they have the disease. But once prostate cancer "wakes up" and begins to spread, it is dangerous. Although the disease tends to progress slowly, it is generally fatal if it spreads beyond the prostate gland itself.

More than half of diagnosed cases originate in the prostate's posterior section, nearest the rectum. A few rare types originate in the anterior section nearest the urethra. A malignant tumor may grow directly through the prostate gland and spread cancer cells to surrounding tissue, including the rectum and bladder. Cancer cells may also invade the lymphatic system or bloodstream, travel to nearby lymph nodes, and then spread to the bones, liver, lungs, and other organs.

Doctors treating prostate cancer have long been frustrated by not knowing which prostate cancers will remain dormant and which will spread and become life-threatening. Identification of a protein called KAI-1 (named for the gene that controls its production) may make this dilemma obsolete. This protein appears to serve as a "marker" for metastatic, or spreading, prostate cancers. If high levels of KAI-1 are found in can-

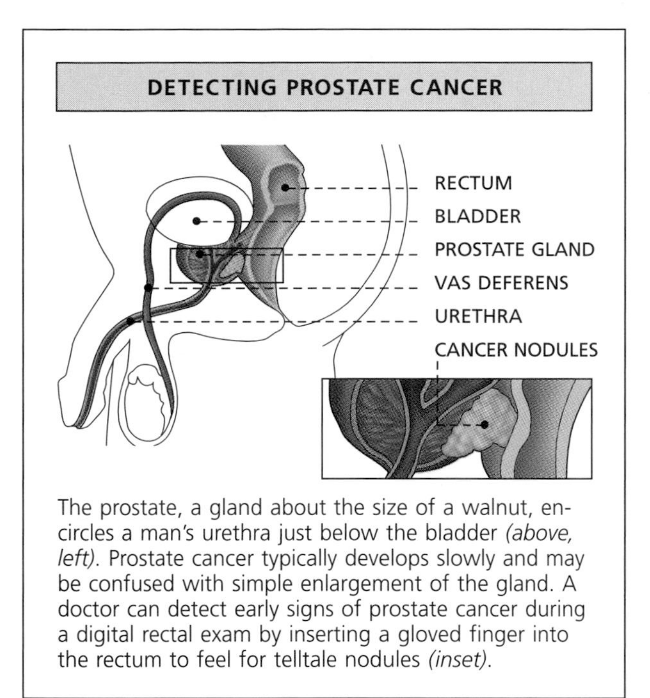


The prostate, a gland about the size of a walnut, encircles a man's urethra just below the bladder *(above, left)*. Prostate cancer typically develops slowly and may be confused with simple enlargement of the gland. A doctor can detect early signs of prostate cancer during a digital rectal exam by inserting a gloved finger into the rectum to feel for telltale nodules *(inset)*.

cerous tissue samples, the prostate cancer is unlikely to spread, or metastasize; if the protein is absent, the cancer is likely to spread.

Cancer that has not spread beyond the prostate gland can be cured. Fortunately, more than half of American men with prostate cancer are diagnosed when the disease is in its early stages. Cancer that has spread beyond the prostate to nearby tissues is rarely curable, but it often can be controlled for years with treatment. Once the cancer becomes widespread, life expectancy ranges from 2 to 3 years. With improved detection and treatment of prostate cancer over the past 30 years, the overall 5-year survival rate has increased from 50 percent to nearly 80 percent.

## CAUSES

Prostate cancer affects mainly elderly men. Four out of five cases are diagnosed in men over 65, but less than 1 percent in men under 50. Men with a family history of prostate cancer are three times more likely to die of it than is the general population. On a case-by-case basis, doctors cannot say with certainty what causes prostate cancer, but experts generally agree that diet contributes to the risk. Men who consume great amounts of fat—particularly from red meat and other sources of animal fat—are most likely to develop symptoms of advanced prostate cancer. The disease is much more common in countries where meat and dairy products are dietary staples than in countries where the basic diet consists of rice, soybean products, and vegetables.

The underlying factor linking diet and prostate cancer is probably hormonal. Fats stimulate production of testosterone and other hormones, and testosterone acts to speed the growth of prostate cancer. Theoretically, high testosterone levels spur dormant prostate cancer cells into activity. Some findings suggest that high testosterone levels also influence the initial onset of prostate cancer. Eating meat may be risky for other reasons: Meat cooked at high temperatures produces carcinogens that directly affect the prostate. A few other risk factors have been noted. Welders, battery manufacturers, rubber workers, and workers frequently exposed to the metal cadmium seem to be abnormally vulnerable to prostate cancer.

Researchers know more about what will not cause prostate cancer than what will. No proven link exists between prostate cancer and an active sex life, masturbation, use of alcohol or tobacco, circumcision, infertility, infection of the prostate, or a common noncancerous condition called **benign prostatic hyperplasia (BPH)** that involves an enlarged prostate gland. Most elderly men experience BPH to some degree. The theory that men who have vasectomies are at slightly increased risk for prostate cancer remains unproved.

### DIAGNOSTIC AND TEST PROCEDURES

Because most malignant prostate tumors originate in the part of the gland nearest the rectum, many cancers can be detected during routine rectal examinations. Men over 50 should have a rectal exam annually, and most doctors recommend that the exam be supplemented by a prostate-specific antigen (PSA) blood test. PSA is a protein whose concentration tends to increase in the presence of prostate cancer, making it twice as effective as a rectal exam in detecting early prostate cancer; together the two measures offer the best chance of catching prostate cancer while it is localized and most treatable. Prostate cancer may also be discovered incidentally during treatment for urinary problems.

If routine screening arouses suspicion, a doctor will inspect the prostate visually using transrectal ultrasonography. X-rays of the urinary tract, along with blood and urine studies, are performed routinely to aid diagnosis. Performing a biopsy will confirm cancer diagnosis: Guided by ultrasound images, the doctor inserts a needle into the prostate and extracts a small tissue sample from the tumor. A pathologist then studies the sample under a microscope to determine whether cancer cells are present. KAI-1 protein levels and other indicators can determine whether the cancer is likely to spread. If a diagnosed cancer is thought likely to spread, doctors may arrange CT scans, bone scans, chest x-rays, or other imaging tests to determine whether the disease has spread beyond the prostate.

## TREATMENT

Now more than ever, doctors have the information necessary to make informed decisions about which early prostate cancers require prompt treatment. Once the decision is made to treat a cancer, other factors, such as a patient's age and general health, affect the type of treatment given. Because decisions about how to treat this cancer are complex, patients should seek a second opinion from a specialist at a major cancer center and should participate in the treatment decision.

### CONVENTIONAL MEDICINE

Depending on when the disease is diagnosed, conventional treatment includes some combination of radiation therapy, surgery, and hormone therapy. Localized prostate cancer usually can be cured with conventional surgery, radiation therapy, or cryosurgery—freezing malignant cells with liquid nitrogen. The choice is made on a case-by-case basis and depends on many factors.

The standard operation—a radical prostatectomy—involves the removal of the prostate and nearby lymph nodes. In many cases surgeons can remove the gland without cutting nerves that control penile erection or bladder contraction, making such complications as impotence or incontinence less common than in the past. After surgery most men experience some degree of incontinence but eventually regain complete urinary control. Postop patients can manage impotence or incontinence resulting from surgery in a variety of ways. Impotence can be overcome with penile implants or other devices. Incontinence can be managed with special disposable underwear, condom catheters, or penile clamps; in three cases out of four, incontinence can be eliminated altogether with surgically inserted sphincter implants in the urethra.

Radiation therapy may be given as an alternative or follow-up to surgery for cancer that has not spread. If cancer has spread to nearby tissue, radiation is the preferred treatment; it is also used in advanced cases to relieve pain from the spread of cancer to bones. Even advanced cases that cannot be cured may be controlled for years with hormone therapy, sometimes supplemented by other treatments. Hormone therapy slows the cancer's growth by cutting off the testosterone supply, although the treatment's effectiveness may decrease over time. Testosterone can be removed from the bloodstream by surgically removing the testicles or by administering female hormones such as estrogen or other drugs that block testosterone production. Men generally prefer the testosterone-blocking drug treatment because it is effective, less invasive, and causes fewer side effects than surgery or hormone drugs. If the testicles are removed, the scrotum can be left intact with implants to conceal disfigurement.

If treatment is effective, prostate cancer goes into remission and may never return. All prostate cancer survivors should be examined regularly and have their PSA levels monitored closely. As with other types of cancer, new therapies are being developed for the treatment of advanced prostate cancer. Researchers are using radiation and hormone therapy in innovative ways and are testing the effectiveness of chemotherapy on patients who do not respond to other treatments.

## AN ESSENTIAL BLOOD TEST

*A tumor marker blood test is designed to measure a specific chemical that often is elevated in the presence of a specific cancer. In this case, the chemical is a protein called prostate-specific antigen (PSA) and the malignancy is prostate cancer. While most tumor marker tests are used to measure the response of various cancers to treatment, the PSA test is considered reliable enough to use in diagnosis.*

*But as useful as it is, the PSA test is not infallible and therefore cannot be the sole basis for a diagnosis. A man's PSA level tends to rise whenever the prostate becomes enlarged, but the enlargement may or may not be caused by cancer. This means that a higher-than-normal test reading can raise unnecessary alarm—a so-called false-positive reading. A PSA test may also indicate that cancer is not present when in fact it is. Because of its uncertainty, experts recommend that the PSA test be given along with the conventional gloved-finger rectal exam.*

*The PSA test is easy to give, relatively cheap, and has improved detection of early prostate cancer dramatically. Coupled with rectal exams and the newly developed KAI-1 tumor marker test, the PSA test enables doctors to detect and treat threatening prostate cancers at a very early stage. The American Cancer Society recommends that all men over 50 have an annual PSA test; for information about your local screening site, call 1-800-ACS-2345.*

See Cancer for more information on treatments such as radiation and chemotherapy.

### COMPLEMENTARY THERAPIES

Because excess dietary fat appears to promote prostate cancer, reducing fat may help slow the disease's progress. Anyone who has been diagnosed with early prostate cancer should maintain a low-fat, high-fiber, moderately reduced-calorie diet. If dietary fat is shown to play a role in initiating prostate cancer, cutting fat more severely would clearly be an advisable preventive measure for young and middle-aged men, particularly those with a strong family history of the disease.

Studies indicate that men with chronic deficiencies of vitamin A or selenium are more likely to develop advanced prostate cancer. Both nutrients can be toxic when taken in excess, so be sure to consult a doctor before taking dietary supplements. Good natural sources of vitamin A include most green and yellow fruits and vegetables, as well as liver, lamb, and turkey.

### AT-HOME CARE

Radiation therapy for treating localized prostate cancer is generally well tolerated. Some men, however, may experience fatigue, diarrhea, uncomfortable urination, dry skin, nausea, and other unpleasant side effects. Doctors can prescribe medication and suggest other ways to minimize side effects, including those things you can do for yourself. Rest whenever you feel the need, eat light snacks throughout the day rather than having three large meals, and avoid clothes that irritate your skin. For more information, see Cancer.

## PREVENTION

To lower your dietary fat, eat more fish, poultry, fresh vegetables, fruits, and low-fat dairy products. In general, eat less red meat; remove skin from poultry before cooking; and cut down on butter, margarine, and oils. To avoid carcinogens created when cooking meats, try poaching or roasting, not frying or barbecuing. ■

# PROSTATE PROBLEMS

## SYMPTOMS

**For an enlarged prostate:**
- difficulties in urination, including a weak or intermittent stream, unusual frequency (especially at night), straining, dribbling, or inability to empty the bladder.

**For acute prostatitis:**
- frequent, difficult urination.
- a burning sensation when urinating.
- sudden fever, chills.
- pain in the lower back and the area behind the scrotum.
- blood in the urine.

**For chronic prostatitis:**
- frequent, difficult urination.
- pain in the pelvis and genital area.
- painful ejaculation, bloody semen, or sexual dysfunction.

## CALL YOUR DOCTOR IF:

- your symptoms lead you to suspect an enlarged or infected prostate. If allowed to progress, prostate problems can lead to bladder stones, generalized infection, or kidney failure.

In addition, an enlarged prostate can be a sign of cancer. *(See Prostate Cancer.)*

P

The prostate is a walnut-sized gland that surrounds the male urethra—the tube that transports urine from the bladder through the penis. Its primary function is to produce an essential portion of the seminal fluid that carries sperm; the prostate also controls the outward flow of urine from the bladder. Because of this dual role, signs of prostate trouble can include both urinary and sexual difficulties.

Prostate problems occur in two principal forms: **enlargement of the prostate,** called BPH (for benign prostatic hyperplasia); and **prostatitis,** a bacterial infection, which may be either sudden and severe **(acute prostatitis)** or milder but persistent or recurrent **(chronic prostatitis).** A chronic infection may follow an acute one.

The signs of **prostate enlargement** generally appear after the age of 45. Typically, the first indication is a need to urinate at night, with the urge gradually increasing over time. Other urination problems may develop: a difficulty or hesitancy in initiating the urine stream; an inability to empty the bladder completely; and dribbling at the end of urination. These signs all have a common origin—the narrowing of the urethra because of growth of the glandular tissue surrounding it. Although the problem varies in severity, few men escape it altogether: Prostate enlargement affects 50 percent of those over 50 and a somewhat astonishing 90 percent of those over 80.

**Prostatitis** is less common and can occur in younger men or without symptoms of enlargement. While some of the signs resemble those of BPH, others are more typical of infection. **Acute prostatitis** may produce fever, chills, and lower back pain. **Chronic prostatitis** generally brings milder versions of those symptoms and may also cause painful ejaculation, urethral discharge, or sexual dysfunction.

Many men are reluctant to seek treatment for BPH or prostatitis, especially if their discomfort is minor. If either condition progresses toward severe symptoms, the danger can increase sharply. With prostatitis, the infection may reach the testicles and epididymis (a long, coiled tube behind each testicle through which sperm is transported from the testicles). It can also spread to a sexual partner. With BPH, the bladder may eventually

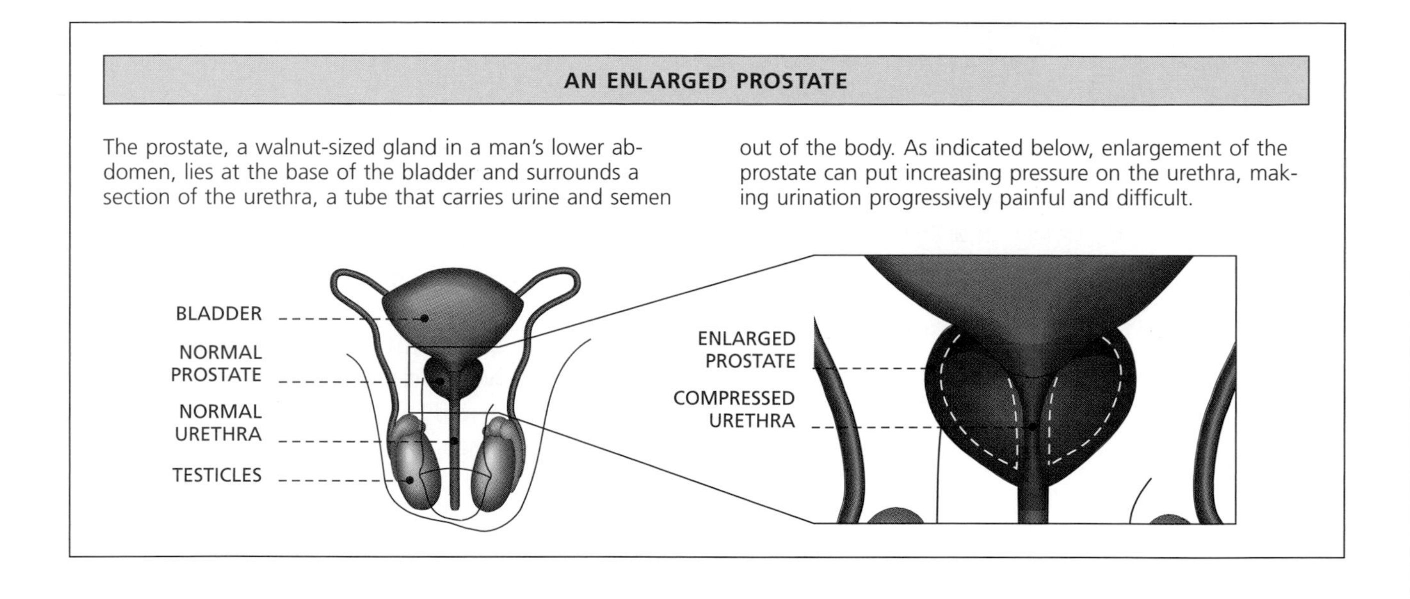


**AN ENLARGED PROSTATE**

The prostate, a walnut-sized gland in a man's lower abdomen, lies at the base of the bladder and surrounds a section of the urethra, a tube that carries urine and semen out of the body. As indicated below, enlargement of the prostate can put increasing pressure on the urethra, making urination progressively painful and difficult.

be unable to empty itself, and the lingering pools of urine become sites of infection or stone formation. Such urine retention is very painful and should be treated as a medical emergency. If the outflow of urine is blocked, pressure within the bladder may back up to the kidneys, eventually leading to permanent damage.

As the average age of the U.S. population rises, so does the number of men who seek relief from prostate problems. But with BPH, some aspects of the condition, including the chances of its worsening, are still poorly understood. As a result, the field is alive with controversy over when to take medical action and also over the relative merits of standard surgery and newer forms of medical treatment.

## CAUSES

Although the molecular mechanisms underlying **prostate enlargement** remain uncertain, the condition seems to stem from age-related changes in hormone balance that begin when a man is in his forties. Testosterone levels in the blood decrease, while other hormone levels rise; the net effect is the increase of a testosterone derivative that stimulates cell growth in the prostate. This results in enlargement and consequent stricture of the urethra within the gland. **Prostatitis** is usually the result of a urinary tract or bladder infection that has spread into the prostate gland. The infection can be sexually transmitted.

### DIAGNOSTIC AND TEST PROCEDURES

If symptoms indicate **prostate enlargement,** a physician will want to determine whether the growth of the gland is benign (BPH) or malignant (prostate cancer). The physician will insert a gloved finger into the rectum to feel the prostate for hardness or nodules, which can indicate malignancy. A urine sample is taken to detect infection and/or chemical indicators of cancer cells. (In 10 to 20 percent of benign cases, the prostate also harbors such cells.) Ultrasound imaging of the bladder and prostate is usually performed, and the bladder may be examined with a cystoscope. If symptoms suggest **prostatitis,** a urine test will identify the infectious agents. A rectal exam will find the prostate to be very tender and sensitive and will provide a check for coexisting conditions.

## TREATMENT

For **prostate enlargement,** be sure that you and your doctor consider the whole range of treat-

### SELF-MONITORING

*A primary goal in treating prostate enlargement is to reverse the growth of the prostate so the bladder can be emptied and the frequency of urination decreased. In gauging the success of treatment, your physician may suggest that you monitor the rate of urine flow on a regular basis. A reduced flow indicates that prostate growth is further constricting the urethra; an increased flow is evidence that the treatment is working.*

*Flow-rate monitoring is a simple chore involving a watch and a container calibrated in cubic centimeters. Calculate the flow rate by measuring the volume of urine voided and the time in seconds it takes to empty your bladder. For example, if the volume voided is 200 cc and the time taken to empty the bladder is 10 seconds, the flow rate is 20 cc per second. A normal flow rate for a man over 50 years of age is at least 15 cc per second.*

ment options. Just a few years ago, many physicians felt that surgery was the only solution; today, researchers are proposing an array of new treatment choices, from hormone-blocking drugs to lasers that can remove prostatic tissue without hospitalization.

## CONVENTIONAL MEDICINE

**Enlarged prostate:** When BPH symptoms are mild to moderate, medication may be the appropriate therapy. Two recently approved prostate drugs, terazosin and prazosin, relax the smooth muscles at the bladder neck and urethra, easing urination. Another new medication, finasteride, has shown some ability to gradually reduce prostate size and symptoms, though noticeable improvement may take three to six months.

When symptoms are severe or there is evidence of cancer, surgery is usually recommended. About 85 percent of patients experience marked relief of symptoms. In the most common surgery, the patient is placed under anesthesia, but no incision is needed. A small cutting instrument called a resectoscope (*resect* means to remove part of an organ) is passed through the penis and into the prostate by way of the urethra. Using an electrical apparatus at the end of the scope, the surgeon carves away the inner prostate, leaving a hollow shell through which the urine can flow. This procedure is known as TUR, or transurethral resection.

In about 15 percent of cases, TUR can have complications, including possible impotence and urinary incontinence; some patients experience infection or bleeding, and others require a second operation to reopen the urinary tract. For these reasons, and because of the desire of patients to avoid surgery, there is much enthusiasm for nonsurgical resectioning methods. Several kinds of laser resecters, which can be used for outpatients, have shown good results. The instrument is passed through the urethra, as in TUR; the laser is then fired, and the heat quickly coagulates and vaporizes excessive prostate tissue.

Microwave devices, similarly inserted, have been widely employed in Europe and Canada for nearly a decade; in the U.S., however, they have not yet been approved by the FDA and are available only at selected centers. Like laser resections, they can be done in an outpatient setting.

If the prostate is too large for TUR or other methods, the surgeon may recommend open prostatectomy, the removal of the prostate gland via surgical incision.

**Prostatitis:** A prolonged course of antibiotics is usually successful in eliminating the infection. Stool softeners, sitz baths, and nonsteroidal anti-inflammatory drugs (NSAIDs) are prescribed for discomfort. If an infection is neglected too long, antibiotics may not be effective—and it may be difficult to remove the infection even by surgery without causing further complications.

## ALTERNATIVE CHOICES

### AYURVEDIC MEDICINE

A practitioner may prescribe herbal remedies and exercises to increase circulation and relieve congestion in the prostate.

### CHINESE MEDICINE

**Prostatitis** and urethritis are considered conditions of damp heat and would be treated accordingly by a practitioner.

### HERBAL THERAPIES

An extract of the berries of the saw palmetto *(Serenoa repens),* a scrubby tree of the American Southeast, is said to shrink an enlarged prostate and relieve symptoms. Other remedies include Asian ginseng *(Panax ginseng),* flower pollen, horsetail *(Equisetum arvense),* nettle *(Urtica dioica),* true unicorn root *(Aletris farinosa),* and the powdered bark of pygeum *(Pygeum africanus),* an evergreen tree.

For **prostatitis,** pipsissewa *(Chimaphila umbellata)* and horsetail are used to treat chronic infection. Thuja *(Thuja occidentalis)* and pasqueflower *(Anemone pulsatilla)* are also suggested for inflammation of the prostate.

### HOMEOPATHY

Numerous medications are available to the homeopathic practitioner for treating prostatic enlargement and prostatitis, among them Berberis vulgaris and Staphysagria.

### NUTRITION AND DIET

**Prostate enlargement** may respond to nutritional support. In addition, if surgery is elected, good nutrition afterward will speed recovery.

Zinc, which is involved in many aspects of hormonal metabolism, is thought to promote prostate health and reduce inflammation; rich sources of zinc are oysters, wheat bran, whole oatmeal, pumpkinseeds, and sunflower seeds. Vitamins C and E may promote prostate health. The amino acids glycine, alanine, and glutamic acid are said to alleviate symptoms. The prostate may also benefit from large amounts of essential fatty acids, as found in flaxseed oil, walnut oil, sunflower oil, soy oil, and evening primrose oil.

### YOGA

See the positions illustrated above.

**YOGA**

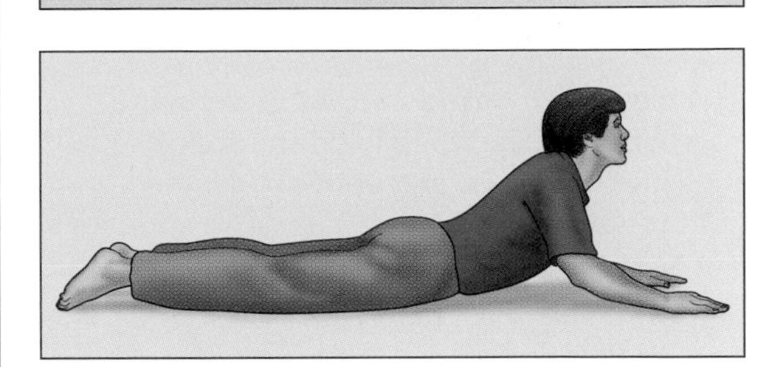

**1** Try the **Cobra** for an enlarged prostate. Place both forearms on the floor, elbows directly under your shoulders. Inhale and push your chest up while pressing your pelvis against the ground *(above).* Hold for 15 seconds, breathing deeply, then slowly relax.

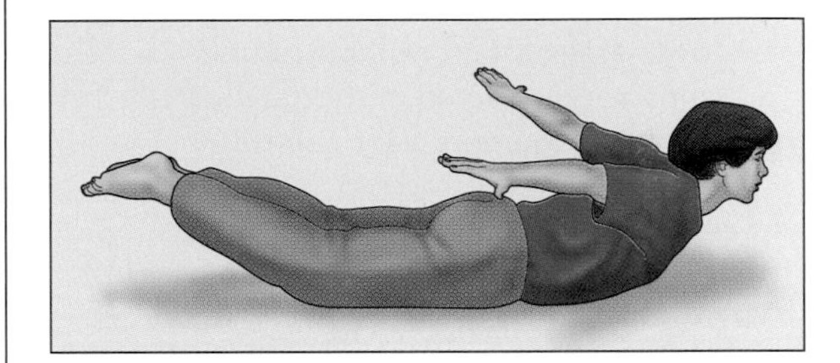

**2** Lie on your stomach for the **Boat.** Inhale as you lift your head, chest, arms, and legs off the floor. Stretch your arms behind you and hold the position for 15 or 20 seconds, then exhale as you relax back onto the floor. Do once or twice a day.

## PREVENTION

To prevent a recurrence of **chronic prostatitis** and promote prostate health:

- Take warm sitz baths.
- Drink more water; dehydration stresses the prostate.
- Avoid prolonged bicycle riding, horseback riding, or other exercises that irritate the region below the prostate.
- Take supplements of zinc and vitamin C. ■

# PSORIASIS

## SYMPTOMS

- deep pink, raised patches of skin with white scales, typically on the scalp, knees, elbows, and upper body; mild to severe itchiness.
- pitting, discoloring, and thickening of the fingernails and toenails. If psoriasis develops on the nails, they may separate from underlying skin.
- Red, scaly, cracked skin on the palms of the hands signals **palmar psoriasis;** on the soles of the feet the same condition is **plantar psoriasis.** These forms of psoriasis affect only those areas; the condition can become very inflamed and ooze fluid, making movement very painful.

See also the Visual Diagnostic Guide.

## CALL YOUR DOCTOR IF:

- your psoriasis becomes worse after you stop taking heavy doses of corticosteroid for this or another ailment. You may need a different course of medical treatment.
- your skin inflammation does not respond to any form of treatment; you need to be checked for the possibility of a more serious underlying ailment.

Unpredictable, intractable, and unsightly, psoriasis is one of the most baffling and persistent of skin disorders. It is characterized by skin cells that multiply up to 10 times faster than normal, typically on the knees, elbows, and scalp. As underlying cells reach the skin's surface and die, their sheer volume causes raised, white-scaled patches. **Palmar** or **plantar psoriasis,** which affects only the hands or feet, tends to be much more painful and often blisters and oozes.

Though not contagious, psoriasis tends to run in families. Fair-skinned people aged 10 to 40 are particularly susceptible, especially those with a blood relative who suffers from the disorder. Psoriasis is extremely rare among people with dark skin. Outbreaks are triggered by the immune system and can affect other parts of the body, particularly the joints, in which case the condition is called **psoriatic arthritis**. Although psoriasis may be stressful and embarrassing, most outbreaks are relatively benign. With appropriate treatment, symptoms generally subside within weeks.

## CAUSES

A variety of factors, ranging from emotional stress to a streptococcal infection, can precipitate an episode of psoriasis. As many as 80 percent of patients suffering a flareup report a recent emotional trauma, such as a new job or the death of a loved one. Many doctors believe such external strains serve as triggers for an inherited defect in skin-cell production.

Injured skin, obesity, and certain drugs—including the painkiller ibuprofen and the antimalarial medication chloroquine—can aggravate psoriasis. The disease often appears two to three weeks after an infection such as strep throat. Alcohol consumption clearly makes psoriasis worse, as does a diet high in protein and low in fiber.

## TREATMENT

Despite the fact that psoriasis is technically incurable, it responds well to most treatments for dermatitis. In addition to the conventional therapies below, **light therapy** *(page 708)* is accepted and practiced by conventional doctors.

## CONVENTIONAL MEDICINE

A standard treatment recommended by many doctors is to soak in a warm bath for 10 to 15 minutes, then immediately apply a topical ointment such as petroleum jelly, which helps your skin retain moisture. Some doctors recommend salicylic acid ointment, which smooths the skin by promoting the shedding of psoriatic scales. Steroid-based creams are effective; however, because they can have harmful side effects, psoriasis sufferers should be especially careful not to overuse them.

Treatment with capsaicin, a component of cayenne *(Capsicum frutescens),* may also be effective. Available as an over-the-counter ointment for treating shingles, it causes the body to block production of an inflammation-causing chemical found in psoriatic skin. It also prevents the body from building blood vessels to the affected area, thereby stemming the abnormal growth of psoriasis. Because capsaicin can burn and severely damage the skin if used incorrectly, try this only under a doctor's supervision.

A topical ointment containing calcitriol, which is related to vitamin D, has proved as effective as hydrocortisone creams for treating psoriasis and has fewer side effects. Coal-tar ointments and shampoos can alleviate symptoms, but many psoriasis patients seem vulnerable to the side effects—in particular folliculitis, a pimple-like rash affecting the hair follicles. Some studies also indicate that continued use of such coal-tar products may increase the risk of skin cancer.

Anthralin therapy is generally reserved for severe forms of psoriasis. Anthralin salve is carefully applied to the affected areas and removed after 30 to 60 minutes. All the white scales should be gone, revealing an underlying layer of fresh, normal skin. If not properly applied by a trained therapist, however, anthralin may irritate healthy skin and leave stains that can last several weeks. For persistent, difficult-to-treat cases of psoriasis, many medical doctors also recommend and prescribe **light therapy.**

**WHERE PSORIASIS STRIKES**

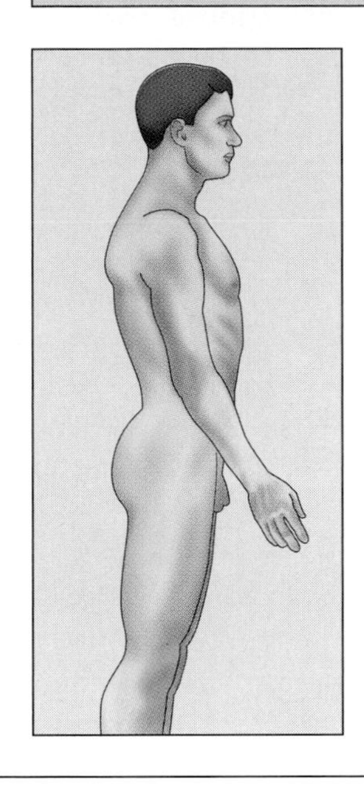

The thick, dry, scaly patches associated with the skin disorder psoriasis can vary greatly in size and appear just about anywhere on the body. The condition most frequently affects the scalp, elbows, and knees, shown in pink at left.

## ALTERNATIVE CHOICES

If conventional treatments for psoriasis are not working for you, ask your doctor about the potential benefits of the following alternatives.

### AROMATHERAPY

As an alternative to coal-tar shampoos for psoriasis on your scalp, mix together 4 drops of essential oil of cedarwood and 2 drops of juniper *(Juniperus communis)* or lemon in 1 tbsp almond or olive oil. Apply the mixture to your scalp and leave it on overnight under a shower cap. Shampoo and rinse thoroughly in the morning. Repeat three times a week until the symptoms clear. Since some people are sensitive to essential oils, place a drop on your skin for 30 minutes to be sure you have no adverse reactions.

### CLIMATOTHERAPY

Climatotherapy is based on the idea that specific climatic conditions can help or even heal certain diseases. For psoriasis, spending time in the sun can be beneficial. Special facilities at Israel's Dead Sea or other resort locations offer treat-

**C A U T I O N !**

**Many psoriasis patients choose corticosteroid treatments, to avoid the messiness and potential skin-damaging side effects of coal-tar products. Remember that steroid medicines can have serious and far-reaching side effects, too. Excessive or long-term use of steroidal ointments can thin the skin and cause white spots, acne, and permanent stretch marks. Used extensively around the eyes, steroidal ointments can, in rare cases, lead to glaucoma. Oral corticosteroid treatment may cause psoriasis to flare up again after treatment stops.**

**People whose psoriasis stubbornly resists conventional treatment should know that the sudden onset of psoriasis may indicate a human immunodeficiency virus (HIV) infection, a precursor to AIDS.**

ment designed for people suffering from psoriasis and other skin disorders. The combination of sunlight, relaxation, and mineral baths seems to have a therapeutic effect for many people.

### HERBAL THERAPIES

Burdock *(Arctium lappa)* root, dandelion *(Taraxacum officinale)* root, and Oregon grape *(Mahonia aquifolium)* are said to help reduce symptoms of psoriasis. Simmer 1 tbsp of any of these dried herbs in a cup of boiling water for 10 minutes; strain and drink hot, up to three cups a day. You may also take up to 1½ tsp fluidextract of burdock or dandelion root daily.

Evening primrose oil *(Oenothera biennis)* may soothe itching associated with psoriasis. Some doctors believe it's as effective as corticosteroids with fewer side effects, although people with liver disease or high cholesterol should use it only under medical supervision; pregnant women should not use it, because it can affect their hormone levels. The recommended dose of two 500-mg capsules a day can be costly; flaxseed and borage oils are less expensive alternatives.

Mix tinctures of burdock, skullcap *(Scutellaria lateriflora)*, sourdock *(Rumex crispus)*, and cleavers (*Galium* spp.) in equal parts; take 1 or 2 tsp a day. Or steep 1 tbsp of fresh nettles *(Urtica dioica)* and fresh cleavers in 1 cup boiling water for 10 minutes, strain, and drink two or three cups a day.

A rinse made of dried rosemary *(Rosmarinus officinalis)* and sage *(Salvia officinalis)* offers an alternative to tar-based shampoos. Pour a pint of boiling water over 1 oz of each of the herbs and let the mixture steep overnight. Strain and use daily as a hair rinse after each shampoo.

### HOMEOPATHY

Don't try to choose homeopathic remedies on your own to treat a chronic, systemic condition such as psoriasis. A homeopath assesses many variables, including the site of the inflammation, as well as the patient's family history and reaction to stress. Remedies homeopaths recommend for psoriasis include Sulphur, Graphites, Lycopodium, and Arsenicum album.

### LIGHT THERAPY

Like other serious or chronic skin disorders, psoriasis may respond to light therapy, or phototherapy. Patients receive timed exposure to ultraviolet radiation, in some cases after taking an oral medication called psoralen. The treatment is repeated several times a week for up to eight sessions per month. Although many doctors and patients report positive results, the treatments can have serious short- and long-term side effects; the drug psoralen is not recommended for pregnant women, because of the potential risk to the developing fetus. While light therapy may not be right for every psoriasis sufferer, it may be worth discussing with your doctor. *(For more on light therapy, see Dermatitis.)*

### MIND/BODY MEDICINE

The skin, the largest organ in the body, often mirrors turmoil within, so it's no surprise that many psoriasis patients have a history of high anxiety, low self-esteem, and stress-related problems. Many mind/body techniques help psoriasis patients by addressing the psychological roots and consequences of the disease. In particular, **hypnotherapy, guided imagery,** any of a number of **relaxation** techniques, **biofeedback,** and psychotherapy may be effective.

You can train yourself to relax by trying anything from a brisk half-hour walk every day to self-hypnosis, in which you focus your attention to block out irritating stimuli. If you think internal stress contributes to your condition, make a relaxation technique part of your daily schedule.

### NUTRITION AND DIET

Fish oil high in eicosapentaenoic acid (EPA), from such fish as mackerel, herring, and salmon, may help reduce inflammation and itching. Because you would have to eat up to two pounds of fish a day to get enough EPA, try a 1,000-mg fish-oil capsule containing EPA four times a day; or try 1 tbsp cod-liver oil, also high in vitamin A, once a day.

Vitamin A plays a vital role in the growth and maintenance of skin; when an outbreak of psoriasis occurs, take a megadose of up to 100,000 IU a day for a month under a doctor's supervision, then return to maintenance levels not exceeding 50,000 IU a day. A daily 400 to 1,000 IU of vitamin D may also help with healing. To avoid the risk of overdose, particularly of these fat-soluble vitamins, ask your doctor to monitor your progress. Always check dosages carefully before giving megasupplements to children.

Vitamin B complex containing vitamin $B_5$ and vitamin $B_1$ may promote healthy skin; to help fight psoriasis, the suggested dosage is 50 mg three times a day. Rubbing concentrated vitamin E ointment into your scalp two or three times a week can deter skin damage.

Some research has suggested that eating too much citrus fruit can aggravate psoriasis, and that psoriasis patients, like eczema patients, cannot metabolize fatty acids. To help prevent flare-ups, adopt a diet high in fish and raw vegetables, and low in fatty meats and acidic fruits.

### AT-HOME REMEDIES

- For mild forms of psoriasis, try a warm bath followed by an application of topical ointments that help the skin retain water and soothe inflammation. Use ordinary petroleum jelly or vegetable shortening, an over-the-counter corticosteroid cream, or a salicylic acid ointment. Make sure none of these topical preparations contains additives, preservatives, or perfumes.
- For scalp psoriasis, wash your hair with a coal-tar shampoo or with a mixture of cedarwood and juniper or lemon oils. A rinse with a rosemary-sage solution may also be helpful.
- Sunbathe. Expose areas of inflamed skin, but cover the rest of your body with sunscreen. Avoid overexposure.
- Start a regular exercise or relaxation routine. Allot at least 15 minutes four to five days a week to some activity that relieves stress. ■

## PSORIATIC ARTHRITIS

*In a trait unique among skin ailments, psoriasis can lead to a complication called psoriatic arthritis, most notably in the joints of the fingers and toes. It afflicts some 5 percent of psoriasis sufferers, with joint inflammation developing shortly before or after the emergence of skin lesions. Symptoms resemble those of rheumatoid arthritis, but patients test negative for that disease.*

*Doctors frequently treat the skin problem first, because the joint inflammation will usually subside when the skin inflammation is brought under control. Psoriatic arthritis responds well to aspirin and nonsteroidal anti-inflammatory drugs (NSAIDs), but patients should avoid the heavy doses of steroids used to treat other forms of arthritis. As with other skin ailments, psoriatic skin lesions can become much worse when steroid dosages are reduced or stopped.*

P

# PUPIL DILATION

*Read down this column to find your symptoms. Then read across.*

| SYMPTOMS | AILMENT/PROBLEM |
|---|---|
| ◆ one pupil is dilated and responds to light less than the other pupil, with no other symptoms. | ◆ Holmes-Adie syndrome (a harmless condition in which the pupils respond to light at different rates) |
| ◆ enlarged pupils of equal size that are fixed (do not change in size with changes in light), following a visit to a doctor who put drops in your eyes. | ◆ Temporary effect of eye drops specially formulated to temporarily dilate your eyes for an examination |
| ◆ fixed pupils of different sizes, or enlarged pupils of the same size, after taking drugs for any reason. | ◆ Side effect of many illegal recreational, over-the-counter, and prescription drugs—especially those containing epinephrine, such as bronchodilators |
| ◆ one pupil is larger than the other and fixed; the eye may constantly turn outward; double vision; drooping eyelid. | ◆ Third nerve palsy—the third cranial nerve is not functioning properly; often a side effect of diabetes, lead poisoning, alcohol abuse, or possibly a brain tumor |
| ◆ one pupil is smaller than the other and fixed; eye pain, redness, and/or swelling; tearing; blurred vision. | ◆ Uveitis (inflammation of the iris) |
| ◆ over time, one pupil becomes larger than the other and fixed; throbbing eye pain; loss of peripheral vision; seeing halos around lights; possible nausea. | ◆ Glaucoma |
| ◆ change in pupil size, or pupil asymmetry, anywhere from a few days to a few weeks after an injury to your head; headache; nausea; drowsiness; dizziness; inability to move arms or legs. | ◆ The effects of a head injury, either with or without concussion |
| ◆ pupils of different sizes; fever, vomiting; headache that is worse upon leaning forward; neck stiffness or pain, especially when tilting the chin toward the chest. | ◆ Meningitis, or possibly encephalitis (an infection of the brain) |
| ◆ pupil dilation accompanied by a sudden, severe headache that may radiate into the neck. | ◆ A brain aneurysm or a migraine headache |

| WHAT TO DO | OTHER INFO |
|---|---|
| ◆ The first time you experience this, **get emergency medical care;** a single dilated pupil can indicate serious illness, such as stroke or brain injury. | ◆ Holmes-Adie syndrome has no known treatment, but it does not lead to more serious problems. |
| ◆ Pupils should return to normal within a few hours; if they haven't contracted in 24 hours, call your ophthalmologist. | ◆ Wear sunglasses or stay in a darkened room if light bothers your eyes. |
| ◆ Ask your doctor about this symptom and your medication regimen; you may need to change. | ◆ Your pupils should return to normal as the drug effects wear off. |
| ◆ See your doctor. Treatment depends on the cause of the palsy, and may include antibiotics, exercises, and possibly surgery. | |
| ◆ See your doctor without delay; without proper treatment (rest, corticosteroid eye drops, and possibly other medications), uveitis can cause blindness. | ◆ Uveitis may occur suddenly, or it may come on gradually over time. |
| ◆ **Get emergency care immediately.** Acute glaucoma can cause blindness in a matter of days; other forms may be managed with surgery and/or medication. | |
| ◆ **Call your doctor now;** you may need emergency treatment for bleeding or blood clotting that is occurring between your skull and brain. | ◆ A serious head injury is not always accompanied by unconsciousness. Reduce your risk by using a helmet while riding a bike or motorcycle or while playing contact sports, and by wearing your seat belt in the car. |
| ◆ **Get emergency care immediately.** Without proper treatment, either of these infections can cause death. | ◆ One form of meningitis, aseptic meningitis, has identical symptoms but is not serious. A doctor's diagnosis is required. |
| ◆ Call your doctor without delay, unless you have a history of migraines with this symptom; only a physician can tell for sure the difference between migraine and aneurysm. | ◆ An aneurysm can be a medical emergency, or it may be treated with medication over the long term. |

# RABIES

## SYMPTOMS

After an incubation period typically of one to three months:
- pain, followed by tingling at the site of the animal bite.
- sensitive skin.

Up to 10 days after the above symptoms appear:
- drooling.
- inability to swallow liquids.
- rage, alternating with periods of calm.
- convulsions.
- paralysis.

## CALL YOUR DOCTOR IF:

- you are bitten by a wild or unimmunized animal, or any animal whose immunization status is uncertain. **Call or go to a hospital now;** immediate treatment is vital.
- you are bitten and experience any of the symptoms listed above. **Call or go to a hospital now.**
- you plan to travel to a country where rabies is common; ask your doctor to vaccinate you against rabies.

Rabies is a viral brain disease that is almost always fatal if it is allowed to develop and is not prevented with prompt treatment. You may develop it if you are bitten by an infected animal. Carriers of rabies include dogs, cats, bats, skunks, raccoons, and foxes; rodents are not likely to be infected. About 70 percent of rabies cases develop from wild animal bites that break the skin.

The disease is also called hydrophobia (meaning fear of water) because it causes painful muscle spasms in the throat that prevent swallowing. In fact, this is what leads to fatalities in untreated cases: Victims become dehydrated and die.

The incubation period for symptoms can range anywhere from 10 days to two years, but the typical time between the bite and the first appearance of symptoms is one to three months. The first symptoms include a tingling, itching, or cold sensation at the site of the bite, a low fever, and a general sense of illness. This may be followed by chills, difficulty swallowing liquids, restlessness, outbursts of rage, extreme excitability, muscle spasms, and drooling.

A bite from a rabid animal does not guarantee that you will get rabies; only about 50 percent of people who are bitten and do not receive treatment ever develop the disease. But don't take chances. If you are bitten by or have any exposure to an animal that may have rabies, go to the hospital immediately. Treatment virtually ensures that you will not come down with the disease. But any delay could diminish the treatment's effectiveness.

## CAUSES

Rabies is caused by a virus that infects the central nervous system—the brain and spinal cord. The virus enters through the skin or mucous membranes, then travels to the brain, where it multiplies and migrates through nerves to other tissues.

### DIAGNOSTIC AND TEST PROCEDURES

If you are bitten, your doctor will need to know what kind of animal bit you, and under what circumstances. If the animal is found to be healthy, or if its owner can prove it has been vaccinated

CAUTION!

**See a doctor immediately after you have been bitten by an animal that may have rabies. The longer you wait to get treatment, the greater your risk of developing the disease.**

for rabies, you probably won't need treatment, except to cleanse the wound. But if you're unsure of the animal's health, your doctor should give you the shots that prevent rabies without waiting for any confirmation that the animal was infected.

## TREATMENT

As soon as possible after you are bitten, clean the wound thoroughly with soap and water; give it a second scrubbing with an antiseptic, such as hydrogen peroxide. If the wound is superficial and you know the animal has been vaccinated, that's all you'll have to do. Otherwise, call ahead to the nearest hospital and go there immediately.

### CONVENTIONAL MEDICINE

Victims of animal bites used to undergo up to 25 painful injections of rabies vaccine in their abdomen. Now treatment consists of a single dose of rabies immunoglobulin and five injections of human diploid cell rabies vaccine given over 28 days. You may also need a shot to prevent tetanus from setting in.

### ALTERNATIVE CHOICES

If you are bitten by an animal that may have rabies, it is imperative that you receive the rabies vaccine. You may try alternative methods in conjunction with conventional medicine to speed healing and reduce discomfort.

#### AROMATHERAPY

Oil of myrrh *(Commiphora molmol)* is antiseptic and astringent. Aromatherapists recommend that you apply it directly to a wound to help cleanse it.

#### CHINESE HERBS

For centuries, doctors of Chinese medicine used skullcap *(Scutellaria baicalensis)* to treat rabies-related convulsions. Today a qualified practitioner would send you to the emergency room of the nearest hospital. After you received the vaccine, the practitioner might suggest an herbal formula to strengthen your entire system.

#### HERBAL THERAPY

A compress of lavender *(Lavandula officinalis)* may help your wound heal faster.

#### HOMEOPATHY

A homeopathic practitioner may give you a remedy to speed wound healing. Echinacea is believed to strengthen the immune system to help you recuperate.

### AT-HOME CARE

- Cleanse your wound with soap and water, followed by hydrogen peroxide.
- Speed healing by using herbal compresses and aromatic oils.
- Cleanse your system by drinking lots of fruit and vegetable juices.

## PREVENTION

- Stay away from strange animals.
- Insist that neighbors obey leash laws.
- If you plan on traveling to an area where rabies is common in domestic animals (India, parts of South America), develop immunity to the virus by getting injections of human diploid cell rabies vaccine. Ask your doctor for details. ■

# RASHES

*Read down this column to find your symptoms. Then read across.*

| SYMPTOMS | AILMENT/PROBLEM |
|---|---|
| For itching skin that is not accompanied by a rash, see Itching Skin. See also the Visual Diagnostic Guide. | |
| ◆ scaly, itchy, red rash between the toes; may also cause unusual flaking on the soles of the feet; may affect toenails. | ◆ Athlete's foot |
| ◆ rash—either localized or diffuse—in an otherwise healthy person. | ◆ Contact dermatitis; allergies; stress; dietary deficiency |
| ◆ rash that progresses rapidly from a simple red flush to small bumps, then a crusted, pimplelike inflammation; extremely itchy. | ◆ Chickenpox |
| ◆ red rash in a baby's diaper area. | ◆ Diaper rash |
| ◆ tiny pink bumps usually found on the back of the neck and upper back that itch and sting; usually associated with hot, humid weather. | ◆ Heat rash |
| ◆ red rash that may resemble a bull's-eye and that fans out several inches from the bite mark; rash is not always obvious; followed by fever, headaches, lethargy, and muscle and joint pain. | ◆ Lyme disease |
| ◆ red rash that spreads from face downward and is preceded by fever, cough, and inflamed nasal passages. | ◆ Measles |
| ◆ rash that looks similar to the measles rash but is less extensive, lasts for a shorter period of time (usually only three days), and is not accompanied by cough. | ◆ German measles |
| ◆ distinctive red, scaly, round or oval patches with normal skin in the center; patches gradually get larger. | ◆ Ringworm |

R

| WHAT TO DO | OTHER INFO |
| --- | --- |
| ◆ When you bathe, wash and dry your feet thoroughly, and use an antifungal powder. Keep your feet exposed to the air as much as possible. | ◆ Tea tree oil (*Melaleuca* spp.) ointment may also be effective. |
| ◆ See your doctor to treat severe cases. Consider mind/body techniques, such as guided imagery, to alleviate stress. Consult a nutritionist; a zinc deficiency may cause a rash. | ◆ Stress can play a role as a catalyst for many skin disorders. |
| ◆ Keep a child at home to recuperate and to avoid spreading the disease. Chickenpox is more serious in adults; call your doctor. | ◆ The same virus that causes chickenpox causes shingles. |
| ◆ For most cases, use an over-the-counter zinc ointment; consult your pediatrician about more severe or longer-lasting cases. | ◆ Diaper rash can be treated with a variety of at-home remedies and alternative therapies. Changing a diaper as soon as it is soiled will help your baby's skin heal. |
| ◆ Cool your body in a cold bath; wear light, loose clothes; avoid excessive heat; avoid activities that cause you to sweat. | ◆ Heat rash is caused by blocked sweat glands. Sometimes it affects babies who are overdressed or who have a fever. |
| ◆ Call your doctor if you think you have been bitten by a tick. Get tested for Lyme disease and Rocky Mountain spotted fever. Treatment involves antibiotics. | ◆ If Lyme disease is not treated in its earliest stages with antibiotics, complications of the heart and nervous system may develop. |
| ◆ Call your child's pediatrician. Keep your child at home to recuperate and to avoid spreading the disease. | ◆ Serious complications of measles include encephalitis and pneumonia. |
| ◆ Keep your child at home to recuperate and to avoid spreading the disease. If you are pregnant and have been exposed to the virus, call your doctor. | ◆ The rubella virus can cause birth defects if transmitted by an infected mother to her unborn child. |
| ◆ Try a topical antifungal drug such as miconazole or clotrimazole. See the Visual Diagnostic Guide. | |

| SYMPTOMS | AILMENT/PROBLEM |
| --- | --- |
| ◆ pink rash that starts near the wrists and ankles and spreads to the face, torso, palms, and soles of the feet; often accompanied by fever, chills, and severe headaches. | ◆ Rocky Mountain spotted fever |
| ◆ light pink, short-lived rash on torso, face, and extremities in children under three years old; occurs three to four days after a fever, lasts less than 48 hours, and does not itch. | ◆ Roseola |
| ◆ rash, especially between the fingers and on the wrists, that consists of reddish spots and tiny, grayish lines—the burrows caused by a mother mite digging in with her eggs; extremely itchy. | ◆ Scabies |
| ◆ pinpoint lesions on the torso and extremities; raised spots on the tongue; rash peels in five to seven days; sometimes accompanied by fever, headache, vomiting, and chills. | ◆ Scarlet fever |
| ◆ painless ulcers on the genitals and sometimes in the mouth, later followed by red, circular, nonitching lesions on the skin, especially on the palms and soles. | ◆ Syphilis |
| ◆ bright red rash in a baby's diaper area that does not respond to treatment for standard diaper rash; possibly, white patches in the mouth that leave red sores when wiped away. | ◆ Thrush |
| ◆ extremely itchy raised skin lesions with white centers and red rims anywhere on the body; usually part of an allergic reaction to something, such as penicillin or food; extreme heat or cold can also cause an outbreak. | ◆ Hives |

| WHAT TO DO | OTHER INFO |
| --- | --- |
| ◆ Call your doctor if you suspect you have been bitten by a tick. Get tested for Rocky Mountain spotted fever and Lyme disease. Spotted fever is life-threatening in adults. Antibiotics are almost always required. | ◆ Despite its name, Rocky Mountain spotted fever is most common in southeast and south-central states. |
| ◆ Allow the rash to run its course without interference from ointments or medication. | ◆ Caused by a virus, roseola occurs most often in the spring and fall. The rash usually follows a very high fever (103°F to 105°F). By the time the rash appears, the child is almost fully recovered. |
| ◆ Call your doctor for treatment to kill the mites that cause the disease. | ◆ Scabies is highly contagious. |
| ◆ Call your child's pediatrician without delay. | ◆ Scarlet fever can cause any of a number of serious complications and can be life-threatening. |
| ◆ Call your doctor. Penicillin in high doses is usually required. Discontinue all sexual relations until treatment is completed. | ◆ Syphilis is usually transmitted through sexual intercourse or oral sex; it can also be transmitted from an infected mother to her unborn baby through the placenta. |
| ◆ See Yeast Infections. | ◆ Newborns can contract thrush while passing through the birth canal. It can also be a side effect of several long-term diseases, such as diabetes and leukemia, or can appear following an aggressive course of antibiotics. |
| ◆ Oral antihistamines may provide relief; avoid applying topical ointments since they may obstruct pores. | |

# RAYNAUD'S SYNDROME

## SYMPTOMS

- sudden coldness, numbness, or prickly pins-and-needles sensation in the fingers, and possibly toes, when exposed to even a mild drop in temperature—as when walking into an air-conditioned room, for instance. The same symptoms might also be triggered by emotionally stressful situations.
- dramatic color changes in the fingers: When first exposed to cold, fingers turn white, then blue; when rewarmed, they quickly turn red and may throb uncomfortably.

## CALL YOUR DOCTOR IF:

- Raynaud's episodes become more intense. Irreversible damage to fingers or toes—a loss of feeling, for example—can occur in serious cases.
- skin ulcers, sores, or discoloration appears on your fingers or toes. These signs suggest that extremities are being severely deprived of blood. In rare cases, gangrene may result.

Raynaud's syndrome, which may afflict up to 1 in 20 Americans, is a circulatory disorder of blood vessels of the extremities. Constriction of those vessels is a normal physiological response to low temperatures, helping the body conserve heat. In Raynaud's syndrome, named for a French physician who first described the condition more than a century ago, nerve receptors in the extremities are overly sensitive to stimulation. Even a slight temperature drop—perhaps the faint chill produced by opening a refrigerator door—will cause a spasmodic closing of the small arteries in the fingers (and sometimes in toes). Typically fingers turn white, then blue, then red, indicating a progression from total blood deprivation to limited blood flow to sudden infusion of oxygenated blood as blood vessels suddenly dilate. Episodes are brief, usually lasting only a few minutes.

The syndrome takes two forms. About 90 percent of cases are of the type called **Raynaud's disease** or **primary Raynaud's**—an isolated condition with no connection to other medical problems. It most often affects women and usually sets in before the age of 40. The remaining 10 percent of cases are termed **Raynaud's phenomenon** or **secondary Raynaud's.** This version, which tends to start later in life, is connected to other medical factors—an underlying disease, for instance, or the long-term use of such vibrating tools as a chain saw or jackhammer.

For most sufferers, Raynaud's syndrome is a mild but maddening condition. Ordinarily, its most serious consequence is a loss of sensitivity in the affected extremity. Very rarely, a severe case results in tissue death and gangrene.

## CAUSES

The underlying causes of **Raynaud's disease** are unknown. It afflicts women disproportionately; men account for only about 1 case in 5. It is not thought to be an inherited condition, but it frequently affects more than one family member.

**Raynaud's phenomenon** has many causes, including such connective-tissue diseases as scleroderma, rheumatoid arthritis, and lupus; exposure to certain chemicals and drugs, such as beta-adrenergic blockers (used to treat high blood pressure) or ergotamine (used to treat migraines); and use of vibrating machinery.

## TREATMENT

Relief from Raynaud's is linked to improved circulation. Some exercises may help by forcing blood into the extremities, but relaxation techniques can also work. Of course avoiding triggers—such as cold or nicotine—will decrease the number of attacks.

### CONVENTIONAL MEDICINE

For most people, Raynaud's syndrome is not disabling enough to merit prolonged medical care. If attacks are frequent or severe, calcium channel blockers or other medications—angiotensin-converting enzyme (ACE) inhibitors, for example—may be prescribed, but many people find drugs ineffective. A simple exercise—swinging your arms around like a windmill—will force blood into your extremities and may be as effective as drug therapy.

### ALTERNATIVE CHOICES

In addition to trying the treatments discussed below, you might seek professional help from an **acupuncturist, chiropractor, homeopath, osteopath,** or **massage** therapist.

#### CHINESE HERBS

The most common Chinese herbal prescription for Raynaud's syndrome is peony *(Paeonia lactiflora).* Dong quai *(Angelica sinensis)* might also be prescribed for cold extremities. Consult a practitioner for dosages.

#### NUTRITION AND DIET

Simple changes in diet, along with nutritional supplements, can significantly moderate Raynaud's syndrome. Consuming more vitamin E, magnesium, and fish oils may help reduce blood vessel spasms in the fingers and toes. Fruits, vegetables, seeds, and nuts contain vitamin E. Magnesium is found in seeds, nuts, dark green vegetables, fish, and beans.

### AT-HOME REMEDIES

You can train your fingers to resist chills. Starting in a warm room, place your hands in a warm bowl of water for 5 minutes; then move to a cold room or outdoors and again place your hands in warm water, now for 10 minutes. Repeat the procedure several times a day for as many days as necessary. Eventually, this will produce a conditioned reflex that is the very opposite of the normal one: When exposed to cold, the blood vessels in the fingers will open up rather than close down—without the aid of warm water.

Avoid substances that make you vulnerable to chill. These include nicotine, caffeine, birth-control pills, and most over-the-counter decongestants, cold remedies, or diet pills.

Treat finger or toe infections without delay. When circulation is impaired, even minor infections can become a problem.

## PREVENTION

Devise ways to stay warm in your own home or office. Always carry a sweater. Use insulated glasses. Keep fingers and toes dry with talcum powder. Wear socks and mittens to bed. Outdoors, wear loose layers of blended fabrics; shoes made of breathable materials; a hat and, perhaps, earmuffs; and mittens rather than gloves. If you plan to be outside for several hours, try chemical "heaters" in your socks and mittens. ■

# RESPIRATORY PROBLEMS

## SYMPTOMS

- wheezing and breathing with effort.
- cough that may bring up phlegm.
- chills and fever.
- fatigue.

Respiratory problems may be accompanied by:

- rapid breathing and rapid heartbeat.
- shortness of breath.
- pain in the chest.
- slight headache.
- overall malaise.
- common cold symptoms: runny nose, sore throat, and sneezing.

## CALL YOUR DOCTOR IF:

- you have a common cold or cough that lasts for more than 7 to 10 days and that is not relieved by over-the-counter medications.
- you have a feeling of fullness in your face, pressure behind your eyes, postnasal drip, and a foul smell in your nose. These are symptoms of sinusitis.
- you have had a cough for a long time, are coughing up colored phlegm, or are short of breath. These may be signs of chronic bronchitis, emphysema, or lung cancer.
- you have a high fever (101°F or more), chills, pain in your chest, and a cough that brings up bloody phlegm. These may be signs of pneumonia or other serious illness.
- you have enough trouble breathing to cause you worry or distress; many diseases can make breathing difficult.

Respiratory problems can be divided into three categories: infections of the upper and lower respiratory tracts, such as the common cold, sinusitis, pneumonia, and tuberculosis; chronic obstructive lung diseases, such as asthma, bronchitis, and emphysema; and occupation-related lung diseases, such as asbestosis and coal miner's disease.

## CAUSES

Respiratory infections, which can range from mild to extremely serious, are caused primarily by viruses or bacteria settling in your airways. Your ability to handle these infections depends on such factors as age, the presence or absence of other underlying diseases, and whether or not you smoke.

Chronic obstructive diseases have multiple causes. The chronic inflammation of lung tissue characteristic of asthma, for example, can be brought on by pollen, irritants, or exercise. The destruction of lung tissue that is the result of emphysema is caused by excessive smoking or a hereditary enzyme deficiency.

Occupation-related lung diseases can be brought on by an individual's hypersensitivity to work-site substances or by the inhalation of particulate foreign matter, such as asbestos fibers, coal dust, and stone dust (which causes silicosis).

### DIAGNOSTIC AND TEST PROCEDURES

Physicians use a variety of diagnostic tests and techniques to evaluate problems in your respiratory tract, including chest x-rays, lung scans, CT scans, analysis of a sputum specimen, and pulmonary function tests.

Invasive tests may be used when specific information is required. An ABG (arterial blood gas) test, for example, measures oxygen and carbon dioxide levels in the blood; a lung biopsy provides tissue samples that can be examined under a microscope.

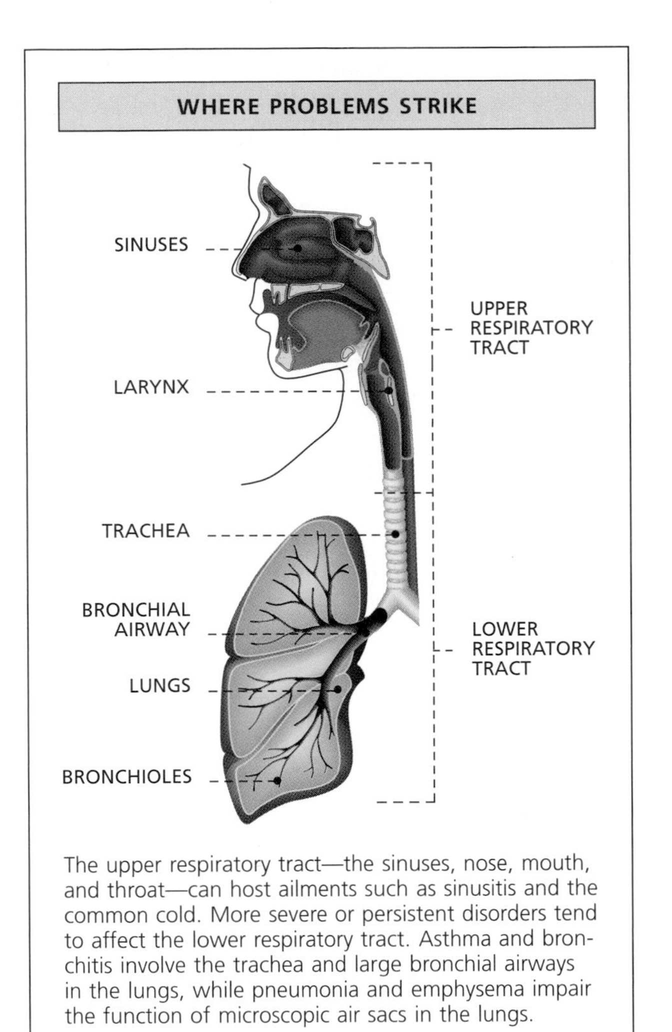


The upper respiratory tract—the sinuses, nose, mouth, and throat—can host ailments such as sinusitis and the common cold. More severe or persistent disorders tend to affect the lower respiratory tract. Asthma and bronchitis involve the trachea and large bronchial airways in the lungs, while pneumonia and emphysema impair the function of microscopic air sacs in the lungs.

## TREATMENT

Many respiratory infections usually go away on their own in a week to 10 days. Conventional and alternative therapies offer a range of simple treatments to relieve discomfort.

### CONVENTIONAL MEDICINE

If you have a bacterial respiratory infection, your doctor will probably prescribe an appropriate antibiotic. For the common cold, sinusitis, and acute bronchitis, you can make yourself more comfortable with bed rest, plenty of liquids, increased humidity (or steam), and medications for fever or pain. If you smoke, you will be advised to quit. Inhaled medications may help for chronic obstructive diseases such as asthma and emphysema. There is no effective treatment for the occupation-related lung diseases asbestosis and silicosis, except to avoid further exposure to respiratory irritants—including secondhand smoke—and if you smoke, to quit.

### ALTERNATIVE CHOICES

Alternative therapies may be helpful in relieving symptoms of respiratory problems. Consult an aromatherapist or herbal therapist for advice on using essential oils and herbs for massages and steam inhalation that may help reduce congestion and soothe inflammation. A practitioner of Chinese medicine might recommend **acupuncture, acupressure,** or various **Chinese herbs. Homeopaths** prescribe a wide range of medications for respiratory problems. Most practitioners agree that your immune system can be strengthened and maintained through good nutrition and healthful dietary practices. Try the recommended daily dosages of vitamins A, B complex, C, and E, and the minerals zinc and selenium.

### AT-HOME REMEDIES

During the typical 7- to 10-day course of a respiratory infection, the best remedies for alleviating symptoms are bed rest, plenty of liquids, humidity or steam, and fever or pain medications. ■

# RESTLESS LEG SYNDROME

## SYMPTOMS

- a distinctive tingling or crawling sensation deep in the legs, accompanied by an irresistible urge to move the legs to relieve the sensation.
- occurring most frequently at night, disturbing sleep; during the day, the feeling may prevent you from sitting or standing still for any length of time.
- usually strikes people over the age of 30; becomes more common as people grow older.

## CALL YOUR DOCTOR IF:

- you are experiencing any of the above symptoms for the first time; your doctor needs to rule out the possibility of more serious problems, such as kidney disease, diabetes, Parkinson's disease, deep vein thrombosis *(see Phlebitis)*, sciatica, or other neurological disorders.

Restless leg syndrome is a neurological disorder that has long baffled doctors and for which a cure remains elusive. People who suffer from the syndrome feel a tingling or crawling sensation deep in their legs and have an overwhelming need to move their legs to relieve the discomfort. Sometimes the arms are also affected. The symptoms often worsen at night, leading some experts to cite this condition as a major cause of insomnia and other sleep disorders.

Although restless leg syndrome is not health-threatening, it can be uncomfortable and even painful at times. Both drug therapy and simple lifestyle changes offer ways for sufferers to cope. But probably the greatest peace of mind for people with the syndrome comes from knowing that they are not imagining their discomfort.

## CAUSES

Restless leg syndrome is believed to be a genetic neurological condition brought on by a chemical imbalance in the brain. Research shows that caffeine can increase the symptoms. The syndrome has also been linked to iron or folic acid deficiencies, especially in people with kidney disease.

## TREATMENT

Drug therapy helps many sufferers, so consulting a physician is an important part of treatment.

### CONVENTIONAL MEDICINE

Your doctor will want to examine you to rule out other causes for your distress. If you are otherwise in good health, you will probably be started on a course of drug therapy. The principal medicine offering relief is clonazepam, which acts to stabilize the conduction of nerve impulses. Other drugs that may bring relief include the combination product of carbidopa and levodopa, a medication used to treat Parkinson's disease, and the sedatives methadone and codeine, which are usually prescribed as a last resort because they can be habit-forming. Because all these drugs can produce undesirable side effects and because most people eventually build a tolerance to them, which reduces their effectiveness, your doctor will want to closely monitor your progress while you are receiving drug therapy.

## ALTERNATIVE CHOICES

Some sufferers have found that alternative therapies can help lessen or relieve the physical discomfort associated with the condition.

### ACUPRESSURE

Applying pressure to Bladder 57 and Stomach 36 in succession may help relieve the tingling sensations of restless leg syndrome. Also try Spleen 6 and Gall Bladder 39. *(See pages 22–23 for information on point locations.)*

### HERBAL THERAPIES

Herbs with strong sedative qualities may be effective in reducing muscle tension and relieving pain. Such herbs include passionflower *(Passiflora incarnata),* valerian *(Valeriana officinalis),* and black cohosh *(Cimicifuga racemosa).* Cramp bark *(Viburnum opulus),* an antispasmodic, may also help relax muscles. Seek help from a medical herbalist for appropriate remedies and dosages.

### HOMEOPATHY

Homeopathic practitioners frequently treat restless leg syndrome and the insomnia often associated with it with Rhus toxicodendron and Causticum. Consult an experienced practitioner.

### NUTRITION AND DIET

To help correct nutrient deficiencies that may be contributing to your symptoms, take vitamin E, a multivitamin with iron, or a B-complex vitamin supplement in standard over-the-counter doses. To offset a folic acid deficiency, a nutritionist might advise you to take folic acid supplements (400 to 1,000 mcg). Some nutritionists also recommend supplementing the diet with a general food concentrate, such as blue-green algae, which may help correct unidentified nutrient deficiencies. You may also find it helpful to avoid such stimulants as caffeine and decongestants.

### LEG MASSAGE

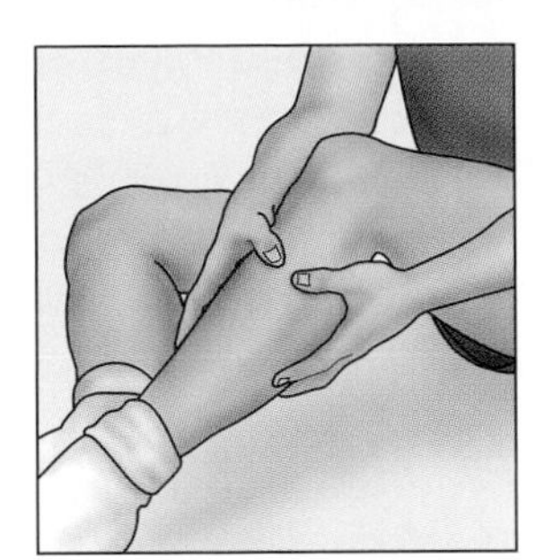

**1** Sit on the floor and bend one knee, keeping your foot flat. Grasp your calf in both hands and use your thumbs to find the muscle that runs along the outside of the shinbone below the kneecap. Massage the muscle with your thumbs all the way down to the anklebone.

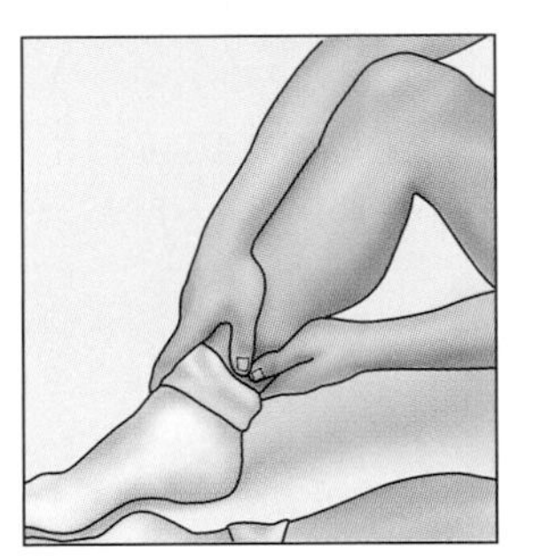

**2** Place both thumbs on the inside of your leg near the anklebone. Keeping your hands around your calf for support, massage the inside of the leg vigorously with your thumbs, moving from the ankle up to the knee.

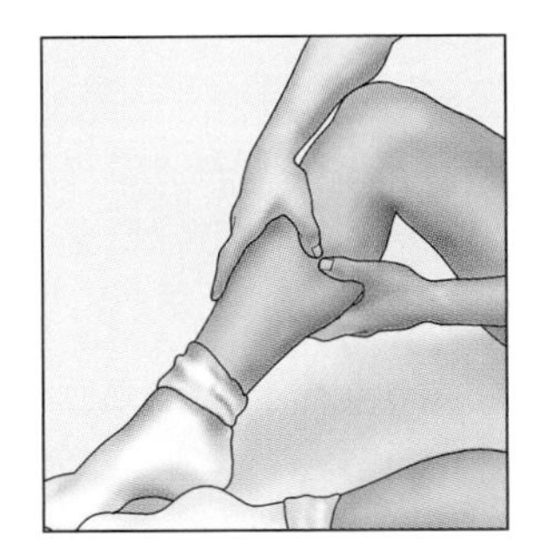

**3** Finally, use the thumbs and fingers of both hands to knead the back and sides of your calf muscle. Work from the knee down to the ankle. When you finish massaging one leg, repeat the entire process on the other. Alternately massage both legs several times.

## AT-HOME REMEDIES

- Avoid stimulating activities up to three hours before bed; this includes exercising and eating a heavy meal.
- Keep your bedroom quiet and cool; an overly warm room appears to aggravate restless leg syndrome.
- To reduce stress, which can trigger symptoms, practice **relaxation** techniques such as **yoga, biofeedback,** or **meditation.**
- Soak your feet in cool water, which is also said to be effective in bringing relief. Never use ice water, because it can cause nerve damage. ■

R

# RHEUMATIC FEVER

## SYMPTOMS

- fever.
- a red, raised, latticelike rash, usually on the chest, back, and abdomen.
- swollen, tender, red, and extremely painful joints—particularly the knees or ankles.
- nodules, or small bony protuberances, over the swollen joints.
- sometimes, weakness and shortness of breath.
- sometimes, uncontrolled movements of arms, legs, or facial muscles.

These symptoms often begin one to six weeks after a strep throat infection has appeared to clear up. Sometimes, however, people with rheumatic fever do not recall having had a sore throat.

## CALL YOUR DOCTOR IF:

- you are experiencing the symptoms listed above, particularly if you remember having recently had a sore throat; you may have rheumatic fever and should receive medical attention.
- you have a sore throat without other cold symptoms, accompanied by a fever higher than 101°F; you may have strep throat and should receive medical attention.
- you experience sudden and unexplained joint pain after recovering from strep throat; the strep infection may have spread and should be medically treated.

A rare but potentially life-threatening disease, rheumatic fever is a complication of untreated strep throat, caused by streptococcus A bacteria. The main symptoms—fever, muscle aches, swollen and painful joints, and in some cases, a red latticelike rash—typically begin one to six weeks after a bout of strep, although in some cases the infection may have been too mild to have been recognized. Rheumatic fever can also cause a temporary nervous system disorder once known as St. Vitus's dance. Today it is called chorea. People with mild cases of chorea may find it difficult to concentrate or write. More severe cases can cause the muscles of the arms, legs, or face to twitch uncontrollably.

The joints most likely to become swollen from rheumatic fever are the knees, ankles, elbows, and wrists. The pain often migrates from one joint to another. However, the greatest danger from the disease is the damage it can do to the heart. In more than half of all cases, rheumatic fever scars the valves of the heart, forcing this vital organ to work harder to pump blood. Over a period of months or even years—particularly if the disease strikes again—this damage to the heart can lead to a serious condition known as rheumatic heart disease, which can eventually cause the heart to fail. *(See Heart Disease.)*

Because of antibiotics, rheumatic fever is now rare in developed countries. In recent years, though, it has begun to make a comeback in the United States, particularly among children living in poor inner-city neighborhoods. The disease tends to strike most often in cool, damp weather during the winter and early spring. In the United States, it is most common in the northern states.

## CAUSES

Rheumatic fever results from an inflammatory reaction to certain streptococcus A bacteria. The body produces antibodies to fight the bacteria, but instead the antibodies attack a different target: the body's own tissues. The antibodies begin with the joints and often move on to the heart and surrounding tissues. Because only a small fraction (fewer than 0.3 percent) of people with strep ever contract rheumatic fever, medical experts believe that other factors, such as a weakened immune system, must also be involved in the development of the disease.

### DIAGNOSTIC AND TEST PROCEDURES

To determine the presence of streptococcus bacteria, your doctor will do a throat culture. This uncomfortable but painless procedure involves swabbing out a sample of throat mucus for laboratory analysis. It usually takes 24 hours to grow and analyze the culture.

Your doctor will also give you a complete examination, listening to your heart for signs of inflammation and looking for other telltale symptoms, such as arthritis in more than one joint and the small bony protuberances, or nodules, that often appear over the swollen joints.

## TREATMENT

Appropriate, often long-term, conventional treatment can greatly lessen the risk of heart disease and other health problems associated with rheumatic fever. Alternative treatments serve as complements to conventional care—helping to ease symptoms of the illness and strengthening the immune system to help avoid recurrent attacks.

### CONVENTIONAL MEDICINE

Your doctor will prescribe bed rest and penicillin to get rid of the streptococcal organisms. To prevent a recurrence of the illness, you may be put on a long-term prescription of antibiotics. For fever, inflammation, arthritic joint pain, and other symptoms, you may be given aspirin or an aspirin substitute and perhaps a corticosteroid. If you have developed rheumatic heart disease, surgery may be necessary to repair damage to the heart.

### ALTERNATIVE CHOICES

Your alternative-care practitioner, in consultation with your medical doctor, can provide treatments to supplement the antibiotics prescribed for rheumatic fever. Alternative medicine may also help you boost your immune system and reduce the likelihood of recurrent infections.

#### HERBAL THERAPIES

To help fight the strep infection behind rheumatic fever, herbalists recommend several herbs with antimicrobial properties. Garlic *(Allium sativum)* is considered a particularly effective natural antibiotic. Take three cloves a day. If garlic smell becomes a problem, you can try three garlic oil capsules instead.

Teas made from either goldenseal *(Hydrastis canadensis)* or echinacea (*Echinacea* spp.) can also be effective. Drink the brew at least three times a day.

Boneset *(Eupatorium perfoliatum),* sometimes called feverwort, can help relieve the fever and other discomforts of rheumatic fever. Make a tea from the herb; drink it hot and as often as every half-hour.

As a safe heart tonic that helps minimize any long-term damage rheumatic fever may have caused, drink hawthorn *(Crataegus oxyacantha* or *Crataegus monogyna)* tea daily. Or you can take 30 to 40 drops of hawthorn tincture twice a day.

#### HOMEOPATHY

After you have recovered from the first attack of rheumatic fever, homeopaths recommend various treatments to avoid further attacks. Remedies include Aconite, Mercurius vivus, Bryonia, and Pulsatilla. Consult an experienced homeopath.



**CAUTION!**

**Pay attention to sore throats, especially in children. If your child has a severe sore throat without other cold symptoms, accompanied by a fever higher than 101°F, or a milder sore throat that persists for more than two or three days, see a doctor. It may be strep throat, which can be treated with antibiotics.** ■

# ROCKY MOUNTAIN SPOTTED FEVER

## SYMPTOMS

- moderate to high fever with chills.
- abrupt and severe headache.
- aching muscles.
- pinkish spots (about one-eighth inch) beginning around wrists or ankles, and spreading to torso, developing on about the fourth day of fever.
- nausea.
- vomiting.
- loss of appetite.
- fatigue.
- abdominal pain.
- hypersensitivity to light.

## CALL YOUR DOCTOR IF:

- you develop the symptoms above and you know or suspect that you have been bitten by a tick. Rocky Mountain spotted fever is potentially fatal and must be treated promptly with antibiotics. Treatment is much less effective if delayed by more than three days.

Although Rocky Mountain spotted fever (RMSF) was named in the West, this tick-borne illness occurs in most states and is most prevalent in southeast and south-central states. While most cases of RMSF are mild and disappear within two weeks, the disease is fatal in up to 20 percent of patients who are not treated; the elderly are especially vulnerable. For those who are diagnosed within a day or two of the appearance of symptoms, antibiotics provide effective treatment.

RMSF is caused by bacteria that are transmitted by the brown dog tick in the East, the Rocky Mountain wood tick in the West, and the lone star tick in the Southwest. Only adult ticks pass this disease to humans. In most tick populations, 1 to 5 percent of ticks harbor the disease.

A tick may spend up to 24 hours on your clothing before biting. It may then feed for several days before dropping off. Because ticks inject an anesthetic similar to lidocaine into the skin, you seldom feel a tick bite.

Symptoms begin 3 to 10 days after the bite. The rash usually begins as very small pinkish spots that turn white when pressed. Later, a tiny red dot that does not whiten when pressed may form at the center of the rash. Initial spots may merge and darken into purplish patches. If the disease is not treated, you may get chills, abdominal pain, nausea, intense headache, mental confusion, and eventually gangrene (tissue death).

When treatment is delayed more than three days after the first symptoms, the death rate is above 6 percent; when started within three days, it is 1.3 percent. Dark-skinned patients have a higher death rate because the rash may be invisible. At greatest risk are campers, dog owners, foresters, children who play outside, and others who spend time outdoors. Almost all cases occur in spring or early summer; some 1,500 cases occur annually. The disease isn't contagious person-to-person.

## CAUSES

The organism that causes RMSF, *Rickettsia rickettsii,* is released from a tick's salivary glands 6 to 10 hours after the tick begins feeding. The bacteria then invade human blood-vessel cells and in-

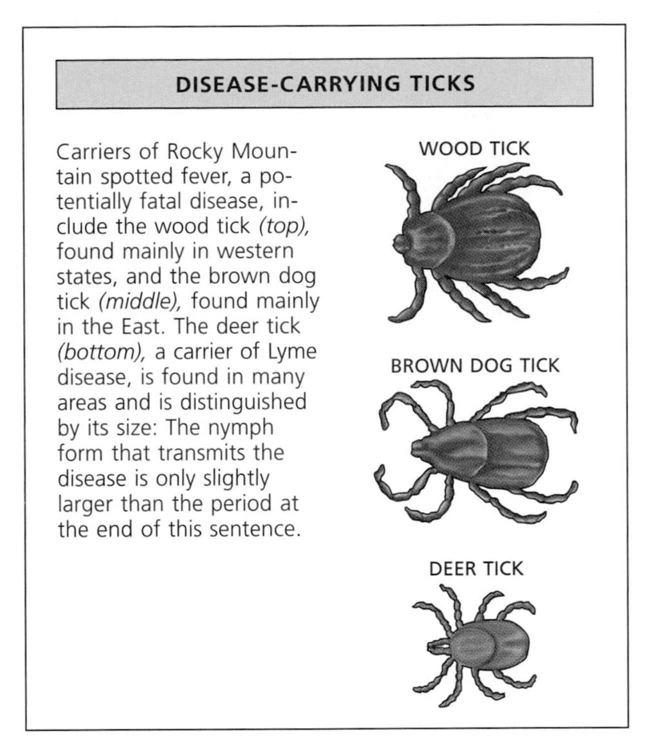


**DISEASE-CARRYING TICKS**

Carriers of Rocky Mountain spotted fever, a potentially fatal disease, include the wood tick *(top)*, found mainly in western states, and the brown dog tick *(middle)*, found mainly in the East. The deer tick *(bottom)*, a carrier of Lyme disease, is found in many areas and is distinguished by its size: The nymph form that transmits the disease is only slightly larger than the period at the end of this sentence.

terfere with blood clotting throughout the body.

The rash, as well as damage to organs and tissues, is caused by leakage of blood from blood vessels. Vulnerable areas include the lungs, gastrointestinal tract, heart, brain, eyes, and kidneys.

### DIAGNOSTIC AND TEST PROCEDURES

In the absence of a known tick bite, RMSF is difficult to diagnose. As many as half of all sufferers do not recall a tick bite. The rash helps distinguish the disease, but it does not appear immediately. Eventually, blood tests that measure antibodies can confirm a diagnosis. But this does not help with early diagnosis, since antibodies are seldom detectable for 10 to 14 days.

During the earliest stage, the rash may be mistaken for measles, but unlike measles, the rash seldom appears on the face.

## TREATMENT

Early identification of the disease is critical. The later the diagnosis, the more difficult it is to control the infection.

### CONVENTIONAL MEDICINE

Most sufferers can be treated with oral tetracycline or doxycycline. Because tetracycline stains developing teeth, pregnant women and patients younger than eight years old may be given oral chloramphenicol, but this treatment may produce anemia and bone-marrow suppression. Symptoms usually begin to subside within 36 to 48 hours.

## PREVENTION

Avoidance, or early removal, of ticks is the best way to prevent RMSF. Take care if you are camping, mowing, gardening, or walking in fields or woods where ticks live. Most ticks live near the ground, so wear shoes and long pants tucked into socks. Spray insect repellent on clothing. Frequent mowing helps suppress tick populations. Inspect ankles, waistline, and hair thoroughly several times a day and at bedtime. Ticks show up best against light-colored clothing, although the color white, heat, and perspiration odor may attract them. Fit your dog or cat with a flea collar.

### REMOVING A TICK

*If you find a tick on your skin, do not rub or crush it, as this may lead to infection. Some physicians advocate coating the tick first with vegetable or mineral oil, kerosene, or alcohol, which may interfere with its breathing and cause its grip to loosen. Others suggest simply grasping the tick with blunt tweezers (or gloved fingers) as close to the mouthparts as possible and pulling gently upward and outward until it lets go. Do not twist or puncture the tick if possible. After removal, disinfect the attachment site and wash your hands in soap and water.* ■

# SCABIES

## SYMPTOMS

- intensely itchy rash with red patches generally located between the fingers, around the wrists, and on the elbows, navel, nipples, lower abdomen, and genitals. The face and scalp are rarely affected.
- pencil-thin lesions that mark where the scabies mites have burrowed into the skin; visible in only about 25 percent of cases.
- itching that is most severe at night.
- scabs that tend to form over scratched areas.

See also the Visual Diagnostic Guide.

## CALL YOUR DOCTOR IF:

- you suspect you have scabies; you and anyone else you may come in direct physical contact with need to be treated with a pediculicide (an insecticide that kills mites and lice).
- your lesions appear to ooze or show other signs of infection; the chief complication of scabies is secondary bacterial infections, especially strep and staph.
- you develop an additional rash or have any other adverse reaction after applying the treatment gamma benzene hexachloride (more commonly known as lindane). In rare instances this pediculicide, especially when applied too liberally, has been shown to damage the central nervous system and even cause death.

The contagious skin disease known as scabies can be traced to the insidious action of the mite *Sarcoptes scabiei*. The primary symptom—incredibly itchy, red lesions—results when the female mite burrows into the skin and deposits eggs and feces. Long considered a problem only of the unclean and poor, scabies is actually quite common at all socioeconomic levels. Closed environments such as nursing homes and childcare centers provide ideal breeding grounds for the parasite, which needs a human host to survive. An estimated 300 million new cases spring up each year worldwide. The number of cases in the United States is currently on the rise, probably because more children under the age of five are being cared for in centers.

## CAUSES

Scabies mites can survive for only two to three days without a human host, but if they do infest you, it can be very difficult to get rid of them. Transmission almost always occurs through direct person-to-person contact. The telltale red, itchy, pencil-thin lesions usually appear two to three weeks after infestation; the sores are caused by the body's allergic reaction to the mites and their feces.

Since the distinguishing burrow lines show in only about 25 percent of patients, you may have to rely on other signals to determine whether you have been infested. If you find yourself overcome with an overwhelming need to scratch particular areas of your body, especially at night, check with your doctor. People with flaking skin disorders, such as eczema and psoriasis, need to be especially vigilant. Because they already tend to have itchy, red skin, they may not notice symptoms until the infestation is widespread.

Contrary to common assumptions, it is highly unlikely that you would contract scabies from your pet; indeed, human skin will not sustain the type of mite often found on dogs, and the pimplelike rash you might get from a canine mite not only is less itchy but may actually clear up on its own.

## TREATMENT

To get rid of scabies, those people who are infected and everyone they came in contact with must be treated at the same time. Since the mites can survive for two or three days on almost any surface, including tables and countertops, toys, and linens, all areas must be thoroughly vacuumed and washed. Items that may be difficult to clean, such as stuffed animals, should be bagged and stored for a week.

There has been some controversy about the dangerous side effects of some pediculicides, which kill mites and lice. Several alternatives exist, including herbal remedies, for those who want a more benign (though also potentially less effective) solution.

### CONVENTIONAL MEDICINE

A bath with soap and hot water will wash away some of the mites and their debris, but this step alone will not get rid of all the parasites. Most doctors prescribe a pediculicide, which you apply to your skin from the neck down. You may need some assistance with this treatment since you must be certain to cover all areas. Leave the lotion on the skin for 8 to 12 hours and then wash it off. Do not reapply the lotion without your physician's approval.

Gamma benzene hexachloride was at one time the most commonly prescribed pediculicide, but if used improperly, it can attack and permanently damage the central nervous system. Multiple applications, especially in young children, have led to brain damage, paralysis, and seizures. In 1990 the FDA approved the use of permethrin, a cream that works well against scabies without the potent side effects. Permethrin has quickly become the treatment of choice of most dermatologists.

After you rid your skin of mites, you can take an antihistamine for the itch (which can still rage for days after treatment because of feces left in the burrows) and apply corticosteroid creams to reduce inflammation.

### ALTERNATIVE CHOICES

Like their conventional counterparts, many alternative remedies for eradicating scabies mites are potent and even toxic if taken internally, but many herbs do offer safe relief from itching and inflammation. If mites return after you try an herbal parasiticide, you may want to use the more conventional preparations. The longer the parasites live in your skin, the greater your risk of infection.

#### HERBAL THERAPIES

Larkspur *(Consolida regalis),* the most effective herbal parasiticide, is poisonous if taken internally. Consult an herbalist for treatment.

#### HOMEOPATHY

For relief of itching, try taking Sulphur (6x) every eight hours for up to three days.

### AT-HOME REMEDIES

- To relieve itching, add a cup of oatmeal or cornstarch or a pinch of chickweed to your bath; soak in hot water and scrub with soap, but avoid overscrubbing, which can lead to a skin condition called eczematous scabies.
- Rubbing lavender *(Lavandula officinalis)* oil into your sores can also help relieve itching.

## PREVENTION

The best way to prevent getting scabies is to avoid contact with the mite. For some people, especially those who work in hospitals, day-care centers, and other crowded conditions, that may be difficult. If you contract the parasite, take basic steps to avoid reinfection and infecting others:

- Apply a pediculicide from the neck down and leave it on for at least eight hours; ensure anyone who had physical contact with you also applies it, even if they do not show symptoms.
- Wash all linens, towels, and clothes in hot water; store stuffed animals and other hard-to-wash items in bags for at least a week.
- Wash all tables, chairs, and floors, and vacuum all rugs. ■

# SCARLET FEVER

## SYMPTOMS

Scarlet fever occurs most frequently in children. Its symptoms include:

- bright red or scarlet rash, usually beginning on the neck or chest.
- high fever.
- sore throat.
- tongue coated with red spots.
- swollen glands in neck.
- vomiting.

## CALL YOUR DOCTOR IF:

- your child develops symptoms of scarlet fever, especially if the child has recently had strep throat. Left untreated, scarlet fever may have serious complications affecting the heart, kidneys, and other organs.

Scarlet fever is one of those childhood diseases that have been tamed by antibiotics. Once a common and dangerous illness, today it is rare and easily managed.

The disease occurs mostly in children between the ages of 2 and 10. After an incubation period of two to five days, it typically starts with a very high fever of up to 104°F. Anywhere from 12 to 48 hours later, a distinctive scarlet rash appears, first on the neck and chest and then all over the body. The rash feels like sandpaper and is most prevalent above the armpits and at the groin. The tongue also becomes swollen and turns bright red. After three days the rash and fever usually disappear, but the tongue may remain swollen for several more days.

Unlike certain other childhood diseases such as German measles and measles, scarlet fever cannot be left to run its course; it must be treated or it can lead to arthritis, jaundice, kidney problems, and rheumatic fever.

## CAUSES

Scarlet fever is a contagious infection that is caused by streptococcal bacteria and spread by contact with an infected person or inhalation of the bacteria. Once inside the pharynx or throat, the bacteria multiply and produce a toxin that circulates in the blood and causes the symptoms.

### DIAGNOSTIC AND TEST PROCEDURES

Your pediatrician will inspect your child's throat, take a culture, and examine it for the presence of streptococcal bacteria.

## TREATMENT

Unless treated with antibiotics, scarlet fever can have serious complications. Call your pediatrician immediately if you think your child has the disease. Along with taking antibiotics, your child

## CAUTION!

**Although scarlet fever is easily controlled with antibiotics, it may lead to serious complications if left untreated. Be sure to see your doctor or pediatrician without delay if you think your child may have contracted scarlet fever.**

should get plenty of bed rest and drink lots of fruit juice to flush out his system. Cool baths may reduce the fever, and acetaminophen will help relieve pain. Caution: Don't use aspirin, which has been associated with Reye's syndrome, a sometimes fatal brain disease whose cause is unknown.

### CONVENTIONAL MEDICINE

Your pediatrician will prescribe an antibiotic, such as penicillin. If your child is allergic to penicillin, he'll be given an alternative, such as erythromycin. The medicine must be taken for at least 10 days, even if the symptoms disappear sooner. Other family members should also be examined and treated if necessary. Before the advent of antibiotics, households were quarantined because of scarlet fever, but this is no longer necessary.

### ALTERNATIVE CHOICES

A child with scarlet fever must take an antibiotic to kill the infection. Alternative therapies may be used together with antibiotics to accelerate healing and reduce discomfort.

#### ACUPRESSURE

Ask a qualified practitioner to recommend acupressure massages that will boost your child's immune system and will also help fight the infection more quickly.

#### AROMATHERAPY

For scarlet fever, aromatherapists recommend inhaling the vapors of eucalyptus *(Eucalyptus globulus)* oil, which may help antibiotics destroy bacteria. Place a few drops on a handkerchief and inhale through your nose.

#### CHINESE HERBS

A practitioner of Chinese medicine may prescribe an herbal formula to eliminate toxins and strengthen your child's ability to fight off disease.

#### HERBAL THERAPIES

Catnip (*Nepeta cataria*) contains chemicals that are thought to reduce fever. Herbalists recommend taking 2 or 3 drops of the extract in a glass of water three times a day.

Echinacea (*Echinacea* spp.) may help combat the bacteria, ease the rash, and help clear chest congestion. After your child's fever has abated, give him a tea three times a day made with 2 tsp of the powdered root simmered in 1 cup of water for 15 minutes.

#### HOMEOPATHY

A homeopath may prescribe a remedy to help your child fight off the infection and heal faster. Homeopathic remedies to treat scarlet fever may include Ferrum phosphoricum (for sore throat and shivering associated with early stages of scarlet fever) and Kali muriaticum (for skin rash and white tongue).

#### NUTRITION AND DIET

Proper nutrition boosts the body's immune system and helps it fight infection. If your child becomes ill, make sure he drinks plenty of fluids to help flush out toxins and prevent dehydration. Citrus juices are a good choice.

## PREVENTION

- Stay away and keep your child away from people who have scarlet fever.
- Stay healthy by eating balanced meals and getting plenty of sleep and exercise. ■

# SCHIZOPHRENIA

## SYMPTOMS

A diagnosis of schizophrenia is considered when a person experiences at least two of the following symptoms:

- delusions.
- hallucinations.
- disorganized speech.
- irrational or catatonic behavior, such as stupor, rigidity, or floppiness of limbs.
- negative symptoms, such as inaction, silence, loss of will.

These symptoms are usually accompanied by a substantial decrease in the ability to interact with others.

## CALL YOUR DOCTOR IF:

- you or someone you know experiences the above symptoms. Schizophrenia can be a devastating disorder, and medical care is vital. Be aware that it may not be easy to persuade someone who is becoming mentally ill to acknowledge symptoms or see a physician.

While schizophrenia literally means "split mind," it should not be confused with a "split," or multiple, personality. It is more accurately described as a psychosis—a cluster of severe and prolonged mental disturbances that disrupt normal thought, speech, and behavior.

The onset of schizophrenia is usually characterized by the psychotic symptoms listed at left or by bizarre behavior. But many patients show "negative" symptoms, such as decreased emotional arousal, mental activity, and social drive.

It is seldom useful to talk about subcategories, such as paranoid schizophrenia or catatonic schizophrenia, since individual patients commonly exhibit a variety of symptoms and therapists make different diagnoses. But most schizophrenics do share a range of similar symptoms. For example, they often report a sense of strangeness and confusion about the source of their sensations. They feel great loneliness, anxiety, and an overwhelming sense of being disconnected from others.

A schizophrenic person may think and communicate by private rules, jumping from one idea to another, using vague or repetitive words, or mixing a "word salad" of new words or jumbled phrases. It is common for schizophrenics to be suspicious and resentful. They may sense that their thoughts are stolen, broadcast, or replaced by new information from strangers seeking to control their behavior. They may describe voices that speak directly to them or criticize their behavior.

Schizophrenia normally appears in men when they are in their teens, and in women in their twenties, but the prevalence is about the same. About 1 in 100 people will be treated at some time for schizophrenia. Some patients experience only a single episode and remain symptom free afterward. More commonly, the course of illness fluctuates over several decades, with each recurrence leading to increasing impairment.

## CAUSES

Most specialists agree that symptoms are provoked by chemical disturbances of brain function, but no exact mechanism is known. Schizophrenia seems to be a syndrome of multiple causes and types. Genetics seems to play a role, but there is no single "schizophrenia gene." While it is clear that a supportive family can be helpful in preventing relapse, it is also agreed that family strife does not cause schizophrenia.

## TREATMENT

The goals of conventional treatment include helping patients toward normal interactions with others, enabling patients to live in the community, and controlling the illness through the smallest effective dosage of medication. A combination of medication and psychotherapy is usually required.

### CONVENTIONAL MEDICINE

The modern era of medical treatment for schizophrenia began in 1952 with the use of the tranquilizer chlorpromazine. This drug (and modern relatives like haloperidol) for the first time controlled acute symptoms, reduced hospitalization from years to days, and lowered the rate of relapse by more than 50 percent. However, not everyone responds to these drugs. Long-term control is less successful than short-term alleviation. Also, prolonged medication may bring harmful side effects, especially the neurological muscle disorder known as tardive dyskinesia (TD), which causes involuntary facial movements, such as grimacing and sucking motions.

Clozapine, approved in the U.S. in 1990, has been helping many people unresponsive to other antipsychotic medications without causing TD; it does, however, cause a serious decline in white blood cells in 1 percent of patients, so weekly blood tests are required. A new drug, risperidone, appears to relieve symptoms without this complication. For most patients, lifelong use of antianxiety drugs is necessary to prevent relapse. Additional drugs, such as antidepressants, may be used to treat side effects or related symptoms, including stiffness, tremors, and depression.

Psychotherapy by itself is of little value without medication. However, supportive and sympathetic psychotherapy is needed to help the patient diagnosed with schizophrenia understand the disease and reenter society and family life.

### ALTERNATIVE CHOICES

Because schizophrenia is such a serious and complex disorder, few therapies are known to be effective. However, research interest in schizophrenia has grown rapidly in recent years.

#### NUTRITION AND DIET

There is some good evidence that folic acid (a B-complex vitamin) is helpful as an adjunct to treatment. Also, vitamin C raises the potency of the antipsychotic haloperidol, and vitamin E may relieve the symptoms of tardive dyskinesia, especially in its early stages. More controversial is the possibility that zinc, manganese, and niacin are of benefit.

### HELP FOR THE SCHIZOPHRENIC

*Accepting, nonjudging friends and relatives can help reduce anxiety and the severity of symptoms. Schizophrenics tend to be easily upset by "expressed emotion"; researchers advise family members to reduce criticism and to be as unobtrusive as possible.*

*Also, sympathetic family members who encourage patients to be active in their own care can help reduce the sense of helplessness. Patients who are in a supportive environment are more likely to accept their medication and to avoid relapses.*

*Some patients react better to a certain drug, or simply prefer its "feel." It is important to respond to these preferences when possible, and to reinforce efforts toward independence.* ■

# SCIATICA

## SYMPTOMS

- pain radiating through your buttock, down the back of your thigh and leg, often to your foot. The pain can be sharp or dull, shooting or burning, intermittent or continuous. It usually affects just one side of the body. Coughing, sneezing, bending, or lifting may make it worse.
- in some cases, numbness and weakness of the affected area.

## CALL YOUR DOCTOR IF:

- the pain is severe and doesn't respond to over-the-counter analgesics; your physician may prescribe a stronger painkiller and other therapy.
- the pain persists for more than three or four days and is accompanied by leg or foot weakness; this may indicate a more serious neurological problem.

Sciatica, characterized by pain radiating into one or both buttocks and descending the back of the leg, results from compression of the sciatic nerve at the base of the spine. This nerve (one for each side of the lower body) is the longest in the peripheral nervous system, extending through the buttocks and down as far as the foot. The pain can occur along its entire length.

## CAUSES

Pressure on a sciatic nerve may be due to poor posture, muscle strain, pregnancy, being overweight, wearing high heels, or sleeping on a too-soft mattress. It can also result from a slipped disk *(see Pinched Nerve, Back Problems, and Disk Problems)* or inflammation of the sciatic nerve, in some cases caused by osteoarthritis *(see Arthritis).*

### DIAGNOSTIC AND TEST PROCEDURES

Your doctor may use the so-called straight-leg-raising test—lifting your leg to a 45-degree angle—to help locate the point of pain. Other tests include an x-ray, or an MRI or CT scan.

## TREATMENT

### CONVENTIONAL MEDICINE

Your physician may prescribe muscle relaxants, nonsteroidal anti-inflammatory drugs (NSAIDs), systemic painkillers, narcotics, or corticosteroids. Physical therapy is often recommended, once acute inflammation and pain have subsided. A nutritionist may suggest daily doses of the amino acid DL-phenylalanine taken every other week to help alleviate pain.

### ALTERNATIVE CHOICES

#### BODY WORK

The **Alexander technique,** a system of posture retraining, can teach correct methods of sitting, standing, and moving to prevent future attacks.

S

#### CHIROPRACTIC
Soft-tissue and vertebral manipulation may reduce pressure on a sciatic nerve.

#### HERBAL THERAPIES
Teas made from white willow *(Salix alba)* bark or meadowsweet *(Filipendula ulmaria)* may relieve joint pain; try black cohosh *(Cimicifuga racemosa)* for muscle spasms.

#### HOMEOPATHY
For stiffness that is worse in the morning and at night but improves with heat, try Rhus toxicodendron. For severe shooting pain extending from your lower back to your ankles that worsens with motion, consider Bryonia. Consult a practitioner for proper dosages and courses of treatment.

#### NUTRITION
High doses of calcium (1,000 mg) and magnesium (400 mg) at bedtime, along with vitamin C (500 mg), may be beneficial. Taking 50 mg of vitamin $B_6$ three times a day for one week only may also help. Consult a nutritionist for further guidance on taking supplements.

#### OSTEOPATHY
Slipped disks might benefit from the soft-tissue massage and positioning that osteopaths use to relieve pressure on the sciatic nerve. Consult an osteopath if your sciatica is associated with a strain or muscle injury and improves with exercise but is unrelieved by rest.

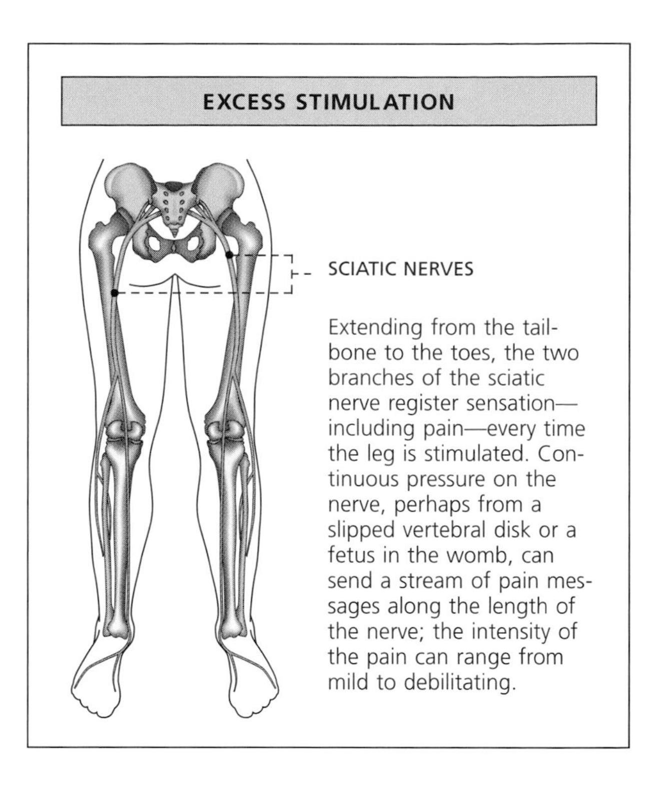


**EXCESS STIMULATION**

Extending from the tailbone to the toes, the two branches of the sciatic nerve register sensation—including pain—every time the leg is stimulated. Continuous pressure on the nerve, perhaps from a slipped vertebral disk or a fetus in the womb, can send a stream of pain messages along the length of the nerve; the intensity of the pain can range from mild to debilitating.

### AT-HOME REMEDIES
The following remedies might help reduce pain.

- Apply ice to the affected area for 30 to 60 minutes as soon as pain starts. Do this several times a day for two or three days. Thereafter, apply a hot-water bottle at the same intervals.
- Try the following self-massage technique: Lie on your back with your knees bent; relax for several minutes; take a sock containing two soft rubber balls and position them on either side of your spine in the small of your back; allow your body weight to sink into the floor, over the balls. Remove the balls and relax for a few more minutes. Follow the same procedure for your buttocks. If you're having disk problems, check with your doctor before attempting this technique.
- During periods of acute pain, don't pick up anything heavier than 10 pounds, and take the weight of lifted objects in your bent legs and arms, not in your back. Push rather than pull heavy objects.

## PREVENTION

- Sleep on a firm mattress on your back or side with your knees bent; avoid sleeping on your stomach. During acute attacks only, sleep with a pillow under or between your knees.
- Adjust the height of your chair so your feet are flat on the floor and your knees are a little higher than your hips; make a habit of sitting with both feet flat on the floor instead of crossing your legs.
- Make sure your chair has firm back support, and sit with your back straight against it. ■

# SCOLIOSIS

## SYMPTOMS

Scoliosis, an abnormal sideways curvature of the spine, may be present if, looking from the rear:

- the entire body seems to tilt to one side.
- the shoulders appear uneven, with one shoulder blade more prominent than the other.
- one leg seems longer than the other.
- the hips appear to be at uneven heights or look as if they have shifted to the right or the left.
- the back looks crooked on bending forward.
- from the front the ribs appear more prominent and spaced more widely apart on one side than the other.

## CALL YOUR DOCTOR IF:

- you see any of the symptoms described above. Be especially vigilant if you have a family history of scoliosis. The condition may worsen over time and must be evaluated and treated by a physician in order to arrest its progress.

Scoliosis is a progressive lateral, or sideways, curvature of the spine. People with scoliosis have backs that take on a distinct C- or S-shaped curve that deviates markedly from the normal vertical alignment of the spine *(right)*. Scoliosis is sometimes present at birth, although it most often appears between the ages of 10 and 14, becoming increasingly severe as the child grows. The disorder occurs in both boys and girls but tends to be more serious and progress more dramatically in females.

Because scoliosis itself does not generally cause pain, it is sometimes referred to as a "silent" condition. However, if untreated, it may eventually cause painful secondary problems such as disk problems, sciatica, or arthritis. In severe cases, the torso may become so twisted and distorted that the heart and lungs are affected, causing chronic fatigue and shortness of breath.

## CAUSES

The causes of scoliosis are poorly understood. Doctors suspect that there is a genetic component to scoliosis, although the cause of most cases is unknown. Children who have suffered from diseases of the muscles, bones, or nervous system, such as polio or cerebral palsy, may also develop scoliosis. And in both children and adults, scoliosis may occur following traumatic injuries such as a fractured back, or as a result of conditions that affect the nervous system.

## TREATMENT

The standard treatments for scoliosis are exercise, orthopedic bracing, and in severe cases, surgery. For the most part, bracing can only halt the progress of the condition rather than correct any curvature that has already occurred; so it is important to begin early. Scoliosis generally progresses most rapidly during early adolescence, when a youngster's bones are growing at their peak rate. The earlier a child develops scoliosis, the more extensive the curvature will be if it is left untreated.

CURVATURE OF THE SPINE

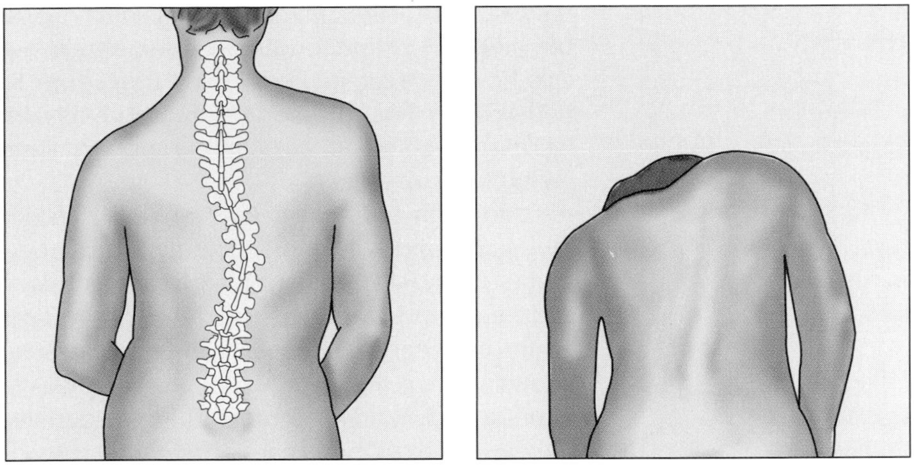

Scoliosis, or sideways curvature of the spine, distorts the carriage of the shoulders and hips by forcing the spine out of its normal alignment *(above, left)*. One shoulder rises higher than normal, while the opposite hip is more prominent. On bending forward *(above, right)*, the back may appear to have a hump on the side of the affected shoulder.

## CONVENTIONAL MEDICINE

The treatment a doctor prescribes for scoliosis depends on the patient's degree of spinal curvature. A mild curve of less than 25 degrees can usually be controlled by an exercise program designed to strengthen the torso. Orthopedic body braces, molded to fit the individual's torso and hold it erect, are usually prescribed to manage curves of 25 to 30 degrees or greater. For children and adolescents, the brace is adjusted as the patient grows. It is worn until the skeleton stops growing—at around 16 in most girls and 17 to 18 in most boys.

Curves of 40 degrees or more may call for surgery. Typically, metal rods are implanted alongside the spine, providing an internal splint that corrects the curve. The surgeon also fuses several vertebrae together to straighten and immobilize that section of the spine.

## ALTERNATIVE CHOICES

The only proven means of treating scoliosis is conventional medical therapy. There is no reliable evidence to show that alternative methods such as acupressure, acupuncture, or manipulation by a chiropractor or osteopath will control progressive spinal curvature. However, such treatments may reduce the discomfort of muscular pain or disk problems.

## AT-HOME CARE

Consistent long-term care is essential in treating scoliosis. Patients must exercise conscientiously, and those who wear a brace must stick to the prescribed schedule for its use. Typically, a brace is worn 23 hours a day and removed only for bathing and physical therapy—requirements that youngsters find particularly onerous. To help a child cope with a brace, try the following:

- Enlist family, friends, and teachers to provide emotional support.
- Seek the assistance of physicians, orthopedic surgeons, and physical therapists in developing an appropriate exercise program. Encourage your child to engage in activities such as running, fast walking, and dance, all of which can be done while wearing the brace. Exercise won't correct the curvature, but it will improve your child's overall health and muscle tone.
- Watch carefully for signs of chafing and skin breakdown. Have your child wear a snug T-shirt under the brace and use rubbing alcohol to toughen skin that comes in contact with the frame. ■

S

# SEASONAL AFFECTIVE DISORDER

## SYMPTOMS

Some or all of these symptoms are present during the fall and winter. Occasionally, seasonal affective disorder (SAD) occurs in summer, but with diminished rather than increased eating or sleeping symptoms.

- depression, difficulty enjoying life, pessimism about the future.
- loss of energy, inertia, apathy.
- increased sleep, difficulty getting up in the morning.
- impaired functioning: difficulty getting to work on time; tasks that are normally easy seem impossible.
- increased appetite, weight gain.
- carbohydrate cravings.
- desire to avoid people.
- irritability, crying spells.
- decreased sex drive.
- suicidal thoughts or feelings.

**For children and adolescents:**

- feeling tired and irritable.
- temper tantrums.
- difficulty concentrating.
- vague physical complaints.
- marked cravings for junk food.

## CALL YOUR DOCTOR IF:

- you or your child suffers some of these symptoms with the onset of fall and winter and they seem to diminish or dissipate as spring and summer approach.

Seasonal affective disorder (SAD) is an extreme form of the "winter blues," bringing lethargy and curtailing normal functioning. It was only recently recognized as a specific disorder, but since 1982 much has been learned about it and how to treat it. People suffering from SAD undergo extreme differences in mood, as if they were split between a "summer person" and a "winter person."

Although a different kind of SAD can occur in the summer, its most common form begins gradually in late August or early September and continues until March or early April, when the symptoms begin to dissipate. Sufferers have been known to increase their sleep by as many as four hours a night and gain more than 20 pounds as they attempt to "hibernate" the winter away.

Research suggests that SAD may affect 11 million people in the United States each year, and that an additional 25 million suffer a milder form that is indeed called the winter blues. Four times as many women suffer from SAD as men, and it tends to run in families.

As might be expected, geographical location plays the largest role in susceptibility to SAD; the nearer one lives to one of the poles, the greater the incidence. People in Canada or the northern United States are eight times more likely to fall victim to SAD than those living in sunny southern areas like Florida or Mexico.

## CAUSES

Researchers are still far from agreement about the precise cause of SAD and suggest it may have more than one cause. Currently, the most likely explanation involves the neurotransmitter serotonin, which during the short days of winter reaches its lowest concentrations in key parts of the brain, causing depression. Whatever the chemical constituents, SAD is triggered by inadequate outdoor light and exacerbated by stress.

For children, the fall onset of SAD comes at the time that school starts, and it is difficult to sort out SAD from other possible reasons for mood changes. Often overlooked by doctors and parents, SAD should be considered a possibility.

### DIAGNOSTIC AND TEST PROCEDURES

Because no laboratory test exists for SAD, diagnosis is made on the basis of the patient's history and should be made by a psychiatrist experienced with the disorder. Illnesses with similar symptoms that must be ruled out are underactive thyroid function, chronic viral infections, and chronic fatigue syndrome. In children, abuse and separation anxiety should also be considered, and in adolescents, substance abuse and anxiety disorder.

## TREATMENT

The most effective treatment for SAD is light therapy, sometimes combined with antidepressant drugs or psychotherapy or both.

### CONVENTIONAL MEDICINE

**Light therapy** can be used in different ways and may employ different types of light boxes, light visors, and lamps. All are designed to bring in extra light to the eyes. Check to be sure a light box filters out harmful ultraviolet light.

In the most common form of light therapy, you sit before a light box of strong fluorescent light (10,000 lux—about 10 to 20 times brighter than ordinary indoor light) for periods varying from 15 minutes to 1½ hours a day. You place the box on a table or desk where you can do paperwork, read, or make phone calls.

Other light sources include larger boxes that stand on the floor, visors with lights attached, and dawn simulators—lights programmed to turn on by your bed on winter mornings before dawn.

Light boxes can be bought for several hundred dollars at special stores. Experts warn against constructing your own light box because of possible damage from ultraviolet light.

Since SAD is a form of depression, many different types of antidepressants have been used. The preferred drugs at the present time are the selective serotonin reuptake inhibitors (SSRIs), because they regulate the brain levels of serotonin and have fewer side effects than many other antidepressants.

### ALTERNATIVE CHOICES

Exercise and many other mind/body therapies for depression can be helpful with SAD. **Massage** may also be a useful adjunct to other therapies. Try three or four massage sessions to see if it works; one session is not enough to judge.

For many centuries, healers believed that certain electrical emissions in the atmosphere—negative ions—improve a person's mood and health. In the last 30 years, scientists have developed small devices that emit negative ions into the atmosphere of a room. The negative ionizer seems particularly helpful for people with SAD (one study showed a 58 percent reduction of depression) and may be a good supplement to light therapy and medications.

#### NUTRITION AND DIET

People with SAD are apt to overeat in the winter, with special cravings for sweets and starches. One SAD expert recommends that patients avoid snacking on carbohydrate-rich foods and instead recommends balancing carbohydrates with protein or restricting carbohydrate-rich food to a single balanced meal a day.

### AT-HOME REMEDIES

- Take a walk at lunchtime when the sun is high. Be outdoors as often as you can.
- Exercise as much as you are able.
- Take winter vacations in places with long days.
- Increase the natural light in your home by trimming low-lying branches near the house and hedges around windows.
- Paint your walls with lighter colors.
- Keep warm and enjoy the fun aspects of winter—such as wood fires, books, music.
- If all else fails and you can manage it, move to a sunnier climate. ■

# SEXUAL DYSFUNCTION

## SYMPTOMS

Sexual dysfunction is broadly defined as the inability to fully enjoy sexual intercourse.

**For men, you may have a sexual problem if you:**

- ejaculate before you or your partner desires (premature ejaculation).
- do not ejaculate, or ejaculation is delayed (retarded ejaculation).
- are unable to have an erection sufficient for pleasurable intercourse; see Impotence.
- feel pain during intercourse.
- lack or lose sexual desire.

**For women, you may have a sexual problem if you:**

- lack or lose sexual desire.
- have difficulty achieving orgasm.
- feel anxiety during intercourse.
- feel pain during intercourse.
- feel vaginal or other muscles contract involuntarily before or during sex.
- have inadequate lubrication.

## CALL YOUR DOCTOR IF:

**you or your partner has**

- concerns about your sexual life.
- pain during intercourse. This may indicate infection or illness.
- been exposed to chemicals or sexually transmitted diseases.
- been sexually abused or assaulted.
- a prolonged erection unaccompanied by sexual desire. This condition, called priapism, is serious and requires immediate medical attention.

For couples of any age, sexual dysfunction—the inability of both partners to fully enjoy sexual intercourse—can be an obstacle not only to having children but also to maintaining a positive and loving relationship. Problems of this kind are common, affecting more than half of all couples at some time, according to some studies. While sexual dysfunction rarely threatens physical health, it can take a heavy psychological toll, bringing on depression, anxiety, and debilitating feelings of inadequacy. Problems may be difficult to resolve without expert help, especially because misinformation is one of the leading causes of sexual dysfunction.

One example of misinformation is that impotence is an unavoidable consequence of aging. In reality, healthy men can enjoy sexual intimacy well into their senior years. Achieving an erection may take 5 to 15 minutes of genital stimulation, however.

Another erroneous belief is that women have no interest in sex after a hysterectomy. Although there may be a decrease in vaginal lubrication if the ovaries are removed along with the uterus, libido (the sex drive) remains intact—and, because any worries about pregnancy are gone, it may even increase.

As people live longer and attitudes change, more older couples desire to prolong the years of healthy sexuality. Sex in old age was at one time thought to be inappropriate and even immoral; now, both physical and emotional intimacy are seen as important to well-being throughout life. Although sexual desire and the frequency of intercourse decline with age, sexual enjoyment and satisfaction do not. For couples in good health, sexual activity, which includes touching and caressing, may continue into the eighties and even nineties.

Sexual dysfunction takes different forms in men and women.

**Men:** In the male partner of a couple, dysfunction is often associated with anxiety. If a man operates under the misconception that all sexual activity must lead to intercourse and to orgasm by his partner, and if the expectation is not met, he may consider the act a failure. Such an attitude can be a self-fulfilling prophecy.

The most prevalent physical dysfunction in men is premature ejaculation, in which orgasm occurs before or immediately after the penis enters the vagina. This problem, especially common among young men, can lead to performance anxiety, frustration for one's partner, doubts about one's masculinity, and perhaps impotence—itself a common dysfunction.

A more unusual problem is retarded ejaculation, in which orgasm is delayed so long that it satisfies neither partner. A few men experience retrograde ejaculation—in which the semen, rather than emerging from the end of the penis, moves backward into the bladder during orgasm. Rarer still is priapism, a prolonged erection unaccompanied by sexual desire. This condition is potentially dangerous and requires prompt medical attention.

**Women:** The inability to experience sexual pleasure, known as arousal dysfunction, is one of the most common dysfunctions for a woman. It is difficult to treat and should be discussed with a professional, as well as with her partner.

Some women become aroused but are unable to achieve an orgasm. The fact is that only about one in three women reaches a climax regularly through intercourse alone, without additional stimulation of the clitoris. About 10 percent of women never achieve orgasm. But it is possible and even common to have a pleasurable sex life without orgasm. Lack of orgasm might be considered a dysfunction only if it represents a change or causes anxiety.

Pain during intercourse (dyspareunia) can occur for a variety of reasons, from a simple anatomical problem or vaginal infection to complex and deep-rooted fears, and it can increase at the time of menopause, when there is decreased lubrication of the vagina. If pain persists, it may cause vaginal muscles to contract involuntarily before intercourse, a response known as vaginismus. In some women, this contraction is triggered by the knowledge that sexual activity is about to begin .

Homosexual men and women are also at risk for sexual dysfunction. Knowledge about AIDS, the difficulties of striving for "safer sex," and the psychological effects of discrimination are just a few of the factors that can give rise to anxieties that depress sexual function.

## CAUSES

Many factors, of both physical and psychological natures, can affect sexual response and performance. Injuries, ailments, and drugs are among the physical influences; in addition, there is increasing evidence that chemicals and other environmental pollutants depress sexual function. As for psychological factors, sexual dysfunction may have roots in traumatic events such as rape or incest, guilt feelings, a poor self-image, depression, chronic fatigue, certain religious beliefs, or marital problems.

**Men:** With premature ejaculation, physical causes are rare—although the problem is sometimes linked to a neurological disorder, prostate infection, or urethritis. Possible psychological causes include anxiety, guilt feelings about sex, and ambivalence toward women.

When men experience painful intercourse, the cause is usually physical—an infection of the prostate, urethra, or testes, or an allergic reaction to spermicide or condoms. Infections can be initiated by sexually transmitted diseases, such as chlamydia and genital herpes. Painful erections may be caused by Peyronie's disease, fibrous plaques on the upper side of the penis that often produce a bend during erection. Cancer of the penis or testis and arthritis of the lower back can also cause pain.

Retrograde ejaculation occurs in men who have had prostate or urethral surgery, take medication that keeps the bladder open, or suffer from diabetes—a disease that can injure the nerves that normally close the bladder during ejaculation.

**Women:** Dysfunctions of arousal and orgasm may have similar causes. They can be physical (drugs, illness, hormonal deficiencies, gynecologic factors, inadequate stimulation) or psychological (stress, fatigue, depression, performance anxiety, relationship problems). Among the most common are day-to-day discord with one's partner and inadequate stimulation by the partner. Finally, sexual desire can wane as one ages, although this varies greatly from person to person.

Pain during intercourse can occur for any number of reasons, and location is sometimes a clue to the cause. Pain in the vaginal area may be due to infection, such as urethritis; also, vaginal tissues may become thinner and more sensitive during breast-feeding and after menopause. Deeper pain may have a pelvic source, such as endometriosis, pelvic adhesions, or uterine abnormalities. Pain can also have a psychological cause, such as fear of injury, guilt feelings about sex, fear of pregnancy or injury to the fetus during pregnancy, or recollection of a previous painful experience.

Vaginismus may be provoked by these psychological causes as well. Or it may begin as a response to pain, and continue after the pain is gone. Both partners should understand that the vaginal contraction is an involuntary response, outside the woman's control.

Similarly, insufficient lubrication is involuntary, and may be part of a complex cycle: Low sexual response may lead to inadequate lubrication, which may lead to discomfort and then an even worse response, and so on.

## TREATMENT

No matter which partner experiences a sexual dysfunction, it is important for both to understand it. Both may contribute to the problem—and to the solution.

**Men:** Premature ejaculation is commonly curbed by the "squeeze" technique, a kind of biofeedback. This method has a high success rate, and repeated practice usually leads to better natural control. When you feel that orgasm is imminent, withdraw from the woman's vagina, or signal her to stop stimulation. You (or she) then squeezes gently on the head of the penis with the thumb and forefinger, halting the climax. After 20 or 30 seconds, begin lovemaking again. After several cycles, proceed to ejaculation.

Note that premature ejaculation may signal a more complex disorder whose psychological aspects should be explored in therapy. To rely only on physical control may mask the symptom without resolving the cause.

Retarded ejaculation is often treated by reducing anxiety and learning to control the timing of ejaculation. The sensate focus exercises described in the box at the end of this entry may help; you should withhold penetration until you sense that ejaculation is inevitable.

Retrograde ejaculation may be corrected through surgery that allows the valve at the base of the bladder to close. But it is basically a harmless disorder, causing a problem chiefly if children are desired; in such situations, it may be possible to retrieve sperm from the bladder for artificial insemination *(see Infertility)*.

When a man lacks sexual desire, the cause may be physical illness, hormonal abnormality, or medications that affect libido. There may also be psychological causes, including depression or interpersonal problems, which a therapist may help identify.

**Women:** Arousal problems may be difficult to resolve if sexual satisfaction has never been experienced. Therapies are designed to help the patient relax, become aware of feelings about sex, and eliminate guilt and fear of rejection. The sensate focus exercises described at the end of this entry may also help.

In postmenopausal women, scant lubrication can easily be corrected with over-the-counter vaginal lubricants, egg white, or saliva. (Keep in mind that oil-based products can cause infection, however.) Inadequate lubrication in a healthy, premenopausal woman may reflect either a muted sexual response or inadequate arousal by the partner. Explore feelings about sex and seek to eliminate guilt and fear of rejection. Extended foreplay, masturbation, and relaxation techniques may help.

For inability to achieve orgasm, the communication of your desires about sexual foreplay and intercourse to your partner is an essential first step toward satisfaction. Although such treatments as experiential therapy, psychoanalysis, or behavior modification can be beneficial, you must realize that orgasms (let alone simultaneous orgasms) are not necessary to a good sexual relationship.

For pain during intercourse, first make sure there is adequate stimulation and lubrication. A physical exam may reveal a need to medicate for infection, remove scars around the hymen, or gently stretch painful scars at the vaginal opening. Endometriosis and pelvic adhesions can often be treated by laser to relieve so-called deep pain. Problems related to menopausal change may be relieved with **hormone replacement therapy** *(see Menopausal Problems).* If pain persists, psychotherapy may uncover hidden fears about intercourse. Sensate focus exercises can teach appropriate foreplay and de-emphasize intercourse until both partners are ready. Education can reduce fears of pregnancy or of harm to the fetus.

Vaginismus is difficult to reverse without help. The vaginismus support group, Resolve, recommends psychotherapy or group therapy. If you have a partner, seek therapy together in a safe and supportive environment. To accustom your body to the feeling of penetration, a therapist may recommend inserting a series of vaginal dilators, each slightly larger than the last. You advance at your own pace until you are comfortable inserting a dilator the size of your partner's erection. Contraction and relaxation exercises can teach control of the vaginal muscles and increase sexual responsiveness. Psychotherapy may also increase desire, improve communication skills, and resolve underlying conflicts about sexuality. With therapy and a supportive partner, the improvement rate is good.

## ALTERNATIVE CHOICES

Some problems with sexual function are normal. For example, women starting a new or first relationship may feel sore or bruised after intercourse; use an over-the-counter lubricant or egg white. For relaxation, soak in a warm bath; add 5 drops of essential oil of lavender or clary.

**Yoga** and **meditation** provide needed mental and physical relaxation for several conditions, such as vaginismus. **Relaxation** facilitates therapy and relieves anxiety about the dysfunction. **Massage** is extremely effective at reducing stress, especially if performed by the partner.

### SENSATE FOCUS EXERCISES

*The following exercises are valuable not only for dysfunction but also for revitalizing sexual interest and renewing sexuality following a period of inactivity. Remain in each focus area until you are satisfied.*

***Focus 1.*** *With the partners taking turns, one is totally receptive for about 15 minutes while the other explores, stimulates, and caresses all parts of the body except genital areas and breasts. The manual stimulation should range from light touch to stroking and rubbing. Lips or other parts of the body may also be used.*

***Focus 2.*** *Continue the various forms of stimulation and expand them to include the genital areas and breasts. The receptive partner should provide feedback on what is most pleasurable. Oral-genital contact is permitted, but hold back from penetration and orgasm.*

***Focus 3.*** *As stimulation continues, proceed to penetration and activities leading to orgasm.* ■

# SEXUALLY TRANSMITTED DISEASES

## SYMPTOMS

Especially if you are a woman, you may experience no symptoms until you have developed serious complications, or you may notice:

- a vaginal, anal, or urethral discharge; the color may be white, yellow, green, or gray, or the discharge may be blood-streaked, and it may have a strong odor.
- genital and/or anal itching or irritation.
- a rash, blisters, sores, lumps, bumps, or warts on or around the genitals.
- burning during urination.
- swollen lymph glands in the groin.
- pain in the groin or lower abdomen.
- vaginal bleeding.
- testicular swelling.
- flulike symptoms.
- painful intercourse.

See also AIDS, Chlamydia, Genital Herpes, Genital Warts, Gonorrhea, Hepatitis, Syphilis, Trichomoniasis.

## CALL YOUR DOCTOR IF:

- you have any of the above symptoms. Sexually transmitted diseases are contagious and may result in serious complications or death if left untreated.

Sexually transmitted diseases (STDs), once called venereal diseases, are among the most common contagious diseases. One in four American adults has a sexually transmitted disease, and each year 12 million new cases are reported.

As the name of this group of diseases implies, these infections can be contracted by means of vaginal, anal, or oral sex. You are at high risk if you have more than one sex partner and/or you don't use a condom when having sex.

You are also at high risk for some of these diseases—notably AIDS and hepatitis B—if you share needles when injecting intravenous drugs.

Except for AIDS and hepatitis B, sexually transmitted diseases can be cured or managed if they are treated early. But you may not realize you have an STD until it has damaged your reproductive system, vision, heart, or other organs. Also, having an STD weakens the immune system and leaves you more vulnerable to other infections. Pelvic inflammatory disease is a complication of many STDs that can leave women unable to have children and can even be life-threatening. If you pass an STD to your newborn, the baby may die or suffer blindness and organ damage.

## CAUSES

Bacterial STDs include chlamydia, gonorrhea, and syphilis. Viral STDs include AIDS, genital herpes, genital warts, and hepatitis B. Trichomoniasis is caused by a parasite. The microbes that cause STDs are found in semen, blood, vaginal secretions, and sometimes saliva. Most of the organisms are spread by vaginal, anal, or oral sex, but some, such as those that cause genital herpes and genital warts, may be spread through skin contact. You can get hepatitis B by sharing personal items, such as razors, with someone who has it.

### DIAGNOSTIC AND TEST PROCEDURES

If you are in a high-risk group, ask your doctor to test you for STDs during your annual physical even if you have no symptoms. If you test positive, your sexual partners will require treatment too. STDs may be detected during physical

## How to Put On a Condom

***Male condom:***

- *Always put the condom on before you allow the penis to touch the vagina, mouth, or anus. Always use a latex condom; animal-skin condoms are more porous and may allow microbes to pass. Use water-based lubricants; oil-based lubricants such as petroleum jelly may eat through a condom.*
- *Hold the condom by the tip to squeeze out air. Leave space at the end for semen to accumulate.*
- *Unroll the condom over the erect penis.*
- *Withdraw if the condom breaks or slips off during intercourse; put on a new condom.*
- *After sex, hold the condom at the rim and pull it off slowly, while the penis is still erect.*
- *Use a new condom every time you have sex.*

***Female condom, or "pouch":***

- *Always insert the polyurethane pouch in the vagina before the penis touches it. Put a water-based lubricant in the pouch.*
- *Squeeze the inner ring of the pouch. Insert the pouch in the vagina as you would a diaphragm.*
- *Using your index finger, push the inner ring as far as it will go; the outer ring stays outside the vagina.*
- *Guide the penis into the pouch. If it slips out of the pouch during sex, guide it back in.*
- *After sex, remove the pouch gently before standing up.*
- *Use a new pouch every time you have sex.*

examination; through Pap smears; and in tests of blood, urine, and genital and anal discharges.

## TREATMENT

Don't try to treat an STD yourself. These diseases are contagious and serious. You must see a doctor.

### CONVENTIONAL MEDICINE

Bacterial STDs can be cured with antibiotics if treatment begins early enough. Viral STDs cannot be cured, but you can manage symptoms with medications. There is a vaccine against hepatitis B, but it will not help if you already have the disease.

### ALTERNATIVE CHOICES

See entries for specific sexually transmitted diseases for information on alternative therapies.

### AT-HOME REMEDIES

- Douche with vinegar, yogurt, or lemon juice solutions to relieve vaginal distress.
- Take zinc and vitamins A, C, and E to boost your immune system and to help treat some skin infections, such as herpes.
- Practice relaxation techniques to ease stress and speed healing.
- Take warm baths and analgesics such as aspirin, ibuprofen, or acetaminophen for pain.
- Ask your doctor or pharmacist about other over-the-counter remedies.

## PREVENTION

Always avoid sex with anyone who has genital sores, a rash, a discharge, or other disease symptoms. If you are in a high-risk group you should:

- Use latex condoms and water-based lubricants. Remember that condoms are not 100 percent effective at preventing disease.
- Avoid sharing towels or clothing.
- Wash before and after intercourse.
- Get a vaccination for hepatitis B. ■

# SHINGLES

## SYMPTOMS

- slight fever, malaise, chills, upset stomach.
- bruised feeling, usually on one side of your face or body.
- pain (often in the chest) that is followed several days later by tingling, itching, or prickling skin and an inflamed, red skin rash.
- a group or long strip of small, fluid-filled blisters.
- deep burning, searing, aching, or stabbing pain, which may be continuous or intermittent.

*(See also the Visual Diagnostic Guide.)*

## CALL YOUR DOCTOR IF:

- you suspect an outbreak is beginning; antiviral drugs taken in the early stages may shorten the course of the infection.
- shingles on your face spreads near your eye; get treatment to avoid possible cornea damage.
- the affected area becomes secondarily infected with bacteria (indicated by spreading redness, swelling, a high fever, and pus); antibiotics can help halt the spread.
- your rash lasts longer than 10 days without improvement; get treatment to avoid potential nerve damage.
- the pain becomes too great to bear; your doctor may prescribe stronger analgesics or a nerve block.

Shingles is a reactivation of the herpes zoster virus in which painful skin blisters erupt on one side of your face or body. Typical shingles begins with a general feeling of malaise accompanied by a slight fever and a tingling sensation or pain on one side of your body. Within days a rash appears in that same area in a line along the affected nerve, and a group of small, fluid-filled blisters crops up. Typically, this occurs along your chest, abdomen, back, or face, but it may also affect your neck, limbs, or lower back. The area can be excruciatingly painful, itchy, and tender. After one to two weeks the blisters heal and form scabs, although the pain continues.

The deep pain that follows after the infection has run its course is known as postherpetic neuralgia. It can continue for months or even years, especially in older people. Shingles usually occurs only once, although it has been known to recur in some people.

## CAUSES

Shingles arises from the same virus, herpes zoster, that causes chickenpox. Following a bout of chickenpox, the virus becomes dormant in the spinal nerve cells, but it can be reactivated at a time when the immune system is suppressed—by physical or emotional trauma or a serious illness. Medical science doesn't understand why the virus becomes reactivated in some people and not in others.

## TREATMENT

No treatment has yet been discovered to prevent or halt shingles, and although steps can be taken to shorten its duration, frequently the virus must simply run its course. Because the pain following shingles is difficult to manage and can last so long—months or, in rare cases, years—the best approach is early and immediate treatment. Also, early medical attention may prevent or reduce the scarring that shingles can cause.

## CONVENTIONAL MEDICINE

Your doctor may suggest medications to reduce inflammation and help you cope with the pain. Analgesics such as aspirin or acetaminophen can alleviate mild pain. Oral, topical, or intravenous use of acyclovir, an antiviral drug, may help stop progression of the rash. A short course of corticosteroids either taken orally or applied as a cream can reduce inflammation. Vidarabine monohydrate is another prescription medication that prevents blisters from spreading; it also helps decrease pain and speed healing. Benzoin, available over the counter, may protect irritated skin when applied to unbroken lesions. If the area becomes infected by bacteria, antibiotics can keep the infection under control. For the pain that lingers after lesions have healed, your doctor may prescribe a tricyclic antidepressant, which in small doses helps relieve pain.

## ALTERNATIVE CHOICES

In addition to the remedies mentioned below, you might want to consult an **acupuncturist** or a **homeopath** for treatments to speed healing or shorten the duration of the disease.

### HERBAL THERAPIES

Dabbing or sponging lesions with a solution of lemon balm *(Melissa officinalis)* or calendula *(Calendula officinalis)* may reduce inflammation. Make a 50-50 mixture of tincture and boiled, then cooled, water. You can also try three daily applications of a commercially prepared gel made from an extract of licorice *(Glycyrrhiza glabra)*, which appears to interfere with virus growth. An over-the-counter cream made from cayenne *(Capsicum frutescens)* might decrease the pain of shingles, but it is extremely hot and should be applied only after blisters have healed and never on broken skin.

### NUTRITION AND DIET

For relief of postherpetic pain, take 1,200 to 1,600 IU of vitamin E daily, but for no more than two weeks, only under a doctor's care, and only if you don't have high blood pressure. To alleviate symptoms once the disease has begun, take 500 mg one to three times a day of the amino acid L-lysine, but only for one week. Studies have shown that this works best if you avoid foods containing the amino acid arginine, such as chocolate, cereal grains, nuts, and seeds.

## AT-HOME REMEDIES

- Keep the affected area clean, dry, and exposed to air (without clothes covering it) as much as possible. Don't scratch or burst the blisters. If the pain keeps you from sleeping, snugly bind the area with an elastic sports bandage.
- For the first three or four days, try ice for 10 minutes on, 5 minutes off, every few hours. Later, apply cool, wet compresses soaked in aluminum acetate, available over the counter in the form of astringent solution, powder packets, or effervescent tablets.
- To desensitize nerve endings, crush two aspirin, mix them with 2 tbsp rubbing alcohol, and apply the paste to lesions three times a day. To cut down on itching, ask your pharmacist to mix 78 percent calamine lotion with 20 percent rubbing alcohol, 1 percent phenol, and 1 percent menthol. You can apply this mixture continuously until your blisters scab over. Other remedies for itching include frequent applications of vitamin E oil, gel from the aloe vera plant, or fresh leeks that have been chopped in a food processor. Dusting colloidal oatmeal powder where clothes rub against your skin can reduce pain.

# PREVENTION

Because shingles comes on suddenly, with scarcely any warning, there is little you can do in the way of prevention, but your doctor may be able to avert the pain that follows. Some pain experts have had success using a nerve block during the acute phase of the disease. Administered on an outpatient basis in a hospital to deaden pain and shrink inflammation at the nerve root, a nerve block may act as a preemptive strike against later development of postherpetic neuralgia. ■

# SHIN SPLINTS

## SYMPTOMS

Shin splints are characterized by pain, aching, and occasionally, swelling anywhere in the lower leg. However, the pain is most often in the locations described below:

- on the front of the leg, toward the inside.
- on the inner side of the leg, toward the back.

## CALL YOUR DOCTOR IF:

- you have a hard swelling, numbness, tingling, and severe pain in your lower leg. You may have ruptured a tendon, a condition requiring immediate medical attention.
- you feel pain concentrated in a small area anywhere along the inside part of the lower leg bone. The area is sensitive to the touch and does not seem to "warm up" with sports activity. This could mean that you have a stress fracture, which requires medical evaluation.
- your symptoms persist or worsen after three to seven days. You may have muscle or tendon damage that requires the attention of a doctor.

Shin splints, one of the most common ailments of active people, is a general term referring to pain in the lower leg. Experts differ when explaining what the exact condition is, although most agree that it involves the two muscles that run from the knee to the ankle and the side of the foot, swathing the tibia, or shinbone. These muscles point the foot up and down, and support the arch and the front of the foot to keep it from slapping while walking and running. Injuries that result in small tears in the fibers of these muscles bring on shin splints.

Shin splints may also be related to a condition known as **compartment syndrome,** in which a muscle grows too large for its outer sheath. Stress fractures of the tibia and irritation to the nerves in the shin are also associated with shin splints.

## CAUSES

Any unusual or repetitive stress to the lower leg can bring on shin splints. Seasoned athletes and novices alike suffer from the ailment, with runners, cyclists, skiers, and aerobic dancers being especially vulnerable. People who have flat feet, knock-knees, or bowlegs place abnormal stress on their legs and are likely to suffer from shin splints. Poorly cushioned shoes, exercising on unyielding surfaces such as concrete, and poor posture can contribute to the condition.

## TREATMENT

Most approaches focus on ensuring adequate rest to allow for healing, followed by a program of strengthening exercises designed to ward off recurrences. It is important to start treatment when the condition first makes itself evident. Ignoring

### CAUTION!

**If you suffer from circulatory problems, diabetes, or heart disease, avoid massage and applications of heat or cold until you consult your doctor.**

S

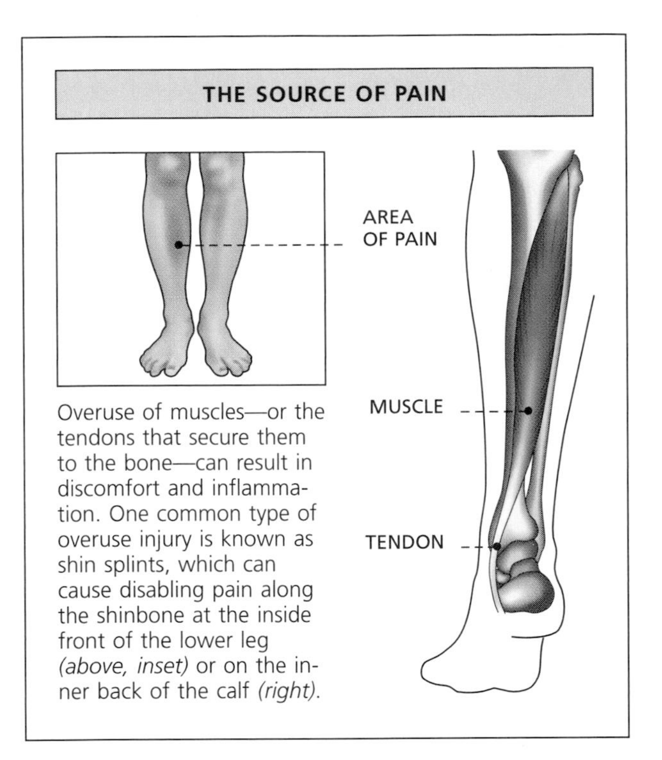

Overuse of muscles—or the tendons that secure them to the bone—can result in discomfort and inflammation. One common type of overuse injury is known as shin splints, which can cause disabling pain along the shinbone at the inside front of the lower leg *(above, inset)* or on the inner back of the calf *(right).*

the early nagging pain—or attempting to tough it out—will only worsen shin splints.

## CONVENTIONAL MEDICINE

Doctors usually recommend the sports medicine therapy RICE (rest, ice, compression, and elevation) as initial treatment for shin splints. *(See box on page 770.)* They often prescribe crutches to keep weight off the injured leg, and aspirin or ibuprofen to reduce inflammation and pain. Your doctor may recommend that you see a physical therapist for an exercise program and may suggest ultrasound treatment to relax the muscles, improve circulation, and promote healing.

## ALTERNATIVE CHOICES

There are a number of alternative treatments that complement the conventional therapies described above. Many employ massage.

### ACUPRESSURE

After gently massaging the affected area, apply gradual, steady pressure to Stomach 36, four finger widths below the kneecap, one finger width outside the shinbone. (The muscle you press is the one that flexes as you move your foot up and down.) The pressure should not cause pain. Try for three minutes, three times a day. *(See pages 22–23 for more information on locating this point.)*

### CHINESE HERBS

A Chinese herbal practitioner might apply a poultice of gardenia *(Gardenia jasminoides),* flour, and wine to reduce swelling and to promote healing. Practitioners also may recommend moxibustion, in which a smoldering piece of mugwort leaf *(Artemisia argyi)* is held about an inch above the affected area. The process is thought to increase circulation and promote healing. Also perhaps helpful is a massage technique in which the ball of the thumb is used to alternately press hard and rub lightly on the sore area.

## AT-HOME REMEDIES

Other than treatments from a physical therapist, you can apply all of the standard conventional and alternative therapies for shin splints at home. Remember RICE. Keep off your feet to rest your legs. Apply ice in alternating intervals, 10 minutes on, 10 minutes off. Wrap your leg in an elastic sports bandage to compress the tissues and counteract swelling. And keep your legs elevated to reduce blood pressure in the inflamed tissues.

# PREVENTION

The key to preventing shin splints is finding as many ways as possible to cut down on the stresses that tend to cause the injury. Wear supportive shoes, and check with a podiatrist about inserts to help correct postural difficulties that may contribute to shin splints. Stretching exercises for the muscles in the toes, heel, knee, and lower leg can help condition the muscles and make them more resistant to injury. Be sure to exercise on resilient surfaces such as wood or earth, not on unyielding concrete. ■

# SHOULDER PAIN

*Read down this column to find your symptoms. Then read across.*

| SYMPTOMS | AILMENT/PROBLEM |
|---|---|
| ◆ pain in the shoulders and possibly other joints that begins after taking a new medication. | ◆ Common reaction to medications such as oral contraceptives, penicillin, and some antianxiety drugs |
| ◆ pain, stiffness, and swelling in both shoulders; worst upon awakening and dissipates during the day or with rest; may be accompanied by similar symptoms in other joints (especially the fingers); fatigue; possibly, persistent low-grade fever, insomnia, weight loss. | ◆ Arthritis |
| ◆ pain at the top, outer part of the shoulder that is worst upon awakening and may subside with normal activity but increases with stretching or exertion; inflammation; redness. | ◆ Bursitis of the shoulder joint |
| ◆ painfully tender and stiff shoulder that hurts more at night and may interrupt sleeping; shoulder may tingle, feel numb, or appear swollen. | ◆ Tendonitis |
| ◆ shoulder pain in a specific spot that is worse with movement and follows injury, overexertion, or heavy lifting. | ◆ Strained, inflamed, or torn tendon or ligament; torn muscle |
| ◆ moderate to severe shoulder pain and stiffness that has worsened over several weeks; difficulty moving the arm in any direction. | ◆ Frozen shoulder (a severe inflammation of the shoulder joint) |
| ◆ sudden pain in the shoulder joint that accompanies flu or another infection. | ◆ Side effect of an infection |
| ◆ sudden, intense shoulder pain; inflammation; shoulder feels hot to the touch, but there is no fever. | ◆ Accumulation of crystals in the shoulder joint |
| ◆ a painful, possibly misshapen shoulder that is impossible to move; usually caused by an accident. | ◆ Fractured bone or dislocated shoulder joint |

| WHAT TO DO | OTHER INFO |
|---|---|
| ◆ Ask your doctor about possible alternative medications. | |
| ◆ A nonsteroidal anti-inflammatory drug (NSAID) or aspirin, combined with applied heat, can relax muscles and reduce pain and inflammation. Get adequate rest and regular, gentle exercise (such as swimming) to expand your shoulder's range of motion and help suppress symptoms. | ◆ Your doctor or chiropractor can suggest many other drugs and procedures that may alleviate pain and inflammation. |
| ◆ Immobilize the shoulder as much as possible. Take nonsteroidal anti-inflammatory drugs (NSAIDs) or aspirin to reduce pain and inflammation. | ◆ If bursitis does not heal itself in a few days, call your doctor. |
| ◆ Aspirin, ibuprofen, or other nonsteroidal anti-inflammatory drugs (NSAIDs) may relieve pain and swelling. Follow the RICE regimen: rest, ice, compression, and elevation. | ◆ Wearing a triangle-shaped sling immobilizes your arm and helps rest your shoulder to promote healing, and is especially helpful when sleeping. |
| ◆ To minimize inflammation and pain, use the RICE regimen: rest, ice, compression, and elevation. *(See Tendonitis.)* Call your doctor if pain does not lessen in 24 hours; a torn muscle may require prompt surgery. | ◆ Supporting the arm in a sling takes weight off the shoulder and can dramatically reduce pain. See also Sprains and Strains. |
| ◆ Treat as you would bursitis. | ◆ Be patient; frozen shoulder can last for six months to several years. |
| ◆ Nonsteroidal anti-inflammatory drugs (NSAIDs) may lessen the pain. | |
| ◆ See Gout. Call your doctor. Left untreated, gout can lead to kidney damage. | ◆ Gout is caused by uric acid crystals. A related condition, pseudogout, is caused by a type of calcium crystal. |
| ◆ **Seek medical care immediately.** Do not move the arm or shoulder. Whatever its position, stabilize it. *(See Emergencies/First Aid: Fractures and Dislocations.)* | ◆ Expect to wear a cast or splint for a few weeks to allow healing. |

S

# SICKLE CELL ANEMIA

## SYMPTOMS

- episodes of severe pain, primarily at the joints, in the abdomen, or along the arms and legs.
- fatigue, pallor or jaundice, and rapid heartbeat, indicating anemia.
- susceptibility to infections.
- in affected children, delayed growth and development, including delayed sexual maturation.
- priapism, a painful, persistent erection; sometimes experienced by affected teenage and adult males.

## CALL YOUR DOCTOR IF:

- your infant's hands or feet swell and the baby shows signs of anemia; such symptoms are often the first indication of the disease.
- your affected child has a fever of 101°F or higher, often an indicator of a bacterial infection (which can quickly become fatal); or the child has seizures, becomes irritable, or is lethargic—symptoms of a neurological problem. **Seek emergency medical care immediately.**
- your affected child's abdomen is distended and rigid, and the child shows signs of anemia; this might indicate pooling of blood in the spleen, a life-threatening situation. **Seek emergency medical care immediately.**
- painful episodes persist more than several hours; intramuscular or intravenous pain relievers, or perhaps hospitalization, may be necessary.

Sickle cell anemia is one of the most common forms of an inherited blood disorder called sickle cell disease. People of African descent are at greatest risk. To develop sickle cell anemia, a person must inherit two sickle cell genes. When only one gene is present, a person has another form of sickle cell disease known as sickle cell trait. People with sickle cell trait do not generally experience symptoms except occasionally under low-oxygen conditions, such as when scuba-diving or at high altitudes. They can also pass on the gene, and possibly the disease, to their children.

In addition to having the symptoms of anemia, people with sickle cell anemia may also experience episodes known as crises, which affect various parts of the body. How often these crises occur varies from person to person. Repeated crises can lead to organ failure and even death.

The vaso-occlusive, or painful, crisis is by far the most common. It causes mild to severe pain in oxygen-deprived tissues, organs, or joints. A painful crisis can be triggered by dehydration, infection, stress, trauma, exposure, lack of oxygen, or strenuous physical activity.

Aplastic and hyperhemolytic crises can lead to severe anemia. In aplastic crises, the bone marrow temporarily stops producing red blood cells. In a hyperhemolytic crisis, the red blood cells break down too rapidly to be replaced adequately. The fourth type of crisis, splenic sequestration, is usually a childhood difficulty that occurs when blood becomes trapped in the spleen, causing the organ to enlarge and possibly leading to death.

Because this disease can be life-threatening, early diagnosis and treatment is vital.

## CAUSES

People with sickle cell disease receive a gene for abnormal hemoglobin (the oxygen-carrying protein in red blood cells) from each parent. Red blood cells are normally round and flexible. Cells with abnormal hemoglobin are crescent shaped and less flexible, causing them to break down rapidly, leading to anemia. Viral infections can trigger aplastic and hyperhemolytic crises. Painful crises are caused by the sickled cells becoming trapped in smaller blood vessels and preventing oxygen from reaching surrounding tissues.

### DIAGNOSTIC AND TEST PROCEDURES

Sickle cell screening of newborns is required in 30 states. A blood test can identify people with the trait or the disease. Prenatal tests can detect the disease in unborn babies. Genetic testing is available for couples who plan to become parents.

## TREATMENT

At present, no cure exists; but with proper management, people with the disease can lead productive lives. If you or your child has sickle cell anemia, be sure to choose a doctor who is very familiar with the disease and its complications.

### CONVENTIONAL MEDICINE

It is important to protect an affected child from infections, which can lead to dangerous complications—including death. Because their spleens do not function properly, children with sickle cell anemia are at great risk for such serious infections as meningitis, hepatitis, peritonitis, osteomyelitis (bone infection), and pneumonia. In addition to standard immunizations, your child should also receive vaccines for influenza and pneumococcus. Your child's pediatrician will probably also prescribe a preventive course of penicillin by mouth daily from the age of two months to five years. You will be advised of other preventive steps you can take to avoid crises *(see Prevention, below)*. In addition, you and your family may be referred to a counselor to deal with the emotional issues of this disease.

During crises, hospitalization will probably be required. Hydroxyurea, a drug used to treat other blood disorders, is being tested in the management of sickle cell anemia in adults; it seems to reduce the severity of painful crises.

**ABNORMAL BLOOD CELLS**

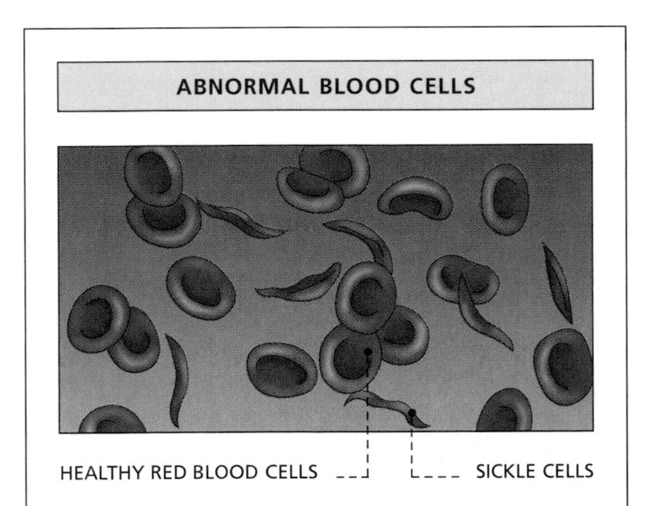


As they deliver oxygen to body tissues, normal, round red blood cells slip easily through tiny capillaries. Cells carrying abnormal hemoglobin—the oxygen-transporting protein in blood—tend to collapse into a crescent, or sickle, shape. Because narrow capillaries cannot accommodate the oddly shaped cells, blood flow is impaired and surrounding tissue is starved of oxygen.

### ALTERNATIVE CHOICES

Not much is known about the effectiveness of various alternative treatments for sickle cell anemia. **Acupuncture** may be able to help mitigate painful crises. Seek professional advice.

### LIFESTYLE

Sickle cell crises can disrupt personal and family life. Parents will want to help an affected child grow up as normally as possible. Let teachers know of your child's illness and teach them how to deal with a crisis; ask them to provide assignments when your child is homebound.

## PREVENTION

Avoiding the triggers that can precipitate crises is an important preventive step. Maintaining a good diet, drinking plenty of fluids, taking regular, moderate exercise, and getting enough sleep will help prevent dehydration and fatigue and keep the body strong. To guard against infection, take care of wounds, practice good oral hygiene, and have regular checkups. Children with the disease should be current with all immunizations. ■

# SINUSITIS

## SYMPTOMS

- feeling of fullness in the face.
- pressure behind the eyes.
- nasal obstruction, difficulty breathing through the nose.
- postnasal drip.
- foul smell in the nose.
- fever (possibly).
- toothache (possibly).

## CALL YOUR DOCTOR IF:

- sinusitis develops into an inflammation around the eye (orbital cellulitis), which could cause damage to the eye and facial nerves.
- the condition does not improve within seven days.
- sinusitis recurs more than three times in a year, and periods between bouts grow shorter; you may have a chronic infection that could become serious.

Sinusitis is an infection or inflammation of the sinuses, the air-filled pockets in the bones of the face. One of the most common healthcare complaints in the United States, sinusitis affects as many as 30 to 50 million Americans a year. Some researchers estimate that as much as 14 percent of the country's population suffers chronic (long-term) sinusitis.

Of all the human body's mysterious components, the sinuses are among the most puzzling. Some scientists believe that the sinuses function mainly as mucus factories for the nose and throat. Others say these hollow chambers help warm the air we breathe, still others that they exist merely to lighten the skull.

All humans have four pairs of sinuses *(below, right),* which connect to the nasal passages through a series of holes and interconnections. Mucus forms on the surfaces of the sinuses, which are also covered with tiny hairs called cilia. When we breathe, the mucus traps dirt brought in by the air; then the cilia push the mucus out through tiny openings that serve as drains. These openings, known as ostia, are very small, in some cases measuring only a few millimeters across. While the frontal, sphenoidal, and ethmoidal sinuses have ostia at the bottom, the maxillary sinuses have their ostia at the top. Consequently, mucus has to drain upward from these cavities, against the pull of gravity. Given that humans walk erect, it's not surprising that sinus problems are common.

## CAUSES

Sinusitis occurs when the mucus-producing linings of the sinuses become inflamed, and by far the most frequent cause of this condition is blockage of the ostia. Once these openings are clogged, foreign material can't get out, oxygen levels drop, and bacteria in the nasal cavity slither into the sinuses, causing the sinus walls to swell and fill with pus. If the infection doesn't go away, the body sends in disease-fighting cells to kill the bacteria. Unfortunately, these well-intentioned bodyguards can themselves do considerable damage to the sinus walls. Defender cells can damage the cilia, the hairlike structures that help expel foreign matter. Furthermore, scarring caused by the cells' battles can result in the formation of sores. Large, mushroom-shaped growths called nasal polyps can also appear inside the nose, interfering with breathing and setting the stage for other problems. Almost invariably, the invading bacteria seek out and colonize adjacent sinuses. More than 40 percent of all sinusitis patients, in fact, are affected in more than one pair of sinuses.

The most common cause of blockage of the ostia is an upper respiratory tract viral infection, such as a common cold or the flu. These conditions increase secretions in the nasal passageways, provoke swelling of the sinus walls, and cause the cilia to malfunction. Allergic reactions can have the same effect. Hay fever often leads to sinusitis, but allergies to dust, animal dander, foods, smoke, and other pollutants can also trigger reactions that result in blocked sinuses.

In some cases, the ostia are blocked by unusual anatomical features—preexisting nasal polyps, a deviated septum, foreign bodies, or tumors, for example. Certain diseases, including diabetes and HIV infections, can create a predisposition to sinusitis. And people with poorly working mucus and ciliary functions, such as patients with cystic fibrosis, have a better-than-average chance of coming down with the condition. Sinusitis is also common among people with chronic tonsillitis and adenoid problems.

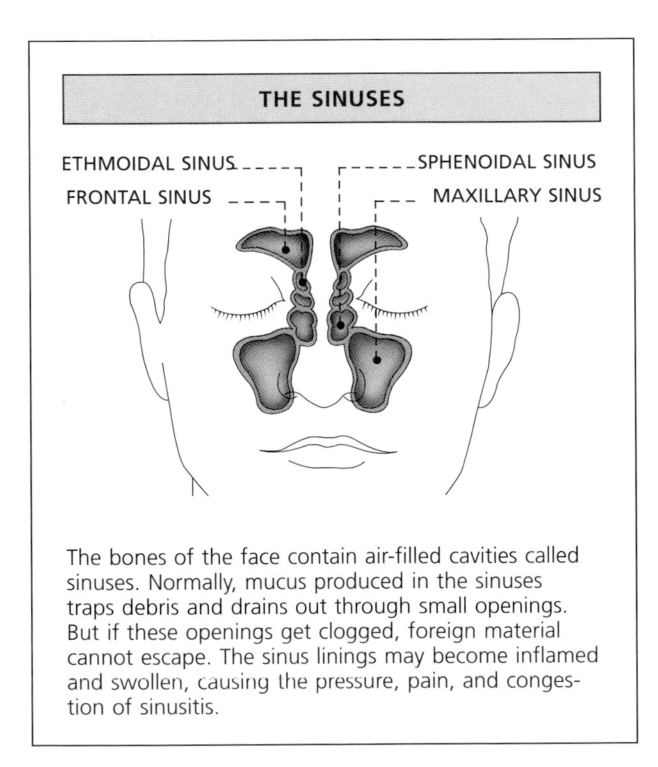


The bones of the face contain air-filled cavities called sinuses. Normally, mucus produced in the sinuses traps debris and drains out through small openings. But if these openings get clogged, foreign material cannot escape. The sinus linings may become inflamed and swollen, causing the pressure, pain, and congestion of sinusitis.

### DIAGNOSTIC AND TEST PROCEDURES

In most cases, doctors diagnose sinusitis based on their "clinical impression," or the sum total of your symptoms, medical history, and the results of a physical examination. Some doctors prefer to verify this impression with a test called transillumination. In this procedure, the doctor shines a special flashlight into your nose and examines the roof of your mouth for signs of sinus congestion. Unfortunately, transillumination might not pick up an infection in a deep, distant sinus. Your doctor may also order an x-ray of your sinuses, but even this technique may not be sensitive enough to detect a deep infection.

Doctors often go ahead and assume you have sinusitis and prescribe medications accordingly. If your body doesn't respond after several attempts, they begin other tests. An otolaryngologist (ear, nose, and throat doctor) may insert a tiny tube into your nose and examine the sinuses directly, a technique known as an endoscopy. A CT scan can show swelling in the deep sinuses and reveal any anatomic abnormalities, but even these scans are not always reliable.

## TREATMENT

The goal of most treatments is to open up the sinuses and restore proper drainage. If the sinuses are infected with bacteria, it is important to kill the disease organisms before they cause further damage or spread to other sinuses.

### CONVENTIONAL MEDICINE

Before you start treating sinusitis, make sure you actually have it; sinusitis can be hard to distinguish from an upper respiratory tract infection, dental disorder, asthma, or even a headache.

ACUPRESSURE

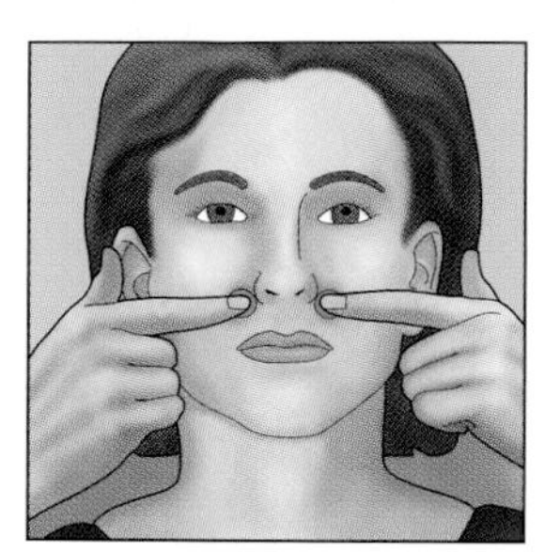

**1** Pressing LI 20 may help relieve the pain, congestion, and swelling of sinusitis. Using the index fingers, gently press the points on either side of your nose. Apply pressure upward, underneath your cheekbones. Breathe deeply and hold for one minute.

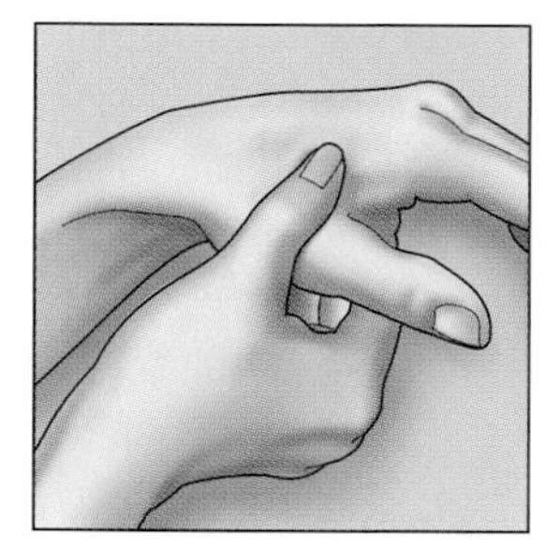

**2** To ease headache pain and congestion, try pressing LI 4. With your right thumb, press into the webbing between the thumb and index finger of your left hand. Hold for one minute, then repeat on the other hand. (Do not use if you are pregnant.)

The bugs that most often invade the sinuses are frequent residents of the nose and throat—*Streptococcus pneumoniae* and *Hemophilus influenzae (H. flu).* These pathogens usually respond to such tried-and-true antibiotics as ampicillin and amoxicillin. However, because certain strains of *H. flu* have developed resistance to amoxicillin, some doctors prescribe other medications, such as sulfamethoxazole and trimethoprim, cefaclor, and amoxicillin and clavulanate. More-expensive choices are loracarbef, azithromycin, and clarithromycin.

Treatment usually lasts 7 to 14 days for acute cases, and from 2 to 3 weeks for chronic or recurrent cases. CAUTION: Stopping the antibiotic treatment prematurely may increase the infection's duration or severity.

Besides antibiotics, many doctors prescribe inhaled steroids such as beclomethasone or triamcinolone to reduce inflammation and open the sinuses so they can drain. Decongestants can also reduce swelling and help unclog the sinuses. Most doctors prefer oral decongestants, including pseudoephedrine, over nose sprays like oxymetazoline because sprays can become habit-forming if used for more than three days.

Drugs containing guaifenesin are used to break up hard, encrusted mucus, but they generally don't work very well. Antihistamines are not usually prescribed for sinusitis because they tend to make mucus thicker and less able to drain from clogged sinuses. Antihistamines may provide some relief, however, if your condition is caused by allergies.

When sinusitis becomes chronic and other remedies fail, physicians may suggest a sinus washout or surgery. Washout procedures, in which the doctor uses a sterile saline solution to clean out the nasal passages, are rarely performed today. Instead, surgeons prefer surgical techniques such as antrostomy, which involves drilling a hole at the bottom of the frontal sinus to improve drainage. In another procedure, called endoscopic sinus surgery, physicians insert a tiny scope through the nose. Not only does the scope allow doctors to see the insides of the nasal cavities, but it also serves to open clogged passageways and remove dead cells from the sinus wall. Between 80 percent and 90 percent of patients report moderate to complete relief of symptoms with endoscopic surgery. Extremely rare side effects of this procedure include meningitis, blindness, or double vision *(see Vision Problems).*

## ALTERNATIVE CHOICES

Many alternative therapies are attempts to relieve the pain of sinusitis and open the sinuses for drainage. Others aim to fight infection by boosting the immune system.

### ACUPRESSURE

Applying gentle pressure to the face and hands can help ease the pain of sinusitis *(see the illustration above, left).*

### ACUPUNCTURE

An acupuncturist will apply medium stimulation to various ear points—adrenal, forehead, internal nose, lung, and near the sinuses—to help drain the sinuses.

### AROMATHERAPY

Inhalants of eucalyptus, pine, or thyme may help break up your clogged sinuses. You may also alleviate the symptoms by holding menthol or eucalyptus packs over your sinuses. Other suggestions: Gently swab your nasal passages with oil of bitter orange, or massage your face with essence of lavender mixed into vegetable oil.

### CHINESE HERBS

The exact makeup of a prescribed mixture depends on whether the sinusitis is "hot" (acute or infectious) or "cold" (chronic or allergic). Either way, the preparation may include the Chinese herb ephedra *(Ephedra sinica),* a decongestant. (Do not use ephedra if you have hypertension or heart disease.) A number of other Chinese herbs are also helpful in relieving sinusitis symptoms. These include honeysuckle *(Lonicera japonica),* fritillary bulb *(Fritillaria cirrhosa),* tangerine peel *(Citrus reticulata),* xanthium fruit *(Xanthium sibiricum),* and magnolia flower *(Magnolia liliflora).*

### HERBAL THERAPIES

Bromelain tablets have been shown in controlled studies to reduce inflammation, nasal discharge, headache, and breathing difficulties. You can give your immune system a boost with echinacea (*Echinacea* spp.), goldenseal *(Hydrastis canadensis),* or garlic *(Allium sativum),* preferably raw. Breathing the steam of clove *(Syzygium aromaticum)* tea or ginger *(Zingiber officinale)* root tea also provides some relief. To combat excessive mucus production, herbalists suggest elder *(Sambucus nigra)* flower, eyebright *(Euphrasia officinalis),* marsh mallow *(Althaea officinalis),* or goldenrod *(Solidago virgaurea).*

### HOMEOPATHY

Homeopaths recommend specific remedies for various types of sinusitis discomfort. For acute sinusitis with thick, stringy mucus and pain in the cheeks or the bridge of the nose, use Kali bichromicum (30c) once or twice a day. For sinusitis with intense facial pain, alternating chills and sweat, and yellow-green discharge from the nose and mouth, use Mercurius vivus (30c) twice a day. For acute sinusitis with a clear, thin discharge, sneezing, headache, and a stopped-up nose at night, use Nux vomica (30c) twice a day. For sinusitis with light yellow or green nasal discharge accompanied by low spirits and lack of thirst, use Pulsatilla (30c) twice a day. If symptoms linger for more than two days, seek the advice of a professional homeopath.

### NUTRITION AND DIET

A good healthful diet including fruits and raw green vegetables can help stimulate secretions and break up sinusitis. Nutritionists also suggest the following supplements to the diet: vitamin C, 500 mg every two hours; bioflavonoids, 1 gram per day; beta carotene (vitamin A), 25,000 IU per day; and zinc lozenges, 23 mg every two waking hours for up to one week. Stay away from foods that you suspect may trigger an allergic reaction.

## AT-HOME REMEDIES

- Inhale steam from a vaporizer, a humidifier, a mixture of hot water and vinegar, or even a cup of tea or coffee. Steam is one of the best and least-expensive remedies for unclogging sinuses.
- Use warm compresses on your nose to help open your sinuses.
- Drink plenty of liquids.

## PREVENTION

It's difficult to prevent sinusitis, but you can reduce your chances of having your sinuses become infected. First, avoid allergenic substances. Allergens that people don't often think of include the dust in their beds and certain foods, such as dairy products and wheat. Whenever possible, avoid cigarette smoke. Note: People with diabetes, cystic fibrosis, and certain other diseases may be prone to sinusitis. For help in preventing respiratory infections, see Common Cold and Flu. ■

# SKIN CANCER

## SYMPTOMS

**The general warning signs of skin cancer include:**

- any change in size, color, shape, or texture of a mole or other skin growth.
- an open or inflamed skin wound that won't heal.

**Melanoma, the most dangerous type of skin cancer, may appear as:**

- a change in an existing mole.
- a small, dark, multicolored spot with irregular borders—either elevated or flat—that may bleed and form a scab.
- a cluster of shiny, firm, dark bumps.

**Basal cell carcinoma (BCC) may appear on sun-exposed skin as:**

- a pearly or flesh-colored oval bump with a rolled border, which may develop into a bleeding ulcer.
- a smooth red spot indented in the center.
- a reddish, brown, or bluish black patch of skin on the chest or back.

**Squamous cell carcinoma (SCC) may appear on sun-exposed skin as:**

- a firm, reddish, wartlike bump that grows gradually.
- a flat spot that becomes a bleeding sore that won't heal.

*(See also the Visual Diagnostic Guide.)*

## CALL YOUR DOCTOR IF:

- an existing mole changes size, shape, color, or texture; or you develop a very noticeable new mole as an adult.
- a new skin growth or open sore does not heal or disappear in a few weeks.

All skin cancers originate in the outer layer of skin known as the epidermis. In the normal course of skin rejuvenation, basal cells located at the base of the epidermis move upward to replace dead cells constantly being shed from the skin's surface. Along the way, the round basal cells are transformed into flat squamous cells. Throughout the epidermis are melanocytes, cells that produce a protective pigment called melanin.

Skin cancers fall into two major categories: **melanoma** and **nonmelanoma. Melanoma** is cancer of melanocytes, affecting about 1 in 10 skin cancer patients. It can start in heavily pigmented tissue, such as a mole or birthmark, as well as in normally pigmented skin. Melanoma usually appears first on the torso, although it can arise on the palm of the hand; on the sole of the foot; under a fingernail or toenail; in the mucous linings of the mouth, vagina, or anus; and even in the eye. Melanoma is an extremely virulent, life-threatening cancer. It is readily detectable and always curable if treated early, but it progresses faster than other types of skin cancer and tends to spread beyond the skin. Once this occurs, melanoma becomes very difficult to treat and cure.

The two most common skin cancers, **basal cell carcinoma (BCC)** and **squamous cell carcinoma (SCC),** are **nonmelanomas,** which are rarely life-threatening. They progress slowly, seldom spread beyond the skin, are detected easily, and usually are curable. **BCC,** which accounts for nearly 3 out of 4 skin cancers, is the slowest growing; **SCC** is somewhat more aggressive and more inclined to spread. In addition, there are a few rare nonmelanomas, such as **Kaposi's sarcoma,** a potentially life-threatening disease characterized by purple growths and often associated with AIDS.

Some technically noncancerous skin growths have the potential to become cancerous. The most common are **actinic keratoses**—crusty reddish lesions that may scratch off but grow back on sun-exposed skin. Another precancerous skin growth, **cutaneous horns,** appears as funnel-shaped growths that extend from a red base on the skin.

Every malignant skin tumor in time becomes visible on the skin's surface, making skin cancer the only type of cancer that is almost always detectable in its early, curable stages. Prompt detection and treatment of skin cancer is equivalent to cure.

Skin cancer is by far the most common cancer in the world. Most cases are cured, but the disease is a major health concern because it affects so many people. Over 700,000 cases of nonmelanoma skin cancer are diagnosed annually in the United States alone, and about 32,000 cases of melanoma. Of the 9,000 or so deaths from skin cancer in the U.S. each year, about 7,000 are from melanoma. Skin cancer tends to strike people of light skin color; dark-skinned people are rarely affected, and then only on light areas of the body such as the soles of the feet or under fingernails or toenails. An estimated 40 to 50 percent of fair-skinned people who live to be 65 will develop at least one skin cancer. The incidence of skin cancer is predictably higher in places with intense sunshine, such as Arizona and Hawaii; it is most common in Australia, settled largely by fair-skinned people of Irish and English descent.

**TWO SKIN CANCERS**

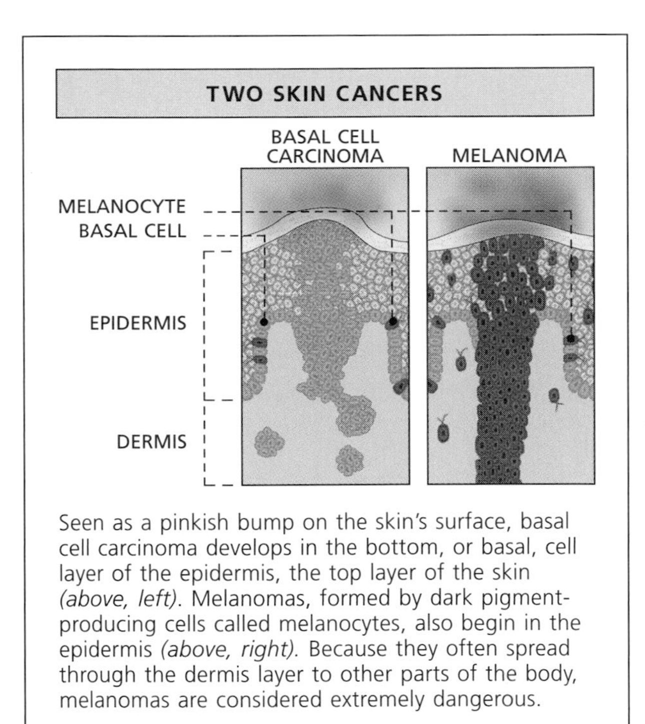


Seen as a pinkish bump on the skin's surface, basal cell carcinoma develops in the bottom, or basal, cell layer of the epidermis, the top layer of the skin *(above, left)*. Melanomas, formed by dark pigment-producing cells called melanocytes, also begin in the epidermis *(above, right)*. Because they often spread through the dermis layer to other parts of the body, melanomas are considered extremely dangerous.

## CAUSES

Excessive exposure to sunlight is the main cause of skin cancer. Sunlight contains ultraviolet (UV) rays that can alter the genetic material in skin cells, causing mutations. Sunlamps, tanning booths, and x-rays also generate UV rays that can damage skin and cause malignant cell mutations. **BCC** and **SCC** have been linked to chronic sun exposure, typically in fair-skinned people who work outside. **Melanoma** is associated with infrequent but excessive sunbathing that causes scorching sunburn. One blistering sunburn during childhood appears to double a person's risk for developing melanoma later in life. *(See Sunburn.)*

Fair-skinned people are most susceptible because they are born with the least amount of protective melanin. Redheads, blue-eyed blonds, and people with pigment disorders such as albinism bear the greatest risk. But people with many freckles or moles, particularly abnormal-looking ones, may also be vulnerable to melanoma. Workers regularly exposed to coal tar, radium, inorganic arsenic compounds in insecticides, and certain other carcinogens are at slightly higher than normal risk for nonmelanoma skin cancer.

The incidence of skin cancer is rising, even though most cases could be prevented by limiting skin's exposure to ultraviolet radiation. Skin cancer is about three times more common in men than in women, and the risk increases with age. Most people diagnosed with skin cancer are between ages 40 and 60, although all forms of the disease are appearing more often in younger people. If you or any close relatives have had skin cancer, you are more likely to get the disease.

### DIAGNOSTIC AND TEST PROCEDURES

If you are in a high-risk group for skin cancer or have ever been treated for some form of the disease, you should familiarize yourself with how skin cancers look *(see the Visual Diagnostic Guide)*. Examine your skin from head to toe every few months, using a full-length mirror and hand mirror to check your mouth, nose, scalp, palms, soles, backs of ears, genital area, and between the buttocks. Cover every inch of skin and pay special attention to moles and sites of previous skin cancer. If you find a suspicious growth, have it examined by your doctor or dermatologist.

All potentially cancerous skin growths must be biopsied to confirm a cancer diagnosis. Depending on the suspected type of skin cancer, the biopsy techniques vary slightly but crucially. Any potential **melanoma** requires a surgical biopsy, in which the entire growth is removed with a scalpel. A pathologist then studies the sample under a microscope to determine whether cancer cells are present. If cancer exists and it is melanoma, grains of melanin will be visible in the cancer cells. Skin growths that may be melanoma tumors should never be removed by shaving, burning, or freezing because those techniques do not allow pathologic examination of the growth. Eye melanomas usually are not biopsied because they are virtually unmistakable to an experienced ophthalmologist. If melanoma is diagnosed, other tests may be ordered to assess the degree of cancer spread. Skin growths that are most likely **BCC, SCC,** or other forms of **nonmelanoma** can be biopsied in various ways. Part or all of the growth can be taken with a scalpel, or a thin layer can be shaved off for examination under a microscope.

## AND THIS LITTLE PIGGY HAS NONE!

*Each of us is defended by an army of immune cells that protect the body from attack. Some immune cells target invaders such as bacteria and viruses; others—including killer T cells—target cancer. T cells easily find and neutralize lone cancer cells that occasionally appear in the body. But if cancer cells begin to multiply faster than T cells can kill them, the T cells appear to surrender, runaway cancer cells continue to multiply, and a tumor develops.*

*But can T cells be reinforced to counterattack a barrage of malignancy? In the case of melanoma in Sinclair swine, a breed of miniature pigs, the answer seems to be yes. Some 85 percent of Sinclair swine develop melanoma tumors within the first six weeks of life, but over the next month the tumors disappear. Researchers attribute this seemingly miraculous recovery to a special kind of T cell identified in the pigs. By isolating and studying these uniquely endowed killer T cells, researchers hope to develop melanoma treatments that will work in humans.*

## TREATMENT

Most skin cancers are detected and cured before they spread. Melanoma that has spread to other organs presents the greatest treatment challenge.

### CONVENTIONAL MEDICINE

Standard treatments for localized **basal cell** and **squamous cell carcinomas** are safe and effective and cause few side effects. Small tumors can be removed with electric current, frozen with liquid nitrogen, or killed with low-dose radiation. Applying an ointment containing a chemotherapeutic agent called 5-fluorouracil to a superficial tumor for several weeks may also work. Larger localized tumors are removed surgically.

In rare cases where BCC or SCC has begun to spread beyond the skin, tumors are removed surgically and patients are treated with chemotherapy, radiation, or immunotherapy. Some patients with advanced SCC respond well to a combination of retinoic acid (a derivative of vitamin A) and interferon (a type of disease-fighting protein produced in laboratories for cancer immunotherapy). Retinoic acid also seems to inhibit cancer recurrence in patients who have had tumors removed.

**Melanoma** tumors must be removed surgically, preferably before they spread beyond the skin into other organs or glands. The surgeon excises the tumor fully, along with a safe margin of surrounding tissue and possibly nearby lymph nodes. Neither radiation nor chemotherapy will cure advanced melanoma, but either treatment may slow the disease and relieve symptoms. Chemotherapy, sometimes in combination with immunotherapy—using interferon—is generally preferred. If melanoma spreads to the brain, radiation is used to slow the growth and control symptoms.

Immunotherapy is a relatively new field of cancer treatment that attempts to target and kill cancer cells by manipulating the body's immune system. Some of the most promising developments in the field of immunotherapy have sprung from efforts to cure advanced melanoma. Some researchers are treating advanced cases with vaccines, while others are using drugs such as interferon and interleukin 2 in an effort to stimulate immune cells into attacking melanoma cells more aggressively. Genetic manipulation of melanoma tumors may make them more vulnerable to attack by the immune system. Each of these experimental treatment approaches aims to immunize a patient's body against its own cancer—something the body cannot do naturally. *(See box at left.)*

People who have had skin cancer once are at risk for getting it again. Anyone who has been treated for skin cancer of any kind should have a checkup at least once a year. About 20 percent of skin cancer patients experience recurrence, usually within the first two years after diagnosis.

See Cancer for more information on treatments such as chemotherapy and radiation.

### COMPLEMENTARY THERAPIES

Once skin cancer is diagnosed, the only acceptable treatment is medical care. Alternative approaches may be useful in cancer prevention and in combating nausea, vomiting, fatigue, and headaches from chemotherapy, radiation, or immunotherapy used to treat advanced skin cancer.

#### NUTRITION AND DIET

Skin experts know that the mineral zinc and the antioxidant vitamins A (beta carotene), C, and E can help repair damaged body tissue and promote healthy skin. Now researchers are trying to determine whether these and other nutrients might protect skin from the harmful effects of sunlight. To test the theory, selected skin cancer patients are given experimental supplements of these vitamins in the hope of preventing cancer recurrence.

#### HERBAL THERAPIES

Following the advice of a local herbalist, some light-skinned Zimbabweans have used a crude ointment from the root and bark of the African sausage tree *(Kigelia pinnata)* to treat skin cancer. While initial research indicates that kigelia extract can kill melanoma cells, further study is needed to determine whether or not a kigelia-based drug will effectively treat melanoma in humans.

## PREVENTION

If you are susceptible to skin cancer, take the following precautions whenever possible:

- Avoid intense sun exposure by staying out of it from late morning through early afternoon.
- Outside, wear a hat, long sleeves, trousers, and sunglasses that block UV radiation.
- Use a sunscreen with a sun protection factor of 15 or higher whenever you are outside.
- Consider taking a B-complex vitamin; B vitamins contain a compound called PABA, the active ingredient in many sunscreens.
- Report suspicious skin lesions to a doctor at once, especially if you have abnormal-looking moles or a family history of melanoma.
- Check skin medications with your dermatologist; they may cause increased sun sensitivity.

C A U T I O N !

**CHILDREN AND SKIN CANCER**

**Protect infants from direct sunlight at all times. Start teaching children early about the potential hazards of summer sun and the importance of sun protection. The effects of sun on skin accumulate over a lifetime, and one bad sunburn during childhood significantly increases the risk for melanoma. Women diagnosed with melanoma should not become pregnant until they are completely cured: In rare instances, melanoma cells have spread from a mother to her unborn child.** ■

# SNEEZING

## SYMPTOMS

- A sneeze is usually set off by an irritated nose or a tickling sensation deep in the nasal passages that is relieved by an explosive involuntary expulsion of air.
- Sneezing can itself be a symptom—along with other symptoms such as an itchy, runny, or congested nose or itchy, watery eyes and mouth breathing—of either a head cold *(see Common Cold)* or an allergy.

## CALL YOUR DOCTOR IF:

- you begin sneezing and experience other allergy symptoms, such as those of asthma or eczema; you may have developed a sensitivity to certain irritants that you previously tolerated.

Sneezing is the body's way of eliminating irritants or a foreign object from the nasal passages. People sneeze for four basic reasons. They sneeze when they have a cold, to help clear the nose. They also sneeze when they have allergic rhinitis, or hay fever, to eliminate allergens from the nasal passages. People with vasomotor rhinitis, a condition characterized by a chronic runny nose, also sneeze occasionally. (The sneezing results from the blood vessels in the nose becoming supersensitive to humidity and temperature, and even to spicy foods.) The fourth common cause of sneezing is nonallergic rhinitis with eosinophilia syndrome, or NARES. People with this condition have the symptoms of chronic rhinitis but do not test positive for allergens. Instead, for some unknown reason, their bodies seem to release histamine, a chemical that produces allergy symptoms such as sneezing.

An occasional sneeze is nothing to worry about. Sneezing that is part of a cold will go away with the cold, usually in about a week. However, persistent sneezing or sneezing accompanied by other allergy symptoms—a runny or congested nose, a sore throat, or itchy, watery eyes—may be worth a trip to the doctor.

## CAUSES

Sneezing is caused by an irritant in the nasal passages—anything from ground pepper and tiny foreign objects to pollen, mold, and other allergens.

## TREATMENT

Most allergy-related sneezing can be successfully treated with over-the-counter antihistamines and by home care focused on reducing such allergens as dust, mold, and pet dander. If you have hay fever, you can also reduce your discomfort by taking appropriate precautions before going outside.

### CONVENTIONAL MEDICINE

Your doctor will examine you and discuss your symptoms. You may be referred to an allergist for skin tests. Allergy shots, to desensitize you to a specific allergen, may be recommended. The first line of defense for persistent sneezing is home management and use of over-the-counter or non-sedating prescription antihistamines to dry the mucous membranes, or decongestants to shrink swollen blood vessels blocking the nose. Cromolyn sodium, usually prescribed as a nasal spray, helps allergy sufferers by preventing histamine from being released in the body. Cortisone nasal sprays, which reduce inflammation, may also bring relief and are effective for NARES sufferers.

## ALTERNATIVE CHOICES

### ACUPRESSURE

Steady pressure on the following points may help control sneezing: Triple Warmer 5, Gall Bladder 20, Large Intestine 20, and Large Intestine 4. In addition, pressing your finger across your upper lip, the point of Governing Vessel 26, may help you stop a sneeze. See the illustration above, right, and pages 22–23 for more information on point locations.

### ACUPUNCTURE

For chronic sneezing, you may wish to consult an acupuncturist, who will examine you and target appropriate points based on the exam.

### HERBAL THERAPIES

Hot teas made from either red clover *(Trifolium pratense)* or nettle *(Urtica dioica)* are thought to relieve allergy symptoms and make breathing easier by reducing inflammation.

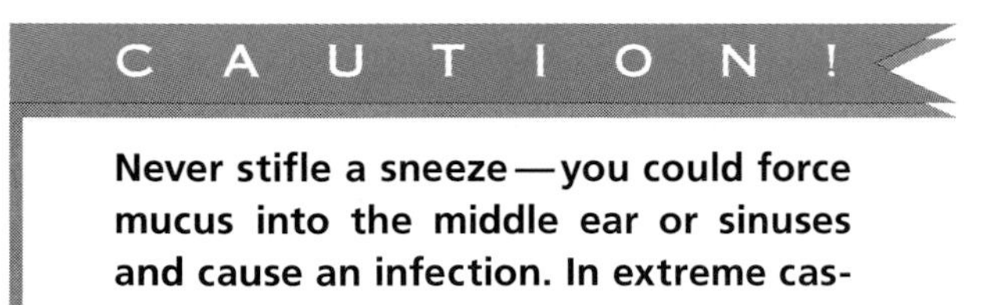


**Never stifle a sneeze—you could force mucus into the middle ear or sinuses and cause an infection. In extreme cases, you could burst an eardrum from backed-up air pressure.**

**ACUPRESSURE**

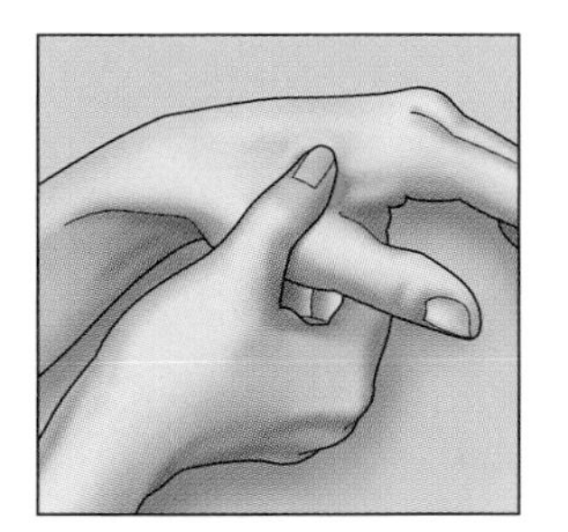

**1** To help stop fits of sneezing, press Large Intestine 4, located in the web between the thumb and index finger. Squeeze the web of each hand with the thumb and index finger of the other for one minute. Do not press this point if you are pregnant.

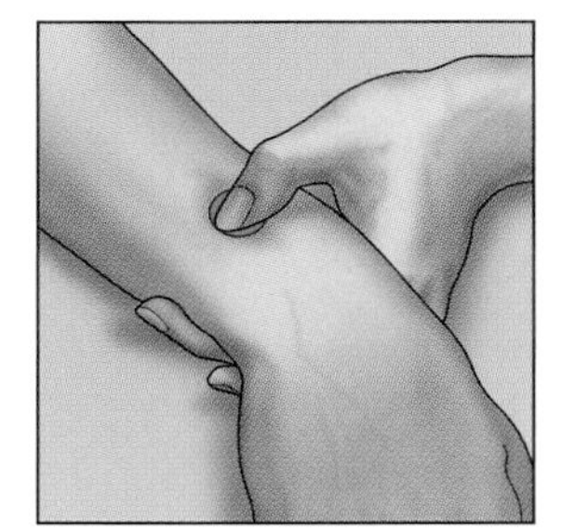

**2** Pressing Triple Warmer 5 may help reduce allergic sensitivity. Center your thumb on the top of your forearm, two thumb widths above the wrist joint. Press firmly for one minute, then repeat on the other arm. Do two or three times.

### HOMEOPATHY

Depending on your specific symptoms, a homeopathic physician may prescribe one of the following remedies: Nux vomica, Pulsatilla, or Natrum muriaticum. Remedies that are derived from pollen or other allergens may also work. For acute sneezing episodes, you may be prescribed Arsenicum album, Sabadilla, Euphrasia, Allium cepa, or Dulcamara.

### NUTRITION AND DIET

You will want to seek professional help for allergies. Food allergies may aggravate hay fever. Try eliminating dairy products, food additives, and foods containing chemical residues such as pesticides or steroid hormone residues (often found in meats). Some nutritionists recommend high doses of vitamin C (3,000 to 6,000 mg, spread evenly throughout the day) as a natural antihistamine.

## AT-HOME REMEDIES

Eliminating allergens in the home is one of the surest ways to alleviate chronic sneezing. Follow the suggestions listed for hay fever. ■

# SNORING

## SYMPTOMS

- rough, hoarse, fluttering noise when breathing during sleep, varying in frequency, pitch, and intensity.

## CALL YOUR DOCTOR IF:

- you live with a snorer and note that his or her snoring is very loud or marked by intervals of no breathing at all. The person may have obstructive sleep apnea, a serious respiratory condition.
- you are frequently very sleepy and tired during the day. You could have obstructive sleep apnea, a serious condition that is preventing you from getting enough oxygen during sleep.
- you frequently fall asleep in inappropriate settings, such as at the office or while eating. You could have obstructive sleep apnea or narcolepsy, a disorder that causes sufferers to fall asleep during normal waking hours.

Snoring is usually not a serious problem. Men are 50 percent more likely to snore than women, but most people snore occasionally. Chronic snorers tend to be overweight and middle-aged.

Sometimes, though, snoring can point to a dangerous medical condition. The most serious is obstructive sleep apnea, in which the snorer stops breathing for anywhere from several seconds to two minutes. This results in decreased oxygen in the blood, which leads to fatigue at best and sudden death at worst. If you think you have this disorder, you must seek conventional treatment.

Other potentially troubling problems are also indicated by regular—often loud—snoring that falls into one of two types: moderate (snoring every time a person sleeps, but which may be intermittent or occurs only when the person lies on his back) and heavy (loud snoring throughout sleeping, no matter what position). Fortunately, there are a variety of remedies that can lessen the intensity of snoring, if not eliminate it entirely.

## CAUSES

Snoring is caused by vibration of the soft palate (the soft part of the mouth's roof) as the lungs strain to inhale oxygen through obstructed airways. Typically this occurs when the muscles that keep these airways open become too lax; any condition or substance that promotes muscle relaxation—including alcohol; medications such as sleeping pills, cold medicines, or antihistamines; an overly soft or large pillow; sleeping on one's back; poor muscle tone; or obesity—can have this effect. Obstruction can also be caused by nasal deformities, such as an excessively long soft palate or uvula, or a deviated septum. In children, enlarged adenoids or tonsils often cause snoring. Any ailment that makes bronchial airways constrict, such as asthma, can lead to obstruction and snoring; smoking, which irritates the passageways, can also make snoring worse.

### DIAGNOSTIC AND TEST PROCEDURES

First, your physician will ask about any allergies you may have, as well as about your eating patterns, what drugs you take, and whether you drink alcohol or smoke. If these are not the culprits, your doctor may examine your throat and nasal passages for any signs of nasal deformities.

If your doctor suspects that you have obstructive sleep apnea, your partner may be asked to keep a diary noting your sleeping patterns, or you may be enrolled in a sleep-monitoring study, which will analyze when and how often you stop breathing during sleep.

## TREATMENT

In most cases, snoring requires no medical treatment; going on a diet and cutting out smoking and alcohol usually clear up the problem. Alternative therapies can also help. In more serious cases, however, surgery may be necessary.

### CONVENTIONAL MEDICINE

If snoring is light, no treatment may be necessary. If allergies are the cause, your physician will likely prescribe antihistamines or a nasal decongestant. Snoring caused by nasal deformities may require corrective surgery to open up the airways. If it is determined that you have obstructive sleep apnea, your doctor will pursue treatment more aggressively, because of the potentially dangerous consequences of the condition.

### ALTERNATIVE CHOICES

If your snoring is due to allergies, asthma, bronchitis, or emphysema, there are a number of alternative remedies that may help you open up your airways and sleep more peacefully. Refer to the listed ailment entries for treatment advice.

## PREVENTION

- Consider losing some weight: Most snorers tend to be overweight, and shedding excess fat has been shown to substantially decrease—if not eliminate—snoring.
- Avoid midnight snacks and alcoholic beverages: Drinking alcohol or eating heavily before going to sleep causes muscles to slacken.
- Avoid sleeping pills or other sedatives: Although they put you to sleep, they relax your neck muscles, making your snoring worse.
- Stop smoking: Smoking causes nasal and bronchial congestion, a major cause of snoring.
- Sleep on your side: While heavy snorers will snore in any position, moderates tend to snore only when sleeping on their backs. One way to avoid this is to sew a pocket onto the back of your nightclothes and insert a tennis ball, which will make it uncomfortable for you to lie on your back and prompt you to turn on your side during sleep.
- Sleep without a pillow: By putting a kink in your neck, pillows can contribute to airway obstruction. ■

### OBSTRUCTIVE SLEEP APNEA

*Between 1 and 5 percent of adults suffer from a snoring disorder that is no joke: obstructive sleep apnea. The condition, which generally targets men (a reported 9 out of 10 sufferers are men), occurs when breathing stops 30 or more times, for 10 or more seconds in each incident, during a 7-hour sleep period. People with serious cases of the disease may not breathe at all for up to three-quarters of the time that they are asleep. The result is not only oxygen deprivation but also high blood pressure; in the very worst cases, the condition can be fatal. If you are a loud, heavy snorer, you may have sleep apnea and should consider enrolling in a sleep-study program, which will monitor your sleep patterns and help develop therapies for your recovery.*

# SORE THROAT

## SYMPTOMS

The classic symptoms of a sore throat include a burning sensation or "scratchiness" in the back of the throat; pain, especially when swallowing; and, perhaps, tenderness along the neck. These symptoms may be accompanied by:

- sneezing and coughing.
- hoarseness.
- runny nose.
- mild fever.
- general fatigue.

## CALL YOUR DOCTOR IF:

- you also have a fever higher than 101°F without other cold symptoms; this may indicate a case of strep throat that needs treatment.
- you also have flulike symptoms that don't get better after a few days; this may indicate infectious mononucleosis.
- any hoarseness lasts longer than two weeks; this could be a sign of throat cancer or oral cancer.
- your sore throat persists for more than a week and is accompanied by postnasal drip; this may be a sign of allergies that require medical attention.
- your sore throat is accompanied by drooling, or you experience difficulty swallowing or breathing; this may indicate an inflamed epiglottis, the structure that overhangs the opening to the larynx, or an abscess in the back of the throat; these two uncommon conditions require medical attention.

Everyone knows what a sore throat feels like. It is one of the most common health complaints, particularly during the colder months of the year, when respiratory diseases are at their peak. Typically the raw, scratchy, burning feeling at the back of your throat is the first sign you'll have of a cold or the flu on the way. But a sore throat can also presage more serious conditions, so you should watch how it develops, and call your doctor if there are any signs that you have more than the run-of-the-mill type.

## CAUSES

At least 90 percent of sore throats are caused by inflammation of throat tissue, often triggered by viral infections, including the common cold, flu, measles, chickenpox, herpes, and infectious mononucleosis. Bacterial infections, such as whooping cough, can also lead to a sore throat. The streptococcus bacterium, which produces the illness known as strep throat, is most commonly at fault, but the bacterium responsible for gonorrhea can also cause sore throats among people who engage in oral sex.

Living in a dusty or very dry environment can cause a raw and painful throat, as can overuse (or misuse) of the voice, or habitual use of tobacco or alcohol. People who suffer from allergies, persistent coughs, or chronic sinusitis are also prone to sore throats.

In rare cases, a persistent sore throat may be a sign of a potentially cancerous growth in the throat or mouth.

### DIAGNOSTIC AND TEST PROCEDURES

If it appears that your sore throat may be the result of a bacterial rather than a viral infection, your doctor may do a throat culture. This painless procedure involves swabbing out a sampling of throat mucus for laboratory analysis. Your doctor's office may be equipped to analyze the culture within a few minutes, or you may have to wait a day or two while the sample is sent to an outside laboratory.

For persistent throat pain, or if other symp-

## Curing Morning Sore Throat

*Some people wake up regularly with a sore throat, which then goes away as the day progresses. This "morning-only" sore throat is often caused by sleeping with your mouth open but can also result from a backup of stomach acids into your throat during the night.*

*If you think your sore throat may come from sleeping with your mouth open, try a bedroom humidifier or vaporizer (be sure to follow directions for cleaning a humidifier carefully).*

*If you believe the soreness may be due to a backup of stomach acids, try sleeping on a tilted bed frame. Place bricks or boards under your bed so that the head of the bed is four to six inches higher than the foot. Piling pillows under your head will not help because they will cause your body to bend in a way that will put even more pressure on your esophagus and make the problem worse. Also, avoid eating or drinking anything for an hour or two before going to bed.*

toms are present, your doctor may order additional tests to check for other conditions.

## TREATMENT

Most sore throats are self-limiting, which means they usually go away on their own without any kind of treatment. In the absence of other symptoms, therefore, you may first want to try alternative treatments for a painful throat. However, if the pain persists or worsens after a few days, you should see your doctor. If left untreated for too long, strep throat may lead to rheumatic fever, which can damage the heart, or to acute nephritis, which can damage the kidneys.

### CONVENTIONAL MEDICINE

For a bacterial throat infection, such as strep throat, your doctor will probably prescribe penicillin—or, if you are allergic to penicillin, some other antibiotic such as erythromycin—for 7 to 10 days. To avoid a recurrence, it is very important that you complete the entire course of the antibiotic, even after symptoms have gone away.

Antibiotics are not effective for sore throats caused by viral infections. Your doctor will most likely recommend that you simply rest, drink plenty of liquids, gargle with salt water, and take aspirin or acetaminophen if needed for pain relief. Over-the-counter throat lozenges containing a mild anesthetic can also provide relief. CAUTION: Do not give aspirin to a child or young adult with a sore throat, as it may lead to Reye's syndrome, a rare but very serious illness.

### ALTERNATIVE CHOICES

See the illustrations on the following page for **acupressure** techniques that may help relieve the pain of a sore throat. In general, alternative therapies are geared toward symptom relief, although in some cases they also address the actual cause of the sore throat.

#### ACUPUNCTURE

Acupuncture can be very helpful in relieving the pain and reducing the inflammation of a sore throat. A professional acupuncturist will stimulate points along the kidney, large intestine, and stomach meridians. *(See pages 22 and 23 for information on point locations.)*

#### AROMATHERAPY

To increase blood circulation and improve fluid drainage in sore areas, massage your throat and chest with a lotion made with 2 drops each of eucalyptus *(Eucalyptus globulus)* and peppermint *(Mentha piperita)* in 2 tsp of a carrier oil such as vegetable or almond oil.

#### HERBAL THERAPIES

To help fight the infection causing a sore throat, herbalists recommend several herbs with antimicrobial properties. At the first sign of soreness, take three raw cloves of garlic *(Allium sativum)* a day. (Garlic is a natural antibiotic and antiseptic.) If garlic smell becomes a problem, try four garlic oil capsules instead. Teas made from either goldenseal *(Hydrastis canadensis)* or echinacea (*Echinacea* spp.) may also be effective. To make goldenseal tea, pour 1 cup boiling water over 1 tsp powdered herb; let it steep for 10 to 15 minutes, strain, then drink. Repeat three times a day. To make echinacea tea, put 1 to 2 tsp of the root in 1 cup water and bring slowly to a boil; reduce heat and let the tea simmer for 10 to 15 minutes. Cool the tea to a comfortable temperature and drink; repeat three times a day.

Or try a tea made from licorice *(Glycyrrhiza glabra),* which may help enhance the immune system's defenses against bacteria. Put 1 tbsp of the root in 3 cups water; simmer for 10 to 15 minutes. Drink three times a day. CAUTION: Some forms of licorice affect high blood pressure. Use licorice for no longer than one week unless under the care of a health practitioner.

To ease the discomfort of a sore throat, drink teas made from sage *(Salvia officinalis)* or chamomile *(Matricaria recutita).* A simple lemon tea can also be very soothing. Squeeze the juice of one lemon in 8 oz warm water, add honey to taste, and drink.

A traditional Native American treatment is drinking a tea made from the inner bark of the slippery elm *(Ulmus fulva).* Put 2 tsp powdered bark in 1 cup water. Bring to a boil and simmer for 10 to 15 minutes.

#### HOMEOPATHY

Homeopaths prescribe several remedies for sore throats. Consult a homeopathic practitioner or try those listed here.

- If the pain comes on suddenly and is accompanied by great thirst and hoarseness, try Aconite (6c) three times a day.
- If the pain comes on suddenly and is accompanied by fever, headache, and restlessness, use Belladonna (6c) three times a day.

#### ACUPRESSURE

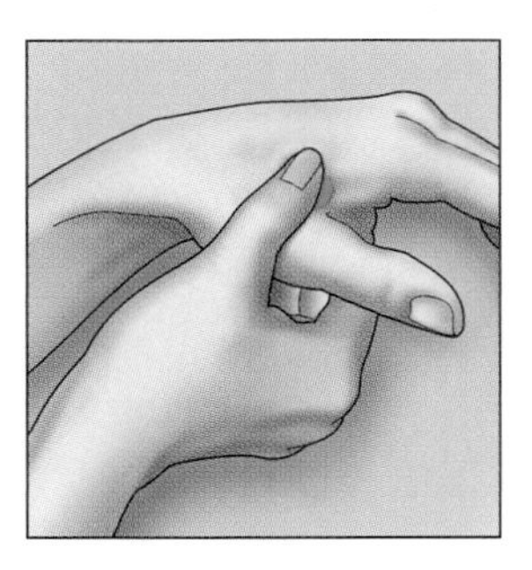

**1** For a sore throat from a cold or the flu, try pressing your right thumb into LI 4, between the thumb and index finger of your left hand. Apply firm pressure against the bone above your index finger for one minute, then repeat on the other hand. Do not use during pregnancy.

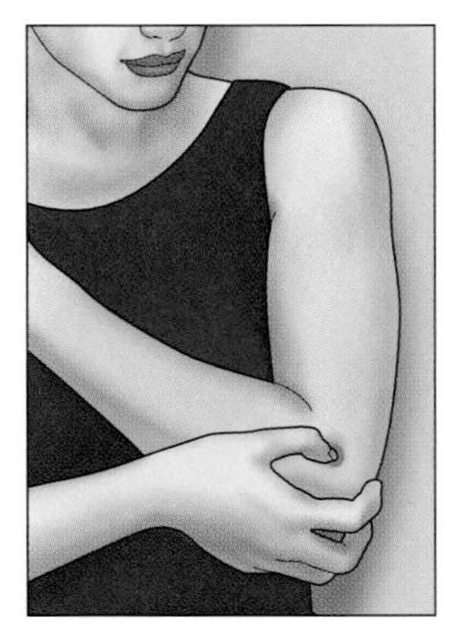

**2** Acupressure may help ease the symptoms of a fever due to a cold. Apply pressure with your thumb to LI 11, located at the outer end of the elbow crease on your left arm. Hold for one minute and repeat on the right arm.

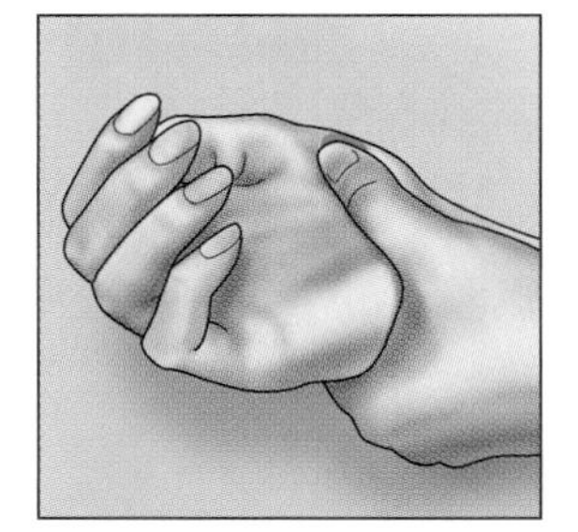

**3** To help relieve the discomfort of a sore and swollen throat, try pressure at LU 10. Using your left thumb, apply pressure to the center of the pad at the base of your right thumb. Hold for one minute and repeat on the other hand.

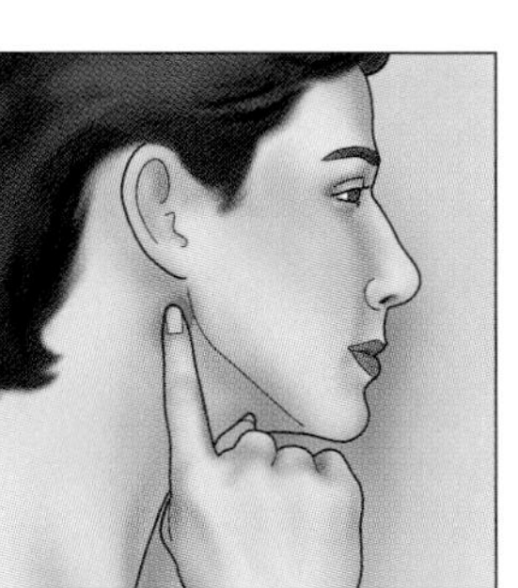

**4** To relieve an irritated throat, place your index fingers on SI 17, in the indentations at both corners of your jawbone just below your earlobes. Breathe deeply and press on both sides gently for one minute. These points are very sensitive, so apply pressure slowly and carefully.

- If your sore throat has come on gradually and is accompanied by fatigue, try Ferrum phosphoricum (6c) three times a day.
- If the back of your throat is red and swollen

and the pain is relieved by cold water or ice, try Apis (6c) three times a day.

- ◆ If your sore throat is accompanied by flulike symptoms, extreme sluggishness, and weakness, use Gelsemium (6c) three times a day.

#### NUTRITION AND DIET

At the first sign of soreness, take 500 to 6,000 mg of vitamin C daily to help fight the cold or other viral infection causing it. CAUTION: Unless your body is accustomed to megadoses of vitamin C, it cannot absorb more than about 1,000 mg every two hours; the excess will be passed off in your urine or, in some cases, result in diarrhea. Also, if you take a dose at the higher end of this range, drink plenty of fluids to keep the vitamin C from concentrating in your kidneys.

Some practitioners of **naturopathic medicine** attribute repeated sore throats to a zinc deficiency. Try a daily supplement of 20 to 40 mg.

If you have frequent sore throats, especially ones associated with ear infections, you may have a food allergy. Consult a healthcare practitioner who specializes in food allergies.

### AT-HOME REMEDIES

- ◆ Get plenty of rest and drink a lot of fluids.
- ◆ Take aspirin or other over-the-counter medication for pain relief.
- ◆ Suck on a zinc lozenge—about 23 mg of zinc—every four hours. Zinc can relieve sore throats and other cold symptoms.
- ◆ To help relieve the pain, apply a warm heating pad or compress to your throat. You can also try a warm chamomile poultice: Mix 1 tbsp dried chamomile flowers into 1 or 2 cups boiling water; steep for five minutes, then strain. Soak a clean cloth or towel in the tea, wring it out, then apply to your throat. Remove the cloth when it becomes cold. Repeat as often as necessary.
- ◆ A salt plaster may also help provide relief. Mix 2 cups sea salt with 5 to 6 tbsp lukewarm water; the salt should be damp, but not wet. Place the salt in the center of a dishtowel, then roll the towel along the longer side. Wrap the towel around your neck; cover it with another dry towel. Leave on for as long as you wish.
- ◆ Try steam inhalations to ease the pain. Run very hot water in a sink. With a towel draped over your head to trap the steam, lean over the sink while the water is running. Breathe deeply through your mouth and nose for 5 to 10 minutes. Repeat several times a day.

#### HOMEMADE GARGLES

To wash away mucus and irritants and bring relief from the pain of a sore throat, try any of the following gargles:

- **Salt water:** Mix ½ tsp salt in 8 oz warm water.
- **Sage:** Put 1 to 2 tsp dried leaves in 1 cup boiling water; steep for 10 minutes, then strain and cool until lukewarm.
- **Chamomile:** Steep 1 tsp of the dried herb in 1 cup warm water.
- **Apple cider vinegar:** Mix 2 tsp vinegar in 1 cup warm water.
- **Lemon:** Mix the juice of one lemon in 8 oz warm water.
- **Horseradish:** Mix 1 tbsp pure horseradish, 1 tsp honey, and 1 tsp ground cloves in 8 oz warm water.
- **Raspberry:** Put 1 to 2 tsp raspberry leaf in 1 cup boiling water; steep for 10 minutes, then strain and cool until lukewarm.
- **Cayenne pepper:** Mix the juice of half a lemon, 1 tbsp salt, and ¼ tsp cayenne pepper (or more if you can tolerate it) in ½ cup warm water. The cayenne pepper temporarily reduces the amount of pain-causing chemicals produced by nerve endings in the throat.
- **Aspirin:** Dissolve two tablets crushed aspirin in 1 cup warm water.
- **Hydrogen peroxide:** Make a mixture of half hydrogen peroxide and half warm water.

## PREVENTION

If you tend to get recurrent sore throats, replace your toothbrush every month; bacteria can collect on the bristles. Also, be sure to toss an old toothbrush once you've recovered from a sore throat to avoid reinfecting yourself. ■

# SPRAINS AND STRAINS

## SYMPTOMS

Sprains, which affect joints, and strains, also called muscle pulls, usually occur after a fall or sudden movement that pulls or twists a part of the body violently.

**For a sprain:**

- pain in the affected joint.
- rapid swelling of a joint, often accompanied by bruising.
- stiffness and difficulty moving a joint.

**For a strain:**

- sharp pain at the site of an injury, followed by stiffness, tenderness, and in some cases, swelling.

## CALL YOUR DOCTOR IF:

- the pain, swelling, or stiffness does not improve in two to three days.
- you feel a popping sensation when you move a sprained joint; this may indicate a serious injury that requires immediate medical treatment.
- you can't move or bear weight on an injured joint. You may have a broken bone.
- the bones in an injured joint don't seem to be aligned properly. The ligaments that hold the joint together may be badly torn, requiring surgical repair.
- an injured muscle does not move at all; it may have torn completely through and may require immediate medical attention.
- you have repeated sprains or strains, indicating a chronic weakness that should be evaluated by a physician.
- you have difficulty moving or walking after straining any back muscle. You may have nerve damage *(see Back Problems).*

Sprains and strains are among the most common injuries, ranging from twisted ankles to aching backs. A **sprain** injures ligaments, the tough, fibrous bands of tissue that connect bones to one another at a joint. A **strain** damages muscle tissue, leaving muscles, or the tendons that attach muscle to bone, stretched or torn.

Given adequate time and rest, most sprained joints or strained muscles will heal themselves. But severe tearing or complete rupture of the affected tissues usually requires surgical repair. And damage caused by a sprain can leave the bones in the affected joint improperly aligned, or the ligaments so stretched and weakened that the joint is particularly vulnerable to future injury. *(See also Muscle Pain, Tendonitis, Groin Strain, Hamstring Injury.)*

## CAUSES

Anything that places sudden or unaccustomed stress on joints or muscles may cause a sprain or strain. Falls, lifting heavy objects, and the exertion of an unfamiliar sport are common culprits. Being overweight, inactive, or in poor physical condition boosts the likelihood of injury.

### THE RICE TREATMENT

*Doctors, physical therapists, and athletes all swear by RICE—rest, ice, compression, and elevation—as the standard treatment for the first 48 to 72 hours in muscle, tendon, or ligament injuries. Rest the area immediately to avoid further injury. Apply ice, alternating 10 minutes on, 10 minutes off, to reduce swelling and inflammation. Use elastic bandages to compress the area and reduce swelling. And keep the injured area elevated to promote drainage of fluid.*

S

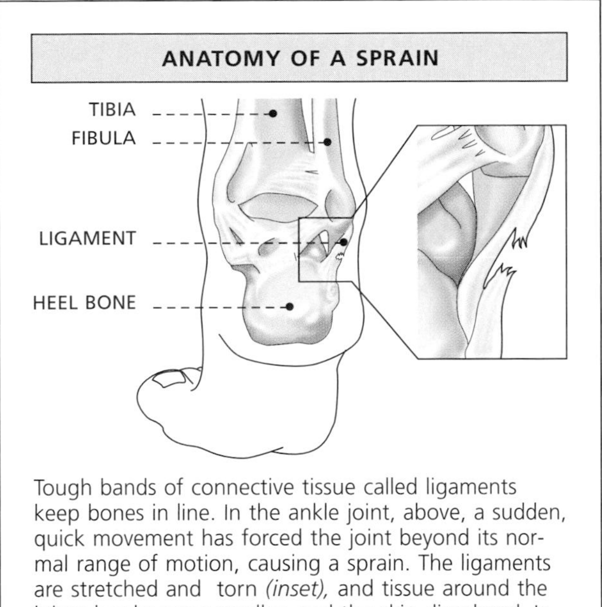


Tough bands of connective tissue called ligaments keep bones in line. In the ankle joint, above, a sudden, quick movement has forced the joint beyond its normal range of motion, causing a sprain. The ligaments are stretched and torn *(inset)*, and tissue around the injury has become swollen and the skin discolored. In most cases, a sprained joint will still function but can be painful to use.

### DIAGNOSTIC AND TEST PROCEDURES

Your doctor may order x-rays to rule out fracture, or an MRI scan to check for ruptured tissues.

## TREATMENT

Treatment of both sprains and strains focuses on control of the initial pain and swelling, followed by adequate rest to allow healing.

### CONVENTIONAL MEDICINE

Most sprains and strains heal in two to three weeks. Doctors routinely prescribe rest, ice, compression, and elevation immediately following the injury, along with aspirin or ibuprofen to reduce inflammation and pain. Elastic bandages may then be used to support or immobilize the injured area while it heals, and a sprained ankle or knee often calls for crutches to keep weight off the joint. To speed healing, your doctor may also recommend heat or infrared treatments from a physical therapist.

### ALTERNATIVE CHOICES

Alternative therapies can help relieve the pain and swelling associated with sprains and strains.

#### CHINESE HERBS

A practitioner of Chinese medicine may use a poultice of gardenia *(Gardenia jasminoides)*, flour, and wine to reduce swelling and promote healing. Massage with the extracted oil of safflower flower *(Carthamus tinctorius)* is believed to improve circulation, which encourages healing.

#### HOMEOPATHY

The anti-inflammatory action of homeopathic preparations of Arnica (6x to 30c), taken orally, may relieve pain.

#### NUTRITION AND DIET

Research indicates that vitamin supplements may help heal sprains and strains. If your doctor approves, take daily supplements of vitamin C (1,000 mg), beta carotene (vitamin A) (10,000 IU), zinc (up to 60 mg), vitamin E (400 IU), and selenium (50 mcg).

### AT-HOME REMEDIES

Once the initial swelling has subsided and you are no longer in acute pain—usually after 48 to 72 hours—you may use a heating pad to relieve soreness and stimulate circulation in the injured area. Massaging the area with an over-the-counter topical cream containing aspirin or another analgesic can also alleviate lingering soreness or tenderness.

## PREVENTION

The best way to prevent sprains or strains is to keep yourself in good physical shape, so that your muscles, ligaments, and tendons are strong and flexible enough to resist trauma. To prevent recurring injury, ask your doctor for exercises designed to rehabilitate the muscles in the injured area. If you are overweight, ask about an appropriate diet and a general conditioning program. ■

# STAPH INFECTIONS

## SYMPTOMS

- pain and swelling around a cut or scraped area of skin.
- boils or small, white-headed pimples around hair follicles.
- in infants and young children, blistering and peeling skin.
- swollen lymph nodes in the neck, armpits, or groin.

## CALL YOUR DOCTOR IF:

- any pain, swelling, or pus forms around a cut or scraped area of skin; the infection may spread into the bloodstream.
- the lymph nodes in your neck, armpits, or groin become swollen; this can also be a symptom of a variety of other illnesses, including mononucleosis, tuberculosis, and cancer.
- you have a boil that is very tender, particularly if it has red lines radiating from it, or if you have fever and chills; the infection may have spread.
- you have a boil or **carbuncle** on or near your lip, nose, cheeks, forehead, or spine; the infection can spread into your brain or spine.
- you have recurrent boils; they may be a sign of diabetes.

Staph infections can invade and attack any part of your body, from your skin, eyes, and nails to the inner lining of your heart. Symptoms vary, depending on where the infection develops. Staph infections usually enter the body through an open cut or wound. The infection can spread to adjacent tissue or, through the bloodstream, to distant internal organs, such as the heart or kidneys, where it can become life-threatening. People with a chronic illness, such as diabetes, cancer, or chronic liver or kidney disease, are particularly susceptible to severe staph infections.

Staph infections are known by a variety of names, many of which are also used to describe strep infections. **Folliculitis** is a superficial infection of the hair follicles that produces small, white-headed pustules. Shaving the skin or friction from clothing rubbing against the skin can injure the follicles and cause the infection to erupt. The area where the pustules appear may itch for a day or two beforehand.

Sometimes a staph infection invades the deepest part of the hair follicle, resulting in a large, painful, pus-filled inflammation known as a boil. Although boils can form anywhere on the body, they are found most frequently on the face, neck, buttocks, and armpits. If one appears on the eyelid, it is known as a sty. When several separate boils occur simultaneously on the body, the condition is called **furunculosis.**

A **carbuncle** is a cluster of connected boils deep under the skin. Carbuncles are usually found on the upper back or nape of the neck and are more common in men than in women.

Another common staph infection of the skin is impetigo, characterized by small patches of tiny blisters and pustules that become crusty after breaking open. Less common, but potentially more serious, is **cellulitis,** which occurs in the deeper layers of the skin. It usually begins with a tender swelling and redness around a cut or sore, then gradually spreads into nearby tissue. Red lines may radiate from the infected area to nearby lymph nodes, which may also become infected and swell to two or three times their normal size—a serious condition called **lymphadenitis.**

Infants and young children sometimes develop **scalded skin syndrome,** a staph infection characterized by a blistering, peeling rash. Another staph infection that afflicts mostly children is conjunctivitis; this causes the eyes to redden and to weep a yellow, watery pus that forms a crust overnight during sleep. **Blepharitis,** a staph infection that involves the edges of the eyelids, can also result in red, crusty eyes. When a staph infection forms around the edges of fingernails, causing swelling and pus-filled blisters, the condition is known as **paronychia.**

A staph infection called **mastitis** can enter the breasts of nursing mothers through cracked, sore nipples, resulting in painful breast abscesses. Menstruating women who use tampons are at risk of developing a potentially life-threatening staph infection, toxic shock syndrome.

Staph infections sometimes spread through the bloodstream to the bones and joints—particularly those of the arms, legs, and spine—where abscesses may then form. The affected joint swells and fills with pus. Left untreated, it may become arthritic and permanently stiff.

If a staph infection spreads to the lungs, staphylococcal pneumonia can occur; if it spreads to the kidneys, a kidney infection may develop. Both conditions can be life-threatening. A spreading staph infection can also attack the endocardium, or inner lining of the heart, resulting in bacterial **endocarditis,** a serious condition that can cause permanent damage to the heart. (This condition occurs primarily in intravenous-drug users.) The colon can also become a target of a staph infection, particularly among people who are taking an antibiotic for other ailments. The drug may kill off other kinds of bacteria in the colon, enabling staphylococci to multiply freely.

## CAUSES

Staph infections are caused by *Staphylococcus aureus,* a type of bacterium commonly found in the nose, mouth, rectum, or genital area. In fact, at any one time, about 30 to 40 percent of people carry staphylococci in their noses without any symptoms of illness. The bacteria are harmless until they enter the body through a cut, scrape, or other break in the skin. Once they invade the body, the bacteria form pus-containing abscesses. Bacteria that enter the body on contaminated food can cause food poisoning.

### DIAGNOSTIC AND TEST PROCEDURES

Your doctor will examine the infection and perhaps take a sample of pus for laboratory analysis to determine if its cause is staphylococci or another kind of bacterium. If your doctor suspects that the infection has spread to other areas of your body, further tests, such as a blood analysis or a lymph node culture, may also be done. If you have recurrent boils or sties, your doctor may take a nasal culture to determine whether your nose is harboring staphylococci.

## TREATMENT

In mild cases, such as boils or **folliculitis,** you can clean the infected area yourself with antibacterial soap and apply some of the topical treatments mentioned under At-Home Remedies. If the infection persists or worsens, however, you should see your doctor for antibacterial medications to make

### STAPH INFECTIONS IN HOSPITALS

*Staph infections are easy to pick up in a hospital after a surgical procedure, despite the best efforts of nurses, doctors, and others to keep the hospital a germfree environment. For this reason antibiotics are often prescribed to patients for a full 24 hours following surgery. In cases when the risk is especially high—when the patient is having intestinal surgery, for example—antibiotics are administered before the operation as well as after it.*

sure the infection does not lead to serious complications. Alternative treatments to strengthen your immune system can help prevent a recurrence.

## CONVENTIONAL MEDICINE

Your doctor will probably give you an oral antibiotic, such as erythromycin or dicloxacillin, to clear up the infection. If you have a skin infection, you may be prescribed an antibiotic cream to apply to the infected area. In recurrent cases of boils or sties, when a nasal culture has revealed the presence of staphylococci, an antibiotic cream is inserted directly into the nostrils.

Some abscesses must be surgically drained for the infection to heal completely. Your doctor may refer you to a surgeon for this procedure, which can usually be done, using a local anesthetic, right in the surgeon's office. If the infection is severe, you may be hospitalized so that antibiotics can be administered intravenously.

## ALTERNATIVE CHOICES

Your alternative medical practitioner can provide comprehensive treatment for your staph infection. Alternative medicine can also help you to strengthen your immune system so that you can avoid recurrent infections. However, if the infection does not respond to these treatments and worsens or spreads, you should seek conventional treatment with antibiotic medications.

### ACUPUNCTURE

In Chinese medicine, any kind of boil is believed to be caused by excess heat in the body. Treatment therefore consists of stimulating points on the body that can dissipate that heat. Consult a professional acupuncturist.

### HERBAL THERAPIES

Several herbs have antibacterial properties that are believed to be helpful in fighting staph infections. They include:

- Garlic *(Allium sativum):* Take three cloves a day at the first sign of infection; if garlic smell becomes a problem, try three garlic oil capsules instead.

### YOGA

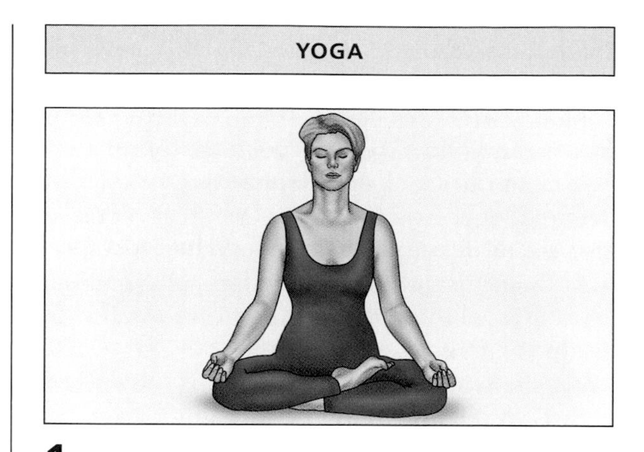

**1** To help boost your immune system, try the **Half Lotus:** Bend your left leg and bring the foot close to your body. Bend your right leg and place the foot high on the left thigh. Ideally, your knees should touch the floor. (For **Full Lotus,** place each foot on the opposite thigh.) Hold for five minutes, breathing deeply.

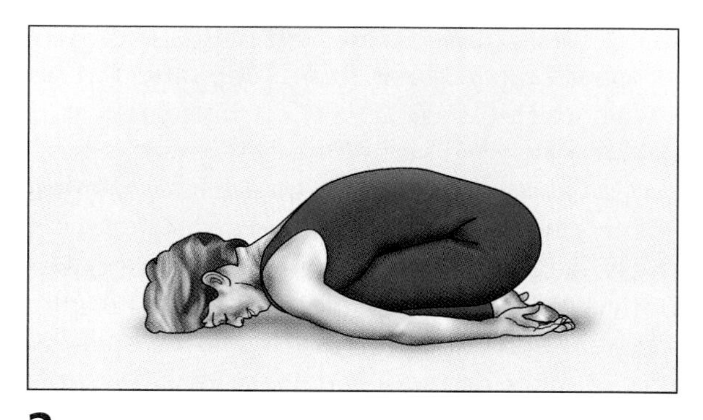

**2** The **Child** may help stimulate your immune system by relaxing your body. Sit on your heels, thighs together. Exhale slowly while bending forward from your hips. Move your forehead to the floor. Breathe deeply for 20 seconds, then inhale as you arise. Do once.

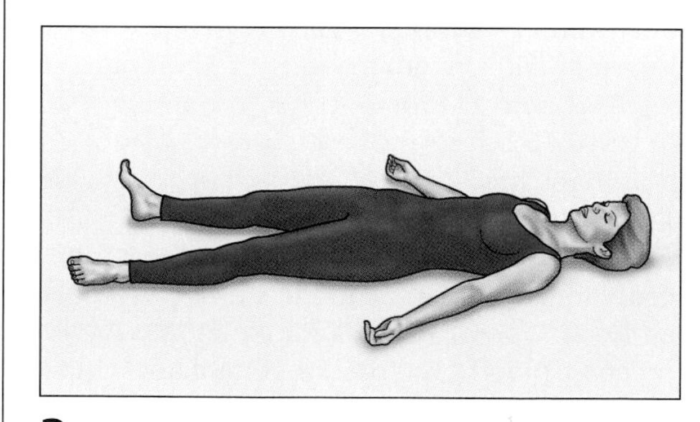

**3** Another position that promotes relaxation is the **Corpse.** Lie on your back, with your feet about 18 inches apart and turned out slightly. Place your hands about 6 inches from your hips, palms up. Close your eyes; breathe deeply for 8 to 10 minutes.

S

- Goldenseal *(Hydrastis canadensis):* Make a tea from the powdered herb and drink three cups a day.
- Echinacea (*Echinacea* spp.): Make a tea from the root and drink three cups a day.

To help heal staph abscesses and reduce any swelling of the lymph nodes, use cleavers *(Galium aparine),* an anti-inflammatory herb believed to be a tonic for the lymphatic system. Make a tea from the dried herb and drink three cups a day; if you prefer, take 2 to 4 ml of a tincture of the herb three times daily.

See also At-Home Remedies.

#### HOMEOPATHY

Staph infections are treated with remedies designed to boost your body's immunity to the infection. Treatments vary according to the type of infection and where it appears on the body. Consult an experienced homeopath.

#### NUTRITION AND DIET

To help rid your body of the infection and restore your natural immunity, eat plenty of green, orange, and yellow vegetables, which are rich in beta carotene (vitamin A), and drink 8 to 10 glasses of water each day. To activate your immune system and help your white blood cells fight the infection, take zinc supplements (30 to 50 mg) daily. In addition, supplements of vitamin C (1,000 to 5,000 mg spread evenly throughout the day) and bioflavonoids (300 to 2,000 mg daily) may help fight the infection. Recurrent boils or other staph infections can be signs of a poor diet. Consult a nutritionist.

### AT-HOME REMEDIES

- To speed healing, place a warm compress such as a warm, wet washcloth on a boil or sty for 20 to 30 minutes, three or four times a day. To help prevent scarring, add a few drops of thyme oil, lavender, or bergamot to the water in which the washcloth is soaked. After the boil or sty has ruptured and the pus has drained, clean the area with warm water and lemon juice or Epsom salt. Keep clean until completely healed. CAUTION: Never squeeze or lance a boil or sty; if you do, you may cause permanent scarring or cause the infection to spread.
- Apply a cleavers compress to the staph infection. Chop up the fresh leaves, then soak them briefly in warm water. Squeeze out most of the water and wrap the leaves in gauze. Place on the infected area of skin.
- Apply a paste made from goldenseal root to the infection. Mix goldenseal root powder with enough water to make a paste. Put it directly onto the infected area of the skin, then cover with a clean, nonporous bandage or cloth. Leave the paste on overnight.
- To prevent a staph infection from spreading while it heals, take showers rather than baths.
- If you have **folliculitis** of the beard, use a new razor blade each day for shaving while the infection is healing.
- If you have a staph infection around the edges of a nail, soak the nail in pure tea tree oil (*Melaleuca* spp.) for five minutes twice a day until the infection clears. A drop of tea tree oil can also be applied directly to a boil.
- Always wash your hands thoroughly after treating a staph infection.

## PREVENTION

- Wash all cuts, scrapes, and wounds with antiseptic soap; keep them clean during healing.
- To keep your staph infection from spreading to other members of your household, do not share towels, washcloths, and bed linens. Change these items daily and launder them in hot water and bleach.
- If you are prone to **folliculitis,** wash your skin with an antibacterial soap before you shave. Soak your razor in rubbing alcohol between shaves, and don't let anyone else use it.
- To avoid food poisoning caused by staph (as well as other) bacteria, always wash your hands thoroughly before preparing food. If you are recovering from a staph infection, have someone else prepare food so you do not spread the infection to others. ■

# STOMACH CANCER

## SYMPTOMS

Stomach cancer usually produces no early symptoms other than mild indigestion or loss of weight and appetite, which are symptoms vague enough to be ignored by most people. As the disease advances, the symptoms become more pronounced. Warning signs of stomach cancer may include:

- indigestion, heartburn, abdominal pain, or discomfort aggravated by eating.
- loss of appetite; a bloated or full feeling after eating small amounts of food.
- either diarrhea or constipation; nausea and vomiting after meals.
- general weakness and fatigue.
- dark patches in stool, or blood on stool.
- vomiting blood.

## CALL YOUR DOCTOR IF:

- feelings of indigestion or abdominal discomfort persist for more than a few weeks, or if you experience dark stools, an indication of bleeding in the stomach or intestinal tract. You need a thorough medical examination, by either your primary care physician or a gastroenterologist, to find out whether your discomfort is due to a stomach ulcer, cancer, or some other cause.

S

Before World War II, stomach cancer—also known as **gastric cancer** or **gastric carcinoma**—was a leading cancer killer in the United States. The disease is now much less prevalent in the U.S., but in Japan, Korea, Latin America, and eastern Europe, it remains one of the most common and lethal cancers.

Almost all stomach cancers start in glandular tissue lining the stomach. A tumor may spread along the stomach wall or may grow directly through the wall and shed cells into the bloodstream or lymphatic system. Once beyond the stomach, cancer can spread to other organs. If treated before it spreads, stomach cancer is curable. A patient whose tumor is removed completely has a good chance of surviving at least five years. Unfortunately, by the time most cases of stomach cancer are diagnosed, the cancer has spread to other organs, making it difficult to treat. Fewer than 1 in 5 patients diagnosed with stomach cancer that has spread to other organs survives five years.

## CAUSES

Stomach cancer often originates at the site of an existing stomach ulcer, although ulcers themselves are not thought to cause the disease. While some stomach ulcers turn cancerous, most do not. For stomach cancer to occur, something has to make normal cells mutate, or reproduce abnormally. Certain dietary agents are linked to stomach cancer: The disease is common among people who frequently eat smoked, pickled, salted, and barbecued foods, all of which contain cancer-promoting nitrites or other nitrogen compounds. Aflatoxins—carcinogenic by-products of a fungus that grows in nuts, seeds, and corn, and in other dried foods stored in humid conditions—also seem to promote stomach cancer. *(See Food Poisoning, Liver Cancer.)* Smoking tobacco and drinking alcohol may slightly increase the risk of stomach cancer.

Another suspected promoter of stomach cancer is *Helicobacter pylori*, a bacterium that infects about half of all Americans over the age of 50 and most people in poor regions of Asia and

Latin America. Long-term *H. pylori* infection causes chronic stomach irritation and ulcers and may contribute to the development of some stomach cancers. A few other treatable diseases, including gastritis, gastric polyposis, and pernicious anemia, are also associated with stomach cancer. Worldwide incidence of stomach cancer is notably higher among coal miners and metal refiners, who inhale certain dust and fumes that contain known carcinogens. In the U.S., stomach cancer occurs twice as often in men as in women, strikes African Americans most frequently, and rarely affects people under 50.

### DIAGNOSTIC AND TEST PROCEDURES

When symptoms warrant a thorough examination, a doctor views the stomach with an x-ray or CT scan, or through an orally inserted gastroscope. If a suspicious mass is identified, a biopsy is performed by extracting a tissue sample and studying it under a microscope for cancer cells. If cancer is confirmed, other tests may be run to determine whether the disease has spread.

**TUMORS IN THE STOMACH**

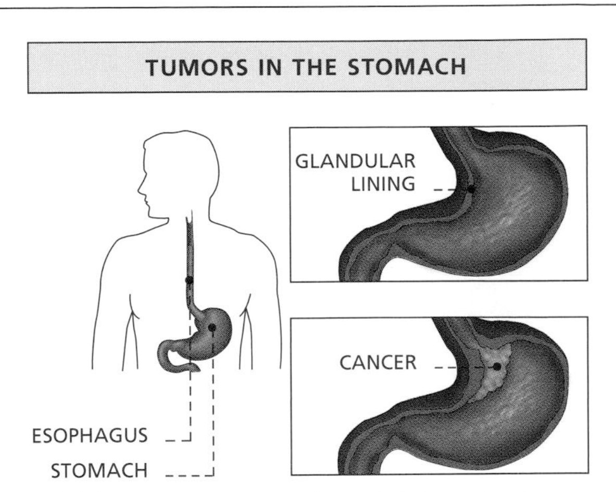


Aided by strong muscles and gastric juices, the stomach blends and liquefies chewed food for absorption by the small intestine. Cancer typically attacks the stomach's glandular lining *(inset, top)*, often at the site of an ulcer. While cancers can form anywhere in the stomach, they tend to start directly below the junction of the esophagus and the stomach *(inset, bottom)*.

## TREATMENT

### CONVENTIONAL MEDICINE

If caught early, stomach cancer is treated surgically, sometimes with radiation or chemotherapy beforehand to reduce the tumor's size. Part or all of the stomach is removed, along with surrounding tissue and nearby lymph nodes. Postop patients typically experience indigestion or diarrhea, but such side effects can be relieved with medication. Patients whose entire stomachs are removed require regular vitamin $B_{12}$ injections, because they cannot absorb the nutrient naturally until their systems adjust to digesting food in the intestines.

Most cases of stomach cancer are too advanced at diagnosis to be cured surgically, but radiation, chemotherapy, or limited surgery can relieve symptoms, slow the disease, and possibly prolong life. See Cancer for more information about treatments.

### COMPLEMENTARY THERAPIES

Patients with advanced stomach cancer typically experience significant pain. While medication can offer partial relief, a variety of complementary therapies may also help. Consider **acupuncture** or activities that promote relaxation such as **yoga, massage,** or **meditation.** *(See Cancer.)*

### AT-HOME CARE

Following stomach surgery, people often experience nausea, vomiting, diarrhea, or dizziness after eating. The symptoms usually go away in a few months, but they can be minimized by eating small meals of soft or semiliquid foods, cutting out sweets, and not drinking liquids with meals.

## PREVENTION

Studies suggest that drinking green tea and eating plenty of fresh fruits, vegetables, and garlic may help protect against stomach cancer. However, nothing is more preventive than cutting out smoked, pickled, salted, and barbecued foods. ■

# STOMACH ULCERS

## SYMPTOMS

- burning upper abdominal pain, particularly between meals, early in the morning, or after drinking orange juice, coffee, or alcohol, or taking aspirin; discomfort is usually relieved after taking antacids.
- tarry, black, or bloody stools.

## CALL YOUR DOCTOR IF:

- you have been diagnosed with a stomach ulcer and begin experiencing symptoms of anemia, such as fatigue and a pallid complexion. Your ulcer may be bleeding.
- you have symptoms of a stomach ulcer and develop severe back pain. Your ulcer may be perforating the stomach wall. **Call your doctor now.**
- you have symptoms of a stomach ulcer and vomit blood or material that looks like coffee grounds, or you pass dark red, bloody, or black stools, or stools that resemble currant jelly. These symptoms indicate internal bleeding; **call 911 or your emergency number now.**
- you have an ulcer and become cold and clammy, and feel faint or actually do faint. These are symptoms of shock, usually resulting from massive blood loss; **get emergency medical treatment.**

There is no clear evidence to suggest that the stress of modern life or a steady diet of fast food causes stomach ulcers, but they are nonetheless common in our society: About 1 out of 10 Americans will suffer from the burning, gnawing abdominal pain of an ulcer sometime in life.

Stomach, or peptic, ulcers are holes or breaks in the protective lining of the stomach, the esophagus, or the duodenum, which is the upper part of the small intestine. The most common type are **duodenal ulcers;** as the name suggests, these affect the duodenum. The second most common are **gastric ulcers,** which develop in the stomach, followed by the comparatively rare **esophageal ulcers,** which form in the esophagus and are typically a result of alcohol abuse.

Duodenal ulcers, whose typical symptoms are recurrent upper abdominal pain and a bloated feeling after eating, are more common in men than women and generally strike between the ages of 40 and 50 years. People between 60 and 70 years old are prime targets for gastric ulcers, whose symptoms are similar to those of duodenal ulcers.

Fortunately, stomach ulcers are relatively easy to treat; in many cases they are cured with antibiotics. Still, the dangers associated with stomach ulcers—such as anemia, hemorrhaging, pancreatic problems, and stomach cancer—are serious, so ulcers should always be monitored by your doctor. There are, however, a variety of self-help and alternative treatments that can aid in relieving pain and in healing ulcers.

## CAUSES

Until the mid-1980s the conventional wisdom was that ulcers form as a result of stress, a genetic predisposition to excessive stomach acid secretion, and poor consumption habits (including overindulging in rich and fatty foods, alcohol, caffeine, and tobacco). It was believed that such influences contribute to a buildup of stomach acids that erode the protective lining of the stomach, duodenum, or esophagus.

While excessive stomach acid secretion certainly plays a role in the development of ulcers, a relatively recent theory holds that bacterial infection is the primary cause of peptic ulcers. Indeed, research conducted since the mid-1980s has persuasively demonstrated that the bacterium *Helicobacter pylori* is present in 92 percent of duodenal ulcer cases and 73 percent of gastric ulcers.

Other factors also seem to contribute to ulcer formation. Overzealous use of over-the-counter analgesics (such as aspirin, ibuprofen, and naproxen), heavy alcohol use, and smoking exacerbate and may promote the development of ulcers. In fact, research indicates that heavy smokers are more prone to developing duodenal ulcers than are nonsmokers, and that people who drink alcohol are more susceptible to esophageal ulcers and those who take aspirin frequently for a long period of time more likely to contract gastric ulcers than those who abstain.

Other studies show that gastric ulcers are more likely to develop in elderly people. This may be because arthritis is prevalent in the elderly, and alleviating arthritis pain can mean taking daily doses of aspirin or ibuprofen. Another contributing factor may be aging ducts that allow excess bile to seep into the stomach and erode the stomach lining. Also, for no known reason, people with type A blood are more likely to develop cancerous gastric ulcers. Duodenal ulcers tend to appear in people with type O blood, possibly because they do not produce antigens that may protect the stomach lining.

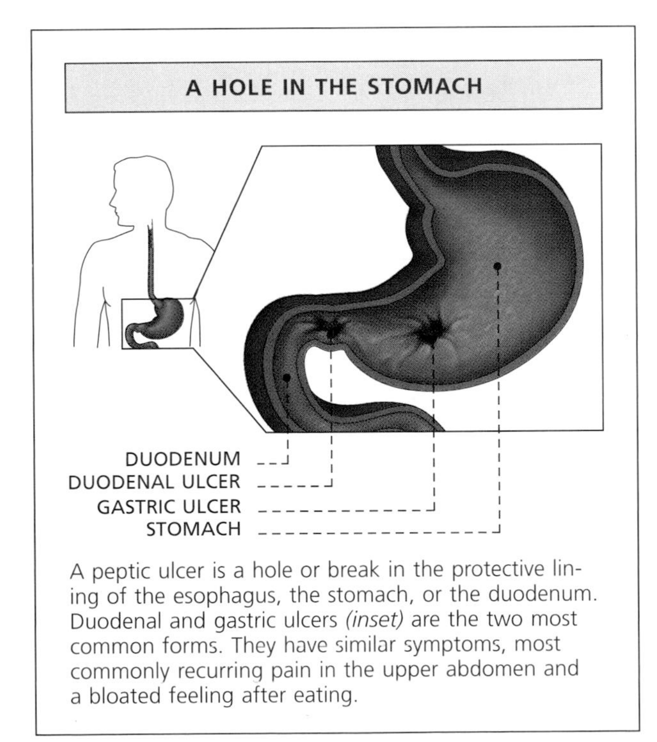


A peptic ulcer is a hole or break in the protective lining of the esophagus, the stomach, or the duodenum. Duodenal and gastric ulcers *(inset)* are the two most common forms. They have similar symptoms, most commonly recurring pain in the upper abdomen and a bloated feeling after eating.

### DIAGNOSTIC AND TEST PROCEDURES

Noting your symptoms may lead your doctor to suspect that you have a peptic ulcer, but it will not likely help determine the type, because the symptoms of gastric and duodenal ulcers are so similar. To make a specific diagnosis, your doctor may administer several tests.

The most common is a barium x-ray, which allows your doctor to spot the ulcer and determine its type and severity. The test requires you to drink a tracing substance called a "barium milkshake," which in an x-ray will highlight the upper digestive tract. You may be asked to eat only bland, easily digestible foods for two or three days before the test. After drinking the chalky liquid you are strapped to a tilting examining table, which evenly distributes the barium around your upper digestive tract and allows the x-ray to capture images at different angles.

If you do not respond to treatment or if you develop new symptoms, your doctor may perform a gastroscopy, or endoscopic examination, in which a flexible tube is inserted down your throat to give the doctor a direct view of the inside of your esophagus, stomach, and duodenum. This allows the doctor to determine the presence and cause of bleeding, and test for any bacterial infection. During this examination your doctor may also conduct a biopsy to check for cancer.

## TREATMENT

Medications are usually used to treat mild to moderate ulcers. If the cause is bacterial, antibiotics can cure the ulcer. For recurrent, severe cases that do not respond to medication, surgery may be necessary.

Although alternative therapies have been

shown to aid in the relief of symptoms as well as in the healing of ulcers, they should be used only as supplements to conventional treatment.

### CONVENTIONAL MEDICINE

The chief goals of treatment are reducing the amount of acid in the stomach and strengthening the protective linings that come in direct contact with gastric acids. This can usually be achieved by taking over-the-counter antacids containing magnesium trisilicate and aluminum hydroxide before meals and at bedtime.

Since long-term use of antacids can interfere with the absorption of nutrients, your doctor may prescribe a class of medications called histamine $H_2$ blockers as an alternative. (The class includes the generic drugs cimetidine, ranitidine, and famotidine among others.) Histamine blockers reduce stomach acids and heal peptic ulcers 80 percent of the time when taken over a period of four to six weeks. Since antacids can reduce the absorption of histamine blockers, your doctor will probably instruct you not to take antacids during this period.

If your ulcer is caused by bacterial infection, your doctor may prescribe a combination of antibiotics, such as amoxicillin or tetracycline with metronidazole, along with a bismuth drug and possibly histamine $H_2$ blockers.

If these treatments are unsuccessful, or if you have developed serious complications as a result of your ulcer, surgery may be necessary. If your ulcer is hemorrhaging, the surgeon will identify the source of the bleeding (usually a small artery at the base of the ulcer) and repair it. Perforated ulcers—holes in the entire stomach or duodenal wall—must be surgically closed. This is an emergency procedure.

In some cases, a surgical procedure that decreases stomach acid secretion is also warranted. Note, however, that peptic ulcer surgery is done only in emergency situations, because there are many potential complications associated with the procedure, including ulcer recurrence, hypoglycemia, hematological complications, and dumping syndrome (chronic abdominal pain, diarrhea, vomiting, and/or sweating occurring an hour after eating).

### CAN YOU CATCH AN ULCER?

*In 1982, two Australian doctors determined that the bacterium Helicobacter pylori played a significant role in the development of peptic ulcers, and further studies have shown antibiotics to be effective in treating ulcers caused by the bacterium. Does this mean that ulcers are contagious?*

*The answer is murky. Not everyone infected with the bacterium develops an ulcer, and certainly other factors—such as heredity and excessive use of aspirin, tobacco, and alcohol—increase the chances of getting one. Still, research has shown that infected children are more likely to transmit the bacterium than adults are, a rate that increases in developing countries, where an estimated 80 percent of children are infected.*

*This does not mean, however, that you should take antibiotics as a preventive measure if you or your child is infected. The best course of action is to consult with your doctor.*

### ALTERNATIVE CHOICES

Although you should be monitored by a doctor if you have a peptic ulcer, alternative therapies can help relieve the discomfort of symptoms.

#### ACUPUNCTURE

Acupuncture targeting the points associated with stress, anxiety, and stomach/gastrointestinal disorders may help with the treatment of peptic ulcers. Consult a licensed acupuncturist.

#### HERBAL THERAPIES

Licorice *(Glycyrrhiza glabra)*, which stimulates mucus secretion by the stomach, is frequently used in herbal treatments of ulcers. To prepare an infusion, add 1 tsp shredded licorice root to 1 cup water and simmer for 15 minutes. Drink hot, three times a day. Alternatively, try drinking ½ tsp licorice extract mixed with 1 cup water three times a day before meals. (Do not use this treatment for more than a few days at a time.)

#### MIND/BODY MEDICINE

**Biofeedback, meditation, massage therapy,** and **yoga** can help you learn how to deal effectively with stress, which increases stomach acid production and irritates ulcers.

#### NUTRITION AND DIET

Some nutritionists recommend increasing your intake of vitamins A and E and zinc, which increase the production of mucin, a substance your body secretes to protect the stomach lining. Another suggestion may include drinking about a quart of cabbage juice daily; its high content of glutamine is thought to expedite the growth of mucin-producing cells.

### AT-HOME REMEDIES

- Cut down on milk. Although it may feel as though milk's coating properties are soothing your ulcer, milk actually stimulates stomach acid secretion, irritating the ulcer.
- Pick appropriate antacids. Like milk, calcium-containing antacids can stimulate stomach acid secretion, so check with your doctor before taking them. Also, don't become dependent on antacids containing a combination of magnesium trisilicate and aluminum hydroxide. These compounds can deplete phosphate levels, causing osteomalacia (bone softening). Experiments suggest that bismuth, an ingredient in some over-the-counter stomach medications, may help destroy the bacterium that causes some peptic ulcers.
- Be cautious when choosing over-the-counter pain relievers. Aspirin and nonsteroidal anti-inflammatory drugs (NSAIDs) such as ibuprofen may not only irritate the ulcer but also prevent a bleeding ulcer from healing. Your best choice may be acetaminophen, which does not cause or promote stomach ulcers.
- Don't overdose on iron supplements. Although people with bleeding ulcers can develop anemia and may need to take iron as a treatment, taking too much can irritate the stomach lining and thus the ulcer. Ask your doctor how much iron you need.
- Learn how to deal with stress. While there is no evidence that stress causes ulcers, it can exacerbate existing ones. Practicing relaxation techniques—including deep breathing, **guided imagery,** and moderate exercise—can help alleviate stress.

## PREVENTION

- Avoid foods that irritate your stomach. Use common sense: If it upsets your stomach when you eat it, avoid it. Everyone is different, but spicy foods and fatty foods are common irritants.
- Eat foods with high fiber content. Fiber has been touted as a cancer-preventing substance, and eating a high-fiber diet can also reduce your chances of developing a duodenal ulcer. Fiber is thought to enhance mucin secretion, which protects the duodenal lining.
- Stop smoking. Heavy smokers are more likely to develop duodenal ulcers than nonsmokers, largely because nicotine is thought to prevent the pancreas from secreting acid-neutralizing enzymes.
- Practice moderation. Heavy consumption of alcohol and aspirin has been shown to contribute to the development of ulcers, so keep your intake to a minimum. ■

# STREP THROAT

## SYMPTOMS

- sore throat that comes on rapidly.
- fever, sometimes greater than 102°F.
- back of the throat that is raw and red.
- white pus on tonsils.
- tender, high lymph nodes in neck.
- absence of cough, stuffy nose, or other upper respiratory symptoms.

## CALL YOUR DOCTOR IF:

- you quickly develop a fever and sore throat simultaneously; these are the hallmark symptoms of strep throat, which in severe cases can develop into rheumatic fever if left untreated.

If you're feeling fine one moment, then suddenly your throat is killing you, you're running a high fever, and all your energy has vanished in a haze of illness, you probably have strep throat.

"Strep," in this case, stands for *Streptococcus pyogenes,* a common strain of bacteria that can live in your throat and nose for months without causing any harm. Tests show that about 18 percent of healthy people have the strep bug living uneventfully in their mouths or throats. Once in a while, however, these bugs turn ugly on you. Maybe you've been under too much stress, or your immune system has been overtaxed with fighting a virus such as a common cold or the flu. Or perhaps you've picked up a bug from an infected person. Whatever the reason, the normally quiet strep organism can suddenly start spewing out toxins and inflammatory substances to bring on the sore throat and other symptoms.

Although strep throat feels awful, it can be cured easily these days with antibiotics such as penicillin or erythromycin. In fact, one of the biggest problems with it is getting people to seek treatment. Because a fever and sore throat are also symptoms of colds and the flu, strep throat is often mistaken for these ailments. But colds and flu normally take several days to develop, and most of the time they are accompanied by a cough, stuffy or runny nose, and headache. A strep throat, by contrast, usually arrives in a hurry and without any other cold or flu symptoms.

Strep throat should never be taken lightly. Untreated, the disease can quickly lead to a more severe illness such as acute nephritis (which can damage your kidneys), meningitis, or rheumatic fever, all of which can be fatal.

## CAUSES

Although by definition strep throat is caused by the *Streptococcus pyogenes* bug, other bacteria can occasionally invade the throat and cause similar symptoms. Other possible invaders: staphylococcus, neisseria, and *Hemophilus influenzae.*

People usually develop strep throat when their immune systems are not functioning at their peak. Stress, overwork, exhaustion, and fights with viral infections can weaken the body's defenses and set up attacks of strep throat. And like other throat infections, strep throat also tends to occur during the colder months.

### DIAGNOSTIC AND TEST PROCEDURES

In the past, when patients displayed the characteristic red, raw throat, spikes in fever, and white spots on the tongue and tonsils, a careful physician would culture a specimen from the patient's throat and wait 24 to 48 hours for the results. If the test indicated streptococcus, the patient could then start taking antibiotics. To avoid this delay—in which the infection often grew worse—most doctors started patients on antibiotics immediately, not waiting for the results of the culture.

Diagnosis has been made much simpler today as a result of the "quick strep" test. Research indicates that this test, which takes about 20 minutes, is just as accurate as the much slower culture analysis. (If the quick test is not clearly negative and your symptoms strongly suggest strep throat, your doctor may also perform a regular culture.) The beauty of the quick test is that you don't need to take antibiotics without confirmation that the strep organism is the culprit.

## TREATMENT

Strep throat is best treated by conventional medicine. For one thing, antibiotics are a quick and surefire cure. Also, the disease can lead to serious complications if left untreated.

### CONVENTIONAL MEDICINE

In most cases, a standard dose of penicillin, taken for 10 days, will eradicate a strep infection without any problems. Most people who are allergic to penicillin can take one of the many kinds of cephalosporins. For patients who are allergic to both penicillin and cephalosporin, the alternative is usually erythromycin. Relief from the sore throat should come within 24 to 36 hours after you start taking antibiotics. Doctors recommend throat lozenges and throat sprays to ease the pain for the first few hours.

Frequently, people on antibiotics notice improvement quickly and stop taking their medications before the course runs out. This practice can have dangerous consequences. Prematurely halting the dosage allows the hardiest strep organisms, those that survived the first doses of antibiotic, to develop resistance to the drug and to bounce back in a more potent form. So even though you may feel better right away, it's important to finish the entire prescription.

### ALTERNATIVE CHOICES

Strep throat is one disease in which conventional medicine clearly excels. However, a number of homeopathic remedies may ease the discomfort of a sore throat and related symptoms.

#### HOMEOPATHY

For a sore throat characterized by a high fever and glassy eyes, use Belladonna 12x (three times a day). WARNING: Exercise extreme caution when using belladonna, a poisonous member of the nightshade family. For a sore throat that's worse at night, accompanied by a coated tongue and bad breath, use Mercurius vivus 12x (three times a day). When the sore throat is worse on the left side, particularly at night, and you have swollen glands and difficulty swallowing, use Lachesis 12x (three times a day). If you feel unusually sensitive to cold and have sharp, sticking pain as well as discharge in the throat, try Hepar sulphuris 12x (three times a day). If you don't feel better in a day, seek the advice of a professional homeopath.

## PREVENTION

The best way to avoid a strep throat is to reduce stress, get plenty of rest, and fortify your body's natural defenses. Nutritional supplements such as vitamin C, beta carotene (vitamin A), and zinc, along with herbs such as echinacea (*Echinacea* spp.), goldenseal *(Hydrastis canadensis),* osha *(Ligusticum porterii),* and garlic *(Allium sativum),* are all thought to boost the immune system. ■

S

## SYMPTOMS

- Physical symptoms may include headache, fatigue, insomnia, digestive changes, neck pain or backache, loss of appetite, or overeating.
- Psychological symptoms may include tension or anxiety, anger, reclusiveness, pessimism, resentment, increased irritability, feelings of cynicism, and inability to concentrate or perform at usual levels.

## CALL YOUR DOCTOR IF:

- you have prolonged or acute symptoms. Excessive stress puts you at risk of other serious disorders, including immune problems, digestive disorders, diabetes, asthma, high blood pressure, migraine headaches, and possibly cancer.
- you have symptoms of stress and any of the following: unusual patterns of sleep, appetite, and moods; physical movement that is unusually agitated or abnormally slow. You may have clinical depression.

Stress is the reaction of our bodies and minds to something that upsets their normal balance. The human response to stressful events is an ancient one, dating back to a time when life was a constant struggle for survival. A good example of stress in action is the way you react when you are frightened or threatened. Your adrenal glands release epinephrine—or adrenaline—a hormone that activates your body's defensive mechanisms: Your heart pounds, your blood pressure rises, your muscles tense, the pupils of your eyes open wide. This cluster of reactions—the fight-or-flight response—concentrates all your body systems on the apparent danger and helps you take the next step, which is either to resist or to retreat.

Of course, not all stressful events are so sudden or so obvious as the threat of bodily harm. Any challenge that overwhelms us—a serious illness, the death of a family member, the loss of a job or a lover—can be stressful to the point of physical and psychological dysfunction. Some of us are especially vulnerable to stressful situations or events, responding in extreme ways to everyday decisions—what to buy at the supermarket, what to wear to the wedding, or how to ask for a raise. But while some people fall to pieces if they are pressed too hard, others are highly productive under pressure. The difference may lie partly in our constitutions, and partly in how we manage our lives.

Continued stress can eventually deplete the body's resources and produce chronic fatigue, loss of appetite or overeating, and other reactions. Coping ability may diminish, causing feelings of insecurity and inadequacy, and possibly leading to depression. At the same time, the body's immune system becomes disrupted, increasing vulnerability to illness and disease. Unrelieved stress—from real or imagined causes—may bring on hypertension, a recognized factor in heart disease and some cancers. Posttraumatic stress disorder, in which symptoms appear immediately or months after a stressful event, can be a protracted and difficult problem.

## CAUSES

Stress occurs when there is an imbalance between the demands of life and our ability to cope with them. Certain work is highly stress producing, especially assembly-line jobs or jobs requiring repetitive tasks with dangerous equipment. Events and situations that are difficult to manage typically bring on stress: burnout on the job, financial problems, the loss of or a threat to your security, bereavement, or divorce. A positive experience, such as marriage or a job promotion, can be equally stressful. Other causes are internal: illness, loneliness, pain, or emotional conflict. The effects of such changes, big and little, are cumulative. We can tolerate only so much stress in a given period of time.

### DIAGNOSTIC AND TEST PROCEDURES

Diagnosing stress is largely a matter of recognizing and understanding the symptoms—both physical and psychological—in yourself or others. Some researchers have developed more objective diagnostic tools. For example, the Holmes-Rahe questionnaire is helpful in identifying potentially stressful events. The questionnaire scale ranks 43 important life events according to their potential stress value. Not all events are considered "bad," but all involve some kind of change, including a new job, a new home, and the birth of a child.

## TREATMENT

You don't have to deal with stress by yourself. A counselor, psychologist, psychiatrist, member of the clergy, or friend can often help you define or resolve a problem that seems unsolvable to you. Developing a stress-abatement routine you trust will help you prepare for an event you know may be stressful.

### CONVENTIONAL MEDICINE

If you have symptoms of stress from a specific event, such as a death in the family, your doctor may prescribe an antianxiety drug, such as diazepam. While such medications are highly effective if taken for brief periods, they can be addictive if taken for more than a few weeks *(see Drug Abuse)*.

Your doctor may suggest psychotherapy to pinpoint events or conditions that are stressful to you, and to devise ways of reducing the stress they cause. Group therapy is often valuable for people who share a stressful life situation. Treatment of posttraumatic stress disorder usually includes counseling and may require antianxiety or antidepressant medications.

### ALTERNATIVE CHOICES

Some treatments once considered alternative are now widely used in the medical community—particularly those designed to promote physical and mental relaxation.

#### AROMATHERAPY

Essential oil of lavender *(Lavandula officinalis)* can help reduce stress: Try 5 or 6 drops in a bath, or put 2 or 3 drops on a handkerchief and inhale from time to time.

#### BODY WORK

By relaxing tense muscles and helping circulation, **massage** helps the mind relax. Between treatments by a trained massage therapist, try self-massaging your temples, neck, shoulders, and face.

#### HERBAL THERAPIES

A traditional response to stress is to drink a cup of hot tea. Some herbalists suggest chamomile *(Matricaria recutita)*, passionflower *(Passiflora incarnata)*, valerian *(Valeriana officinalis)*, or ginseng *(Panax quinquefolius)* tea.

#### LIFESTYLE

Vigorous aerobic exercise can reduce the level of pulse-quickening hormones released during stress and at the same time stimulate a sense of well-being. Even a walk around the block can help reduce anxiety or let off steam. Try to schedule the exercise of your choice—running, swimming, walking—for 30 minutes at least three times a week.

## THE "TYPE A" PERSONALITY

*Some researchers divide people into two classes: the competitive, hard-charging Type A personalities who thrive on challenge; and the less competitive, calmer Type B. Type A people seem to have a higher risk of heart attack. Some studies show that hostility —not just a fast pace—is the quality most strongly linked with heart disease.*

*Some experts think Type A people should try to change their behavior, while others think doing so may simply induce more stress or change an essential personality trait. Many if not most Type A people enjoy life in the fast lane. If you think you are a Type A person, work to control hostility and other negative behavior by trying the following strategies:*

- *Avoid situations you dislike whenever possible.*
- *Schedule true breaks from work.*
- *Manage your time better.*
- *Penalize Type A actions and reward calm, coping actions.*

Stretching exercises can relax tense upper-body muscles that accompany stress and affect breathing. Rotate your shoulders up, back, and then down. Inhale as the shoulders go back; exhale as they go down. Repeat the exercise four or five times, then inhale deeply and exhale. Repeat the cycle.

### MIND/BODY MEDICINE

The **relaxation response** has long been a goal of many Eastern disciplines such as **yoga** and Zen Buddhism. Try this simple routine: Choose a focus word or phrase, for example "peace" or "I'm calm." Sit quietly, relax your body, and breathe slowly and deeply. Say the focus word or phrase each time you exhale. If you lose concentration, simply wait as thoughts pass through your mind, then return to your focus word. Continue for 5 minutes at a time, gradually increasing to 20 minutes. Do the routine at least once a day. Such relaxation exercises, done regularly, can slow your breathing rate, decrease your oxygen consumption, calm your brain-wave rhythms, and lower your blood pressure.

You might also reduce stress through **biofeedback,** identifying the sources of stress and controlling your physical and mental responses. You should learn the proper technique from a professional, then practice at home. Advocates believe that biofeedback can relax specific muscles, alter the brain's electrical activity, reduce heart rate and blood pressure, increase body warmth, and improve gastrointestinal function.

### NUTRITION AND DIET

How well you handle stress can be affected by your diet. Because it is easy to neglect nutrition when you are under stress, make an extra effort to eat a balanced diet—plenty of vegetables and fruit, as well as foods high in complex carbohydrates, moderate in protein, and low in fat. Avoid or reduce caffeine consumption: Excessive caffeine has been shown to increase anxiety.

## AT-HOME REMEDIES

There are many simple, inexpensive ways to manage stress on your own. For many people, a good way to start is by cutting out artificial stress relievers such as alcohol, which can mask symptoms and may become addictive. Try exercise instead. Take walks. Breathe deeply.

In times of stress, social support is crucial. People with close personal relationships are most likely to recover from serious illness or injury, and stress is no different. The ability to form relationships with people—or pets, for that matter—can be a key to good health.

Start taking a **yoga** class and practice by yourself at home. *(See the illustrations opposite.)* Yoga can relax tense muscles, teach you better breathing, lower your blood pressure, decrease your heart rate, and divert your mind from stress.

**Meditation** brings relaxation and increased awareness. When you feel stressed, think affirmations such as "I can face this calmly. I feel sure and confident. I control my own life."

Try visualization or **guided imagery** exercises. Visualizing a pleasant situation can bring physical as well as emotional benefits; combine a visualization session with soothing music. Many excellent teachers, books, and tapes are available to help you learn the technique.

**Hydrotherapy** is easily done at home and highly effective at reducing stress. Soak for 10 to 20 minutes in a tub of very warm water, using half a cup of sea salt and your favorite bath oil.

## PREVENTION

While we can't—and perhaps shouldn't try to—change our personality or avoid stressful situations just because they are stressful, we can take common-sense steps to increase our coping ability. Try the following:

- Practice the relaxation and stress-reduction techniques suggested above.
- Cultivate outside interests and plan occasional diversions to break routine habits.
- Set up a regular sleeping schedule and get plenty of rest—without sleeping pills.
- Exercise regularly and vigorously, as appropriate for your age.
- Avoid the learned behaviors of hurry and worry, which can upset your sleeping, eating, and other schedules. Take time to relax and enjoy your life.
- Make a list of things that trouble you. For each one, ask yourself: What's the worst and the best that can happen? Have I done what I can to prepare myself? Is this problem really worth worrying about?
- Laugh more; avoid self-pity; learn to reestablish equilibrium after a stressful event; make an effort to reach out to people.
- When you're facing a stressful situation, remember a bit of folk wisdom: Count to 10 and take a deep breath before saying or doing anything. A deliberate pause can be an instant tranquilizer.

### YOGA

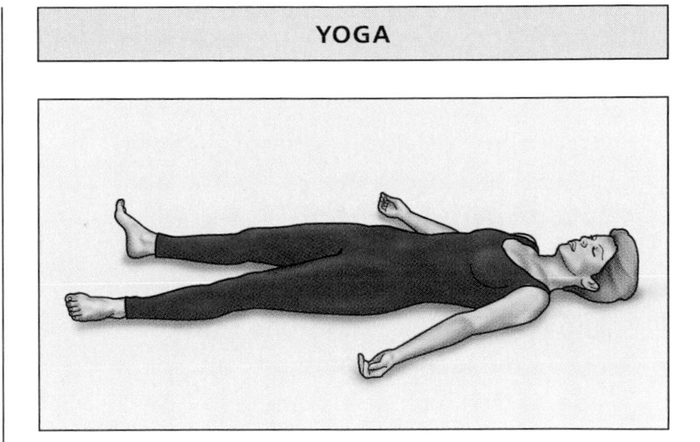

**1** Relaxation exercises are good for stress. For the **Corpse,** you should lie on your back, with your feet approximately 18 inches apart and turned out slightly. With palms up, place your hands about 6 inches from your hips. Close your eyes and breathe deeply for 8 to 10 minutes.

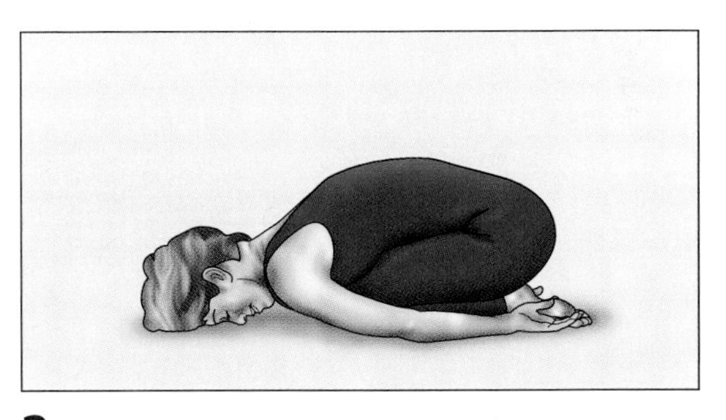

**2** The **Child** relaxes the lower back. Sit on your heels keeping your knees together. Exhale and bend from the hips. Extend your upper body over your knees with arms at your sides, palms up. Move your forehead toward the floor. Breathe slowly, hold for 15 to 20 seconds, then sit up.

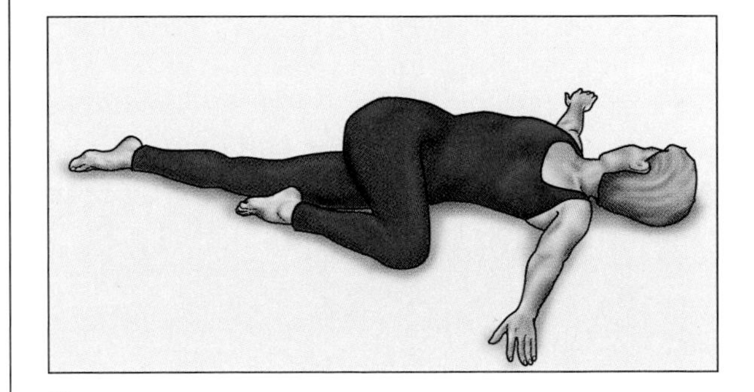

**3** The **Knee Down Twist** also relaxes the lower back. Lie on your back with arms out, inhale, and put your right foot on your left knee. Exhale, turn your head to the right, and move your right knee toward the floor to your left. Hold for 15 to 20 seconds. Repeat on the other side. ■

# STROKE

## SYMPTOMS

- abrupt loss of vision, strength, coordination, sensation, speech, or the ability to understand speech. These symptoms may become more marked over time.
- impairments limited to one side of the body, such as numbness on one side of the face or blindness in one eye.
- sudden loss of balance, possibly accompanied by vomiting, nausea, hiccups, or trouble with swallowing.
- sudden and severe headache followed rapidly by loss of consciousness—indications of a stroke due to bleeding.

## CALL YOUR DOCTOR IF:

- you or someone with you manifests any of the signs of stroke. If the symptoms pass quickly, this may indicate a transient ischemic attack (TIA), a brief blockage of blood flow to the brain that is often a forerunner of stroke. Do not ignore this warning sign; medical intervention is essential.

When the blood supply to the brain is disturbed for any reason, the consequences are usually drastic: Control over movement, perception, speech, or other mental or bodily functions is impaired, and consciousness itself may be extinguished. Disruptions of blood circulation to the brain are known as stroke—a disorder that occurs in two basic forms, both potentially life-threatening.

About three-quarters of all strokes are due to blockage of the oxygen-rich blood flowing to the brain. Called **clot strokes,** they are triggered by either a thrombus (a stationary clot that forms in a blood vessel) or an embolus (a clot that travels through the bloodstream and becomes lodged in a vessel). This type of stroke is often preceded by so-called **transient ischemic attacks,** or **TIAs**—episodes of inadequate blood flow that may produce sudden physical weakness, an inability to talk, double vision, or dizziness. With a TIA, circulation and the vital oxygen supply are quickly restored and lasting neurological damage is avoided. With any stroke, however, the interruption of blood flow lasts long enough to kill brain cells, producing irreversible neurological damage.

The second basic type of stroke is **bleeding stroke,** or **cerebral hemorrhage.** It occurs when a brain aneurysm ruptures or when a weakened or inflamed blood vessel in the brain starts to leak. As blood flows into the brain, the buildup of pressure may either kill the tissue directly or destroy cells by impeding normal circulation to the affected region. This typically produces an excruciating headache, sometimes followed by loss of consciousness. In contrast to clot strokes, which are generally survived, massive bleeding strokes are fatal about 80 percent of the time.

Because of improved treatment and greater public awareness of the dangers of high blood pressure, the overall death rate from stroke is declining. Nonetheless, stroke remains the third leading cause of death in the United States, behind heart disease and cancer. It is also the leading cause of disability and second only to Alzheimer's disease as a cause of dementia.

Recovery from stroke depends on the extent and location of brain damage. Some stroke victims recover fully; but in the vast majority of cas-

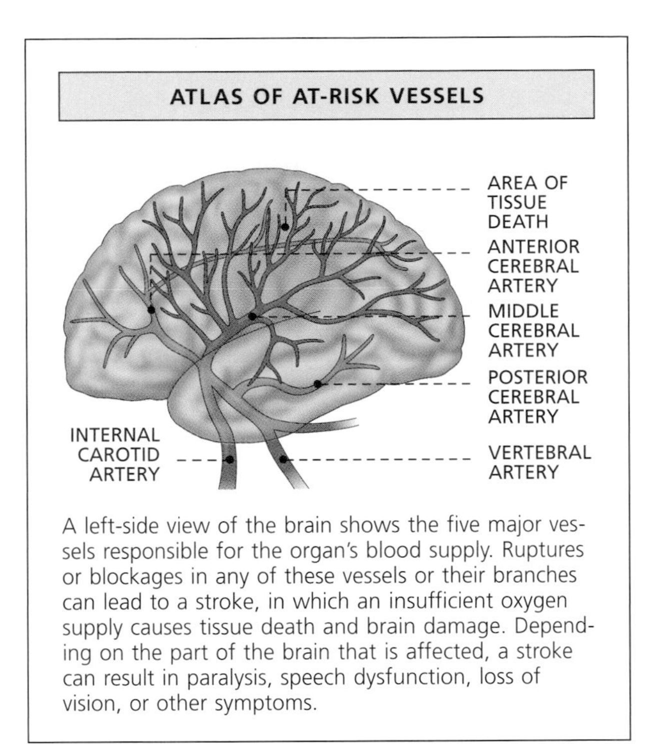


A left-side view of the brain shows the five major vessels responsible for the organ's blood supply. Ruptures or blockages in any of these vessels or their branches can lead to a stroke, in which an insufficient oxygen supply causes tissue death and brain damage. Depending on the part of the brain that is affected, a stroke can result in paralysis, speech dysfunction, loss of vision, or other symptoms.

es, there is lasting physical or mental disability. Weakened stroke victims are also more vulnerable to infectious diseases such as pneumonia. In addition, depression often follows a stroke; unless treated, it can significantly hinder recovery.

## CAUSES

A **clot stroke** occurs when a blood clot obstructs blood flow to a portion of the brain. The blocked vessel is already narrowed by years' worth of plaque buildup due to atherosclerosis. The clot that serves as the final plug may be either a stationary blood clot created on the spot, or an embolus composed of blood, plaque, or some other substance that formed elsewhere and traveled to the site. Stroke-triggering blood clots may be produced when blood flow is sluggish. After a heart attack, for example, clots may form on the damaged heart wall because of slower blood flow there. *(See also Blood Clots.)*

**Bleeding strokes** most often stem from weak arteries or aneurysms in the brain that rupture. Arteries are sometimes congenitally weak, but more often they become weak under the strain of high blood pressure. Bleeding strokes can also result from a leaking **arteriovenous malformation,** a congenital tangle of overgrown blood vessels in the brain.

The vast majority of strokes afflict people over the age of 60. Men are more often affected than women, and African Americans—possibly because of a greater incidence of high blood pressure—more often than Caucasians. A younger person is more apt to have a bleeding stroke, while older people usually suffer clot strokes.

The main controllable risk factors for stroke are high blood pressure, high cholesterol levels (specifically, high LDL cholesterol), a sedentary lifestyle, obesity, the abuse of stimulant drugs such as amphetamines, smoking, use of birth-control pills, and stress.

Incidence of stroke increases among people with a history of TIAs, heart disease (particularly recent heart attack, atrial fibrillation, or mitral valve disease), excessive blood clotting, or diabetes.

### DIAGNOSTIC AND TEST PROCEDURES

When a patient displays strokelike symptoms, a neurologist must not only confirm the symptoms but also identify the type of stroke, its location, and the extent of brain damage. Treatment decisions hinge on all these issues. Testing is typically done quickly, since immediate treatment may limit neurological damage.

The physician first examines the patient and obtains a medical history, if possible. A standard exam includes checking blood vessels in the eyes, listening for unusual noises in the heart and in the prominent carotid arteries of the neck, measuring blood pressure and pulse rate, and testing strength, sensation, and neurological reflexes.

CT or MRI scans are the most critical diagnostic tests for stroke.

## TREATMENT

Acute management of stroke should be left to conventional medicine, but many alternative therapies may contribute to stroke prevention and recovery.

### CONVENTIONAL MEDICINE

Stroke victims are immediately admitted to the hospital and, in many cases, will be given medication to prevent further brain damage. Normally, **clot strokes** are treated with an anticoagulant drug called heparin. Emergency surgery might also be required to drain blood that has hemorrhaged into the brain and perhaps to clip a ruptured artery or aneurysm—blocking off the vessel to halt further bleeding.

Once past the critical phase, a stroke patient remains hospitalized until stable. Upon release, patient and doctor carefully review necessary steps for recovery and prevention of future strokes. Advice will likely involve diet and lifestyle changes, ongoing drug treatment, rehabilitative therapy, and possible surgery for critical arterial narrowing.

People at risk of having **bleeding strokes** need to keep their blood pressure low, if possible through diet and lifestyle changes but, when needed, also with medication. These people are also advised not to take aspirin or ibuprofen. If someone has suffered a bleeding stroke because of an aneurysm rupture, other small aneurysms can sometimes be identified and either removed or clipped. Unfortunately, nothing can be done to reverse congenital arterial weakness.

To prevent **clot strokes,** some patients are first advised to take aspirin. If aspirin proves ineffective, the doctor will probably prescribe ticlopidine, another blood-thinning drug, or warfarin as a last resort. People at particularly high risk for clot stroke because of an existing heart condition would be treated with heparin for acute symptoms and warfarin for long-term therapy. In some patients, surgery to prevent future clot strokes might be recommended. The most favored procedure is endarterectomy, to remove plaque from large carotid arteries leading from the neck into the brain. An experimental technique called cerebral angioplasty is used to widen clogged brain arteries.

Another crucial element of stroke treatment, in addition to emergency and follow-up medical care, is rehabilitation. Immediately after a stroke, other parts of the brain can compensate for areas lost to trauma by forming new neurological pathways. Intensive rehabilitative therapy basically aims to enhance the brain's own recovery efforts. A typical program may involve speech, physical, and occupational therapy.

The psychological well-being of victims, families, and caregivers plays a crucial role in rehabilitation. Successful recovery depends on both the quality of care and the positive mind-set of the victim. Several stroke associations offer psychological support via hot lines, discussion groups, and literature.

### ALTERNATIVE CHOICES

In addition to the therapies described below, you might want to consult a practitioner of **Chinese medicine** or a **homeopathic** physician for treatment of poststroke complications. **Acupuncture,** for example, is endorsed by the World Health Organization as a viable stroke rehabilitation therapy.

#### BODY WORK

Several body-work techniques can help restore mobility, promote circulation, and ease muscle tension and stiffness associated with stroke. Among these are **qigong, shiatsu,** and **massage.**

#### CHIROPRACTIC AND OSTEOPATHY

Chiropractic and osteopathy, two closely related manipulative therapies, can aid stroke recovery in numerous ways. By focusing on realignment of the body's skeletal system, they may be able to reduce muscle spasms and stiffness, improve mobility, alleviate nagging pains, and minimize further neurological damage.

#### HERBAL THERAPIES

A number of scientific studies have shown that ginkgo *(Ginkgo biloba)* increases cerebral blood flow, so it may be helpful in moderating potential complications of stroke such as memory loss, disturbed thought processes, vertigo, and symptoms of depression. Ginkgo also appears to reduce blood-clot formation. Many other herbs are said to be useful in stroke prevention because of their abilities to improve circulation, reduce clot formation, strengthen and tone blood vessels, and combat atherosclerosis. *(See Aneurysm, Atherosclerosis, Blood Clots, Cholesterol Problems, and High Blood Pressure.)*

#### LIFESTYLE

Physical rehabilitation is impossible without regular, gentle aerobic exercise. Swimming in a heated pool is particularly useful for restoring lost motor function and keeping muscles loose.

People at high risk for stroke should not smoke and should eat a low-fat diet. Women at high risk should not take birth-control pills.

#### MIND/BODY MEDICINE

Techniques that teach the body to relax and the mind to focus on healing can help recovering stroke victims; among other benefits, these techniques can increase tolerance to pain and also alleviate the depression or anger that is common in the wake of a stroke. **Hypnotherapy, meditation,** and **yoga** all can be useful. Some stroke victims working to restore lost muscle control and motor function benefit from **biofeedback.**

#### NUTRITION AND DIET

Proper diet has much to contribute to stroke prevention, but it can do little to reverse stroke damage. With prevention in mind, your diet should be rich in vitamins, minerals, and other nutrients that combat high blood pressure, excessive clot formation, and atherosclerosis. Particularly noteworthy stroke-deterring nutrients include potassium, magnesium, vitamin E, and the essential fatty acids contained in fish oils. Some studies suggest that selenium may also protect against stroke. A low-fat diet, however, is probably the best nutrition-related preventive step you can take for both heart attack and stroke.

### A SPIDER-VENOM REMEDY?

*Researchers have discovered that compounds in spider venom may be useful in limiting stroke damage. A spider paralyzes its prey by injecting substances that block the action of a chemical called glutamate, which controls muscle movement in insects. Glutamate also exists in the human brain, serving as an important neurotransmitter when it is present in the right quantities. After a stroke, however, damaged neurons release glutamate in such large amounts that it kills surrounding cells. Hence the interest in spider venom: If the venom compounds manufactured by the spider can halt the workings of glutamate in insect prey, perhaps a version of those same compounds can also limit the cascading neuronal death that occurs during stroke in a human.*

## PREVENTION

Measures that reduce the chances of stroke are the same as those for avoiding heart attack: Adopt habits that promote cardiovascular health and deter atherosclerosis. The essentials of a healthy lifestyle include eating foods that are low in fat, salt, and cholesterol; exercising regularly; controlling weight; monitoring blood pressure and cholesterol levels; and not smoking.

If your risk of stroke is high because of severe atherosclerosis, high blood pressure, or a history of heart disease, TIAs, or previous strokes, you should see a doctor regularly. When clot stroke is the indicated danger, your doctor may advise an aspirin a day to thin blood. ■

# STY

## SYMPTOMS

- **sty:** a red, hot, tender, uncomfortable, and sometimes painful swelling near the edge of the eyelid. *(See also the Visual Diagnostic Guide.)*
- **chalazion:** a relatively painless, smooth, round bump within a fat gland of the eyelid.

## CALL YOUR DOCTOR IF:

- either type of swelling does not subside within a few weeks.
- the swelling interferes with your vision.
- you have pain in the eye.
- you have recurrent sties. A sty can be a symptom of other ailments such as diabetes and chronic skin problems.

A **sty** is a pimple or abscess on the upper or lower edge of the eyelid that signals an infected eyelid gland. Although sties are usually on the outside of the lid, they can also occur on the underside.

An external sty starts as a pimple next to an eyelash. It turns into a red, painful swelling that usually lasts several days before it bursts and then heals. Most external sties are short-lived.

An internal sty (on the underside of the lid) also causes a red, painful swelling, but its location prevents the pus from appearing on the eyelid. The sty may disappear completely once the infection is past, or it may leave a small fluid-filled cyst or nodule that can persist and may have to be cut open.

A **chalazion** is also a sign of an infected eyelid gland, but unlike a sty, it is a firm, round, smooth, painless bump usually some distance from the edge of the lid.

**Sties** and **chalazions** are usually harmless and rarely affect your eye or sight. They can occur at any age and tend to recur elsewhere in the lid.

## CAUSES

**Sties** are usually caused by staphylococcal bacteria, which often live in your nostrils. You can transfer the bacteria to your eyelids just by touching your nose and then rubbing your eyes.

A **chalazion** is caused by the blockage of the tiny gland duct that helps lubricate the eyelid. Bacteria may grow within the blocked gland; the resulting inflammation causes the hard bump.

## TREATMENT

While painful and unsightly, most **sties** heal within a few days on their own or with simple treatment. **Chalazions,** too, often disappear on their own, but it might take a month or more.

### CONVENTIONAL MEDICINE

Typical treatment for a **sty** consists of applying warm compresses to the affected eye for 10 to

15 minutes four times daily for several days. This not only relieves pain and inflammation but also helps the sty ripen faster. Be sure to close your eye while you apply the compresses. When the sty comes to a head, continue applying warm compresses to relieve pressure and promote rupture. Do not squeeze the sty; let it burst on its own.

If sties recur, your doctor may prescribe an antibiotic ointment or solution. Apply it to the eyelid (with your eye closed) as directed.

Sometimes, if there are staphylococcal infections elsewhere in your body as well, your doctor may prescribe an oral systemic antibiotic such as erythromycin. If these conservative treatments fail, surgical removal of the sty may be required.

Minor surgery may also be needed to eliminate the cyst that could result from an internal sty. After using a local anesthetic, your ophthalmologist opens the cyst and removes the contents. The eyelid usually heals quickly.

Although a **chalazion** will often disappear on its own, applying warm compresses and perhaps a corticosteroid ointment will speed the process. The chalazion can also be removed through simple surgery under a local anesthetic. Your doctor then covers the eye for 8 to 24 hours with a pressure patch to control bleeding and swelling.

### ALTERNATIVE CHOICES

Although some alternative treatments may be helpful in relieving and preventing eyelid infections, never put any preparations in the eye itself unless specifically directed by a physician. The surface of the eye is easily damaged by some antiseptics and medications. When applying any lotions or compresses to the eyelid, keep your eye closed.

#### ACUPUNCTURE

In traditional Chinese medicine it is believed that all types of boils, including sties, are caused by heat invasion. To diffuse the heat, a trained acupuncturist may insert needles into BL 54, SP 10, and LI 11 *(see pages 22–23 for point locations).*

#### HERBAL THERAPIES

To help reduce the pain and inflammation of sties, herbalists recommend professionally prepared eye drops made from eyebright *(Euphrasia officinalis).* They may also prescribe an oral preparation of burdock *(Arctium lappa).*

#### NUTRITION AND DIET

If you have recurrent sties and chalazions, a nutritionist may recommend that you take supplements of vitamins A and C, which seem to promote healthy skin. You might also want to try a system-cleansing diet, consuming only raw fruits and vegetables, yogurt, herbal teas, fruit juices, and mineral water for up to a week. Naturopaths believe that this diet, repeated at regular intervals, may keep sties from developing.

### AT-HOME REMEDIES

Apply warm compresses four times daily for 10 to 15 minutes for several days for both sties and chalazions. When the sty has come to a head, it will spontaneously rupture. You can also make a compress by wetting a tea bag with warm water and placing it on your eyelid, with your eye closed, for 5 minutes three to four times a day.

## PREVENTION

If sties tend to recur, you need to cleanse the outside of your eyelids daily. Put a few drops of very mild baby shampoo into a teacup of warm water and stir. Using a cotton swab, gently brush the mixture over your eyelid once a day, keeping your lids closed. It is very important that you avoid contact of the eyelid with cosmetics, dirty towels, or contaminated hands.

Frequent application of warm compresses at the first sign of an infection will prevent further blockage of the lid glands. To keep the infection from spreading to other members of your household, be sure to use a clean, disposable cloth for compresses and do not share washcloths or towels. ■

# SUNBURN

## SYMPTOMS

- mildly reddish to severely red or purplish skin discoloration; skin feels hot and tender. Sunburn appears 1 to 6 hours after exposure to sunlight and peaks within 24 hours, later fading to tan or brown.
- small, fluid-filled blisters that may itch and eventually break; flaking or peeling skin that reveals the tender, reddened underlayer.
- red, blistered skin accompanied by chills, fever, nausea, or dehydration. This severe stage of sunburn is considered a first-degree burn.
- pain and irritation of the eye associated with overexposure to ultraviolet rays from sunlight or other sources.

## CALL YOUR DOCTOR IF:

- your sunburn blisters and is accompanied by chills, fever, or nausea. Severe sunburn requires professional care to limit the risk of infection and to prevent dehydration.
- your eyes are extremely painful and feel gritty. You should have your eyes examined by an ophthalmologist to determine whether the corneas are damaged.

Even though light-skinned people have the highest risk of being sunburned, skin of any color can be damaged by the sun's rays. A sunburn is like any other kind of burn, except that it comes on more slowly. Skin that is reddened and feels hot to the touch can be self-treated and will heal in a matter of days. Sunburned skin that swells or blisters, causing localized pain and overall discomfort, is considered a first-degree burn. A sunburn that results in swelling and extensive blisters may be accompanied by fever, nausea, and dehydration.

Moderate exposure to sunlight simply darkens light skin, but regular tanning over many years can hasten **photoaging,** characterized by leathery skin, dark spotting, and extensive wrinkling. Long-term exposure, especially in Caucasians over 40, is associated with **actinic keratoses,** a precancerous skin condition. Severe sunburn early in life increases the risk of developing malignant melanoma, a type of skin cancer, years later.

## CAUSES

Of the sun's ultraviolet (UV) radiation that penetrates Earth's atmosphere, UVA radiation generally only tans but may also take part in premature aging and wrinkling. UVB rays cause sunburn and the potential for skin cancer. Reflected sunlight from sand, water, or snow is as strong as direct sunlight; shade, clouds, clothes, sunglasses, and sunscreens do not offer complete protection. Certain drugs can intensify the harmful effects of UV radiation; if you are concerned about the potential danger, ask your doctor about photosensitivity.

## TREATMENT

At-home care will alleviate many of the symptoms of sunburn, but no treatment can undo the damage caused by prolonged exposure to the sun.

### CONVENTIONAL MEDICINE

Few cases of sunburn require medical care. If the burn is very painful or widespread, a doctor may prescribe oral corticosteroids to relieve the discomfort. Treatment for extremely severe cases of sunburn—those involving extensive blistering, dehydration, or fever—usually requires bed rest and possibly hospitalization. *(See Burns.)*

## ALTERNATIVE CHOICES

### HERBAL THERAPIES

Lotions, poultices, and compresses containing calendula *(Calendula officinalis)* will reduce inflammation. Echinacea (*Echinacea* spp.) may be used on exposed new skin after peeling or blistering, to help prevent infection. Over-the-counter preparations containing aloe *(Aloe barbadensis)* are excellent for relieving dryness and irritation.

### HOMEOPATHY

Cantharis (12x) taken orally every three to four hours for up to two days is recommended for relieving pain and helping to heal blisters.

### HYDROTHERAPY

A cool bath laced with several tablespoonfuls of baking soda or cider vinegar can relieve the pain, itching, and inflammation of a moderate sunburn.

## AT-HOME REMEDIES

Apply cold compresses or calamine lotion to ease itchiness, take aspirin to relieve pain, and have a cool bath or shower for overall relief. Drink plenty of water, but avoid alcohol, which dehydrates the skin. Do not break any blisters; doing so will slow the healing process and increase the risk of infection. When your skin peels or the blisters break, gently remove dried fragments and apply an antiseptic ointment or hydrocortisone cream to the skin beneath. If you feel feverish or nauseated, drink lots of fluids and see a doctor immediately.

## PREVENTION

The best way to prevent sunburn is to limit your exposure to direct sunlight, especially between 10:00 a.m. and 3:00 p.m. Take a look at your shadow: If it's shorter than your height, stay under cover.

- If you have to be outside in the midday sun, wear loose-fitting clothes, a broad-brimmed hat, and shoes to protect your feet and ankles.
- Note that radiation exposure is greater at higher altitudes and southern latitudes.
- Any water surface reflects the sun's rays and can double the radiation dose. Protect your skin with a water-resistant sunscreen.
- Protect babies' sensitive skin from strong sunlight, and alert older children to the hazards of overexposure.
- Wear sunglasses that are rated for UV protection. In general, gray, brown, and green lenses block out damaging UV rays in that order from most to least effective. ■

### SCREENING THE SUN

*Two types of sunscreens are on the market. Physical sunblocks, such as zinc ointment, protect by creating a barrier between your skin and the sun. They're good for small areas, such as the nose and lips, but not for your whole body. Products containing para-aminobenzoic acid (PABA) block virtually all UVB rays but offer only minimal protection against UVA rays.*

*Sunscreens carry a sun protection factor (SPF); a rating of SPF 15 is recommended for most people, but fair-skinned people who are in the sun all day need more. Apply sunscreen 30 minutes before you go out, and reapply it after a swim. Even if you don't swim, a waterproof sunscreen has more staying power. If PABA gives you a rash, try sunscreens containing cinnamates for UVB protection and avobenzone for UVA protection.*

# SWALLOWING DIFFICULTY

*Read down this column to find your symptoms. Then read across.*

| SYMPTOMS | AILMENT/PROBLEM |
|---|---|
| ◆ Food you swallow feels like it's not going all the way down; possibly, chest pain when you lie down or bend over; possibly, shortness of breath. | ◆ Hiatal hernia; heartburn; side effect of anxiety |
| ◆ difficulty swallowing, possibly accompanied by a sore throat. | ◆ Any of a number of diseases and conditions, including tonsillitis; respiratory allergies; strep throat; laryngitis; sores on the vocal cords; diverticula (small hollow pouches of tissue that form in the esophagus wall and may eventually block the esophagus itself); or a throat abscess |
| ◆ While you are eating, food becomes stuck in your throat, perhaps also causing sharp pain. | ◆ An object is lodged in your throat |
| ◆ swallowing difficulties that are gradually worsening with time; weight loss of 10 pounds or more in the past six months. | ◆ Potentially, throat cancer |
| ◆ sudden, extreme difficulty swallowing; a feeling of drowning or suffocating; quickened pulse; warm and flush skin; possibly, confusion. | ◆ Allergies; possibly, anaphylactic shock (a severe allergic reaction that causes tissues to swell, preventing blood from traveling properly; tissues then become starved for oxygen) |

| WHAT TO DO | OTHER INFO |
| --- | --- |
| ◆ See your doctor if you think you have a hiatal hernia. For heartburn, take over-the-counter antacids and avoid irritants such as fatty and spicy foods, alcohol, tobacco, and caffeine. To alleviate anxiety, find a relaxation technique—such as yoga or meditation—that you're comfortable with and will practice regularly. | ◆ For a hiatal hernia, eat four or five small meals a day instead of three larger ones, and eat slowly. |
| ◆ Consult your doctor. Several of the possible causes of your symptoms require professional medical treatment. | ◆ If you have a bacterial infection, antibiotics may clear up the problem. Vocal cord problems include polyps (swellings on the vocal cord membranes) and singer's nodules (calluslike sores), which are usually the result of repeatedly straining the voice. The best treatment is to rest your voice for several weeks. |
| ◆ If you are choking and cannot breathe, use the Heimlich maneuver. *(See Emergencies/First Aid: Choking.)* If you can't completely remove the object from your throat or if swallowing is still difficult or pain persists after the object is seemingly removed, **see a doctor immediately.** | ◆ If you feel a sharp pain when you try to swallow, do not attempt to "flush" the object down your throat with liquids, because this may damage your esophagus and other tissues. |
| ◆ Call your doctor today. Prompt diagnosis improves the chances of successful treatment. | ◆ Throat cancer most often affects those over 40, especially those with a long history of smoking or heavy drinking. |
| ◆ If you suspect anaphylactic shock, **get emergency medical treatment.** *(See Emergencies/First Aid: Shock.)* While waiting for emergency care, monitor the patient's breathing and pulse, and give nothing to eat or drink. | ◆ The most common cause of anaphylactic shock is sensitivity to the antibiotic penicillin. If you know you have a strong, specific allergy (such as an allergy to bee stings), ask your doctor about preparing an emergency kit to help you prevent anaphylactic shock. |

# SWEATING, EXCESSIVE

*Read down this column to find your symptoms. Then read across.*

| SYMPTOMS | AILMENT/PROBLEM |
|---|---|
| Normal sweating is the body's way of lowering its temperature. Sometimes, however, the body sweats in excess of what is needed for normal cooling. | |
| ◆ chronic sweating and clamminess, especially of the hands, underarms, and feet. | ◆ Hyperhidrosis (chronic sweating) |
| ◆ excessive sweating with chest pain that typically does not recede with rest and lasts a half-hour or more; may be accompanied by nausea, dizziness, or fainting. | ◆ Heart attack |
| ◆ nighttime sweats, weight loss, persistent cough, fever, fatigue, and spitting up blood. | ◆ Possibilities include lung disease, tuberculosis, AIDS, or cancer |
| ◆ sweating with high temperature (over 100°F). | ◆ Breaking fever (defervescence) |
| ◆ sweating, hot flashes, vaginal dryness, or mood swings. | ◆ Menopause |
| ◆ feelings of tension or stress that may cause profuse sweating. | ◆ Anxiety |
| ◆ excessive sweating accompanied by two or more of the following: weight loss, increased appetite, anxiety, insomnia; possibly, rapid heartbeat, muscle weakness, hot skin. | ◆ Hyperthyroidism (overactive thyroid) |
| ◆ sweating when you are taking a prescription, over-the-counter, or illegal drug; going through withdrawal; or drinking excessively. | ◆ Adverse drug reaction; typical effect of drug withdrawal; alcoholism |
| ◆ heat intolerance, increased sweating of the upper body, and decreased or absent sweating of the lower body. | ◆ Diabetes |

| WHAT TO DO | OTHER INFO |
|---|---|
| ◆ See your doctor. In some cases topical aluminum chloride solution is sufficient. For more severe cases, a simple operation severs the nerves that regulate sweating. | ◆ Troublesome residual effects of surgery include compensatory sweating elsewhere on the body and continued underarm sweating. |
| ◆ **Call 911 or your doctor now.** See Emergencies/First Aid: Heart Attack. | |
| ◆ See your doctor without delay. Lung cancer, Hodgkin's disease *(see Lymphoma),* and tuberculosis must all be treated promptly. AIDS patients who seek care early may live for many years. | ◆ Sweating may be the only early symptom of Hodgkin's disease or other lymphomas. People with early HIV infection commonly have sweating, as well as a low fever, fatigue, diarrhea, and mild weight loss. |
| ◆ Take plenty of fluids to prevent dehydration. If fever returns, see your doctor. | ◆ Profuse sweating is often the body's way of quickly returning its temperature to normal. |
| ◆ See your doctor. Sometimes, an antihypertensive drug called clonidine can control abnormal temperature in menopause. See Menopausal Problems. | ◆ Sweating may also occur when estrogen levels decline after childbirth or at the beginning of the menstrual period. |
| ◆ If your sweating causes embarrassment, see your doctor, who will ask about underlying anxiety and may prescribe medication. | |
| ◆ See your doctor. If you are producing too much thyroid hormone, you may require radiation, surgery, or thyroid-blocking drugs. See Thyroid Problems. | ◆ An overactive thyroid causes unpleasant symptoms by speeding up the chemical reactions of your body, both physical and mental. |
| ◆ Discuss these symptoms with your doctor, who may change your prescription medication. See Alcohol Abuse and Drug Abuse. | ◆ Alcohol and large doses of aspirin or other drugs, such as insulin, may cause excessive sweating. *(See Diabetes.)* |
| ◆ See a doctor. This complication of diabetes indicates poor temperature regulation and may lead to hyperthermia and heatstroke. | |

# SWIMMER'S EAR

## SYMPTOMS

Despite its name, you don't have to be a swimmer to get swimmer's ear. The symptoms include:

- itching inside the ear.
- watery discharge from the ear.
- severe pain and tenderness in the ear, especially when moving your head or when gently pulling on your earlobe.
- a foul-smelling, yellowish discharge from the ear.
- temporarily muffled hearing (caused by blockage of the ear canal).

## CALL YOUR DOCTOR IF:

- you are experiencing dizziness or ringing in the ears; such symptoms may indicate a more serious problem that needs medical attention.
- you have severe pain; your doctor can provide medications to relieve it.
- you also notice a rash on your scalp or near your ear; you may have seborrheic dermatitis, for which your doctor can provide treatment.

Known to medical professionals as otitis externa, swimmer's ear is an inflammation of the outer ear canal. Its common name comes from the fact that it often occurs in children and young adults who swim frequently. The inflammation can sometimes lead to an infection that can be very painful.

## CAUSES

Swimmer's ear is often caused by excess moisture in the ear from swimming or even routine showering. The moisture causes the skin inside the ear canal to flake—a condition known as eczema. A break in the skin, which may result from trying to scratch the persistent itch of the eczema, can allow bacteria or (more rarely) a fungus to invade the tissue of the ear canal and cause an infection. Swimming in polluted water, therefore, is a common cause of swimmer's ear; the bacteria in the water find a hospitable home in the moist environment of an inflamed ear canal.

Other skin conditions, such as seborrheic dermatitis and psoriasis, can also lead to swimmer's ear. And another common cause is excessive and improper cleaning of wax from the ears. Not only does wax protect the ear canal from excess moisture, but it also harbors friendly bacteria. Removing this protective barrier—particularly with hairpins, fingernails, or other objects that can scratch the skin—makes it easier for an infection to take hold. Hair spray or haircoloring, which can irritate the ear canal, may also lead to an outer ear infection.

## TREATMENT

Swimmer's ear is usually not a dangerous condition and often clears up on its own within a few days. With mild infections, therefore, you may want to try alternative treatments first. If the pain worsens or does not improve within 24 hours, you should see your doctor. In rare cases, the infection can spread and damage underlying bones and cartilage.

### CONVENTIONAL MEDICINE

Your doctor will probably clean your ear with a cotton-tipped probe or a suction device to relieve irritation and pain. You may be given a prescription ear drop containing a combination of hydrocortisone to help relieve the itching and an antibiotic to fight the infection.

If the pain is severe, your doctor may suggest aspirin, acetaminophen, or some other over-the-counter pain medication. You will also be instructed to keep water out of the infected ear during the healing process. If the infection does not improve within three or four days, your doctor may prescribe an oral antibiotic.

### ALTERNATIVE CHOICES

#### AROMATHERAPY

To improve blood circulation to the area and thus help healing, gently massage the area around the outer ear with an oil made from 3 to 5 drops of either eucalyptus *(Eucalyptus globulus)* or lavender *(Lavandula officinalis)* diluted in 1 tsp olive or other vegetable oil. Rub the oil into the temples and neck and on the earlobe.

#### HERBAL THERAPIES

Mullein *(Verbascum thapsus)* oil, which has anti-inflammatory properties, may help soothe and heal an inflamed ear canal. Put 1 to 3 drops in the infected ear every three hours.

Another useful herb for swimmer's ear is garlic *(Allium sativum),* which has been shown to act as a natural antibiotic. Combine equal parts garlic juice, glycerin, and a carrier oil, such as olive or sweet almond; put 1 to 3 drops in the infected ear every three hours.

#### HOMEOPATHY

Homeopaths prescribe a variety of substances to help relieve the pain of swimmer's ear. Consult a homeopathic practitioner for specific remedies, which may include Aconite, Apis, or Graphites.

### AT-HOME REMEDIES

- Wash the infected ear canal with an over-the-counter topical antiseptic. Or try a homemade solution made from equal parts white vinegar and isopropyl alcohol. Continue to put a few drops of the solution into the ear every two to three hours. Keep the drops in the ear for at least 30 seconds.
- To relieve pain, place a warm heating pad or compress on the infected ear.
- Take aspirin or another analgesic to ease the pain.
- During the healing process, make sure you keep the infected ear canal dry, even while showering. Use earplugs or a shower cap.

## PREVENTION

- Be careful when cleaning your ears. Wipe the outer ear with a clean washcloth. Do not dig into the ear canal, and never use a pointed object.
- Wear earplugs when swimming. Afterward, tilt and shake your head to drain water from your ears.
- Avoid swimming in dirty water.
- Use earplugs or a shower cap to keep your ears dry while showering. Or dry your ears after showering with a hair dryer: Set it on low and hold it about a foot from your ear.
- You can also dry out your ear and help kill germs after swimming or showering by squirting a dropperful of isopropyl alcohol or white vinegar into your ear. Tilt your head so the solution gets to the bottom of the ear canal, then let the liquid drain out.
- To create a protective coating for your ear canal before you go swimming, squirt a dropperful of mineral oil, baby oil, or lanolin into your ear.
- If you wear a hearing aid, take it out as often as possible to give your ear a chance to dry out; a hearing aid can trap moisture in the ear canal. ■

# SYPHILIS

## SYMPTOMS

**There are three stages of syphilis.**

- In the first stage, 10 days to 6 weeks after exposure, painless sores appear on the genitals, rectum, or mouth. Lymph nodes near the groin may be swollen as well.
- In the second stage, one week to six months later, a red rash may appear anywhere on the body. You may have flulike symptoms, such as headache, fever, fatigue, loss of appetite, and pain in bones and joints; symptoms may then disappear, and the disease becomes latent, but the bacteria remain in the body.
- In the third stage, which can start anytime from one year to several decades later, joints may be affected, resulting in arthritis. **Cardiovascular syphilis** develops in approximately 10 percent of patients, causing heart disease. **Neurosyphilis**, which may cause paralysis, blindness, senility, insanity, or loss of sensation in the legs, develops in about 8 percent of patients.

## CALL YOUR DOCTOR IF:

- you experience any of the symptoms above. Syphilis is life-threatening and it's imperative to treat it before it does serious damage to your system.

Syphilis is among the most serious of sexually transmitted diseases. In 1990 some 100,000 cases were reported in the United States—a 40-year high—with the highest incidence occurring in urban populations, among people ages 15 to 39. Epidemiologists attribute the increase to a lack of education about the disease as well as to a rise in the number of prostitutes having unprotected sex. The increase is not reflected among homosexuals or bisexuals, however, presumably because many in that population are using condoms more frequently.

## CAUSES

Syphilis is caused by the spirochete bacterium *Treponema pallidum*, which gains entrance to the body through minor cuts or abrasions in the skin or mucous membranes, most often during sexual intercourse. The disease also may be transmitted from mother to child before or during birth.

### DIAGNOSTIC AND TEST PROCEDURES

Your doctor will be able to determine whether you have syphilis by examining your blood for antibodies to the disease.

## TREATMENT

If caught early, syphilis may be cured with antibiotics. But if you allow the disease to progress to the third stage, you may suffer irreversible damage to your heart or nervous system. If you have

### CAUTION!

**If you are pregnant, get a syphilis test. The life-threatening disease may be passed to your child before or during delivery. Approximately half of all babies infected with syphilis die before or shortly after birth.**

syphilis, you'll require follow-up blood tests at regular intervals for at least a year after treatment.

## CONVENTIONAL MEDICINE

Penicillin is extremely effective in treating the early stages, and fairly effective in treating the later stages, of syphilis. If you are allergic to penicillin, your physician will give you tetracycline or erythromycin.

## ALTERNATIVE CHOICES

Because syphilis is a serious, potentially life-threatening disease, you must see a doctor as soon as you think you have it. Besides taking penicillin or its derivatives, you can use several alternative therapies to speed healing.

### ACUPRESSURE

To treat sexually transmitted diseases, acupressurists work on points that are said to help rid the body of built-up toxins. Several times a day, massage Liver 3, located on top of the foot between the big and second toes, and Liver 8, on the inside of the leg above the knee. Next, press Kidney 3, on the inside of the leg between the anklebone and Achilles tendon. *(See pages 22–23 for more information about point locations.)*

### CHINESE HERBS

A doctor of Chinese medicine will give you a unique herbal formula to help clear toxins from the body. Herbs beneficial in the treatment of syphilis include Chinese foxglove root *(Rehmannia glutinosa)* and dong quai *(Angelica sinensis).*

### HERBAL THERAPIES

Cowboys drank sarsaparilla for a reason: The herb that flavored the popular soft drink was once thought to be the only cure for syphilis, which was rampant in Old West brothels. Sarsaparilla *(Smilax officinalis)* was also used extensively throughout Europe. Trade records from the mid-19th century show that Great Britain alone imported 150,000 pounds a year.

To treat syphilis, some herbalists advocate the following formula: Add 2 tbsp each of sarsaparilla and sourdock *(Rumex crispus)* root to 1 qt boiling water. Simmer for five minutes and add 3½ tsp thyme. Steep covered for one hour. Drink one to three cups per day. Women may use this tea as a douche.

### HOMEOPATHY

In addition to prescribing antibiotics, a homeopathic physician will ask you if any of your ancestors had syphilis or another sexually transmitted disease, on the theory that you could have inherited the tendency to contract syphilis. If so, a homeopath might prescribe a remedy such as Syphilinum, to help stimulate your immune system's response to the disease.

### NUTRITION AND DIET

One thing you can do yourself to alleviate pain and encourage healing is to watch what you eat. Some nutritionists recommend that you cleanse your body of toxins by fasting for one to three days. Always check with your physician before beginning a fast. To stimulate your kidneys and flush out your system, drink the juices of pomegranate and cranberry or a combination of celery, parsley, and cucumber. Eat a balanced diet and avoid high-fat, salty, processed foods, which may make your system too sluggish to fight off disease.

## AT-HOME REMEDIES

- Take a hot bath followed by a cold one to help alleviate the aches and pains associated with syphilis.
- Use acupressure massages, which may help rid your body of toxins.
- Eat a balanced diet to help build up your immune system.

S

# PREVENTION

If you're not in a long-term monogamous relationship, always use a condom when having sex. ■

# TEETHING PROBLEMS

## SYMPTOMS

Although the arrival of your infant's early teeth is a normal development and not an illness, it can be an irritating or painful process for your child and a trying time for you. Indications of teething may include:

- increased fussing, nighttime crying, and clinging from your baby as teeth start pushing out of the gums, usually at about six months.
- drooling and chewing on fingers as more teeth move toward the surface.
- swollen and inflamed gums, especially where a tooth is about to emerge.
- refusal to suck on breast or bottle, because the sucking action hurts inflamed gums.

## CALL YOUR DOCTOR IF:

- your teething baby runs a fever, seems lethargic or irritable, is not responding well to the teething, or has diarrhea while teething; these symptoms may be signs that your child is ill.
- your teething baby has cold symptoms or a fever and clutches an ear or one side of her face; this may signal otitis media.
- no teeth are present by 12 months of age; this could indicate a harmless inherited tendency to late teething, but it might instead mean some metabolic condition that could cause delayed bone development. Your first call should be to your pediatrician, who later might refer you to a pediatric dentist.

Before birth, a baby's teeth have already developed inside the gums. At around four months, the teeth start moving to the surface. By seven months, your infant probably will be actively teething, with most baby teeth in various stages of eruption—or emergence—from the gums. All 20 baby teeth, appearing in the order indicated below, right, are usually in place before the child is three. Heredity determines the speed at which teeth appear; your children probably will share the same teething pattern. Teething is a good time to start a preventive dental program with regular gum cleaning. Dentists also recommend beginning fluoride treatments at around six months, even if teeth are still under the gum. Fluoride strengthens the teeth by bonding with the calcium and phosphorus in their enamel. Good dental habits learned early will be invaluable when your child begins getting permanent teeth by about seven years of age.

## CAUSES

A tooth moving toward the surface of the gum may cause pain and swelling where it will break through. A baby may refuse to suck at this stage because sucking action draws blood to the inflamed area, increasing soreness.

## TREATMENT

Because teething is not an illness, the treatment of it is simply a matter of trying to relieve the child's discomfort.

### CONVENTIONAL MEDICINE

It is not essential to consult your pediatrician unless your baby has symptoms of illness. If you do seek help for a teething infant with persistent discomfort, the doctor may recommend liquid acetaminophen, which should be used sparingly (two to four times a day) but usually provides pain relief. Over-the-counter teething medications with a topical anesthetic such as benzocaine are not recommended, because they can be toxic.

## ALTERNATIVE CHOICES

### ACUPRESSURE

Practitioners suggest gently pressing Stomach 3 and 4 or massaging Large Intestine 4, found between your child's thumb and index finger on either hand. See pages 22–23 for more information on point locations.

### HERBAL THERAPIES

Herbalists recommend marsh mallow *(Althaea officinalis)* root syrup for inflamed gums; use 3 tsp in your child's food or drink daily.

### HOMEOPATHY

Homeopathic teething remedies are available over the counter. If your child's discomfort is not eased within 24 hours, however, you will want to consult a practitioner for advice. Chamomilla is considered one of the most effective homeopathic remedies for teething. Other specific remedies that your practitioner might prescribe include Aconite, Pulsatilla, and Belladonna.

### YOUR BABY'S TEETH

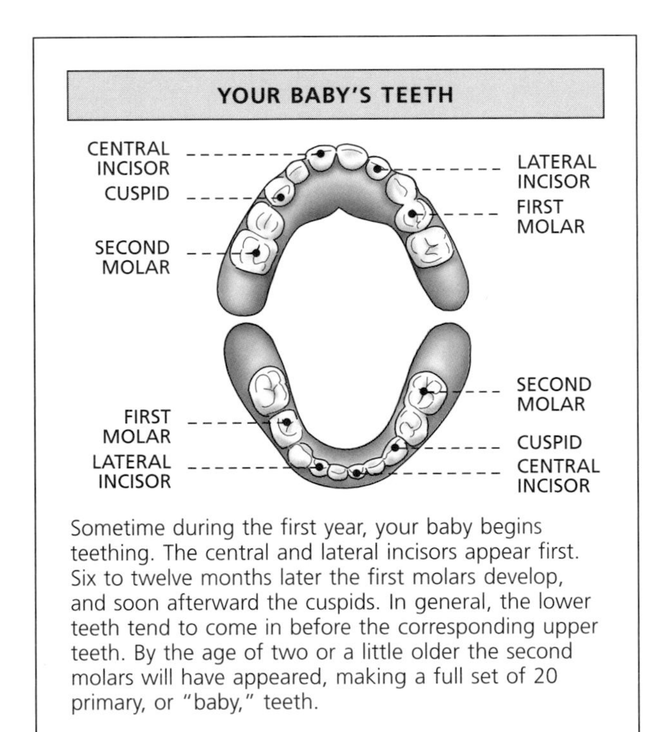


Sometime during the first year, your baby begins teething. The central and lateral incisors appear first. Six to twelve months later the first molars develop, and soon afterward the cuspids. In general, the lower teeth tend to come in before the corresponding upper teeth. By the age of two or a little older the second molars will have appeared, making a full set of 20 primary, or "baby," teeth.

### LIFESTYLE

When your child begins teething, you can start cleaning her gums and teeth daily with gauze or a soft toothbrush. When she is two-and-a-half to three, her motor skills will be more developed and you can start teaching her to brush her teeth. At age four, she is ready for her first dental visit.

### NUTRITION AND DIET

When weaning your teething child, give her easy-to-digest foods such as baby rice or millet; establish regular feeding times and feed slowly, burping after every feeding. Never let your child teethe on or go to sleep with a bottle of milk or juice; the sugars and starches will encourage tooth decay.

## AT-HOME REMEDIES

- A chilled but not frozen teething ring or a chilled wet washcloth can ease soreness and give your child something to chew.
- Wrap an ice cube in a soft cloth and rub it gently on your infant's gums to ease inflammation; keep moving the ice over the gums to avoid damaging tissue.
- Don't let your baby's drooling go unattended; a rash can develop. Put petroleum jelly around your infant's mouth and chin, and use a bib or change the child's clothes if they become saturated from drooling.
- Avoid feeding your child salty or acidic foods, which can aggravate sensitive gums.

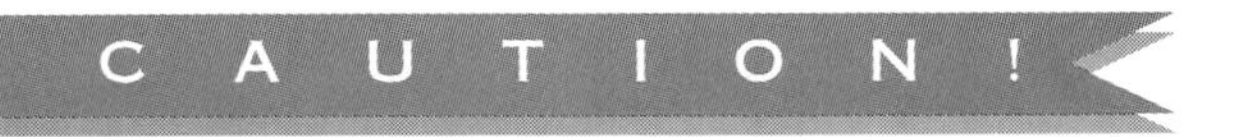


### DANGEROUS OLD REMEDY

**Never rub alcohol on your teething child's gums! In the past, and occasionally today, liquor has been employed to relieve teething pain. Alcohol may momentarily relieve gum discomfort, but alcohol has a direct toxic effect, and even small quantities can lead to severe hypoglycemia and brain damage.** ■

T

# TEMPOROMANDIBULAR JOINT SYNDROME

## SYMPTOMS

- pain in front of the ears, especially upon awakening.
- persistent pain in the facial muscles on one or both sides.
- a clicking or popping sensation when opening the mouth or working the jaw.
- difficulty opening the mouth because it feels locked or painful.
- recurring headaches.

## CALL YOUR DOCTOR IF:

- you have difficulty opening your mouth following an injury or a blow to the face. You may have dislocated or damaged one or both of your temporomandibular joints.
- you have persistent discomfort in your jaw that does not respond to painkillers, heat, massage, or rest. You may need a specialist's diagnosis and advice about more aggressive treatment to relieve both the symptoms and the cause.

The fact that humans need to speak and eat makes the jawbone one of our busiest moving parts. The twin joints that connect the lower jaw, or mandible, to the temporal bones of the skull are relatively simple hinges with small disks of cartilage to protect the bony surfaces that rub against each other. The jawbreaking term for pain or discomfort in this area is temporomandibular joint (TMJ) syndrome, or myofascial pain dysfunction.

As many as two-thirds of Americans exhibit symptoms of TMJ at some point in their lives, when something as simple as a wide yawn or eating a chewy bagel sets off facial pain or jaw popping. This temporary condition usually resolves itself without treatment or responds quickly to rest and painkillers. In some instances, though, patients feel pain that radiates through the face and around the neck and shoulders, a chronic pattern of TMJ that results from other conditions. Most temporary TMJ discomfort can be helped with inexpensive, at-home remedies; but for a few TMJ sufferers, persistent and sometimes unbearable pain is a serious problem requiring medical treatment. Unfortunately, some health insurers insist on labeling TMJ as a dental rather than a medical problem and object to paying for treatment, a fact that can sometimes discourage sufferers from seeking available help and relief.

## CAUSES

Most cases of TMJ are due to excessive strain on the jaw muscles, a displaced disk, or degenerative joint disease—sometimes in combination. The most common cause is strain to the temporalis muscles that open and close the jaw. The strain can stem from unconsciously clenching or grinding the teeth or jutting the jaw forward, as well as from a poor bite caused by misaligned teeth or poorly fitting dentures.

Displacement of one or both of the disks in the jaw's hinges can result from a sudden blow or injury to the head, or simply from hard chewing or a wide yawn. Usually the displaced disk slips back into position without permanently harming the jaw. If such dislocation happens often, however, the jaw may start to pop or click when opened, and the joint may become inflamed, stiff, and painful. The effects of degenerative joint disease are similar: Osteoarthritis or rheumatoid arthritis inflames the joint, causing pain and stiffness. On rare occasions, malnutrition in children can lead to bone deformities that cause TMJ.

## TREATMENT

Taking a painkiller may ease the inflammation and relieve the pain of TMJ but does not get to the underlying cause of the problem. TMJ sufferers need to assess their entire lifestyle—from potentially avoidable day-to-day stresses to eating foods that strain the jaw. In cases where tooth alignment is at fault, you need to see your dentist.

### CONVENTIONAL MEDICINE

Most doctors tell people with mild TMJ to take an over-the-counter analgesic, massage the area, and limit talking and chewing for a few days—resting the jaw by eating soft or liquid foods. More painful or chronic conditions may require treatment by a dentist, physical therapist, orthodontist, oral surgeon, or behavioral specialist.

Some people unconsciously grind their teeth while sleeping, a condition called bruxism. A dentist can diagnose that problem and fit the patient with a bite guard or splint. A doctor who suspects that TMJ is caused by excessive muscle strain may prescribe a muscle relaxant such as diazepam to relieve pain and tension. Since TMJ can be a chronic condition, however, a patient should not rely on such prescription drugs for long-term relief, because of the risk of addiction.

Physical therapy may relieve pain and restore jaw mobility in some cases of TMJ. A physical therapist may recommend massage, moist-heat compresses, ultrasound, or stimulation by interferential electric current to promote circulation and to relieve pain and stiffness. To improve the jaw's range of motion, a therapist may use stretching exercises and may recommend the spray-and-stretch technique, in which the face is sprayed with a numbing coolant and the jaw muscles are stretched. Other physical therapy options include short-wave diathermy and laser treatments. The waves from such treatment reach much deeper than moist-heat applications, and the undulating pressure works like a massage, increasing blood flow to the affected area and reducing inflammation and pain.

Doctors recommend surgery only for extreme cases. The least invasive form, arthroscopy, involves inserting a fiberoptic tube through a small incision and using it to reposition the disk. If arthroscopy fails, open TM joint surgery may be necessary; this entails completely exposing the area and may include a joint replacement. Before making a commitment to surgery, however, a patient should explore all options, potential complications, and side effects and should get a second opinion from another qualified surgeon.

### ALTERNATIVE CHOICES

Various alternative therapies can be effective in treating TMJ. A number of herbal remedies may act as sedatives or relax muscles to ease the pain. Many medical doctors acknowledge **biofeedback**'s success rate for controlling stress-related TMJ.

**THE TEMPOROMANDIBULAR JOINT**

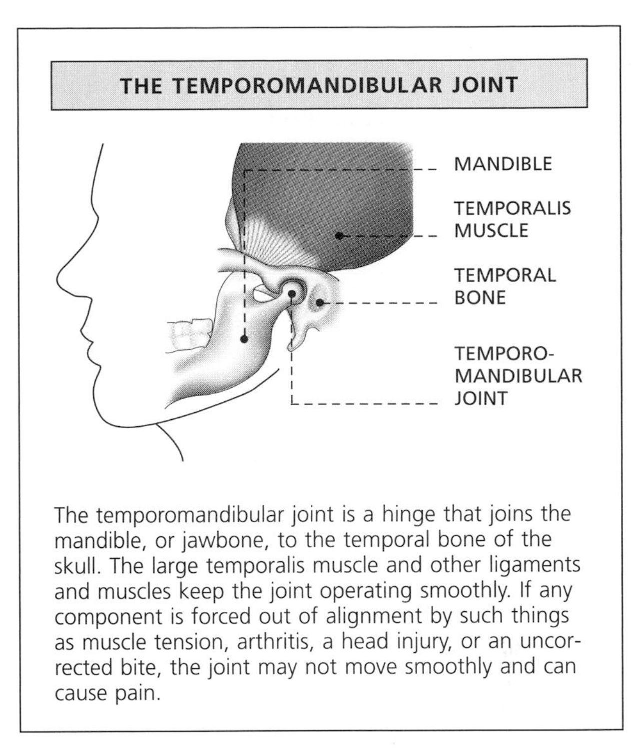


The temporomandibular joint is a hinge that joins the mandible, or jawbone, to the temporal bone of the skull. The large temporalis muscle and other ligaments and muscles keep the joint operating smoothly. If any component is forced out of alignment by such things as muscle tension, arthritis, a head injury, or an uncorrected bite, the joint may not move smoothly and can cause pain.

#### ACUPRESSURE

For patients who feel squeamish about acupuncture needles, acupressure offers a gentle alternative. The acupressure therapist presses points on the stomach meridians, which pass through the area where muscle spasms, stiffness, and pain associated with TMJ are most apt to occur. *(See the illustrations at right.)*

#### ACUPUNCTURE

Acupuncture works by relaxing the muscles, which makes it effective for TMJ symptoms that are caused by stress. Like an acupressurist, an acupuncturist will treat points on the stomach meridians for stress-related TMJ, because those meridians pass through the temporomandibular joints.

#### BODY WORK

When tension is believed to play a role in TMJ, **massage** therapy may provide relief. Two areas can be massaged: One runs from just above and slightly forward of the top of your ear over to your temple; the other is on your jaw about an inch in front of your earlobes. Place a finger on either of these areas, and then open and close your jaw, pressing your teeth together slightly when the jaw is closed. You will feel a muscle pop in and out as it contracts and relaxes. Place your thumb or your index and middle fingers on these areas, and massage lightly in little circles. Doing this for a minute or two at each spot can help relax muscles that cause tension around the joint. For more severe cases of TMJ, consult a professional massage therapist. Techniques that have been reported to help TMJ are deep-tissue **massage,** neuromuscular massage, **Rolfing,** and craniosacral work.

#### CHIROPRACTIC

Chiropractic therapy is recommended for TMJ caused by muscle overuse and strain, rather than by joint damage as in a patient who develops TMJ after whiplash injury in a car accident. A chiropractor not only treats the patient's back and body alignment, but may also use physical therapy, interferential current, ultrasound, or diathermy on the affected joint, any of which can help relax the area and allow the chiropractor to stretch the muscles and manipulate the jaw.

#### ACUPRESSURE

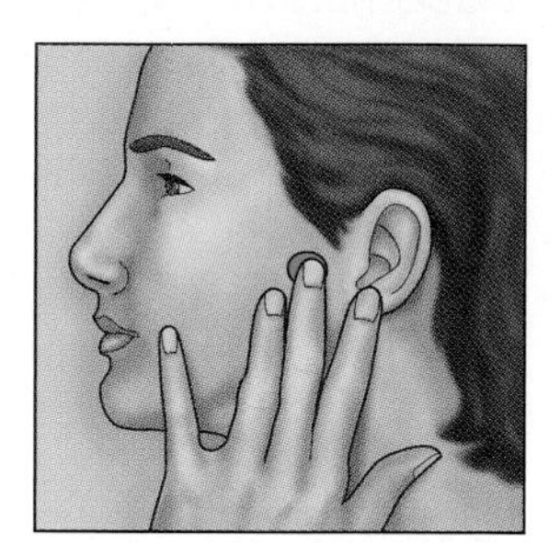

**1** Pressing Stomach 7 may ease tension in the jaw. With your middle fingers, feel on either side of your jaw about one thumb width in front of your ears. Find a slight indentation along the upper jaw line, then press steadily for one minute.

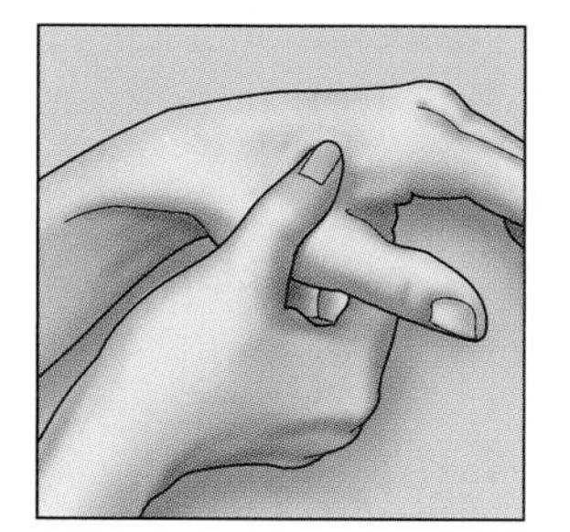

**2** To help relieve facial pain caused by TMJ, press Large Intestine 4, located in the web between thumb and index finger. Squeeze the web of each hand with the thumb and index finger of the other for one minute. Do not press this point if you are pregnant.

#### HYDROTHERAPY

A few drops of the essential oils of lavender *(Lavandula officinalis)* or St.-John's-wort *(Hypericum perforatum)* in warm bathwater may help you to relax. To reduce inflammation of the TM joints, apply hot and cold compresses. Start with a hot towel for three minutes, then switch to a cold towel for half a minute; repeat two or three times a day for chronic conditions, or more frequently if acute.

#### MIND/BODY MEDICINE

While **relaxation** techniques, **hypnotherapy,** and **guided imagery** can all alleviate the symptoms of TMJ, **biofeedback** is the most effective mind/body treatment for TMJ. Biofeedback is a drug-free, noninvasive approach to eliminating tension and controlling stress-related pain, and can be self-administered after training by a professional therapist. Using electrical readings from the muscle that moves the jaw, practitioners can train a patient to control the tension in the overall area. Studies have shown that biofeedback works especially well for chronic TMJ sufferers and may help reduce pain and minimize clicking for a longer time than other treatments.

#### NUTRITION AND DIET

It is important for TMJ sufferers to reduce strain on jaw muscles and joints. Avoid hard foods like raw carrots and apples, and chewy foods like steak and bagels. If the pain in your jaw becomes really unbearable, try fasting or putting yourself on a liquid diet for a day or two; this is especially effective if you also limit talking to when it's absolutely necessary.

From a nutritional standpoint, TMJ patients should consider taking appropriate dosages of bromelain, or the bioflavonoid pyncogenol in combination with vitamin C, to reduce inflammation; calcium/magnesium tablets for muscle spasms; or B-complex vitamins to relieve stress.

#### OSTEOPATHY

Besides recommending proper dental work, physical therapy, or biofeedback, an osteopathic physician may also use hands-on techniques to help increase the range of motion in the head, neck, shoulders, and upper back. You may be able to find an osteopathic doctor who specializes in TMJ.

### AT-HOME REMEDIES

No matter what causes occasional TMJ, you can take aspirin or a nonsteroidal anti-inflammatory drug (NSAID) to relieve the pain. If you have an unexplained, persistent headache that's relieved when you put an ice-cream stick between your teeth, you probably have an alignment problem in your jaw area. Stress-related TMJ usually responds well to at-home remedies. But if your pain is caused by poorly aligned teeth or damage to the joint, don't go on a steady painkiller regimen; see a doctor or dentist. Some other suggestions:

- Massage the band of muscles just above and in front of your temples, as well as the larger muscles along your jaw line. Use small circular motions and repeat as needed.
- Mouth guards for football and hockey players might help mild cases of TMJ due to bruxism (teeth grinding). You'll find the guards in sporting-goods stores. Soften the plastic mouthpiece in warm water, then bite down straight and hard to make an imprint of your teeth. Allow the impression to set, then put the guard between your teeth at night when you sleep. If pain or grinding continues for any length of time, see a doctor.

## PREVENTION

- To prevent TMJ from unconscious muscle strain or uneven pressure on the jaw, don't sleep with your head tilted or with the entire weight of your head concentrated on your chin—a common practice among people who sleep on their stomachs. Try sleeping on your side, or on your back without a pillow.
- Whenever your jaw hurts, stay away from foods that are hard to chew, and minimize talking.
- If you feel tension in your jaw every morning, you may be unwittingly clenching or grinding your teeth. See a dentist or orthodontist about the advantages of being fitted with a bite guard.

### TMJ AND WHIPLASH

*For years doctors have found that people who sustain whiplash injuries in car accidents can develop TMJ. Although debate continues about the precise cause, women seem particularly susceptible, possibly because some women's neck muscles are weaker in relation to head size than they are in men, giving the head-snapping momentum greater impact. Studies have shown that whiplash-related TMJ—which occurs without direct impact or pressure on the jaw—may cause clicking, popping, and on occasion some pain, but almost never persists long-term, if treated.* ■

# TENDONITIS

## SYMPTOMS

- painful tenderness at or near a joint, especially around a shoulder, wrist, or heel (where it is known as Achilles tendonitis), or on the outside of an elbow (where it is called tennis elbow).
- in some cases, numbness or tingling.
- stiffness that, along with the pain, restricts the movement of the joint involved.
- occasionally, mild swelling at the joint.
- persistence of the soreness, which may last or recur long after the tendon has had time to recover from the original injury.

## CALL YOUR DOCTOR IF:

- your pain doesn't ease up in 7 to 10 days. You want to avoid letting chronic tendonitis set in; moreover, you may have another problem such as bursitis, carpal tunnel syndrome, or phlebitis.
- your pain is extremely severe and accompanied by swelling. You may have a ruptured tendon, which requires immediate medical attention.

Tendonitis is an inflammation in or around a tendon, a band of fibrous tissue that connects a muscle to a bone and transmits the force the muscle exerts. Tendons are designed to withstand bending, stretching, and twisting, but they can become inflamed because of overuse, disease, or injuries that leave them with torn fibers or other damage. The pain can be significant and worsens if damage progresses because of continued use of the joint. Most tendonitis heals in about two weeks, but chronic tendonitis can take more than six weeks, often because the sufferer doesn't give the tendon time to heal. Diseases such as diabetes, arthritis, and gout can slow healing.

## CAUSES

Tendons can become inflamed when overstressed from any activity. Weekend athletes, who exercise sporadically rather than regularly, are often laid low by sore tendons. But by far the most common cause is repetitive stress—using the same joints for the same stressful movements again and again. This happens not only in sports but also in many types of office work and other situations.

### DIAGNOSTIC AND TEST PROCEDURES

Your physician may order x-rays and bone scans in order to rule out bone damage. MRI scans can help determine the severity of damage to a tendon.

## TREATMENT

The goals of treatment are to restore movement to the joint without pain and to maintain strength in surrounding muscles while giving the tissues time to heal. Adequate rest is crucial. Returning too soon to the activity that caused the injury can lead to chronic tendonitis or torn tendons.

### CONVENTIONAL MEDICINE

As an immediate treatment for tendonitis, doctors and physical therapists recommend what is known as the RICE program: rest, ice, compres-

T

sion, and elevation *(see At-Home Remedies, below, right).* They may also suggest aspirin or ibuprofen to help reduce inflammation and pain. Ultrasound and whirlpool treatments are employed to relax muscles and tendons, improve circulation, and promote healing. Occasionally, your doctor may prescribe corticosteroids.

Your therapist will probably propose an exercise plan that rests the tendon while strengthening nearby muscle groups and maintaining overall muscle tone. Only gradually will you begin to exercise the tendon itself. Your program may also include "eccentric" exercises, in which you gradually increase use of the injured area, stopping at the first sign of pain. You may work into easy stretching exercises, done several times a day.

### TENDONITIS ON THE JOB

*If your tendonitis is caused by tasks you perform at work and you cannot rest your injuries while keeping up with your duties, ask your supervisor for help in modifying your work habits. You may want to request a work-site inspection by an ergonomics specialist, who can analyze the situation and suggest changes. Try some stretches before and after work, and plan to take a 5- to 10-minute period each hour to rest the injured area by undertaking tasks that do not involve its use.*

## ALTERNATIVE CHOICES

### CHINESE HERBS

Chinese practitioners might prepare a poultice of gardenia *(Gardenia jasminoides),* flour, and wine, which together with tui na—a type of massage that uses the ball of the thumb to manipulate the affected area—may help to reduce swelling and increase circulation.

### HERBAL THERAPIES

For pain, a naturopathic practitioner might suggest white willow *(Salix alba),* the natural form of aspirin, taken orally. Bromelain, an enzyme found in pineapples, is sometimes taken orally with the aim of reducing inflammation in soft tissues.

### HOMEOPATHY

Among the over-the-counter homeopathic remedies suitable for tendonitis symptoms are Arnica (6x to 30c) as an anti-inflammatory and Ruta (6x to 12x) as an antispasmodic.

### NUTRITION AND DIET

Research suggests that vitamin supplements may help heal tendonitis. Ask your doctor about taking daily supplements of vitamin C (1,000 mg), beta carotene (vitamin A, 10,000 IU), zinc (22.5 mg), vitamin E (400 IU), and selenium (50 mcg).

## AT-HOME REMEDIES

Remind yourself of RICE. Rest is mainly a matter of remembering not to use the joint, especially not for the same action that injured it. Ice can be in the form of a bag of frozen vegetables if no ice pack is handy. Compression is best provided by a sports bandage wrapping the area snugly, but not painfully tight. For elevation—to reduce blood pressure in the injured area—put your ankle on a footstool or lift your elbow onto a chairside table.

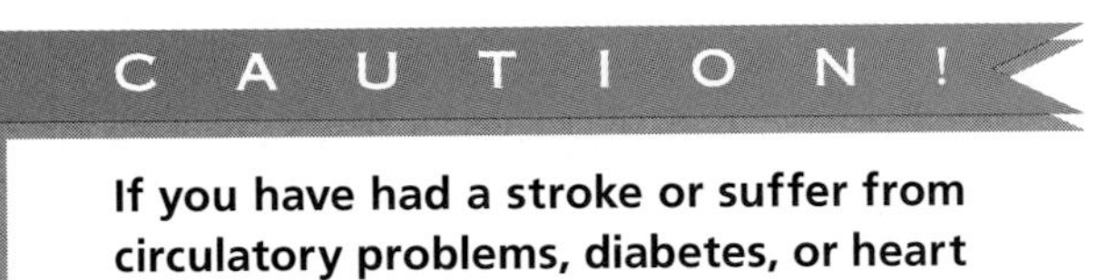


**If you have had a stroke or suffer from circulatory problems, diabetes, or heart disease, avoid massage and applications of heat or cold until you consult your doctor.**

## PREVENTION

Include warmups, cooldowns, and stretches in your exercise routine. Vary your exercises. ■

# TENNIS ELBOW

## SYMPTOMS

- recurring pain on the outside of the upper forearm just below the bend of the elbow; occasionally, pain radiates down the arm toward the wrist.
- pain caused by lifting or bending the arm or grasping even light objects such as a coffee cup.
- difficulty extending the forearm fully (because of inflamed muscles, tendons, and ligaments).
- pain that typically lasts for 6 to 12 weeks; the discomfort can continue for as little as 3 weeks or as long as several years.

## CALL YOUR DOCTOR IF:

- the pain persists for more than a few days; chronic inflammation of the tendons can lead to permanent disability.
- the elbow joint begins to swell; tennis elbow rarely causes swelling, so you may have another condition such as arthritis, gout, infection, or even a tumor.

Doctors first identified tennis elbow (or lateral epicondylitis) more than 100 years ago. Today nearly half of all tennis players will suffer from this disorder at some point, but they account for less than 5 percent of all cases, making the term for this condition something of a misnomer. While people of all ages and races can develop tennis elbow, Caucasian men 30 to 60 years old who work with their hands—carpenters and house painters, for example—are at greatest risk; middle-aged women who do piecework in the garment industry are also highly susceptible.

In recent years cases of tennis elbow have also surfaced in children who play hand-held computer games for extended periods and in office workers who use a computer only rarely but, when they do use one, type intensely for long hours. *(See also Carpal Tunnel Syndrome.)*

## CAUSES

Tennis players with a lazy, late backhand tend to compensate for their poor footwork and timing by snapping the wrist to come around on the ball. This places a great deal of stress on the relatively delicate common extensor tendon, located on the outside of the elbow, and on the extensor carpi radialis brevis muscle, which helps control the wrist. You can cause the same kind of stress by making aggressive twists with a screwdriver or other implement, or by lifting heavy objects with your elbow locked and your arm extended. Younger people with more supple joints can often get away with straining tissues in this way, but the muscles and tendons of people over 30 are more likely to suffer damage.

The damage consists of tiny tears in a part of the tendon and in muscle coverings. After the initial injury heals, these areas often tear again, which leads to hemorrhaging and the formation of rough, granulated tissue and calcium deposits within the surrounding tissues. Collagen, a protein, leaks out from around the injured areas, causing inflammation. The resulting pressure can cut off the blood flow and pinch the radial nerve, one of the major nerves controlling muscles in the arm and hand.

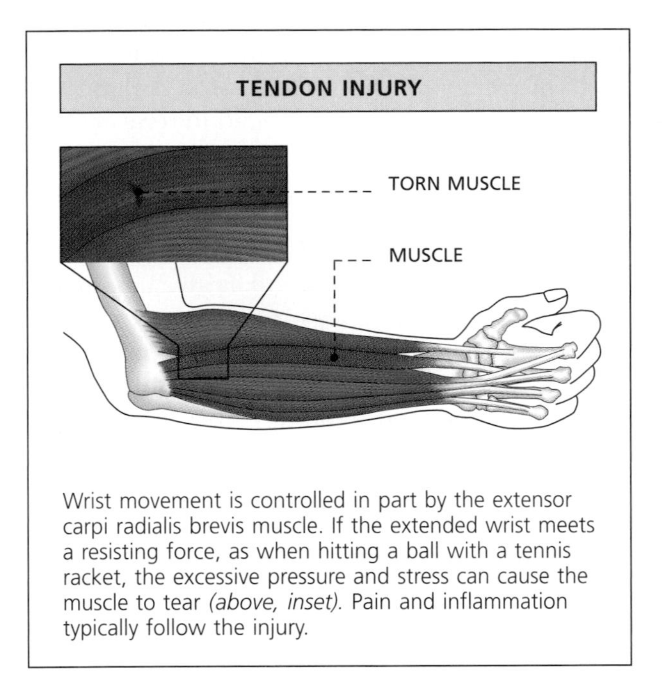


Wrist movement is controlled in part by the extensor carpi radialis brevis muscle. If the extended wrist meets a resisting force, as when hitting a ball with a tennis racket, the excessive pressure and stress can cause the muscle to tear *(above, inset)*. Pain and inflammation typically follow the injury.

Tendons, which attach muscles to bones, do not receive the same amount of oxygen and blood that muscles do, so they heal more slowly. In fact, some cases of tennis elbow can last for years, though the inflammation usually subsides in 6 to 12 weeks.

Many medical textbooks treat tennis elbow as a form of tendonitis, which is often the case, but if the muscles and bones of the elbow joint are also involved, then the condition is called epicondylitis. However, if you feel pain directly on the back of your elbow joint, rather than down the outside of your arm, you may have bursitis, which is caused when lubricating sacs in the joint become inflamed. If you see swelling, which is almost never a symptom of tennis elbow, you may want to investigate other possible conditions, such as arthritis, infection, gout, or a tumor.

## TREATMENT

The best way to relieve tennis elbow is to stop doing anything that irritates your arm—a simple step for the weekend tennis player, but not as easy for the manual laborer, office worker, or professional athlete.

The most effective conventional and alternative treatments for tennis elbow have the same basic premise: Rest the arm until the pain disappears, then massage to relieve stress and tension in the muscles, and exercise to strengthen the area and prevent reinjury. If you must go back to whatever caused the problem in the first place, be sure to warm up your arm for at least 5 to 10 minutes with gentle stretching and movement before starting any activity. Take frequent breaks.

### CONVENTIONAL MEDICINE

Conventional medicine offers an assortment of treatments for tennis elbow, from drug injections to surgery, but the pain will never go away completely unless you stop stressing the joint. Reinjury is inevitable without adequate rest.

For most mild to moderate cases of tennis elbow, aspirin or ibuprofen will help address the inflammation and the pain while you are resting the injury, and then you can follow up with exercise and massage to speed healing.

In some patients the body tries to defend the elbow from further damage by contracting the biceps, which then makes it difficult to extend the arm; the entire area can become quite tight. Gentle massage and careful stretching two to four times a week for several weeks will help offset this problem.

For stubborn cases of tennis elbow your doctor may advise corticosteroid injections, which dramatically reduce inflammation, but they cannot be used long-term because of potentially damaging side effects.

If rest, anti-inflammatory medications, and a stretching routine fail to cure your tennis elbow, you may have to consider surgery, though this form of treatment is rare (fewer than 3 percent of patients). One procedure is for the tendon to be cut loose from the epicondyle, the rounded bump at the end of the bone, which eliminates stress on the tendon but renders the muscle useless. Another surgical technique involves removing so-called granulated tissue in the tendon and repairing tears.

Even after you feel you have overcome a case of tennis elbow, be sure to continue babying your

### SHOULD YOU STRAP IT?

*Many doctors suggest using a strap or band just below the elbow to support the muscles in the area and take stress off tendons, but research has shown that these devices can reduce circulation and actually impede recovery if used for a prolonged period. Sustained pressure on the inflamed arm may also lead to fibrosis, in which excess connective tissue forms, almost like scar tissue; the resulting trauma can impair circulation and result in a permanent weakening of your arm.*

arm. Always warm up your arm for 5 to 10 minutes before starting any activity involving your elbow. And if you develop severe pain after use anyway, pack your arm in ice for 15 to 20 minutes and call your doctor.

## ALTERNATIVE CHOICES

Tennis elbow responds well to a variety of alternative therapies. Some you will be able to try on your own, but you should also consider professional help from a **chiropractor, osteopath,** or a practitioner of traditional **Chinese medicine.**

### ACUPRESSURE

Deep thumb pressure on Large Intestine 11, located on the inside of the elbow, may help relieve pain. See pages 22–23 for more information on locating this point.

### ACUPUNCTURE

Acupuncture has an estimated 60 to 70 percent success rate when used on tennis elbow patients—a record that has helped it gain acceptance even in more conservative medical circles. There are a number of acupuncture points that might prove beneficial, so be sure to seek out an acupuncturist who is experienced in treating this or similar types of conditions.

### BODY WORK

To prevent recurring bouts of tennis elbow, you need to improve your overall body alignment; proper posture and balance may do more for an ailing joint than drug therapies. Consider seeing a body work specialist or an **osteopath** about techniques such as **Rolfing,** the **Feldenkrais method,** and the **Alexander technique**.

### CHIROPRACTIC

Chiropractors, physical therapists, and occupational therapists all commonly use diathermy (a form of electrical stimulation), ultrasound, and **massage** to treat tennis elbow. Electrical and sound currents improve circulation and drainage, which then makes it easier to stretch and massage the affected area. Occasionally, chiropractors and therapists prescribe a splint or band to take stress off the affected tendon or muscle, but be aware that a poor fit or wearing the splint or band for too long can reduce blood flow.

### HERBAL THERAPIES

To help relax a tender arm, massage the affected area with oil of lavender *(Lavandula officinalis)* or eucalyptus *(Eucalyptus globulus)*. Cayenne *(Capsicum frutescens),* which is available in ointment form in most drugstores, as well as prickly ash *(Zanthoxylum americanum)* oil are believed to increase blood flow and speed healing.

### HYDROTHERAPY

If you suffer from recurrent bouts of tennis elbow, consider soaking your arm in warm water for 30 minutes before exercising. Always place the affected joint in ice after a workout.

### MIND/BODY MEDICINE

Several studies have demonstrated that **hypnotherapy** may provide effective relief for pain associated with tennis elbow. Consult an experienced practitioner.

### OSTEOPATHY

A relatively simple osteopathic treatment known as the counterstrain technique can be done at home. Get someone to rotate your arm in a direction opposite from the one that causes you pain, hold it in that position for 90 seconds, and then release it. Repeat several times a day. This exercise is especially helpful for mild to moderate, but not chronic, forms of tennis elbow. You can also consult an osteopath for more specific guidance on this technique.

### AT-HOME REMEDIES

- Take ibuprofen or aspirin, or massage eucalyptus or lavender oil into the joint.
- Keep your arm elevated when possible, to reduce inflammation.
- Alternate hot and cold compresses or apply cayenne or prickly ash to the affected area to increase circulation and speed healing.
- Ask a partner to massage the most painful part of your elbow with the convex side of a spoon; be sure that application is aggressive. This treatment hurts tremendously at first but eventually dulls the nerve endings (and thus the pain) and reduces inflammation.

**CAUTION!**

**PROPER TENNIS TECHNIQUE**

**If you have contracted tennis elbow because you play tennis, consider watching the pros. They almost always correct their position relative to the ball by moving their feet rather than altering their arm motion. Most pros have their racket back before the ball clears the net; the weekend hacker usually does not get into the swing until after the ball has bounced after crossing the net. Avoid the temptation to make up for the lost time by twisting your wrist to bring the racket around to meet the ball, especially on your backhand. Otherwise, chances are good that you'll be using an ice pack for the pain and seeing your doctor soon.**

## PREVENTION

**To prevent tennis elbow:**

- Lift objects with your palm facing your body.
- Try strengthening exercises with hand weights. With your elbow cocked and your palm down, repeatedly bend your wrist. Stop if you feel any pain.
- Stretch relevant muscles before beginning a possibly stressful activity by grasping the top part of your fingers and gently but firmly pulling them back toward your body. Keep your arm fully extended and your palm facing outward.

**To prevent a relapse:**

- Discontinue or modify the action that is causing the strain on your elbow joint. If you must continue, be sure to warm up for 10 minutes or more before any activity involving your arm, and apply ice to it afterward. Take more frequent breaks.
- Try strapping a band around your forearm just below your elbow. If the support seems to help you lift objects such as heavy books, then continue with it. Be aware that such bands can cut off circulation and impede healing, so they are best used once tennis elbow has disappeared. ■

# TESTICLE PROBLEMS

*Read down this column to find your symptoms. Then read across.*

| SYMPTOMS | AILMENT/PROBLEM |
|---|---|
| ◆ pain that gradually increases, tenderness, and swelling behind the testicle, sometimes with painful urination. | ◆ Epididymitis—inflammation of the epididymis, the structure where sperm mature and move from the testicles to the penis |
| ◆ sudden, acute pain and swelling in either testicle; no fever or painful urination, but sometimes nausea and vomiting; often follows strenuous physical exertion, but is usually not related to an injury. | ◆ Testicular torsion—twisting of the spermatic cord |
| ◆ swollen vein or veins in the scrotum, almost always on the left side; usually little or no pain; swelling subsides after lying down. | ◆ Varicocele—varicose veins in the scrotum |
| ◆ pain, swelling, or discoloration after a fall or a blow to the testicles; sometimes accompanied by nausea and vomiting. | ◆ Testicular trauma—a blow or other injury to the testicles |
| ◆ a lump in a testicle that may or may not be painful; when there is pain, it is often worse when lying down. | ◆ Possibly a sign of testicular cancer |
| ◆ impotence; absence of sexual desire; infertility; failure to reach puberty by age 15. | ◆ Hypogonadism—failure of the testicles to produce adequate amounts of the male hormone testosterone |
| ◆ general pain in the scrotum without an obvious cause. | ◆ So-called referred pain from elsewhere in the body |

| WHAT TO DO | OTHER INFO |
|---|---|
| ◆ See your doctor, who may prescribe bed rest, anti-inflammatory medicine, or—if you have a bacterial infection—antibiotics. | ◆ May accompany infection of the prostate or urethra, or may follow heavy lifting or prolonged sitting; usually occurs between ages 20 and 40. |
| ◆ **Get medical help immediately.** A twisted spermatic cord reduces blood supply to the testicles and can cause permanent damage. | ◆ This is a medical emergency, most common in adolescents, often preceded by less severe but similar painful episodes. The spermatic cord must be untwisted by a physician, and surgery may be required to prevent recurrence. |
| ◆ If you have associated pain, see your doctor for an examination. | ◆ Some pain may occur after physical exertion or prolonged standing. About 15 percent of adult men have varicocele, which is a common cause of infertility. |
| ◆ See your doctor. A blood-filled swelling may indicate a ruptured testicle or other injury that should be surgically explored and repaired. | ◆ A ruptured testicle can be diagnosed by ultrasound. If there is no rupture, the cause may be a leaking blood vessel. Sitz baths and bed rest with the scrotum elevated may stop internal bleeding. |
| ◆ See Testicular Cancer. | ◆ Testicular cancer occurs primarily in men under the age of 35. Some kinds of the disease progress extremely rapidly. Treatment depends on the type of tumor. When treatment is begun promptly, prognosis is usually excellent. |
| ◆ See your doctor for hormone testing and sperm count. Hypogonadism is sometimes treated by hormone replacement. | ◆ Infertility may have a genetic cause. Loss of virility after puberty may be caused by drug abuse, damage from radiation therapy or chemical poisoning, or other injury. |
| ◆ See your doctor. Treatment depends on locating the actual source of pain, which may be far from the scrotum. Referred pain is often hard to pinpoint since sensitivity to pain varies from person to person. *(See Pain, Chronic.)* | ◆ Pain may be transmitted to the scrotum from disorders of the colon, kidneys, or other organs. |

# TESTICULAR CANCER

## SYMPTOMS

The earliest warning signs of testicular cancer usually include:

- a change in size or shape of a testicle.
- swelling or thickening of the testicles.
- a firm, smooth, initially painless, slow-growing lump in a testicle.
- a feeling of testicular heaviness.

Other symptoms of testicular cancer may include:

- urinary problems.
- an abdominal mass or abdominal pain.
- persistent coughing, possibly with blood-tinged sputum.
- shortness of breath.
- loss of weight or appetite; fatigue; lower-back pain; tenderness in the nipples or breast enlargement.
- very rarely, infertility.

## CALL YOUR DOCTOR IF:

- you detect any sort of unusual lump or swelling in the scrotum. You should have a thorough physical examination as soon as possible, on the off chance that the abnormality is caused by cancer.

The two testicles, or testes, are glands that produce male hormones and sperm. They hang beneath and behind a man's penis in a pouch called the scrotum. The spermatic cord, composed of the sperm duct, nerves, and blood vessels, connects each testicle to the body. Although testicular cancer is rare, it is the most common type of cancer in men between the ages of 15 and 35. It is much more common in Caucasians than in African Americans and usually is diagnosed when a man is in his mid-thirties.

Almost all testicular cancers are primary—beginning in the testicles themselves. A rare type of testicular cancer arises in the chest or abdomen in traces of embryonic tissue from which the testicles developed in the fetus. Testicular cancer may spread slowly or rapidly, depending on its type, but the path is consistent: Once a malignant tumor penetrates the spermatic cord, cancer cells are free to infiltrate nearby lymph or blood vessels, and they may be carried to abdominal lymph nodes, then to the lungs, then usually to the liver, bones, and possibly the brain.

Thanks to advances in diagnosis and treatment, testicular cancer is among the most curable of cancers, even when advanced, and it is rarely fatal. About 85 percent of patients are diagnosed with localized malignancies that are highly treatable. Improved detection and treatment techniques have raised the overall five-year survival rate above 90 percent. Even if cancer has spread to nearby organs at diagnosis, patients have an excellent chance of surviving at least five years.

## CAUSES

What causes testicular cancer is unknown. Ten percent of testicular cancers occur in men born with an undescended testicle, and many cases of father-son incidence have been reported. Men with fertility problems are more likely to develop benign testicular tumors and may be slightly more prone to testicular cancer. Some research suggests that having a vasectomy increases risk, but other studies do not support this conclusion *(see Testicle Problems).* Other suspected but unproven risk factors include a sedentary lifestyle,

T

early puberty, previous mumps, testicular injury, overexposure to pesticides or radiation, and prenatal conditions related to a mother who was bleeding abnormally, taking estrogen, or taking diethylstilbestrol (DES) during pregnancy. DES was once given to pregnant women to prevent miscarriage but is no longer marketed in the U.S.

### DIAGNOSTIC AND TEST PROCEDURES

Every man should have his doctor explain the steps of testicle self-examination, a simple yet important procedure. He should then physically examine his testicles once a month for signs of abnormality. Any painless lump or swelling in the scrotum may signal cancer. To rule out other possibilities, a doctor may prescribe a course of antibiotics to see if the mass disappears. If it doesn't, ultrasound imaging and chemical analyses of urine and blood are performed. If cancer is suspected, the testicle is surgically removed and a biopsy is performed to determine the presence and type of testicular cancer. If cancer is diagnosed, other tests will determine whether it has spread. Removal of the second testicle is not standard practice because in most cases it remains cancer free. Removing one testicle usually does not cause infertility, but because further treatment may, patients are advised about sperm banking before treatment proceeds.

**WARNING SIGNS**

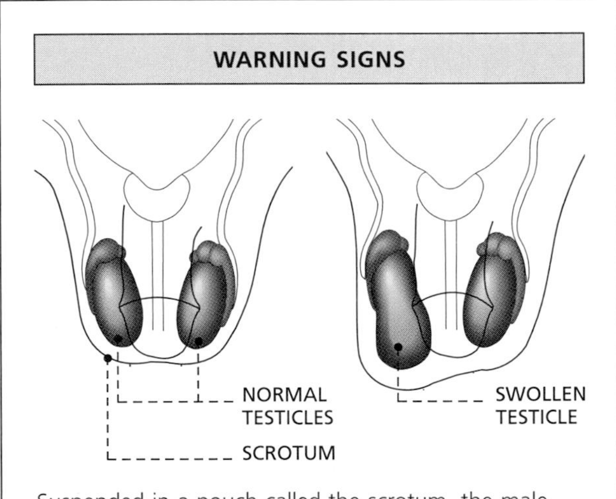


Suspended in a pouch called the scrotum, the male sex glands, or testicles, produce sperm and male hormones. Testicular cancer usually affects only one testicle, typically beginning in the cells that manufacture sperm. Periodic self-examination may detect hard lumps, swelling, or a change in the size or shape of the testicle *(above, right)*—all potential indicators of early testicular cancer.

## TREATMENT

### CONVENTIONAL MEDICINE

Because it is required for diagnosis, surgical removal of a testicle is unavoidable. If cancer is found, a second operation to remove nearby abdominal lymph nodes usually is performed, and these two operations are often enough to cure limited testicular cancer. In addition to surgery, advanced cases are treated with chemotherapy and sometimes radiation. Nearly all testicular cancer patients achieve remission, but they are urged to have frequent follow-up examinations. If cancer recurs, additional treatment frequently produces another remission. If testicular cancer is not cured by conventional chemotherapy, doctors may advise a bone-marrow transplant to allow higher-dose chemotherapy. *(See Lymphoma.)*

See Cancer for more information on treatments such as chemotherapy and radiation.

### COMPLEMENTARY THERAPIES

Although conventional medicine is remarkably successful at curing testicular cancer, simply learning that you have cancer can cause severe emotional distress. Many patients find psychological counseling or support-group therapy helpful in dealing with the emotional consequences.

## PREVENTION

Some studies indicate that young men who exercise regularly are less likely to develop testicular cancer. Other research suggests that correcting an undescended testicle surgically before a boy turns 10 minimizes cancer risk. Most important, however, is regular testicle self-examination. ■

# TETANUS

## SYMPTOMS

You should suspect tetanus if a cut or other wound is followed by one or more of these symptoms:

- stiffness of the neck, jaw, and other muscles, often accompanied by a grotesque, grinning expression.
- irritability.
- uncontrollable spasms of the jaw and neck muscles.
- painful, involuntary contraction of other muscles.

In addition, you may notice restlessness, lack of appetite, and drooling.

## CALL YOUR DOCTOR IF:

- you are bitten by an animal or wounded by an object that might be contaminated with dirt, feces, or dust, and you have not been immunized against tetanus or received a booster within the last 10 years. Tetanus infection can be fatal and should be treated as soon as possible.

Tetanus is a dangerous nerve ailment caused by the toxin of a common bacterium, *Clostridium tetani*. Bacterial spores are found in soil—most frequently in cultivated soil, least frequently in virgin soil. They also exist in environments as diverse as animal excrement, house dust, operating rooms, contaminated heroin, and the human colon. If the spores enter a wound that penetrates the skin and extends deeper than oxygen can reach, they germinate and produce a toxin that enters the bloodstream.

This toxin, tetanospasmin, ranks with botulism toxin as the most potent known microbial poison. It is taken up from the blood by the outermost nerves and moves inward toward the spine at a rate of about 10 inches a day. After 7 to 21 days, it begins to short-circuit nerve signals and block the relaxation of muscles. This results in sustained muscle contractions, notably the lockjaw for which tetanus is nicknamed.

Spasms of the jaw or facial muscles may follow, spreading to the hands, arms, legs, and back and blocking the ability to breathe. Spasms are often precipitated by noise or touch. Once tetanus has spread, the mortality rate is approximately 40 percent, even in modern medical facilities.

An estimated one million infants die of tetanus in developing countries each year because of poor hygiene. Since childhood immunization laws were passed in the United States in the 1970s, only about 50 cases a year are reported in this country; about three-quarters are elderly people or people who have never been immunized.

## CAUSES

Bacterial spores enter the body by way of animal bites, surgical wounds, needle injection sites, burns, ulcers, and infected umbilical cords—and by the proverbial rusty nail. Be particularly suspicious of any wound caused by a dirty or dusty object that has been outdoors or in contact with soil.

### DIAGNOSTIC AND TEST PROCEDURES

Some affected people may experience only pain and tingling at the wound site and some spasms in nearby muscles, but most suffer stiff jaw and neck muscles, irritability, and difficulty swallowing. If muscle spasms develop early, chances of recovery are poor.

It is seldom possible to find either the bacterium or the toxin in a suspected tetanus patient, so diagnosis can be made only on the basis of clinical observations combined with the absence of a history of tetanus immunization.

## TREATMENT

If tetanus does develop, seek hospital treatment immediately. This includes a course of antibiotics and an injection of tetanus antitoxin. You may receive an antianxiety drug such as chlorpromazine or diazepam to control muscle spasms, or a short-acting barbiturate for sedation. You may require the aid of an artificial respirator or other life-support measures during the several weeks needed for the disease to run its course.

## PREVENTION

Tetanus occurs almost exclusively in people who have not been immunized or whose immunization is not adequate. The fact that you are contaminated with tetanus spores by an animal bite or a wound from a dirty object does not mean, however, that you will necessarily contract a tetanus infection. Much depends on how deep the wound is and how well it is cleaned. The toxin-producing bacteria can thrive only when they are protected from the air by a layer of skin or tissue. Because these bacteria do not flourish in oxygen, it is common practice, when possible, to leave a wound open, without stitches and with only a light gauze dressing, so that the entire area is exposed to air.

Most cases of tetanus develop in people who think their wounds are too small to bother with. *(See Cuts, Scratches, and Wounds.)* Even a puncture that barely bleeds can be dangerous; because they are deep, punctures provide a favorable environment for bacteria. Wash the wound thoroughly with soap and a strong stream of water, apply antiseptic solution, and bandage with a sterile gauze pad. Do not tape the wound closed and do not apply antibiotic ointment, both of which keep air from circulating.

If your wound was caused by an object that may have been in contact with soil, especially if the wound has dead, crushed, or infected tissue, see your doctor quickly—within 24 hours, if possible. He will finish cleaning the wound and cutting away any damaged tissue, a procedure known as debridement.

If you haven't had a tetanus booster shot in the last five years, your doctor will probably give you one. If you've never been immunized, your doctor will quickly give you a shot of human tetanus immunoglobulin, which brings immediate protection that lasts a few weeks. Neither the immunoglobulin shot nor the booster will bring enduring immunity, however, so you will still need the full course of immunization shots if you did not receive them in childhood.

Health officials recommend immunization of infants and children with DPT—diphtheria, pertussis (whooping cough), and tetanus—vaccine at the ages of 2 months, 4 months, 6 months, 15 months, and about 5 years. After that, most health experts recommend a tetanus booster every 10 years.

If family members have not been immunized against tetanus, encourage them to have it done. Keep a record of tetanus shots, since booster shots given too frequently may cause allergic reactions.

There is evidence that tetanus immunization remains highly effective for much longer than 10 years. Some experts have suggested that a booster in high school and a second booster at the age of 60 provide adequate protection for life.

The most important preventive measure you can take against tetanus, however, is to acquire the initial immunization series. Any adults who have not done so should see their doctor or health department. ■

# THROAT CANCER

## SYMPTOMS

Initially throat cancer causes no symptoms. The earliest warning signs are likely to resemble symptoms of a chest cold. Symptoms caused by a tumor in the upper or lower throat may include:

- nagging cough, hoarseness, or a mild but persistent sore throat.
- difficulty or pain on swallowing.
- traces of blood in sputum.
- ear pain.
- swollen lymph nodes in the neck.

Additional symptoms that may be caused by a tumor in the region directly behind the nose may include:

- partial hearing loss.
- nasal obstruction or nosebleeds.
- ringing in the ears, or tinnitus.
- symptoms of otitis media, such as pain or pressure in the middle ear.

## CALL YOUR DOCTOR IF:

- symptoms resembling those of an upper-respiratory infection, such as a chest cold, persist for more than two weeks.
- you become suddenly or chronically hoarse for no apparent reason.
- you are a smoker and already have a raspy voice, and you notice another change in your voice.
- lymph nodes in your neck appear swollen.

While any of these symptoms may have other causes, you should have a thorough examination by a nose and throat specialist to get a proper diagnosis.

T

The throat, or pharynx, is a hollow tube through which food and liquids pass from the mouth to the stomach, and through which air travels to and from the lungs. The throat is divided into three distinct sections: the nasopharynx, located directly behind the nose; the oropharynx, directly behind the mouth and including the tonsils; and the hypopharynx, or lower throat *(illustration, right).*

Most primary throat cancers originate from cells that cover the mucous membrane lining the throat. As the cancer grows, it tends to penetrate through the mucous membrane and muscle layers to surrounding tissues. From there the cancer can spread to lymph nodes in the neck, then to the lungs and other organs. A growing tumor may interfere with hearing, smell, taste, speech, or swallowing. Cancers of the nasopharynx and lower throat often spread early, before they cause obvious symptoms. Cancers of the oropharynx tend to stay localized but eventually will spread unless treated successfully.

Throat cancer is seen about three times more often in men than in women and usually does not occur before age 50. Five-year survival rates range from 50 to 90 percent when throat cancer is diagnosed early, and from 5 to 25 percent for cancer that has spread elsewhere in the body.

## CAUSES

Smoking or chewing tobacco and heavy drinking of alcohol cause most cancers of the oropharynx and hypopharynx. Smokers are six times more likely than nonsmokers to develop cancer of these areas, and nearly all people diagnosed with throat cancer are—or once were—smokers. In contrast, the major known risk factor for cancer of the nasopharynx is infection by the Epstein-Barr (E-B) virus, a type of herpesvirus more common in Africa than the U.S.

Inhaling coal or other mineral dust, asbestos, and diesel fumes may increase risk for throat cancer. Poor oral hygiene and regular consumption of salted meats may also contribute. In some cases, throat cancer develops from abnormal tissue growths *(see Oral Cancer).*

POSSIBLE SITES FOR THROAT CANCER

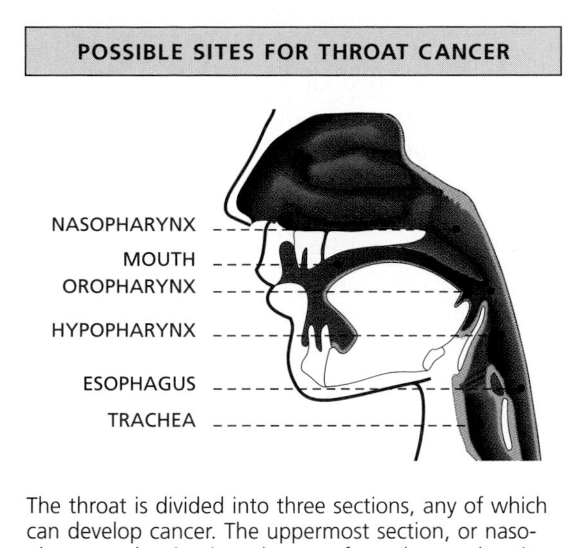


The throat is divided into three sections, any of which can develop cancer. The uppermost section, or nasopharynx, takes in air and mucus from the nasal cavity. Below it lies the oropharynx, a passageway for food and air, and the part of the throat that's visible when you say "aaah." The hypopharynx, or lower throat, delivers food to the esophagus and air to the trachea.

### DIAGNOSTIC AND TEST PROCEDURES

You or your physician may be able to see abnormal growths in your oropharynx but not in the nasopharynx or the hypopharynx, which must be examined with mirrors or a fiberoptic scope. Any suspicious lesion, tumor, or swollen lymph node should be biopsied, or a test for the E-B virus should be made. If cancer is detected, imaging scans can help establish how widespread the disease has become.

## TREATMENT

Provided throat cancer has not spread beyond lymph nodes by the time of diagnosis, treatment removes all traces of the disease, remission is obtained, and in at least half of all cases, the cancer is cured. But treatment for throat cancer is typically risky and complex; depending on a tumor's location and stage of development, doctors must consider the impact of treatment on the patient's speech and other essential functions.

### CONVENTIONAL MEDICINE

Specific treatment for throat cancer depends first on the tumor's location. Patients with cancer of the nasopharynx typically receive high-dose radiation to the head and neck, perhaps following chemotherapy to shrink tumors. This treatment cures more than 80 percent of early cancers and more than half of moderately advanced cases.

Small tumors of the oropharynx usually are treated with radiation in order to avoid disfigurement and other complications. If the cancer does not respond adequately or is too advanced, surgery is indicated, sometimes preceded by chemotherapy or followed by radiation.

Although small tumors of the hypopharynx may be treated with radiation alone, most localized hypopharyngeal cancers require surgery, possibly preceded by chemotherapy or followed by radiation. The cancerous portion of the throat is removed, followed by reconstructive surgery. After throat surgery, many patients need physical therapy to help regain the ability to speak, swallow, and chew. Radiation may be used to relieve symptoms and slow the progress of advanced cancers that cannot be treated surgically.

### AT-HOME CARE

If radiation treatment to the head and neck causes mouth discomfort and a sore and scratchy throat, try the following:

- ◆ Ask your oncologist about appropriate medications and advice on how to ease side effects.
- ◆ Eat soft or semiliquid foods and drink liquids throughout the day to keep your mouth and throat moist.
- ◆ Ask your dentist about proper mouth care during and after treatment. *(See Oral Cancer.)*

## PREVENTION

If you smoke or chew tobacco, stop. If you have a tendency to abuse alcohol, get counseling or medical help to bring the problem under control. ■

# THYROID PROBLEMS

## SYMPTOMS

**Hyperthyroidism:**
- weight loss despite increased appetite.
- increased heart rate, higher blood pressure, and increased nervousness, with excessive perspiration.
- more frequent bowel movements, sometimes with diarrhea.
- muscle weakness, trembling hands.
- development of a goiter.

**Hypothyroidism:**
- lethargy, slower mental processes.
- reduced heart rate.
- increased sensitivity to cold.
- tingling or numbness in the hands.
- development of a goiter.

**Subacute thyroiditis:**
- mild to severe pain in the thyroid gland.
- the thyroid feels tender to the touch.
- pain when swallowing or turning your head.
- appearance of these symptoms shortly after a viral infection, such as the flu, mumps, or measles.

## CALL YOUR DOCTOR IF:

- you are feverish, agitated, or delirious, and have a rapid pulse; you could be having a thyrotoxic crisis, a sudden and dangerous complication of **hyperthyroidism.**
- you feel intensely cold, drowsy, and lethargic; you could be experiencing a myxedema coma, a sudden and dangerous complication of **hypothyroidism** that can cause unconsciousness and possibly death.

Through the hormones it produces, the thyroid gland influences almost all of the metabolic processes in your body. Thyroid disorders can range from a small, harmless goiter that needs no treatment to life-threatening cancer. The most common thyroid problems involve irregular production of thyroid hormones. Too much of these vital body chemicals results in a condition known as **hyperthyroidism.** Insufficient hormone production leads to **hypothyroidism.**

The four parathyroid glands, located at the four axes of the thyroid gland, function independent of the larger gland and are responsible for regulating blood levels of calcium, necessary for the growth and maintenance of bones and teeth. Imbalances in their hormone secretion can result in hyperparathyroidism or hypoparathyroidism, which in turn can adversely affect bone development. Although the effects can be unpleasant or uncomfortable, most thyroid problems are not serious if properly diagnosed and treated.

## CAUSES

All types of **hyperthyroidism** are due to an overproduction of thyroid hormones, and the condition can occur in several ways: In Graves' disease, the release of excess hormones is triggered by an autoimmune disorder *(see Immune Problems).* At other times, nodules called toxic adenomas develop in the thyroid gland and begin to secrete thyroid hormones, altering the normal flow and upsetting the body's chemical balance; certain goiters may contain several of these nodules. In **subacute thyroiditis,** inflammation of the thyroid causes the gland to "leak" excess hormones, resulting in temporary hyperthyroidism. Although rare, hyperthyroidism can also develop from pituitary gland malfunctions or from cancerous growths in the thyroid gland.

**Hypothyroidism,** by contrast, stems from an underproduction of thyroid hormones. Since your body's energy production requires certain amounts of thyroid hormones, a drop in hormone production leads to lower energy production. A common cause of hypothyroidism is Hashimoto's thyroiditis, an autoimmune disorder in which white blood cells gradually replace thyroid tissue, which then comes under attack by immune-system proteins called antibodies. Hypothyroidism can also result when the thyroid gland has been surgically removed or chemically destroyed as treatment for hyperthyroidism. And if you are exposed to excessive amounts of iodide—perhaps from a hidden source such as cold and sinus medicines, or from certain medical tests—you may be at greater risk for developing hypothyroidism, especially if you have had thyroid problems in the past. Untreated for long periods of time, hypothyroidism can bring on a myxedema coma, a rare but potentially fatal condition that requires immediate hormone injections.

Hypothyroidism poses a special danger to newborns and infants, as a lack of thyroid hormones in the system at an early age can lead to the development of cretinism (mental retardation) and dwarfism (stunted growth). Most infants now have their thyroid levels checked routinely soon after birth; if they are hypothyroid, treatment begins immediately. In infants, as in adults, hypothyroidism can be due to a pituitary disorder, a defective thyroid, or lack of the gland entirely. A hypothyroid infant is unusually inactive and quiet, has a poor appetite, and sleeps for excessively long periods of time.

Although cancer of the thyroid gland is the most common endocrine malignancy other than ovarian cancer, it is still quite rare. You might have one or more thyroid nodules for several years before they are determined to be cancerous. People who have received radiation treatment to the head and neck earlier in life, possibly as a remedy for acne, tend to have a higher-than-normal susceptibility to thyroid cancer.

## DIAGNOSTIC AND TEST PROCEDURES

A doctor can diagnose **hyperthyroidism** and **hypothyroidism** by looking at the levels of certain hormones in your blood. Doctors usually take readings of hormones secreted by the thyroid itself, and also of thyroid-stimulating hormone (TSH), a chemical released by the pituitary gland to trigger hormone production in the thyroid.

When you are **hypothyroid,** higher quantities of TSH are circulating in your blood as your body attempts to foster increased production of thyroid hormones; the reverse is true with hyperthyroidism, in which TSH levels are below normal and circulating thyroid-hormone levels are high.

To determine the cause of **hyperthyroidism,** doctors often use radioactive iodide uptake tests, which track the amount of iodide absorbed by the thyroid gland during a set time period. Iodide is a key ingredient in the manufacture of thyroid hormone, so the amount of iodide the thyroid absorbs is a reliable indicator of how much hormone the gland is producing. For this test, you must swallow a small amount of radioactive iodide in liquid or capsule form. After a predetermined wait, the doctor places an instrument over your neck to measure how much of the radioactive iodide has gathered in your thyroid.

If the results of this test suggest that the gland is collecting excessive amounts of iodide, the doctor may then conduct a radioactive iodide uptake scan. In this test, the physician uses a special film to create a picture that shows the exact location of the radioactive iodide in your thyroid gland. The scan will reveal, for example, if the iodide is collecting in adenomas, indicating that the nodules are responsible for the excess hormone. If the scan shows that the iodide is spread equally throughout the tissue, the whole thyroid is involved in the excess production.

Some practitioners believe that blood tests may not be sensitive enough to detect milder forms of **hypothyroidism.** Instead, they advocate monitoring your body's basal (resting) temperature. To track your basal temperature accurately, you must closely follow certain guidelines: Shake the thermometer below 95°F at night and place it where you can reach it without getting out of bed. The following morning, before you get out of bed, take your temperature via your armpit for 10 minutes while staying as still as possible. Keep records of your temperature for at least three days. (Women should do this during the first two weeks of the menstrual cycle, as their basal temperature may rise during the latter half.) Normal body basal temperatures fall between 97.4°F and 97.8°F. If your basal temperature is consistently low, you could be mildly hypothyroid.

If you have one or more adenomas, your practitioner will want to keep careful records of when they were first found and how they develop, since not all adenomas produce excess thyroid hormone. In fact, most of these nodules are not malignant, especially if they remain the same size over long intervals. (Cancerous tissue, by contrast, will undergo noticeable growth.) Nodules that appear suddenly are typically fluid-filled cysts and are often benign. If blood tests indicate that the nodules are producing excess thyroid hormone, and if you have other symptoms, your practitioner will treat you for **hyperthyroidism.**

In any case, you should receive periodic checkups if you have a nodule on your thyroid gland, since you may become hyperthyroid in the future. If your blood tests show elevated hormone levels, your doctor may recommend other tests, including radioactive iodide uptake tests and scans that indicate whether the nodules are "hot" or "cold." Hot nodules, or those that are actively trapping iodide, are rarely cancerous. But cold nodules—those showing low iodide concentrations—indicate a possible malignancy and need to be investigated further.

One type of thyroid cancer can be diagnosed through a simple blood test that measures levels of a hormone involved in bone formation. In most cases, however, doctors check for thyroid cancer by performing a biopsy, which involves drawing cells from the suspect nodule with a fine needle to determine if the tissue is malignant.

## TREATMENT

For thyroid disorders stemming from the over- or underproduction of thyroid hormones, both conventional and alternative treatments offer varied methods to restore hormone levels to their proper balance. Conventional treatments rely mainly on drug therapy and surgery. Alternative treatments attempt to relieve some of the discomfort associated with thyroid conditions, or to improve the function of the thyroid gland through a variety of approaches ranging from diet supplements and herbal remedies to lifestyle changes and special exercises. You should always receive a professional evaluation for any thyroid disorder; most of these conditions require a course of treatment beyond the scope of home care alone.

### CONVENTIONAL MEDICINE

Treating **hyperthyroidism** requires suppressing the manufacture of thyroid hormone, while **hypothyroidism** demands hormone replacement. Conventional medicine offers extremely effective techniques for lowering, eliminating, or supplementing hormone production. Before deciding which therapy is best for you, your doctor will make an evaluation based on your particular thyroid condition as well as your age, general health, and medical history.

Thyroid hormone production can be suppressed or halted completely with a radioactive iodide treatment, antithyroid medication, or surgery. If your doctor decides that radioactive treatment is best, you will be asked to swallow a tablet or liquid containing radioactive iodide in amounts large enough to damage the cells of your thyroid gland and limit or destroy their ability to produce hormones. Occasionally more than one treatment is needed to restore normal hormone production, and many patients actually develop hypothyroidism as a result of this procedure.

If you start using antithyroid medications such as propylthiouracil or methimazole, which are usually administered in tablet form, your hyperthyroid symptoms should begin to disappear in about six to eight weeks, as hormones already in your system run out and the medication starts to impair the thyroid's hormone production. However, you will need to continue taking the medication for about a year. After that time, you will also need to receive periodic medical exams to make sure that the condition has not returned.

Surgery is often recommended for people under 45 when their hyperthyroidism is due to toxic adenomas, since these nodules tend to be resistant to radioactive iodide. Once the tissue is removed surgically, hormone levels typically return to normal within a few weeks.

Although **subacute thyroiditis** can bring on temporary hyperthyroidism, this condition usually does not require medical treatment, and any pain associated with the inflamed thyroid can generally be alleviated with acetaminophen or aspirin. If over-the-counter drugs don't help, a physician may prescribe prednisone or dexamethasone for a short period of time. Since both of these drugs may encourage the development of stomach ulcers and the loss of bone mass, however, ask your doctor if you should also be taking calcium supplements.

**Hypothyroidism** calls for a lifelong regimen of hormone replacement therapy. No surgical techniques or conventional drugs can increase the thyroid's hormone production once it slows down. Although hormones from animal extracts are available, doctors generally prescribe synthetic forms of thyroid hormone, such as levothyroxine. Side effects are rare, but some patients experience nervousness or chest pain while taking these drugs; usually, adjusting the levels of medication will alleviate any unpleasant effects. However, if you are also taking tricyclic antidepressants, anticoagulant drugs, or digitalis, or if you have diabetes, make sure that you and your practitioner discuss any possible interactions or other complications.

Thyroid cancer is usually treated by surgically removing either the cancerous tissue or the whole thyroid gland, a procedure known as a thyroidectomy. If the cancer has spread beyond the thyroid, any other affected tissue, such as the lymph glands in the neck, will also be removed.

## ALTERNATIVE CHOICES

Though the alternative choices available to you for thyroid problems will not completely suppress or replace thyroid hormones, they are often used to strengthen the thyroid itself or to alleviate some of the unpleasant symptoms.

### CHINESE HERBS

Several herbal mixtures may help relieve symptoms in cases of **hyperthyroidism:** baked licorice *(Glycyrrhiza uralensis)* combination, bupleurum *(Bupleurum chinense)* and dragon bone combination, or bupleurum and peony combination. See a practitioner for guidance and supplies.

### HERBAL THERAPIES

For relief from the symptoms of **hyperthyroidism,** try 4 parts bugleweed (*Lycopus* spp.), 2 parts motherwort *(Leonurus cardiaca),* 2 parts skullcap (*Scutellaria* spp.), and 1 part hawthorn (*Crataegus* spp.) in a tincture three times a day.

For insomnia due to **hyperthyroidism,** combine equal parts of valerian *(Valeriana officinalis)* and passionflower *(Passiflora incarnata)* in a tincture and take half an hour before bedtime.

In the case of **hypothyroidism,** you can prepare a tea made from bladder wrack *(Fucus vesiculosus)* to improve thyroid function. Three times daily, pour 1 cup boiling water on 2 tsp bladder wrack and steep for 10 minutes before drinking. Bladder wrack can also be taken in capsule form three times daily.

### LIFESTYLE

Aerobic exercise for 15 to 20 minutes a day is excellent for maintaining good thyroid function. Regular physical activity is especially important if you are hypothyroid. (Check with your doctor before starting an exercise program.)

### NUTRITION AND DIET

For **hypothyroidism,** avoid cabbage, peaches, rutabagas, soybeans, spinach, peanuts, and radishes, as these foods can interfere with the manufacture of thyroid hormones. Supplements of vitamin C, vitamin E, riboflavin (vitamin $B_2$), zinc, niacin (vitamin $B_3$), pyridoxine (vitamin $B_6$), and tyrosine might help boost thyroid production. However, if you have **hyperthyroidism,** eating the foods listed above might help lower your body's production of thyroid hormone.

### YOGA

For many people, the Shoulder Stand position, at least once daily for 20 minutes, can help improve overall thyroid function. Lie on your back and lift your legs up so your hips are off the floor. Supporting your hips with your hands, extend your legs vertically. Slide your hands along your torso toward your shoulders, with your thumbs at the front of your body and fingers at the back. Make sure your body weight is supported by your shoulders, not your head and neck. ■

# TICS AND TWITCHES

## SYMPTOMS

- a brief, flicking sensation confined to a small part of the body, such as the eyelid; usually indicative of a harmless involuntary muscle contraction.
- a repetitive, uncontrollable, purposeless contraction of an individual muscle or group of muscles, typically in the face, arms, or shoulders; may be a sign that you have a tic related to a minor psychological disorder, a condition related to a brain disorder, or trigeminal neuralgia.
- intense, longer-lasting trembling or shaking of a body part or of the entire body; could be symptomatic of caffeine poisoning, alcohol withdrawal, an overactive thyroid gland *(see Thyroid Problems),* or Parkinson's disease.

## CALL YOUR DOCTOR IF:

- your condition consists of unexpected trembling movements that occur only when the affected body part is at rest; you need to be checked for the possibility of Parkinson's disease.
- your tic or twitch is persistent or recurs often; you may be having minor seizures, or you may have a neurological disorder or other condition of a serious nature.

Tics and twitches are defined as involuntary contractions of a muscle or group of muscles. They come in many forms and have a variety of causes—some trivial and some serious.

## CAUSES

Movements such as shoulder shrugging, mouth twitching, and erratic blinking may be signs of a minor psychological disturbance. They most often develop in children ages 7 to 14 as a result of anxiety, and usually stop within a year; some cases may persist into adulthood. The disorder occurs in up to 25 percent of children, and boys

### TOURETTE'S SYNDROME

*Tourette's syndrome is perhaps the best-known involuntary movement disorder. Named after Georges Gilles de la Tourette, the French neurologist who first described the condition in 1885, it usually starts in childhood and persists throughout life. It is a neurological abnormality of unknown cause and is up to four times more common in men.*

*Tourette's can be mild, with only minor involuntary twitches, or more severe and progressive. Symptoms may include continual grimacing, and violent jerking of the head and neck, as well as the arms and legs. As Tourette's progresses, involuntary noises such as grunts, coughing, and barking may occur; in 50 percent of cases, patients occasionally shout out expletives.*

*There is no cure for Tourette's, but some forms can be successfully managed. Antipsychotic drugs such as haloperidol may provide temporary relief from jerking and vocal outbursts.*

exhibit symptoms three times as often as girls.

Caffeine poisoning (which can result from drinking five or more cups of coffee within 12 hours) and alcohol withdrawal may also manifest themselves in involuntary movements, including trembling or shaking. *(See Alcohol Abuse.)*

Tics or twitches are sometimes caused by neurological disorders, in which case they are referred to as dyskinesia. *(See Parkinson's Disease.)* This condition may result from brain damage at birth, head trauma, or use of the antiemetic (vomit suppressant) drug metoclopramide, or drugs to treat psychiatric ailments. Dyskinesia includes muscle spasms, repetitive fidgets, jerking or writhing movements, or a combination of these symptoms.

Other medications, such as phenothiazines and central nervous system stimulants, can also cause temporary twitching, as can fatigue and stress. The condition can also be hereditary.

**ACUPRESSURE**

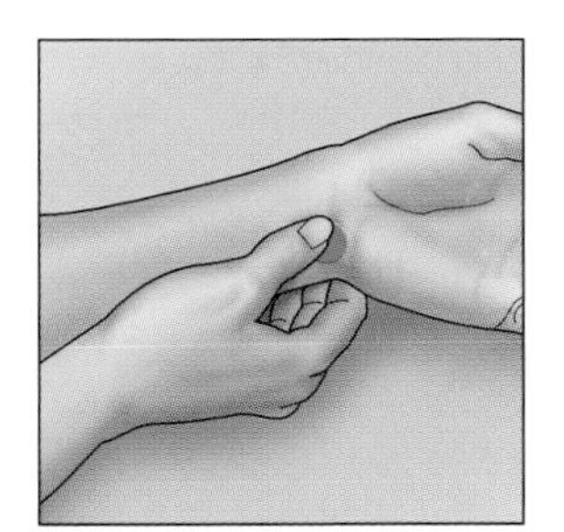

**1** Anxiety-induced sleeping problems may be improved by pressing Heart 7, located along the crease on the inside of the wrist, directly in line with the little finger. Squeeze firmly between thumb and index finger for one minute, then repeat on the other hand.

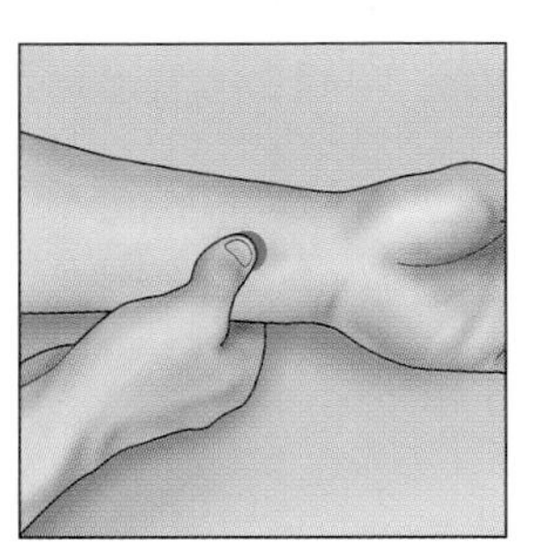

**2** To help calm nerves, press Pericardium 6. Place your thumb in the center of your inner wrist, two finger widths from the wrist crease and between the two bones of the forearm. Press firmly for one minute, three to five times, then repeat on the other arm.

# TREATMENT

## CONVENTIONAL MEDICINE

Tension-related tics or twitches usually disappear on their own, especially if you take steps to reduce stress. Dyskinesia caused by a particular drug may be treated by simply stopping use of the drug. When it is caused by other factors, effective treatment is harder to determine. Your physician will probably have to prescribe a series of drugs before an effective one is found.

If tics are severe and persistent and there is no clear physical cause, your doctor may prescribe antianxiety benzodiazepine drugs or antipsychotic drugs. You can tell whether caffeine may be responsible for your twitching or trembling by not drinking caffeinated beverages for several hours to see if your symptoms disappear. You may need to cut down on your caffeine intake.

## ALTERNATIVE CHOICES

Alternative remedies for various forms of tics and twitches may relieve discomfort as you wait out the symptoms of your disorder, or they may serve as a complement to your physician's prescribed treatment. In addition to the treatments listed below, **acupuncture, acupressure** *(above),* and **massage** may also relieve symptoms.

### HERBAL THERAPIES

Taking a 1-ml dose of hops *(Humulus lupulus)* in tincture form three times a day may relieve symptoms of facial tics and twitches.

### NUTRITION AND DIET

If alcohol abuse has been a problem, it is important to maintain a healthful diet after you stop drinking; a high-dose multivitamin and mineral supplement may also be helpful in easing symptoms of alcohol withdrawal.

## AT-HOME REMEDIES

Avoid fatigue, stress, and caffeine: They can aggravate minor tics and twitches. If your eyelid is twitching, gently massage the area. If caffeine poisoning is a regular concern, replace caffeinated beverages with fruit juices. In addition, herb teas, coffees made from roasted cereal grains and dandelion roots, and carob to replace chocolate in drinks and sweets are viable substitutes. ■

# TINNITUS

## SYMPTOMS

- a noise in the ears, such as ringing, roaring, buzzing, hissing, or whistling; the noise may be intermittent or continuous.
- sometimes, hearing loss.

## CALL YOUR DOCTOR IF:

- you have tinnitus; it could be a symptom of an underlying health problem, such as high blood pressure or an underactive thyroid *(see Thyroid Problems),* that can be treated.
- the noise is accompanied by pain or pus in the ear; these may be signs of an ear infection.
- the noise is accompanied by dizziness; this may be a sign of Ménière's disease or a neurological problem. **Seek medical care immediately.**

Tinnitus, or ringing in the ears, is the sensation of hearing ringing, buzzing, hissing, chirping, whistling, or other sounds. The noise can be intermittent or continuous, and can vary in loudness. It is often worse when background noise is low, so you may be most aware of it at night when you're trying to fall asleep in a quiet room. In rare cases, the sound beats in sync with your heart.

Tinnitus is very common, affecting an estimated 50 million adults in the United States. For most people the condition is merely an annoyance. In severe cases, however, tinnitus can cause people to have difficulty concentrating and sleeping. It may eventually interfere with work and personal relationships, resulting in psychological distress. About 12 million people seek medical help for severe tinnitus every year.

Although tinnitus is often associated with hearing loss, it does not cause the loss; nor does a hearing loss cause tinnitus. In fact, some people with tinnitus experience no difficulty hearing, and in a few cases they even become so acutely sensitive to sound that they must take steps to muffle or mask external noises.

Some instances of tinnitus are caused by infections or blockages in the ear, and the tinnitus often disappears once the underlying cause is treated. Frequently, however, tinnitus continues after the underlying condition is treated. In such a case, other therapies—both conventional and alternative—may bring significant relief by either decreasing or covering up the unwanted sound.

## CAUSES

A wide variety of conditions and illnesses can lead to tinnitus. Blockages of the ear due to a buildup of wax, an infection *(see Otitis Media),* or rarely, a tumor of the auditory nerve can cause the unwanted sounds, as can a perforated eardrum. But perhaps the most common source of chronic tinnitus is prolonged exposure to loud sounds. The noise causes permanent damage to the sound-sensitive cells of the cochlea, a spiral-shaped organ in the inner ear. Carpenters, pilots, rock musicians, and street-repair workers are among those whose jobs put them at risk, as are people who work with chain saws, guns, or other loud devices or who repeatedly listen to loud music. A single exposure to a sudden extremely loud noise can also cause tinnitus.

Certain drugs—most notably aspirin, several types of antibiotics, and quinine medications—can contribute to the condition as well. In fact, tinnitus is cited as a potential side effect for about 200 prescription and nonprescription drugs.

The natural process of aging can result in a deterioration of the cochlea or other parts of the ear and lead to tinnitus. Tinnitus is also associated with Ménière's disease, a disorder of the inner ear, and otosclerosis, a degenerative disease of the small bones in the middle ear. Other medical conditions that can cause ringing in the ears include high blood pressure, allergies, anemia, and an underactive thyroid *(see Thyroid Problems).* Tinnitus can also be a symptom of a disorder of the neck or jaw, such as temporomandibular joint syndrome (TMJ).

For reasons not yet entirely clear to researchers, stress seems to worsen tinnitus.

### DIAGNOSTIC AND TEST PROCEDURES

To determine whether the underlying cause of your tinnitus is a medical condition for which treatment can be prescribed, your doctor will give you a general physical exam, including a careful examination of your ears. Be sure to inform your doctor of all medications you are taking. If the source of the problem remains unclear, you may be sent to an otologist or an otolaryngologist (both ear specialists) or an audiologist (a hearing specialist) for hearing and neurological tests. As part of your examination by these specialists, you may be given a balance test called an electronystagmography. An imaging technique, such as an MRI or a CT scan—which might reveal a structural problem—may also be recommended.

## TREATMENT

Because tinnitus may be a symptom of an underlying medical condition, the first step is to treat that condition. But if the tinnitus remains after treatment or if it results from exposure to loud noise, health professionals recommend various nonmedical options that may help reduce or mask the unwanted noise. Sometimes, tinnitus goes away spontaneously, without any intervention at all.

If you are having difficulty coping with your tinnitus, you may find counseling and support groups helpful *(see the Appendix).* Ask your doctor for a referral.

### CONVENTIONAL MEDICINE

If the cause of your tinnitus is excessive earwax, your physician will clean out your ears with a cotton-tipped probe or a suction device. If you have an ear infection, you may be given a prescription ear drop containing hydrocortisone to help relieve the itching and an antibiotic to fight the infection.

In cases where otosclerosis or a tumor is diagnosed, surgery may be necessary. If your tinnitus is the result of temporomandibular joint syndrome, your doctor will probably refer you to an orthodontist or other dental specialist for appropriate treatment.

For people with chronic tinnitus, drug treatments can offer some success. Lidocaine, a medication used for the treatment of certain types of abnormal heart rhythms, has been shown to relieve tinnitus for some people, but it must be given intravenously and its effect does not last long.

If your tinnitus is accompanied by some hearing loss, a hearing aid may be helpful. Many people have also benefited from tinnitus maskers, devices resembling hearing aids that play a sound more pleasant than the internal noise produced by the tinnitus. A newer device is a tinnitus instrument, which is a combination of hearing aid and masker. Another therapeutic technique, known as auditory habituation, uses a device that generates a certain type of white noise that is quieter than the tinnitus sound; the brain learns to habituate to, or ignore, the tinnitus noise. You must be tested and fitted for any of these devices so that their sounds will cover the particular frequency of noise you hear.

### ACUPRESSURE

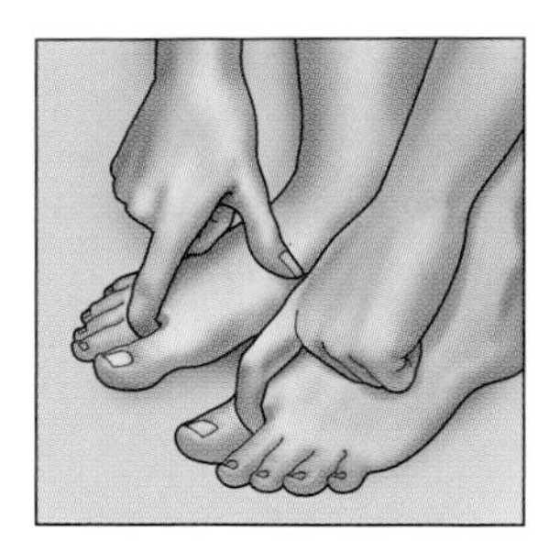

**1** Pressure on Liver 2 may relieve stress brought on by a balance disorder. Press into the web between the big and second toes of both feet, angling the pressure toward the base of your big toe. Press firmly and hold for one minute.

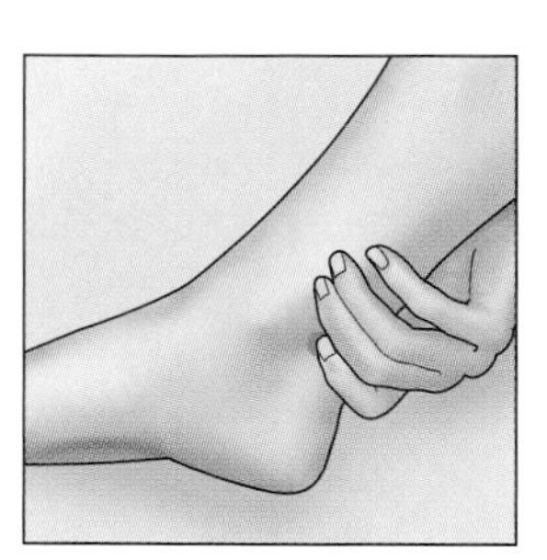

**2** If you have ringing in your ears or earache pain, press the Kidney 3 point, between your Achilles tendon and the inside of your anklebone. Use your index finger to apply firm pressure toward the back of the ankle. Hold for one minute and repeat on the other foot.

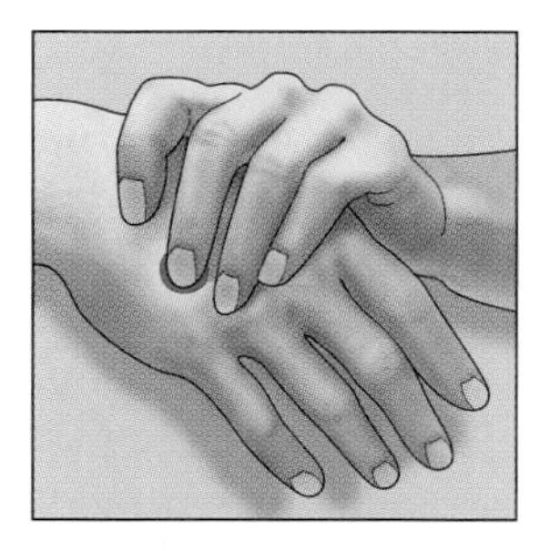

**3** Applying pressure to Triple Warmer 3, in the groove on the back of the hand directly between and behind the fourth and fifth knuckles, may help relieve earache pain. Press gently and hold for one minute, and repeat on the other hand.

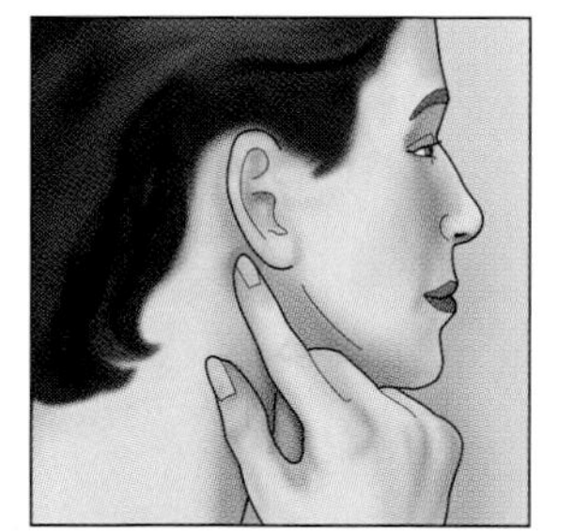

**4** To help relieve ear pain, press your index fingers into Triple Warmer 17, the indentation behind your earlobes. These points may be tender, so press gently. Breathe deeply and hold for two minutes.

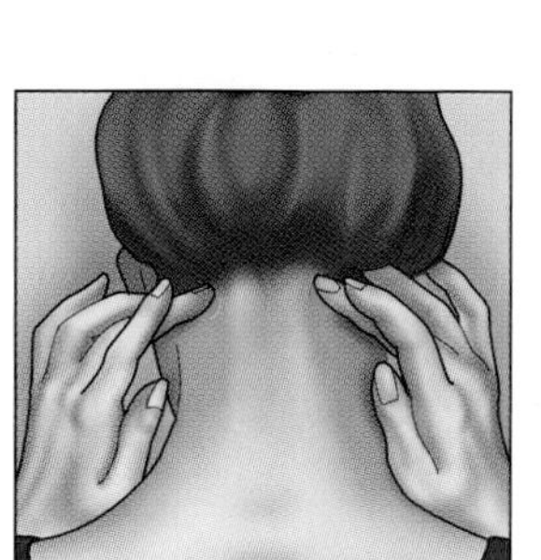

**5** If ringing is worse when your neck is tense, place middle fingers one to two inches apart on Gall Bladder 20, the hollow areas on the sides of the neck at the base of the skull. With eyes closed, breathe deeply and tilt your head back; press up for one to two minutes.

## ALTERNATIVE CHOICES

In addition to the therapies mentioned below, see the illustrations at left for **acupressure** and at right for **yoga** techniques that may help with your tinnitus.

### ACUPUNCTURE

Acupuncture may help decrease the level of the tinnitus sounds you hear. The condition is believed to result from a disturbance in the flow of energy, or chi, to the liver or kidney. Consult a professional acupuncturist for treatment.

### BIOFEEDBACK

Studies have shown that biofeedback can help people cope with their tinnitus, apparently by relieving stress. Patients are trained to relax the forehead muscles, which tighten during times of stress, and to warm their hands and feet. Ask your physician for a referral to a qualified biofeedback practitioner.

### BODY WORK

Practitioners of the **Alexander technique** sometimes use postural training of the neck to help people with tinnitus, particularly in cases accompanied by vertigo. The technique is believed to improve the flow of blood to the ear.

### CHIROPRACTIC

Manipulation that loosens the neck and improves blood supply to the ears may be beneficial in some cases. An **osteopath** can provide similar treatment.

### HERBAL THERAPIES

Ginkgo *(Ginkgo biloba)* has been found useful in minimizing the distress of tinnitus. Take 40 mg of the dried herb or 1 to 2 tsp of the liquid extract three times a day. Don't expect immediate results from ginkgo; you may need to take the remedy for several weeks before experiencing any relief.

### HOMEOPATHY

Several homeopathic remedies are prescribed for tinnitus. A homeopathic practitioner may prescribe one of the following:

**YOGA**

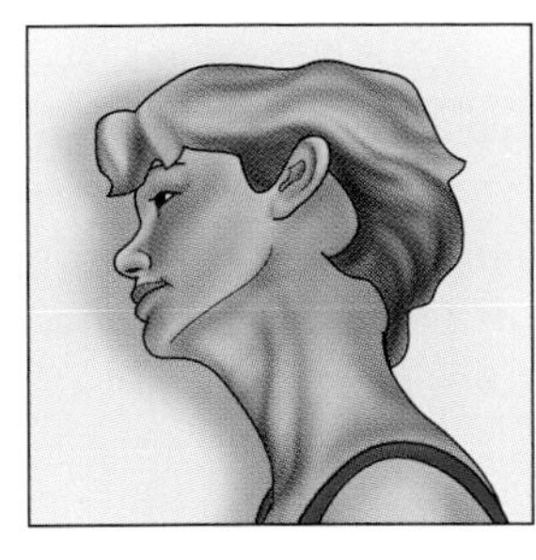

Head movements may help release tension in the shoulder and neck areas. This will expand the neck muscles and increase circulation. Exhale and slowly move your right ear toward your right shoulder and hold for 10 seconds *(top);* inhale and bring your head up, then repeat on the left side. Exhale as you slowly place your chin to your chest and hold for 10 seconds. Lift your head as you inhale, then exhale as you ease your head backward with your chin up *(bottom);* hold for 10 seconds. Inhale as you slowly bring your head back to the starting position. Do twice daily.

- ◆ If the noise is a buzzing or hissing sound, Chininum sulphuricum.
- ◆ If the noise is a ringing sound with no other symptoms, Kali iodatum.
- ◆ If the noise is a roaring sound and is accompanied by some hearing loss, Salicylicum acidum.
- ◆ If roaring sounds are accompanied by a tingling sensation and by the feeling that the ears are blocked, Carboneum sulphuratum.

### LIFESTYLE

Regular exercise that increases blood circulation to the head may help bring some relief from tinnitus. Try running, fast walking, swimming, biking, or some other aerobic activity. Be aware that after beginning an exercise program you may experience a slight worsening of your tinnitus before you notice an improvement.

### MIND/BODY MEDICINE

Some people report that through self-hypnosis they can successfully "turn off" the unwanted sound created by their tinnitus for hours or even days at a time. A trained hypnotherapist may be able to teach you to adjust the volume of your tinnitus using an imaginary dial or other device. This form of **hypnotherapy** works only for people who are able to go into a moderately deep trance.

### NUTRITION AND DIET

To improve blood circulation to your ears, reduce the saturated fat and cholesterol in your diet. Niacin supplements—100 to 6,000 mg a day—can also help lower cholesterol. WARNING: Do not take higher doses of niacin without being monitored by a professional because it can have side effects, such as liver toxicity.

Research has shown that a high percentage of people with tinnitus are deficient in vitamin $B_{12}$. Nutritionists recommend that you get 6 mcg of the vitamin daily. In addition, some evidence indicates that vitamin A supplements (5,000 to 10,000 IU a day) may be at least partially effective against tinnitus.

## AT-HOME REMEDIES

- ◆ Avoid alcohol, smoking, and caffeine; they can make tinnitus worse.
- ◆ Cut down on salt in your diet. Salt can cause fluid to build up in your ears, worsening tinnitus.
- ◆ Avoid loud noises, which can aggravate a case of tinnitus you already have.
- ◆ If you have trouble sleeping because of the noise in your ears, try turning on a radio, which can mask the unwanted sound with soothing music. Or record a "white noise" tape, such as of running water, and play it whenever you need relief.
- ◆ Avoid too much aspirin, which can make tinnitus worse. ■

# TONSILLITIS

## SYMPTOMS

**For tonsillitis**:
- a very sore throat with red, swollen tonsils; there may be a white discharge or spots on the tonsils.
- swollen and tender lymph nodes in the neck under the jaw.
- a low-grade fever and headache accompanying the other symptoms.

**For tonsillar abscess:**
- in addition to inflamed tonsils, severe pain and tenderness around the area of the soft palate, at the roof of the mouth, and difficulty swallowing.
- distinctively muffled speech, as if the child is speaking with a mouthful of mashed potatoes, caused by swelling from the abscess.

## CALL YOUR DOCTOR IF:

- your child has symptoms of tonsillitis.
- your child has tonsillitis and starts drooling or having difficulty breathing, which may indicate a **tonsillar abscess**.
- your child has trouble breathing at night or experiences noisy breathing or episodes of sleep apnea, in which the child stops breathing for brief periods while asleep; these symptoms may indicate adenoid problems or overgrown tonsils.
- your child has recurrent bouts of tonsillitis; surgery may be indicated.
- your child is not responding to antibiotics and has fever or pain, as well as white spots or a discharge on the tonsils; this may indicate mononucleosis or another infection.

The tonsils are masses of lymphatic tissue located at the back of the throat. They produce antibodies designed to help your child fight respiratory infections. When these tissues themselves become infected, the resulting condition is called tonsillitis.

Tonsillitis most commonly affects children between the ages of three and seven, when tonsils may play their most active infection-fighting role. But as the child grows, the tonsils shrink, and infections become less common. Tonsillitis is usually not serious, unless a **tonsillar abscess** develops. When this happens, the swelling can be severe enough to block your child's breathing. Secondary ear infections (otitis media) and adenoid problems are other complications.

## CAUSES

Most tonsil infections and tonsillar abscesses in elementary school-age children are caused by the streptococcal bacterium, the same organism that causes strep throat. Cold or influenza viruses sometimes also cause tonsillitis.

## TREATMENT

To check your child's tonsils, place the handle of a spoon on her tongue and ask the child to say "aaahhh" while you direct a light on the back of her throat. If the tonsils look bright red and swollen, call your pediatrician.

### CONVENTIONAL MEDICINE

Your pediatrician will examine your child's tonsils and take a throat culture to check for strep throat. To check for a **tonsillar abscess,** the doctor will examine the tonsils and soft palate. If he discovers an abscess, he may drain it. For either a strep infection or an abscess, the doctor will prescribe an antibiotic such as penicillin or erythromycin. Be sure to give your child the full course; if unchecked, strep bacteria can cause serious autoimmune disorders such as nephritis or rheumatic fever. To ease pain, the doctor may

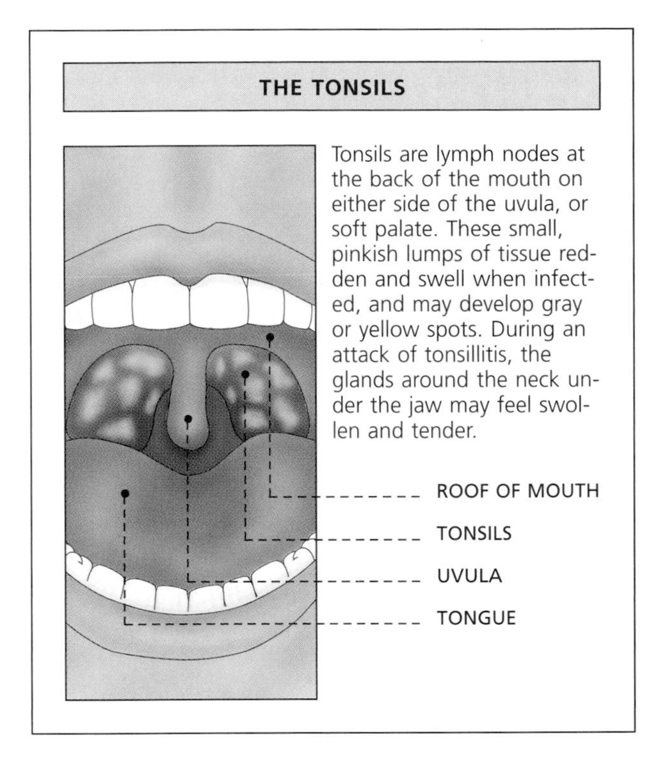


**THE TONSILS**

Tonsils are lymph nodes at the back of the mouth on either side of the uvula, or soft palate. These small, pinkish lumps of tissue redden and swell when infected, and may develop gray or yellow spots. During an attack of tonsillitis, the glands around the neck under the jaw may feel swollen and tender.

also recommend acetaminophen. (Do not give your child aspirin, which has been linked to Reye's syndrome.) Severe cases may warrant a tonsillectomy *(see Prevention, below, right).*

## ALTERNATIVE CHOICES

Some alternative therapies are effective in relieving the symptoms of tonsillitis. But be sure to first get a throat culture to rule out strep throat, which must be treated with antibiotics. A **tonsillar abscess** should be treated by a medical doctor before you start any alternative method.

### CHINESE MEDICINE

A practitioner of Chinese medicine may advise acupressure to relieve a sore throat, or acupuncture to combat chronic tonsillitis. Herbalists may recommend the over-the-counter remedy Honeysuckle and Forsythia Powder, thought to help soothe a sore throat in the early stages of tonsillitis.

### HERBAL THERAPIES

To reduce inflammation, medical herbalists suggest drinking a tea made from cleavers (*Galium* spp.): Add 1 tsp dried herb to 1 cup boiling water. A gargle made from sage *(Salvia officinalis)* is thought to help fight infection: Add 2 tsp to boiling water and steep for 10 minutes. Let your child gargle with the tea (as warm as she can tolerate it) for 5 minutes several times a day.

### HOMEOPATHY

After determining if your child is suffering from acute or chronic tonsillitis, a homeopath may recommend one of the following remedies: for inflamed tonsils, Belladonna, Hepar sulphuris, or Mercurius vivus; for chronic enlarged tonsils, Baryta carbonica or Calcarea carbonica.

### OSTEOPATHY

Osteopaths treat tonsillitis and tonsillar abscesses with the same surgical and drug therapies offered by conventional medical doctors but may also try gentle soft-tissue manipulation techniques to encourage lymphatic drainage.

## AT-HOME REMEDIES

- A saltwater gargle can relieve soreness. Dissolve ½ tsp salt in a glass of warm water and let the child gargle as needed to ease pain.
- Ice cream or frozen yogurt, especially after a tonsillectomy, will relieve soreness and soothe your child.
- A cool-mist humidifier will increase moisture in the room and soothe a child's sore throat. Aim the mist away from your child so that it does not spray directly at her face, and change her clothes if they become damp.

# PREVENTION

Tonsillectomy, the surgical removal of the tonsils, is performed much less frequently today than in years past. Doctors now generally recommend the operation only in serious cases, such as when tonsillar abscess is a recurring problem. If surgery is performed, your child may need to be hospitalized for a day or two and her throat will be sore for four or five days. ■

# TOOTHACHE

## SYMPTOMS

- aching or sharp pain in tooth when biting or chewing.
- soreness in teeth, gums, or jaw.

## CALL YOUR DENTIST IF:

- your gums are painful, red, and swollen; you may have an impacted tooth or a gum disease. *(See Gum Problems.)*
- you experience continuous bouts of throbbing pain in a tooth, or the tooth is extremely sensitive to heat or cold; you may have tooth decay (a cavity) that requires a new or replacement filling. If the decay is advanced, you may need root canal work. You may also have a tooth abscess, a serious infection requiring emergency treatment.
- you have a sharp pain in your tooth, your tooth feels long or loose, and you have a fever. See your dentist immediately; you may have a tooth abscess.

T

A toothache can be caused by something as simple as a piece of food wedged between your gum and tooth—in which case relief involves no more than rinsing or flossing away whatever is causing the pain. But if the pain is not so easily eliminated, you probably have a dental disorder that can cause serious problems if you don't visit your dentist.

Tooth decay cannot be cured, but its progress can be halted through conventional dental care. Other causes of dental pain include impacted teeth—teeth that grow at odd angles—and gum disease, which inflames the area around a tooth so much that you cannot tell if the pain is coming from the tooth or from the tissue around the tooth. *(See Gum Problems.)*

Prevention of tooth decay is the best way to avoid toothaches. Alternative remedies may help alleviate the discomfort of symptoms, but conventional treatment is absolutely necessary to stop decay or infection from spreading.

## CAUSES

The major cause of **tooth decay** is dental plaque—a substance composed of the bacteria, acids, and sugars in your mouth—which corrodes the protective enamel on your teeth. Initially, you may have no symptoms; but as decay develops, you may feel stabbing pain whenever you eat something hot, cold, sweet, or sour.

If decay goes untreated, bacteria infect the underlying dentin and eventually the pulp, or fleshy core, of the tooth. To fight infection, pus floods the pulp, causing a painful abscess. If left untreated, abscesses can damage the jawbone or sinus and lead to generalized blood poisoning.

Impacted teeth are common in people in their late teens and early twenties, who are getting in their third molars, or wisdom teeth. Wisdom teeth are often too big for the jaw and thus do not fully emerge from the gum or grow in at odd angles; they press against neighboring teeth or trap food particles, causing pain and infection.

Toothaches may also be caused by pressure from sinus congestion, by tooth grinding, or by a blow to the face.

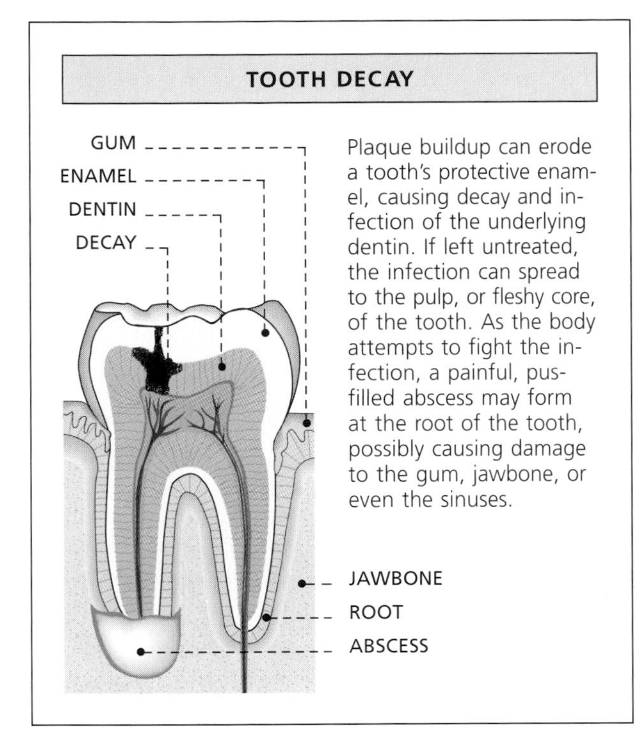


## TREATMENT

### CONVENTIONAL MEDICINE

For most tooth decay, your dentist will remove the decayed portion and fill the cavity with a durable material. If the decay is serious, you may need a root canal, which involves removing the pulp, sealing the opening, and then capping the tooth with a crown. For abscesses, a dentist will likely first prescribe an antibiotic. If damage is so severe that a root canal is impossible, or if a tooth is impacted, extraction is the usual treatment.

### ALTERNATIVE CHOICES

You must see a dentist for aches that you suspect may be related to tooth decay, but alternative treatments may ease the pain in the meantime.

#### ACUPRESSURE

Apply deep pressure to the webbing between index finger and thumb (LI 4) to relieve dental pain; massaging this area with an ice cube may also help. Do not press this point if you are pregnant.

#### HERBAL THERAPY

Rubbing clove oil *(Syzygium aromaticum)* or myrrh *(Commiphora molmol)* on the gum around a painful tooth helps numb it.

### AT-HOME REMEDIES

Try the following remedies to relieve your pain.

- Rinse with salt water; if rinsing doesn't work, floss gently to pry out any trapped particles.
- Numb your gums: Sucking on ice for a minute numbs the gum surrounding a painful tooth.
- Keep cool: Though a hot compress may ease pain, if your toothache is caused by an infection, heat will cause the disease to spread.

## PREVENTION

- Brush and floss after eating; use a nonabrasive, fluoride-based toothpaste. Beware so-called whitening agents; they often contain abrasives that can wear down enamel.
- Cut down on sweets and carbohydrates.
- Get your teeth cleaned professionally every six months, and make sure a dentist examines your teeth annually.

### HYPERSENSITIVE TEETH

*If a tooth reacts just to heat or cold, you could have dentinal hypersensitivity. More than 40 million Americans feel pain caused by the wearing away of enamel and exposure of dentin. It's brought on by age, receding gums, dental surgery, or excessive brushing with whitening toothpastes or hard-bristled brushes. You can help relieve hypersensitivity by using a toothpaste made for sensitive teeth and a toothbrush with soft bristles.* ■

# TOXIC SHOCK SYNDROME

## SYMPTOMS

In a woman who is menstruating or has just completed a menstrual period; or in a new mother or any recent surgery or burn patient:

- high fever—over 102°F.
- vomiting and/or diarrhea.
- a rash resembling a sunburn with peeling skin, especially on fingers and toes.
- dizziness or mental confusion.
- pale and clammy skin, signaling a rapid drop in blood pressure; if toxic shock is left untreated at this stage, it will quickly lead to loss of consciousness, cardiac and respiratory failure, and death.

## CALL YOUR DOCTOR IF:

- you have the symptoms above, which can develop suddenly. Toxic shock can dangerously lower blood pressure, resulting in life-threatening shock *(see also Emergencies/First Aid).* **Seek treatment immediately.**

Toxic shock syndrome is a sudden, potentially fatal condition brought on by the release of toxins from an overgrowth of a bacterium *(Staphylococcus aureus)* commonly found in many women. It is widely known to affect menstruating women, especially those who use superabsorbent tampons. The body responds with the classic symptom of shock: a precipitous drop in blood pressure, which deprives vital organs of oxygen and can lead to death.

This disease reached the headlines in the 1970s after the deaths of several young women who were using a certain brand of superabsorbent tampon; that brand was later removed from the market. Toxic shock syndrome is still primarily a disease of menstruating women who use tampons—especially superabsorbent tampons; however, it has also been linked to the use of menstrual sponges, diaphragms, and cervical caps. A woman who has recently given birth is also at increased risk for developing toxic shock. But the condition is not limited to these factors alone: Its victims also include both men and women who have been exposed to *Staphylococcus aureus* bacteria while recovering from surgery, a burn, or an open wound.

More than a third of all cases of toxic shock involve women under 19 years of age, and up to 30 percent of women who have had the disease will suffer a recurrence. The reason for this is unclear; however, it means that if you have ever suffered toxic shock, you must be especially alert to the symptoms of its onset so that you can get immediate medical care.

People who die from toxic shock are killed by the body's acute response to toxins released by *Staphylococcus aureus* bacteria. Victims suffer what is known technically as **hypotensive shock,** in which the heart and lungs are overburdened to the point that they stop working.

If you are menstruating and have a high fever with vomiting, especially if you have been wearing tampons, you must get medical help right away. If you are wearing a tampon, menstrual sponge, diaphragm, or cervical cap when you are taken sick, remove it immediately, even before calling your doctor.

## CAUSES

The primary cause of toxic shock syndrome is a toxin produced by the bacterium *Staphylococcus aureus*. This organism is one of several related staph bacteria that often cause skin infections in burn victims and hospital patients weakened by surgery. These bacteria are not rare; in fact, *Staphylococcus aureus* is normally—and harmlessly—present in the vagina.

Exactly why and how *Staphylococcus aureus* causes toxic shock syndrome is not completely understood; what is known is that two conditions are necessary. First, the bacteria need an environment in which they can grow rapidly and release toxins. Then the toxins must have a way of getting into the bloodstream, where they trigger serious, life-threatening symptoms.

One theory holds that a tampon saturated with blood can serve as a medium conducive to rapid bacterial growth. What the tampon is made of seems to matter: Polyester foam apparently provides a better growth medium than either cotton or rayon fibers.

In cases that involve the use of menstrual sponges, diaphragms, and cervical caps, either the device had been in the vagina for an exceptionally long time—more than 30 hours—or, in the case of the sponge, pieces of the sponge had been retained in the vagina. (Either situation may provide a favorable environment for growth.)

The way in which bacterial toxins enter the bloodstream may also be related to tampon use. According to researchers, sliding a tampon into place in the vagina may make microscopic tears in its walls, rupturing tiny blood vessels. A superabsorbent tampon—especially if left in overlong, or if used when the menstrual flow is light—can also dry out the vagina, making such tearing even more likely.

Researchers investigating the causes of toxic shock syndrome have ruled out certain factors. Feminine deodorant sprays and douches, underwear, and other clothing do not play a role, and the condition is also unrelated to the victim's menstrual history, drug or alcohol use, cigarette smoking, swimming or bathing, or sexual activity.

## TREATMENT

Toxic shock syndrome requires immediate emergency care in a hospital setting. If you suspect you are suffering an attack, get medical help as soon as possible. If your doctor is not available, call 911 or get to a hospital emergency room right away; have someone take you because you may quickly become too shaky to drive yourself.

### CONVENTIONAL MEDICINE

Treatment for this life-threatening condition must be aggressive. Your doctor or emergency-care specialist should start by giving you antibiotics specific to a staph infection, to kill the bacteria and limit further release of toxins. Other urgent steps—necessary to control your body's response to the toxins and to support vital functions—include blood transfusion and intravenous administration of fluids and electrolytes to stabilize your blood pressure. Some cases call for a ventilator, which will temporarily breathe for you. Caregivers will monitor your vital signs constantly during the acute phase of this disease.

## PREVENTION

Using regular tampons increases your risk of developing toxic shock syndrome far less than using superabsorbent ones. Nevertheless, the most conservative preventive approach would involve switching to sanitary napkins. You may also decrease risk somewhat by taking the following steps:

- Minimize your use of tampons. You might alternate tampons with sanitary napkins during the day, and use napkins at night.
- Use the least absorbent tampon that will control your menstrual flow; change tampons at least every eight hours. Be sure to remove the last tampon when your period is over.
- If you use a menstrual sponge, diaphragm, or cervical cap, remember to remove it when it is not needed. Under no circumstances should you leave any such device in for more than 24 hours. Wash your diaphragm or cervical cap in warm, soapy water after each use. ■

# TREMBLING

*Read down this column to find your symptoms. Then read across.*

| SYMPTOMS | AILMENT/PROBLEM |
|---|---|
| ◆ shaky hands; you regularly drink coffee, colas, or tea. | ◆ Effects of caffeine |
| ◆ trembling (shaking that you cannot control) after taking a new medication. | ◆ Side effects of a medication |
| ◆ trembling; feelings of anxiety, fear, or anger. | ◆ An inherited tendency to tremble in response to stress or other strong emotional states |
| ◆ trembling; hunger; weakness; excessive perspiration; nervousness and confusion; lightheadedness; possibly, headache or irregular heartbeat. | ◆ Hypoglycemia (abnormally low levels of blood sugar) |
| ◆ weight loss despite increased appetite; nervousness; trembling; excessive perspiration; irregular heartbeat; fatigue; protruding eyes; enlarged thyroid gland that you may be able to feel with your fingers. | ◆ Graves' disease |
| ◆ weakness and fatigue; trembling; weight loss; irregular heartbeat; possibly, lack of appetite. | ◆ One of many forms of hyperthyroidism |
| ◆ tremor in your hand, fingers, head, or voice that increases with fatigue or strong emotion, and gradually worsens with time. | ◆ Essential tremor, a harmless but annoying shaking |
| ◆ trembling between bouts of heavy drinking; broken facial capillaries; flushed face; chronic diarrhea. | ◆ Effects of chronic overconsumption of alcohol |
| ◆ trembling accompanied by slow, jerky movements; unsteady balance; indistinct speech; trouble swallowing; age over 50. | ◆ Parkinson's disease |
| ◆ trembling with numbness, tingling; double or blurred vision; weakness; muscle spasms or paralysis; mood swings; incontinence. | ◆ Multiple sclerosis |

| WHAT TO DO | OTHER INFO |
| --- | --- |
| ◆ Reduce your caffeine consumption; talk to your healthcare practitioner if you experience headaches, nausea, irritability, or other withdrawal symptoms. | ◆ Some practitioners believe it is possible to develop a physical addiction to coffee even if you drink only two cups a day. |
| ◆ Many medications, either alone or in combination with others, can cause trembling or other side effects. Check with your doctor or pharmacist about possibly changing your medication. | ◆ Make sure that your doctor and pharmacist have a complete list of all the medications you are taking. |
| ◆ See your doctor soon for an accurate diagnosis. See Anxiety, Panic Attack, Phobias, Stress. | ◆ Try breathing exercises, yoga, and/or aerobic exercise to help you relax and keep emotions from becoming overwhelming. |
| ◆ Eat something sweet; this may boost your blood sugar level in 5 to 20 minutes. | ◆ Eating frequent, small meals that are high in complex carbohydrates yet low in sugar will often keep hypoglycemia attacks at bay. |
| ◆ See your doctor for an accurate diagnosis and treatment. | ◆ Graves' disease is most likely to occur between the ages of 30 and 40. |
| ◆ See your doctor for an accurate diagnosis and treatment. See Thyroid Problems. | ◆ With treatment, most people with hyperthyroidism lead a normal life. |
| ◆ See your doctor about treatment. | ◆ The most common movement disorder in the United States; essential tremor does not lead to more serious problems. |
| ◆ Reduce your alcohol consumption; see Alcohol Abuse. | |
| ◆ See your doctor for an accurate diagnosis and treatment. | ◆ Medication can significantly slow the progress of Parkinson's disease. |
| ◆ See your doctor for diagnosis; the form of the disease will determine treatment. | ◆ Multiple sclerosis can affect every part of the body. Be open to a variety of alternative treatments to see which works best for you. |

# TRICHOMONIASIS

## SYMPTOMS

If you're a woman, you may have no symptoms at all, or you may experience:

- a greenish yellow, frothy vaginal discharge with a pronounced odor.
- vaginal itching or irritation.
- painful intercourse.
- pain in the lower abdomen.
- vaginal bleeding.

If you're a man, you'll probably have no symptoms, or you may experience some discomfort when urinating.

## CALL YOUR DOCTOR IF:

- you experience any of the above symptoms. Trichomoniasis is contagious and can lead to complications. Women shouldn't assume that the problem is simple vaginitis *(see Vaginal Problems).*

Trichomoniasis—a parasitic infection spread primarily through sexual intercourse—is not serious, but it is contagious. In 70 percent of cases, it produces no symptoms, which makes it notoriously difficult to diagnose. In women who do have symptoms, discomfort may persist for a week to several months and may be more pronounced right after menstruation or during pregnancy. Left untreated, the parasite may infect tissues throughout the urinary tract and reproductive system. In women, vulnerable sites for infection include the vagina, urethra, cervix, bladder, and various glands. In men the infection may spread to the urethra, prostate gland, seminal vesicles, and epididymis.

The parasite that causes trichomoniasis likes an alkaline environment. Women have a greater chance of getting the disease if they use oral contraceptives, are pregnant, or frequently use commercial douches, all of which can increase alkaline levels in the body.

## CAUSES

The culprit behind trichomoniasis is a protozoan parasite called *Trichomonas vaginalis.* Usually transmitted through intercourse, the parasite may also be acquired from toilet seats, locker room benches, damp towels, and bathing suits.

### DIAGNOSTIC AND TEST PROCEDURES

Your doctor may want to examine your vaginal or urethral discharge under a microscope or test your urine. Trichomoniasis occasionally shows up on Pap smears in women with no symptoms. Your best bet is to get tested during your annual physical if you think you may have been exposed to the organism.

## TREATMENT

Nine out of ten people with trichomoniasis are cured with a single course of antibiotics. Stubborn cases require larger doses administered over longer periods of time.

## CONVENTIONAL MEDICINE

The drug most commonly used to fight trichomoniasis is metronidazole, which comes in tablet form; few other drugs are as effective. Metronidazole is viewed with caution by some physicians because of test results showing it to cause birth defects and cancer in animals. But no studies have proved it harmful to humans. If you take metronidazole, you may experience side effects such as nausea, vomiting, or a metallic aftertaste. You can minimize discomfort by taking the drug during or immediately after a meal. Also, don't drink alcohol within 24 hours of taking the medicine; if you do, you may experience severe abdominal pain and vomiting.

## ALTERNATIVE CHOICES

Besides taking antibiotics, you can try alternative treatments to help speed healing.

### ACUPRESSURE

A doctor of Chinese medicine may recommend that you flush out toxins by massaging acupressure points Liver 3, between the big and second toes, and Liver 8, on the inside of the leg above the knee. Also try kneading Kidney 3, on the inside of the leg between the anklebone and the Achilles tendon. Use any of these techniques at home several times a day. *(See pages 22–23 for more information about point locations.)*

### AROMATHERAPY

Aromatherapists believe that oil of bergamot *(Citrus bergamia)* may help dry up irritating discharges. Douche with it or add it to your bath.

### CHINESE HERBS

A practitioner of Chinese medicine may prepare a prescription for you with herbs such as gentiana *(Gentiana scabra),* Chinese foxglove root *(Rehmannia glutinosa),* and angelica root *(Angelica pubescens).*

### HERBAL THERAPIES

Herbalists say that you can reduce inflammation and discharges by douching with teas of calendula *(Calendula officinalis),* myrrh *(Commiphora molmol),* and thuja *(Thuja occidentalis).*

### HOMEOPATHY

A homeopathic physician may prescribe a remedy to strengthen your entire system. A complete consultation is necessary to determine which remedy is right for you.

### NUTRITION AND DIET

Antibiotics destroy beneficial as well as disease-causing organisms in your body. Replace the beneficial ones by eating live-culture yogurt or by taking 1 tsp *Lactobacillus acidophilus* supplement and ½ tsp *Bifidobacterium* in a glass of water three times a day.

To promote healing and boost immunity, nutritionists recommend that you supplement a balanced diet with zinc and vitamins A, C, and E.

## AT-HOME REMEDIES

Women who douche frequently with commercial chemical products may raise their risk of developing trichomoniasis. But if you have the infection, use one of the following natural douches once a day, while lying in a warm bath:

- vinegar douche: 1 tsp vinegar to 1 qt warm water.
- live-culture yogurt or a solution of *Lactobacillus acidophilus* (½ tsp to 1 cup of water).

To increase parasite-killing acidity, you may add to either douche the juice of one lemon.
CAUTION: Do not douche if you are pregnant.

## PREVENTION

- Use a condom when having sex.
- Don't share towels or swimsuits.
- Shower immediately after swimming in a public pool.
- Wash before and after intercourse. ■

# TUBERCULOSIS

## SYMPTOMS

- at first, only a mild cough or, often, no symptoms.
- fatigue.
- weight loss.
- cough, with occasional bloody sputum.
- slight fever, night sweats.
- pain in the chest, back, or kidneys, and perhaps all three.

## CALL YOUR DOCTOR IF:

- you exhibit any of the above symptoms, especially if you live in crowded conditions, are malnourished, or have the virus that causes AIDS. (Note: Virtually all of the symptoms of tuberculosis can be confused with those of other diseases; bloody sputum, for example, is also a symptom of pneumonia.)
- you have been exposed to someone with active tuberculosis.

Tuberculosis, commonly referred to as TB, is a chronic bacterial infection that can spread through the lymph nodes and bloodstream to any organ in your body but is usually found in the lungs. In their active state, TB bacteria in essence eat away at the tissue of infected organs, possibly resulting in death. But the organisms usually remain inactive after entering the body; thus, most infected people will never develop the active form of the disease if they receive proper care.

Because the bacteria that cause tuberculosis are transmitted through the air, the disease can be quite contagious. However, it is nearly impossible to catch TB simply by passing an infected person on the street. To be at risk, you must be exposed to the organisms constantly, by living or working in close quarters with someone who has the active disease. Even then, because the bacteria generally stay dormant after they invade the body, only 10 percent of people infected with TB will ever come down with the active disease. The remaining 90 percent will show no signs of infection, nor will they be able to spread the disease to others. Dormant infections can eventually become active, though, so even people without symptoms should receive medical treatment.

Once widespread, TB became relatively rare with the help of antibiotic therapies developed in the 1950s. Today, however, a new and highly resistant form has emerged, creating a public-health hazard in many large cities worldwide. If you have TB—in its active or dormant state— you must seek conventional medical treatment.

## CAUSES

Tuberculosis is generally caused by exposure to microscopic airborne droplets containing the bacterium *Mycobacterium tuberculosis,* also called the tubercle bacillus. The disease is almost never transmitted through clothes, bedding, or other personal items. Because most people with TB exhale only a few of these germs with each breath, you can contract the disease only if you are exposed to an infected person for a long time. If you spend 8 hours a day for six months, or 24 hours a day for two months, with someone with

T

## A RESISTANT MENACE

*Two decades ago, the United States surgeon general announced that tuberculosis was a disease of the past. He spoke too soon: The disease has since resurfaced in a potent new form that has once again turned TB into a public-health hazard. This new form, called multidrug-resistant TB (MDR-TB), is caused by strains of the bacterium M. tuberculosis that, through mutation, have developed the ability to resist two or more antibiotic drugs. Even with treatment, roughly half of all MDR-TB patients die. This mortality rate matches that of patients with regular TB who received no medical care at all.*

an active case of TB, you have a 50 percent chance of acquiring the disease.

People who are malnourished or who live in close quarters stand the greatest chance of contracting tuberculosis. Therefore, the conditions that accompany poverty, although not a cause of tuberculosis, certainly contribute to its ability to spread. Healthcare workers, long-term hospital patients, and prison workers or inmates also face a greater-than-normal risk of becoming infected with TB.

### DIAGNOSTIC AND TEST PROCEDURES

You will generally have no symptoms if you are infected with TB. In fact, you may not even be aware that you have the disease until it is revealed through a skin test, perhaps during a routine checkup. The Mantoux skin test is the most reliable detector of TB. A medical practitioner injects a small amount of liquid material between the top two layers of skin on your arm. If a red welt develops at that site over the next day or so, you are probably infected with TB, though not necessarily in its active form. X-rays of your lungs will usually reveal if the disease has spread.

## TREATMENT

Anyone with tuberculosis must be monitored by a doctor. If you have the infection—but not the active disease—your doctor will probably prescribe an antibiotic drug called isoniazid (INH) as a preventive measure. If you have the active disease, your physician will most likely prescribe broad-spectrum antibiotics.

### CONVENTIONAL MEDICINE

For patients who are infected with tuberculosis organisms but do not have the active disease, doctors usually administer preventive therapy. This usually involves a daily dose of isoniazid and periodic checkups. If you have the active disease, regularly monitored treatment by a doctor is crucial. You will probably be given a combination of several antibiotics, which may include INH, rifampin, pyrazinamide, or ethambutol.

### ALTERNATIVE CHOICES

If you have TB, you must be supervised by a conventional doctor. Alternative therapies may help alleviate some symptoms of the disease, but they cannot replace medical treatment.

#### HERBAL THERAPIES

An herbalist might recommend three cups per day of an infusion from echinacea (*Echinacea* spp.) or pau d'arco *(Tabebuia impetiginosa),* or 20 to 40 drops from a tincture of these herbs three times a day. The plants are thought to have antibacterial properties that guard against further infection.

#### NUTRITION AND DIET

Because malnutrition contributes to the activation of TB bacteria, a balanced diet is essential for people with tuberculosis. Many nutritionists also recommend vitamins A, C, and E, along with the mineral zinc, as these are believed to help keep mucous membranes healthy. ■

# URINARY PROBLEMS

*Read down this column to find your symptoms. Then read across.*

| SYMPTOMS | AILMENT/PROBLEM |
|---|---|
| ◆ pink or red (bloody) urine. | ◆ Any of a variety of diseases and conditions, including prostate problems, kidney stones, kidney cancer, or kidney disease; a reaction to a medication or food |
| ◆ painful urination. | ◆ Any of a variety of diseases and conditions, including bladder infection, kidney stones, urinary blockage, or bladder or prostate cancer |
| ◆ desire to urinate more frequently or with greater urgency than usual. | ◆ Any of a variety of diseases and conditions, including gonorrhea, urethritis (inflammation of the urethra), cystitis (a bladder infection), prostatitis (a prostate problem), kidney stones, or bladder cancer |
| ◆ dwindling amounts of urine or no urine production at all. | ◆ Dehydration; kidney disease |
| ◆ excessive thirst and passing abnormal amounts of urine (more than three quarts a day). | ◆ Any of a variety of diseases and conditions, including a chemical imbalance, diabetes, or psychological problems; a side effect of long-term lithium therapy for manic-depression |
| ◆ cloudy (pus-containing) urine, possibly with a foul odor. | ◆ Cystitis (a bladder infection) |
| ◆ urinary leakage, dripping, or uncontrollable urges to urinate. | ◆ Incontinence |
| ◆ inability or only partial ability to empty the bladder. | ◆ Any of a variety of conditions, including a narrow urethra, an enlarged prostate gland (a prostate problem), bladder or urethral stones, psychological problems, or in children, an impaired urethral valve. |

| WHAT TO DO | OTHER INFO |
|---|---|
| ◆ See your doctor without delay. Although blood in the urine is not always a cause for concern, it may indicate a serious underlying disorder. For more information about treatment, see the various entries listed at left. | ◆ Urine that turns pink or red soon after a sore throat or upper respiratory infection may be a sign of a serious kidney problem. |
| ◆ See your doctor. For more information about treatment, see the various entries listed at left. | ◆ A nonburning pain when urinating may indicate an abnormal blockage within the bladder or urethra, while a burning pain usually indicates a urinary tract infection. |
| ◆ See your doctor. For more information about treatment, see the various entries listed at left. | ◆ How often you need to pass urine each day depends on several factors, including personal habit, the amount of fluid you take in, and the strength of your bladder muscles. |
| ◆ Drink fluids to replenish your body, but avoid drinks containing alcohol or caffeine. If you are not dehydrated but the amount of urine you are passing seems insufficient, your kidneys may be failing. This can be a medical emergency; **call your doctor now.** | ◆ To avoid dehydration, drink plenty of fluids during hot weather, even if you do not feel thirsty. |
| ◆ See your doctor. Depending on its cause, the condition may resolve itself or it may require drug therapy. | ◆ Some types of drugs, particularly diuretics, can cause an increase in urine production. |
| ◆ See your doctor. Cystitis, a bacterial bladder infection, is usually treated with antibiotics. | ◆ Pus is caused by large numbers of white blood cells, an indication of an infection. |
| ◆ See your doctor, who will suggest a remedy. Incontinence is neither a normal nor an inevitable part of aging, and can often be treated successfully. | ◆ Urinary incontinence has several causes, including infection, medications, depression, restricted mobility, and hormone deficiency. Most problems can be corrected by medication or counseling; surgery is sometimes required. |
| ◆ **Call your doctor now.** The inability to urinate even when you feel the urge is a medical emergency. | |

# UTERINE CANCER

## SYMPTOMS

Uterine cancer causes no symptoms at onset. Symptoms usually appear as the malignancy begins to grow, but 5 percent of women with uterine cancer experience no symptoms until the disease spreads to other organs. The most likely symptoms are:

- abnormal vaginal bleeding. Before menopause, this means unusually heavy menstrual periods or bleeding between periods. After a woman enters menopause, this means any vaginal bleeding, unless she is on hormone replacement therapy (HRT). Postmenopausal women on HRT may have monthly bleeding that resembles menstruation and that may mask symptoms of uterine cancer; any unusual or heavy bleeding should be reported to the doctor.
- vaginal discharge that may range from pink and watery to thick, brown, and foul smelling.
- an enlarged uterus, detectable upon pelvic examination.
- unexpected weight loss; weakness and pain in the lower abdomen, back, or legs. This occurs once the cancer has metastasized, or spread to other organs.

## CALL YOUR DOCTOR IF:

- you experience abnormal vaginal bleeding or discharge. Abnormal bleeding is not a symptom of menopause and should not be construed as such. It should be brought to your doctor's attention immediately. Uterine cancer usually doesn't occur before menopause, but it can appear around the time menopause begins.

In women of childbearing age, the uterine lining —the endometrium—thickens each month and prepares to receive a fertilized egg. If no egg is fertilized, the extra layers of tissue and blood are shed and expelled through menstruation. Various conditions—benign and malignant—can affect the uterus. Fibroid tumors on the uterine wall are benign, not precancerous, and women who have them are not at increased risk for uterine cancer. Endometrial hyperplasia is the most serious benign uterine condition, and in some women it evolves into uterine cancer. *(See Endometriosis.)*

Most uterine cancers arise in the endometrium and are called **endometrial cancer** or **endometrial carcinoma.** The more aggressive **uterine sarcoma** arises in the muscular wall of the uterus and accounts for less than 5 percent of all cases. (Only endometrial cancer is addressed here.) If left untreated, endometrial cancer can penetrate the uterine wall and invade the bladder or rectum, or it can spread to the vagina, fallopian tubes, ovaries, and more distant organs. Fortunately, endometrial cancer grows slowly and usually is detected before spreading very far. Of the 32,000 American women diagnosed annually with this cancer, more than 80 percent will be cured.

## CAUSES

High-risk candidates for uterine cancer include postmenopausal women who began menstruating early; went through menopause late; suffer from obesity, diabetes, or high blood pressure; have few or no children; or have a history of infertility, irregular menstrual periods, or endometrial hyperplasia. Women taking the drug tamoxifen to treat breast cancer are at very slightly increased risk, but women who have taken birth-control pills are only half as likely to develop the disease after menopause as those who have not.

Susceptibility to endometrial cancer is linked to how much the endometrium has been exposed to estrogen "unopposed" by progesterone. The reason is simple: With a high level of cell division, the chance of cancerous cell mutation increases, and while estrogen stimulates cell division, progesterone suppresses it. Modern hormone replacement therapy (HRT) for postmenopausal women utilizes low-dose formulations of estrogen combined with progesterone, which pose minimal risk for endometrial cancer. Nonetheless, women on HRT should be examined regularly for signs of uterine cancer.

### DIAGNOSTIC AND TEST PROCEDURES

Pap smears, which screen for cervical cancer, detect a small number of uterine cancers before symptoms develop. Otherwise, uterine cancer is usually diagnosed by the appearance of symptoms. If a tissue biopsy confirms the diagnosis, imaging tests, blood studies, and ultimately surgery can determine the stage of the disease.

## TREATMENT

Conventional medicine successfully cures most women of uterine cancer. Deciding which treatment to use depends on the stage of the cancer as well as on the patient's age and general health.

**WHERE CANCER DEVELOPS**

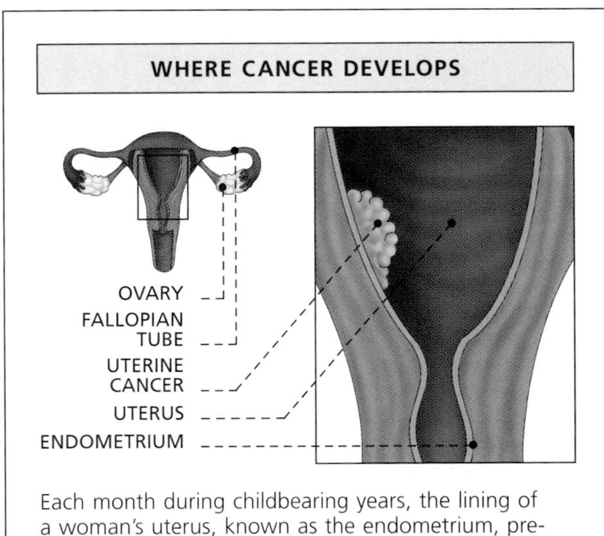


Each month during childbearing years, the lining of a woman's uterus, known as the endometrium, prepares a layer of dense tissue to receive a fertilized egg. If no egg is fertilized, this extra tissue is shed during menstruation. After menopause the endometrial cells are at risk of becoming cancerous *(above, inset)*. Fortunately, most uterine cancers are slow growing and have a high cure rate.

### CONVENTIONAL MEDICINE

Surgery is standard treatment for uterine cancer that has not begun to metastasize, or spread. The preferred treatment for early endometrial cancer is total hysterectomy, in which the uterus, cervix, ovaries, and fallopian tubes are removed. This extensive surgery may be enough to cure early cancer and is most likely to deter recurrence. If the disease has begun to spread beyond the uterus, the patient is given radiation therapy after surgery, in the hope of wiping out the remaining cancer cells. Some doctors also recommend radiation when the cancer has not spread but is already large.

Patients with widespread (metastatic) uterine cancer usually receive hormone therapy to slow the cancer's growth. Chemotherapy or radiation might also be given to reduce the size and number of metastatic tumors. Such treatment is rarely curative but can prolong life and relieve symptoms. If it successfully destroys distant tumors, and the cancer is confined to the urogenital organs, surgery may then be performed.

Patients in remission need checkups every few months for several years. If cancer recurs, it usually happens within three years. Caught early, recurrent cancer may be cured with aggressive radiation therapy or further surgery. *(See Cancer for more information on treatments.)*

### COMPLEMENTARY THERAPIES

To help cope with the emotional difficulties of having uterine cancer, patients might consider joining a support group. Counseling is especially beneficial for premenopausal women who become depressed after a hysterectomy, knowing that they can no longer bear children.

## PREVENTION

Have a Pap smear and pelvic exam annually. If you are of childbearing age, discuss the pros and cons of taking birth-control pills with your doctor. At any age, it pays to control your weight and fitness through exercise and a low-fat diet. ■

# UTERINE PROBLEMS

## SYMPTOMS

- heavy, prolonged, or irregular bleeding, with pain in the lower abdomen or back, which may indicate **fibroids** (benign uterine tumors).
- difficulty urinating and moving bowels, urine leaks when you laugh or cough, backaches; you may have a **prolapsed uterus.**
- bleeding between periods or bleeding after menopause, which may sometimes indicate uterine cancer.
- chronic, abnormal premenopausal bleeding, known as **dysfunctional uterine bleeding.**

## CALL YOUR DOCTOR IF:

- you feel a sharp or chronic pain low in the abdomen. You may have **fibroids** or another serious pelvic disorder such as acute pelvic inflammatory disease or endometriosis. **Call your doctor now.**
- your periods are excessively heavy. This may lead to anemia and may also be symptomatic of **fibroids, dysfunctional uterine bleeding,** uterine cancer, or other uterine problems.

The uterus is a muscular, hollow, pear-shaped organ located in the pelvic cavity behind the bladder and in front of the rectum. The lower portion narrows into the cervical opening, which leads to the vagina. The fallopian tubes are attached on either side of the upper portion of the uterus. The uterus is lined with a mucous membrane called the endometrium, whose state changes with the phases of the menstrual cycle. During normal reproduction a fertilized egg implants itself in the wall of the uterus. It is here that the embryo develops into the fetus, which grows and is nourished until birth.

Normally, the uterus is tipped forward somewhat, but in 20 percent of women it is retroverted (inclined backward). Usually this normal variation in the position of the uterus is present at birth, but changes may be caused by tumors, pelvic inflammatory disease, or endometriosis. A retroverted uterus is usually harmless.

Abnormal endometrial bleeding is referred to as **dysfunctional uterine bleeding.** Such bleeding, which occurs as menorrhagia (heavy menstruation or bleeding longer than 8 days), metrorrhagia (bleeding between periods), or chronic polymenorrhea (a cycle that is less than 18 days), may cause iron deficiency anemia.

A **prolapsed uterus** occurs when the uterus descends from its normal position in the lower abdomen. In severe cases the uterus is visible through the vulva. The disorder is most common in middle-aged women who have had children weighing more than eight pounds at birth, but it may also occur in childless women. In recent years incidents of uterine prolapse have become rarer because women are having fewer children.

Occurring specifically in or on the uterus, **fibroids** are benign tumors, or growths of the muscles and fibrous tissue. Fibroids vary in size, usually grow slowly, and may occur inside the uterus, within the uterine wall, or on the outside surface of the uterus. They occur in more than 20 percent of women over 35 years old. For unknown reasons fibroids are more common in African American women.

Although they are usually not problematic, fibroids may cause enlargement and distortion of the uterus and make it difficult to become preg-

U

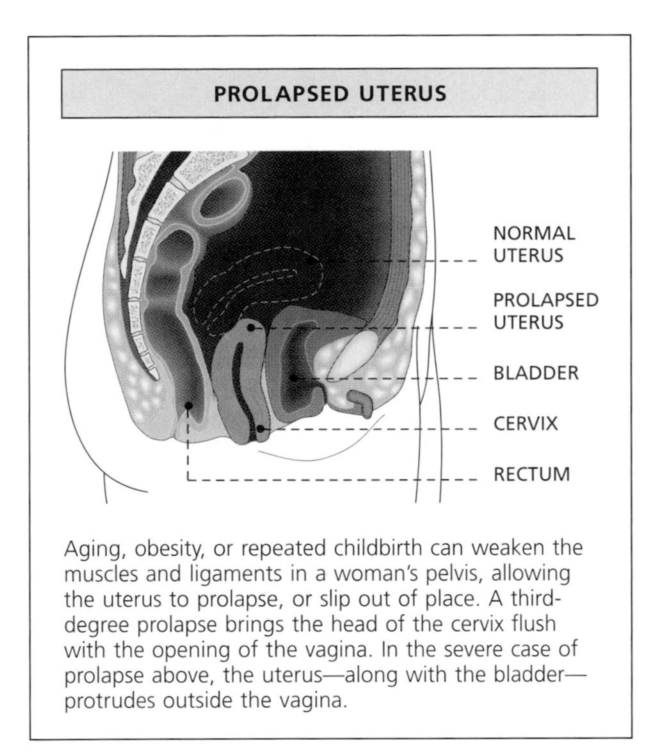


Aging, obesity, or repeated childbirth can weaken the muscles and ligaments in a woman's pelvis, allowing the uterus to prolapse, or slip out of place. A third-degree prolapse brings the head of the cervix flush with the opening of the vagina. In the severe case of prolapse above, the uterus—along with the bladder—protrudes outside the vagina.

nant. Sometimes a fibroid attached to the uterine wall may become twisted or may outgrow its blood supply, causing it to be starved for blood and oxygen. When this happens, you may suddenly feel a sharp pain in your abdomen. See your physician without delay to have this fibroid tumor removed.

Fibroids may cause bladder or bowel pressure or make intercourse painful for you. If they cause your period to become excessively heavy, you could develop anemia. Often, however, there are no symptoms at all. Because fibroids are affected by hormones, they have a tendency to enlarge during pregnancy and, if you are not undergoing estrogen replacement therapy, shrink after menopause.

## CAUSES

Although the cause of **fibroids** is not known, their growth is related to hormones. Because of this, oral contraceptives, estrogen replacement therapy, and pregnancy may cause fibroids to grow and expand.

**Dysfunctional uterine bleeding** occurs when unchecked estrogen stimulation occurs in the endometrium. Several disorders that are characterized by high estrogen levels, including ovarian tumors, obesity, and anovulation (suppressed ovulation) in women in their late thirties and forties, may cause dysfunctional uterine bleeding.

The most common cause of a **prolapsed uterus** is the stretching of the support ligaments that hold it in place. Such stretching often occurs in childbirth. Being overweight may also contribute to and possibly exacerbate the condition.

For more information on the causes and treatment of uterine cancer, see Uterine Cancer.

### DIAGNOSTIC AND TEST PROCEDURES

Often, **fibroids** are brought to your attention only when your physician feels them during a routine pelvic examination. To verify their presence, an ultrasound scan may be performed.

An endometrial biopsy (or, in cases of extremely heavy bleeding, a dilation and curettage) may be performed, which, along with your history, will confirm a diagnosis of **dysfunctional uterine bleeding.**

A **prolapsed uterus** is usually easily identifiable on examination by a physician. A swollen vaginal wall is a telltale sign. During a pelvic exam, when the speculum is inserted, you may be asked to cough, allowing your physician to see the uterus prolapse.

## TREATMENT

Formerly, a physician's all-purpose treatment for uterine disorders was to perform a hysterectomy, but with advances in medicine and growing interest in women's health issues, many other treatment options, both conventional and alternative, are now available.

### CONVENTIONAL MEDICINE

Treatment for **fibroids** varies and should be approached according to your specific medical situation. This is very important because a hysterectomy—removal of the uterus—is commonly recommended to women with fibroids but may not be necessary. If your fibroids are not causing you any problems, you may want to consider doing nothing. Not all fibroids grow. Even large fibroids may not cause any symptoms, and most fibroids shrink after menopause. But you should monitor their growth by having an examination every six months.

To help prevent further fibroid growth, your physician may recommend that you stop taking oral contraceptives or abandon any hormone replacement therapy programs, both of which supply the body with synthetic estrogen. Gonadotropin releasing hormone (GnRH) agonists may be prescribed to shrink fibroids as presurgical treatment, but these drugs are expensive and should not be taken for more than six months to avoid the risk of developing osteoporosis. Also, GnRH agonists may cause early symptoms of menopause, and once use of the drug is stopped, the fibroids are likely to return.

Fibroids may be removed surgically in a procedure known as a myomectomy. Unless your growths are causing severe abdominal pain or you want to have more children, this major surgical procedure is usually not recommended. In 10 to 30 percent of cases the fibroids have been shown to return within five years after a myomectomy is performed.

In most women who suffer from **dysfunctional uterine bleeding**, birth-control pills, which contain hormones, may be prescribed to regulate the menstrual cycle. This treatment does not cure the physical disorder, but it is a comfortable way of eliminating your symptoms and at your physician's discretion may be used up until menopause. Progestins or gonadotropin releasing hormones (GnRH) may also be prescribed to control bleeding, but they take more than 30 days to show any effect and have many side effects.

A hysterectomy may be offered as treatment for severe uterine problems, including uncontrollable heavy bleeding and constant pain or frequent urination caused by fibroids pushing against your bladder.

A procedure known as an endometrial ablation controls bleeding by destroying the endometrium with lasers. Endometrial ablation is a viable alternative to a hysterectomy because it is less invasive.

A vaginal hysterectomy, in which the uterus is removed through the vagina, may be necessary if your **prolapsed uterus** is so displaced that it projects beyond the vulva.

If you prefer not to have surgery, your physician may insert into the vagina a plastic device known as a pessary, which sits in the vagina like a diaphragm to hold the uterus in place. Although a pessary will help support the uterus, it must be replaced every three to six months and is thus not a long-term solution.

## ALTERNATIVE CHOICES

Many of these alternative therapies will ease the symptoms of your uterine disorder, but use them only as a complement to conventional treatment.

### ACUPRESSURE

Cramps that sometimes accompany the menstrual flow and **fibroids** may be treated with a kind of "first aid" acupressure that focuses on specific pressure points for temporary relief of pain. Beneficial points include Spleen 6, Spleen 8, Liver 3, and Conception Vessel 4. See pages 22–23 for point locations.

### BODY WORK

**Massage** and **t'ai chi** may increase energy flow to the pelvis, which may help shrink fibroids.

### HERBAL THERAPIES

Combine equal amounts of the tinctures of blue cohosh *(Caulophyllum thalictroides)*, black cohosh *(Cimicifuga racemosa)*, and chaste tree *(Vitex agnus-castus)*. Take ½ tsp of this mixture three times a day as a tonic thought to improve the vitality of your uterus. For cramping, add 1 part wild yam *(Dioscorea villosa)* to the mixture.

### HOMEOPATHY

Seek treatment from a professional homeopath. Pulsatilla, Belladonna, Sabina, and Sepia are among the remedies that may be prescribed for your uterine disorder.

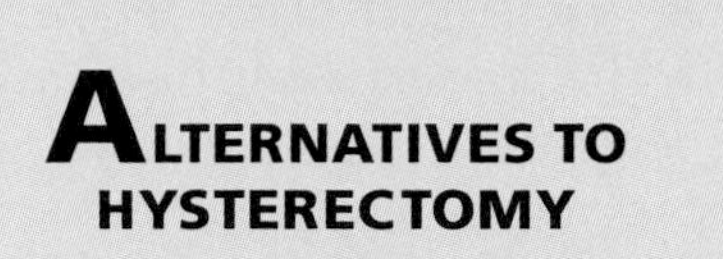

### ALTERNATIVES TO HYSTERECTOMY

*A hysterectomy has traditionally been the indicated treatment for uterine problems, but this procedure is usually necessary only in extreme conditions. The following are alternative choices you should discuss with your physician.*

***For fibroids:***

- *gonadotropin releasing hormone (GnRH) agonist therapy, which shrinks fibroids.*
- *myomectomy, a surgical procedure to remove fibroids; will control bleeding and symptoms of pressure.*

***For prolapsed uterus:***

- *pelvic floor exercises to strengthen the muscles that support the uterus.*
- *a pessary, a plastic device inserted in the vagina to hold the uterus in place.*

***For dysfunctional uterine bleeding:***

- *GnRH therapy and progestins, which may control bleeding.*
- *endometrial ablation, a procedure in which lasers are used to destroy the endometrium to control bleeding.*

#### LIFESTYLE

If heavy bleeding is symptomatic of your **fibroids,** you should try to lighten your daily routine and get more rest during your period.

#### NUTRITION AND DIET

Increasing fiber intake and reducing fat intake will lessen your estrogen production and restore hormone balance, which may effectively combat fibroid growth. Incorporating more vitamin C, bioflavonoids—found in citrus fruits, red onions, and leafy vegetables—and vitamins A and E may also be effective against fibroid growth. A high-fiber diet in the case of a **prolapsed uterus** or **fibroids** will ease difficulty with moving your bowels.

Multivitamin and mineral supplements, along with a high-fiber, low-fat diet that includes vegetables and whole-grain products, may help balance hormone levels that may contribute to uterine problems.

#### AT-HOME REMEDIES

When **fibroids** occur on the outside of the uterus (subserous fibroids), you may become aware of a mass on your abdomen. Lying down and placing a hot pack or hot-water bottle on the lower abdomen lessens pain. The hot packs should be applied three times a week for at least 60 minutes each time. Pelvic floor exercises (also known as Kegel exercises) to strengthen the uterine-support ligaments and to control urination are frequently recommended by physicians to help hold your **prolapsed uterus** in place. You can learn to exercise these muscles by stopping and starting your urine flow. Once you are familiar with the targeted muscles, practice tightening and relaxing them. Initially, 5 sets of the exercises are recommended, 10 times a day. At your own pace you may graduate to 10 sets, 10 times a day.

## PREVENTION

Generally, uterine disorders are not caused by anything in particular that can be avoided. They are, however, closely related to estrogen levels and the phases, or malfunctions, of the menstrual cycle. While maintaining a low-fat, high-fiber diet, getting plenty of rest, and avoiding stress will not render you completely immune to uterine disorders, they are a step in the right direction.■

# VAGINAL PROBLEMS

## SYMPTOMS

- your vulva is inflamed and itches; you may have **vulvitis.**
- the skin of the vulva is thick and has developed white patches; this may indicate a condition called lichen sclerosis or cancer of the vulva. See your doctor for diagnosis.
- increased vaginal discharge with an offensive odor and burning, itching, and pain; you may have **vaginitis.**
- you have been sexually or psychologically abused and experience muscle constriction and pain at any attempt to penetrate the vagina; you may have **vaginismus.**
- an abnormal discharge, bleeding, and/or a firm lesion on any part of the vagina; you may have **vaginal cancer.** *(See Cancer, Cervical Cancer, or Uterine Cancer.)*

## CALL YOUR DOCTOR IF:

- your bleeding is not caused by menstruation. If you are taking oral contraceptives, it may only be breakthrough bleeding. Otherwise, you may have dysfunctional uterine bleeding. *(See Uterine Problems.)* If you are pregnant, there may be a complication in the pregnancy. Postmenopausal bleeding sometimes indicates uterine cancer.
- you have lower-abdominal pain along with fever, menstrual disturbances, abnormal discharge, and/or painful sex. You may have a pelvic infection.
- you use tampons, a diaphragm, or a contraceptive sponge and you develop a high fever or rash. You may have toxic shock syndrome.

The vagina is the part of the female reproductive system that connects the cervix (the entrance to the uterus) with the vulva, the skin folds that enclose the urethral and vaginal openings. This passage, composed of elastic, muscular walls, is lubricated by its own secretions and by mucus-producing glands in the cervix.

The vagina is self-cleaning. As the secretions, or discharge, flow downward, dead cells and other substances are flushed out. The amount and nature of your vaginal discharge will vary at different stages of your menstrual cycle, but some discharge is almost always present. A normal vaginal discharge is clear or white.

**Vaginitis** is an umbrella term meaning inflammation of the vagina. Yeast causes vaginal yeast infections, which are the most common form of the disorder. Other vaginal infections include **bacterial vaginosis** and sexually transmitted diseases such as gonorrhea, trichomoniasis, and chlamydia. Itching, irritation, an abnormal discharge, and inflammation may accompany these disorders. Vaginal infections are very common and treatable.

**Bacterial vaginosis** commonly occurs in the reproductive years. For unknown reasons there may be a change in the balance of naturally occurring bacteria in the vagina that allows disease-causing bacteria to dominate. The predominant sign of this condition is a fishy-smelling discharge, but many women with this infection exhibit no symptoms, which is also true for chlamydia and gonorrhea. To safeguard yourself, you should be routinely tested during your regular gynecological exam.

Overgrowth of fungal yeast cells may also upset your vagina's chemical balance. The result is a vaginal yeast infection, which is generally characterized by itching and soreness and may also produce a white, cottage-cheese-like discharge. Yeast infections are more likely to develop in women who are diabetic, on birth-control pills or antibiotics, or pregnant, but an estimated 75 percent of all women will have a yeast infection at least once in their lifetime. Many will suffer from recurring yeast infections, which are most frequent between the ages of 16 and 35. Vaginal yeast infections may cause pain during

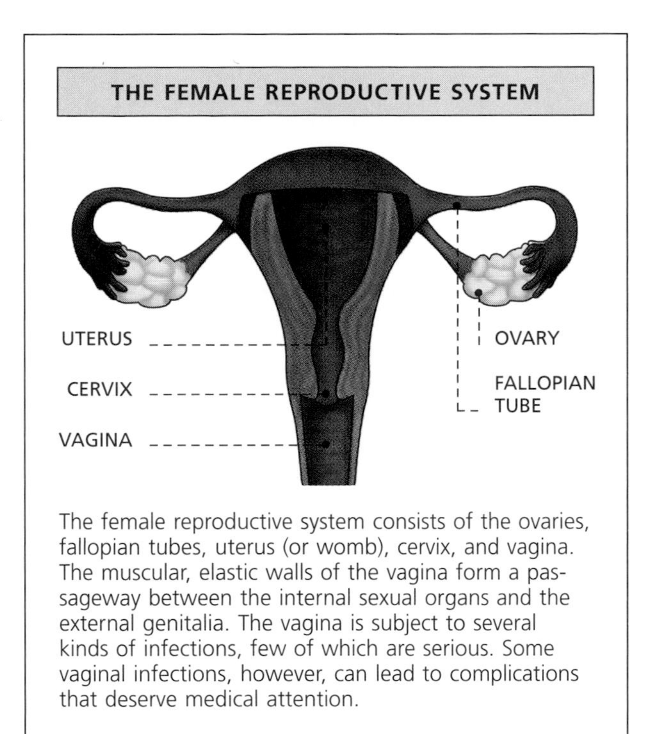


The female reproductive system consists of the ovaries, fallopian tubes, uterus (or womb), cervix, and vagina. The muscular, elastic walls of the vagina form a passageway between the internal sexual organs and the external genitalia. The vagina is subject to several kinds of infections, few of which are serious. Some vaginal infections, however, can lead to complications that deserve medical attention.

urination or during sexual intercourse or both.

Vaginal infections are generally not serious; but, while vaginal yeast infections primarily cause discomfort and annoyance, sexually transmitted infections such as gonorrhea and chlamydia have been found to be associated with an increased risk for pelvic inflammatory disease or other complications. Because of the vulva's proximity to the vagina, **vulvitis** often accompanies vaginitis and the inflammation is usually caused by the same organisms.

Vaginal cancer, accounting for only 2 percent of all gynecological cancers, occurs primarily in women over the age of 50. The severity of vaginal cancer depends on its type and exact location. Varieties include squamous cell carcinoma and clear cell adenocarcinoma. Once cancer appears on the vagina, it may spread to surrounding tissues, including the bladder, rectum, vulva, and pubic bone.

The involuntary constriction of the lower-vaginal muscles is called **vaginismus.** Vaginismus is a sexually related psychological disorder. The spasming of the muscles may be painful, and it interferes with penile penetration or the insertion of other objects such as a speculum or tampon. Sufferers of this disorder usually fear sexual intercourse and associate it with pain.

## CAUSES

**Bacterial vaginosis** is primarily caused by *Gardnerella vaginalis* or *Mobiluncus* dominating the vaginal flora, but several other bacteria may also cause the disease. Stress or a new sexual partner may cause a change in the vaginal flora, which makes this infection more likely.

Vaginal yeast infections are caused by one of four varieties of the *Candida* fungus. Nearly 80 percent of vaginal yeast infections are caused by overgrowth of *Candida albicans.* This unchecked growth may be caused by a significant change in your diet or the use of corticosteroids or antibiotics prescribed to treat another disorder.

**Vulvitis** may be caused by chemical irritation or an allergic reaction to products such as soaps or douches. A viral, bacterial, or fungal infection, decreasing estrogen levels in menopausal women, or cancer may also lead to the disorder.

**Vaginismus** has psychological origins. It occurs most often after sexual trauma such as incest or rape. Negative conditioning with regard to sexuality may also cause the disorder.

Between the 1940s and 1970s, diethylstilbestrol (DES), a synthetic estrogen, was prescribed for women at high risk of miscarriage. (The drug was later found to be ineffective in preventing miscarriage.) Young women whose mothers took DES during pregnancy have an increased incidence of clear cell adenocarcinoma.

### DIAGNOSTIC AND TEST PROCEDURES

A variety of tests may be ordered to diagnose **vulvitis**. Most cases may be identified with a pelvic exam, but a blood test or tests for sexually transmitted disease, if suspected, may also be administered. If your vulvitis persists, a biopsy to test for malignancy may be a necessary precaution.

If **vaginismus** is suspected, your physician will discuss your sexual history with you, paying special attention to psychological factors. A

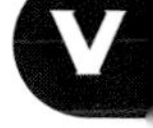

pelvic exam will rule out the possibility of physical disorders and confirm the involuntary constriction of the muscles surrounding the vagina.

Diagnosis of the form of **vaginitis** you may have is made by identifying which organism has caused your infection. This is determined by taking a sample of discharge and viewing it under a microscope. Once you have been diagnosed with a vaginal yeast infection, you can usually recognize the symptoms if it recurs.

The diagnosis of vaginal cancer is usually based on thorough examination with a colposcope and biopsy of any suspicious-looking areas.

## TREATMENT

Whether conventional or alternative, treatment for most vaginal disorders is aimed at maintaining proper bacterial balance and soothing your irritation and discomfort.

### CONVENTIONAL MEDICINE

For postmenopausal cases of **vulvitis** or **bacterial vaginosis** your physician may prescribe antibiotics or estrogen suppositories or topical cream to thicken and lubricate vaginal tissues. For other cases of bacterial vaginosis your physician will prescribe an antibiotic cream such as metronidazole or clindamycin or oral metronidazole. Because an infection commonly passes back and forth between sexual partners, your partner may also need to be treated.

Once your physician diagnoses your vaginal irritation as a vaginal yeast infection, an antifungal drug, such as nystatin, miconazole, or clotrimazole will be prescribed either in a vaginal suppository or as a topical cream. If you suffer from recurring vaginal yeast infections, many over-the-counter treatments are available. These products, which come in vaginal inserts, creams, and suppositories, are, like those prescribed by your physician, either clotrimazole or miconazole.

Because **vaginismus** is of a psychological nature, professional individual and couples' sexual therapy is the best approach.

Cancer can be a life-threatening disease. Your physician's familiarity with your specific case of vaginal cancer will lead to a combination of treatments appropriate for you. In the early stages topical chemotherapy and laser surgery are usually recommended. These treatments are aimed at preserving and maintaining a functional vagina. This is possible, however, only if the condition is caught early. Surgery is primarily recommended when the tumor is extensive. Advanced forms of vaginal cancer are usually treated with radiation therapy. Most cases of vaginal cancer are treated by gynecologists with specialized training in cancer diagnosis and treatment. *(See Cancer for more information on forms of treatment.)*

### ALTERNATIVE CHOICES

The following are supplemental therapies that, along with your physician's prescribed treatment, may ease your recovery.

#### HERBAL THERAPIES

Incorporate fresh garlic *(Allium sativum)* into your diet; it has antibacterial, antifungal, and antiviral properties and may be effective in treating **vaginitis,** including vaginal yeast infections. A fresh, peeled garlic clove wrapped in gauze may be in-

**ATTENTION!**

**PRODUCTS THAT CAN IRRITATE**

**Many women may not be aware that their itching and burning may be caused by irritation from products such as soaps, bath oils and crystals, spermicides, swimming pool chlorine, feminine-hygiene sprays, perfumed douches or lubricants, scented or colored toilet paper, or perfumed pads and tampons. If your physician cannot detect an infection as the cause of your irritation, then an allergy or sensitivity to these commercial products is the likely culprit. Stop using suspect items. Try cool soaks in a tub and add Epsom salt if desired.**

serted in the vagina to help treat **bacterial vaginosis.** This insert should be changed twice daily.

If itching or minor irritation is a symptom of your vaginitis, bathe with an infusion of fresh chickweed *(Stellaria media)* for relief. (Pour 1 cup of boiling water on 1 to 2 tsp of the herb, steep for 5 minutes, and let cool.) To reduce inflammation associated with **vulvitis** and infectious discharge of bacterial vaginosis, an herbal douche may bring relief. To make, pour 1 cup of boiling water over 1 to 2 tsp of calendula *(Calendula officinalis)* and steep for 10 to 15 minutes; let cool before using the tea as a douche.

#### HOMEOPATHY

The following remedies taken three or four times a day for one or two days may be used for minor vaginal problems. A smelly, yellow discharge with severe burning, swelling, and soreness may be treated with Kreosotum (12c); for itching and a white or yellow discharge, Sepia (12c) is recommended; Pulsatilla (12c) may aid in treating a thick, creamy yellow-green discharge. See a professional homeopath if your condition does not clear up.

Many over-the-counter homeopathic mixtures to treat vaginal yeast infections are available under brand names at your local drugstore.

#### LIFESTYLE

If you have recurrent vaginal infections, discontinue use of tampons for six months. In addition, avoid sexual intercourse while your symptoms of vaginal yeast infection or bacterial vaginosis are still apparent.

Wearing cotton panties and avoiding pantyhose and tight clothing will aid in keeping the vagina cool and dry, which may help prevent vulvitis and forms of vaginitis.

#### NUTRITION AND DIET

Monitor your sugar level if you have a vaginal yeast infection. If you are susceptible to these infections, eating yogurt containing active cultures may help to maintain the natural bacterial flora of the vagina.

### AT-HOME REMEDIES

Incorporating *Lactobacillus acidophilus* into your diet may be helpful for treating vaginal yeast infections. A paste can be made from refrigerated capsules, available at health food and nutrition stores. Pour the *Lactobacillus acidophilus* powder into the palm of your hand and add water to create a pasty substance that may be introduced into the vagina using a vaginal applicator or your finger.

Regular sexual intercourse in postmenopausal women may help prevent dryness and thinning of the vaginal walls, which could increase the likelihood of **vaginitis.** The activity stimulates blood flow in the area, which keeps vaginal tissue supple.

Discussing inhibitions with a trained sex therapist may be therapeutic for **vaginismus** sufferers.

Always wipe from front to back to avoid infection from any organisms that may be present in fecal matter.

## PREVENTION

A well-balanced diet always aids in the maintenance of good health. Many women seem to be prone to vaginal infection, while others are rarely affected. Maintaining good hygiene and always using condoms are the best defenses against vaginitis. If you suspect a vaginal infection, do not douche for 24 hours before seeing your physician, as this may wash away secretions that aid in the diagnosis of your disorder.

A true case of **vaginismus** is caused by fear rather than physical abnormality. The best prevention for this disorder is a healthy home environment where sexuality is not made to seem dirty but rather, when appropriate, is discussed in an open, honest, factual manner. If you have suffered sexual abuse or trauma, you should seek professional help. ■

# VARICOSE VEINS

## SYMPTOMS

- prominent dark blue blood vessels, especially in the legs and feet.
- aching, tender, heavy, or sore legs; often accompanied by swelling in the ankles or feet after standing for any length of time.
- Bulging, ropelike, bluish veins indicate **superficial varicose veins.**
- Aching and heaviness in a limb, sometimes with swelling, but without any prominent or visible blue vein, may signal a **deep varicose vein.**
- Discolored, peeling skin; skin ulcers; and constant rather than intermittent pain are signs of **severe varicose veins.**

## CALL YOUR DOCTOR IF:

- swelling becomes incapacitating, or if the skin over your varicose veins becomes flaky, ulcerous, discolored, or prone to bleeding. You may want to have the veins removed to avoid further discomfort and prevent potentially more serious circulatory problems.
- you have red varicose veins. This may be a sign of phlebitis, a serious circulatory condition.
- you cut a varicose vein. Control the resulting burst of blood *(see page 48 in Emergencies)* and have the vein treated to prevent complications.

Varicose veins usually announce themselves as bulging, bluish cords running just beneath the surface of your skin. They can appear anywhere in the body but most often affect legs and feet. Visible swollen and twisted veins—sometimes surrounded by patches of flooded capillaries known as spider-burst veins—are considered **superficial varicose veins.** Although they can be painful and disfiguring, they are usually harmless. When inflamed, they become tender to the touch and can hinder circulation to the point of causing swollen ankles, itchy skin, and aching in the affected limb. *(See also Hemorrhoids.)*

Besides a surface network of veins, your legs have an interior, or deep, venous network. On rare occasions, an interior leg vein becomes varicose. Such **deep varicose veins** are usually not visible, but they can cause swelling or aching throughout the leg. Deep varicose veins may be sites where blood clots can form. Deep vein inflammation, or thrombophlebitis, in the thighs and pelvis may lead to a pulmonary embolism, a potentially fatal condition.

Varicose veins are a relatively common condition, and for many people they are a family trait. Women are at least twice as likely as men to develop them. In the United States alone, nearly 10 percent of all adult men and 20 percent of adult women are affected by them to some degree, bringing the total affecred to more than 20 million people.

## CAUSES

To circulate oxygen-rich blood from the lungs to all parts of the body, your arteries have thick layers of muscle or elastic tissue. To push blood back to your heart, your veins rely mainly on surrounding muscles and a network of one-way valves. As blood flows through a vein, the cuplike valves alternately open to allow blood through, then close to prevent backflow.

Varicosity results from a chronic increase in blood pressure, which dilates the vein. When the vein walls are pushed apart, the valves no longer seal properly, making it difficult for the muscles to push the blood "uphill." Instead of flowing from one valve to the next, the blood begins to pool in the vein, increasing venous pressure and the likelihood of congestion while causing the vein to bulge and twist. Because superficial veins have less muscular support than deep veins, they are more likely to become varicose.

Any condition that puts excessive pressure on the legs or abdomen can lead to varicosity. The most common pressure inducers are pregnancy, obesity, and standing for long periods. Chronic constipation and—in rare cases—tumors also can cause varicose veins. Being sedentary likewise may contribute to varicosity, because muscles that are out of condition offer poor blood-pumping action. The likelihood of varicosity also increases as veins weaken with age. Contrary to popular belief, sitting with crossed legs will not cause varicose veins, although it can aggravate an existing condition.

VALVES IN VEINS

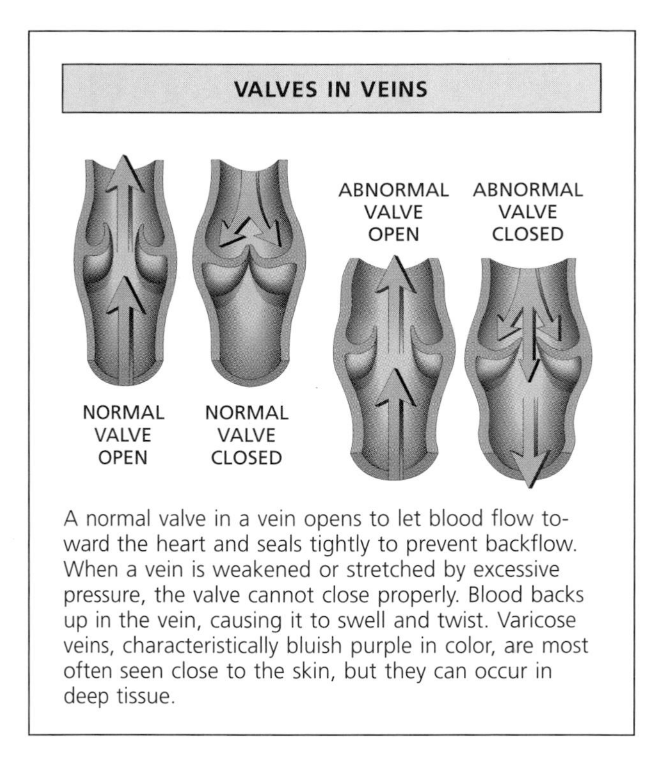


A normal valve in a vein opens to let blood flow toward the heart and seals tightly to prevent backflow. When a vein is weakened or stretched by excessive pressure, the valve cannot close properly. Blood backs up in the vein, causing it to swell and twist. Varicose veins, characteristically bluish purple in color, are most often seen close to the skin, but they can occur in deep tissue.

## TREATMENT

A mild case of varicose veins does not usually require a doctor's care. You can find relief from the discomfort of varicose veins with basic at-home treatment and various alternative remedies.

### CONVENTIONAL MEDICINE

**Superficial varicose veins** normally do not require medical attention, but they should not be ignored. To relieve the discomfort, your doctor may recommend elastic support stockings, which you can buy in most pharmacies and medical supply stores. Support stockings help your leg muscles push blood upward by concentrating pressure near the ankles. Put them on before you get out of bed in the morning. Raise your legs in the air and pull the stockings on evenly; they should not feel tight in the calf or groin. You should wear them all day.

To alleviate occasional swelling and pain, your doctor will probably suggest an over-the-counter anti-inflammatory drug such as aspirin or ibuprofen. If you notice skin around a varicose vein becoming ulcerous or discolored, or if you have continuing pain with no obvious outward signs, contact a doctor at once about the possibility of **deep varicose veins.**

Varicose veins can be eliminated by one of several methods. Spider veins can be removed quite simply through laser treatment. A mild case of **superficial varicose veins** can be treated by sclerotherapy: A chemical known as a sclerosing agent is injected into the vein to collapse its walls so it can no longer transport blood. More severe cases may merit surgical removal, or stripping. Unfortunately, no treatment can prevent new veins from becoming varicose. Before pursuing a particular treatment, discuss all options with a dermatologist or vascular surgeon.

### ALTERNATIVE CHOICES

To cope with varicose veins, try a two-pronged strategy of natural remedies to ease the discomfort and preventive maintenance to keep your body fit and strong.

#### AROMATHERAPY

With numerous oils to choose from, you can tailor aromatherapy to your particular needs. Oil of rosemary *(Rosmarinus officinalis)* massaged gently into an affected area may help stimulate circulation by causing capillaries to dilate. Oils of cypress and chamomile *(Matricaria recutita)* may soothe swelling and inflammation and help relieve pain.

#### BODY WORK

Regular **massage** can significantly alleviate discomfort associated with varicose veins. A trained massage therapist starts at the feet and massages your legs up to the hips and along the lymphatic system, to mobilize congested body tissues. Other techniques, such as **reflexology** and **acupressure,** may also prove helpful in alleviating symptoms of varicose veins.

#### CHIROPRACTIC

To treat varicose veins, chiropractic medicine combines diet and lifestyle therapy with physical manipulation of the skeletal system. Manipulation to relieve strain on the pelvis, for example, is intended to improve the flow of blood and other fluids through the body.

#### HERBAL THERAPIES

Many herbs have long histories of folk use in the treatment of varicose veins, and some have undergone extensive scientific study. Ginkgo *(Ginkgo biloba),* hawthorn *(Crataegus laevigata),* and bilberry *(Vaccinium myrtillus)* are all reported to strengthen blood vessels and improve peripheral circulation. Tinctures or topical ointments of horse chestnut *(Aesculus hippocastanum)* and butcher's-broom *(Ruscus aculeatus)* are also recommended for toning veins while reducing inflammation; butcher's-broom can also be prepared as tea.

For skin irritation associated with varicose veins, try a lotion made of distilled witch hazel *(Hamamelis virginiana).* To disperse buildup of a protein called fibrin that makes skin near varicose veins hard and lumpy, try eating more cayenne *(Capsicum frutescens),* garlic *(Allium sativum),* onion, ginger *(Zingiber officinale),* and pineapple, which contains bromelain, an enzyme that promotes breakup of fibrin.

#### HOMEOPATHY

For long-term treatment of varicose veins, a homeopath may prescribe a constitutional remedy in the potency and dosage best suited to your symptoms. Pulsatilla is one remedy that is commonly prescribed.

For immediate relief from specific symptoms, you can try over-the-counter homeopathic remedies: Hamamelis, or witch hazel, cream in a 6x to 15c solution applied to an area that is bluish and perhaps bruised may relieve soreness. Hamamelis 6x to 15c can also be taken internally as directed on the label for general relief. Belladonna, 12x or 12c potency four times a day, is recommended for red, hot, swollen, and tender varicose veins.

#### HYDROTHERAPY

Sponging or spraying legs with cold water can relieve aches and pain from **superficial varicose veins.** Hot and cold baths may slow the progression of varicose veins on the feet and ankles: Dip your feet in warm water for 1 to 2 minutes, then cold water for half a minute, and alternate for 15 minutes. You might even add an aromatherapy oil to the water.

#### LIFESTYLE

Maintaining your overall fitness—both nutritionally and physically—is most essential to preventing varicose veins from developing. Aerobic exercise totaling 30 minutes a day several times a week will help you keep your weight down while toning and strengthening veins. You might start your morning with a brisk walk, for example, or finish your day with a swim or bike ride.

If you already have varicose veins, you can help control them with a program of specially designed exercises, preferably under the direction of a trained exercise therapist attuned to the condition's particular needs.

#### MIND/BODY MEDICINE

**Yoga**'s stretching and relaxation techniques can be particularly beneficial for varicose veins. Certain positions, such as the Plow, Corpse, and Half Shoulder Stand, promote circulation and the drainage of blood from the legs. The deep-breath-

## Switch Your Bed

*Varicose vein sufferers are told to elevate their feet when resting or sleeping. But before you rush to the bedroom armed with pillows and bricks—or start building a makeshift ramp at the end of your bed—consider changing the bed itself. By switching to a hospital-style adjustable bed, you can keep your feet raised all through the night, and you'll have the added benefit of low back pain relief. Another option—perhaps more attractive to the home decorator—is a well-designed waterbed. Waterbeds adapt their contour to fit your body, minimizing the discomfort to tender veins where they come in contact with the mattress.*

ing exercises you learn to practice in yoga may further alleviate discomfort by getting more oxygen into the bloodstream.

#### NUTRITION AND DIET

Diet plays a critical role in any varicose vein treatment program. Your goals are to promote better circulation and keep weight in check. Extra body fat increases water retention and puts pressure on the legs and abdomen, aggravating varicosity. To decrease body fat, eat foods that are low in fat, sugar, and salt, and high in fiber. To promote a healthy flow of nutrients and waste through the body, make fruits, vegetables, and whole grains the mainstays of your diet, and drink plenty of fluids, especially water.

Certain vitamins and bioflavonoids—natural substances found in many fruits and vegetables—may improve varicose veins; try 500 mg of vitamin C and 400 IU of vitamin E daily. Bioflavonoids are beneficial because they promote the absorption of vitamin E. Among bioflavonoids, rutin is used routinely to treat varicose veins. It is present in many foods, including citrus fruits, apricots, blueberries, blackberries, cherries, rose hips, and buckwheat. A lesser-known bioflavonoid, quercetin, suggests promise in treating varicose veins. You can now buy bioflavonoids as nutritional supplements.

#### AT-HOME REMEDIES

You can minimize the discomfort of varicose veins in your legs. To ease painful swelling and inflammation, rest frequently, wear support stockings, and take one or two aspirin or ibuprofen tablets daily until the condition clears. If you like to sit with your legs crossed, cross them at the ankles rather than the knees for better circulation. Better yet, take a break and put your feet up; periods of rest with your feet a few inches above your heart level let gravity work in your favor, helping pooled blood drain from your legs. To further improve circulation, women should avoid high heels in favor of flat shoes and should wear loose clothing.

## PREVENTION

- Exercise regularly! Staying fit is the best way to keep your leg muscles toned, your blood flowing, and your weight under control.
- Eat foods low in fat, sugar, and salt. Drink plenty of water. Take supplements of vitamins C and E, both critical to blood-vessel health.
- If your daily routine requires you to be on your feet constantly, stretch and exercise your legs as often as possible to increase circulation and reduce pressure buildup.
- If you smoke, quit. Studies show that smoking may contribute to elevated blood pressure, which in turn can aggravate varicosity.
- If you're pregnant, be sure to sleep on your left side rather than on your back to minimize pressure from the uterus on the veins in your pelvic area. This position will also improve blood flow to the fetus. ■

# VISION PROBLEMS

## SYMPTOMS

- Blurred vision when you are looking at distant objects indicates that you are **nearsighted,** or myopic.
- Blurred vision when you are looking at objects nearby indicates that you are **farsighted,** or hyperopic.
- Vertical or horizontal lines that appear blurry or irregular indicate **astigmatism.**
- Flashing-light sensations, tiny objects floating in your eyes, or a sudden loss of central or peripheral vision may indicate **retinal detachment.**
- Difficulty distinguishing between red and green in dim light is a sign that you are **color-blind.**
- Difficulty distinguishing objects in dim light is a sign of **night blindness.**

For symptoms of other vision ailments, see Cataracts, Eye Problems, Glaucoma, and Macular Degeneration.

## CALL YOUR DOCTOR IF:

- you experience symptoms of **retinal detachment;** you need immediate medical treatment to prevent potential blindness.
- you become unusually sensitive to bright light; you may have an inflamed iris.
- you have a foreign object in your eye that will not flush out with water; you risk scarring or infecting the eye.
- your contact lenses become uncomfortable; you may have an infection, abrasion, or foreign body in the eye.
- a cut or blow to your eye affects your vision; you may have internal bleeding or a fracture of the bone around your eye.

Your eyes are your body's most highly developed sensory organs. In fact, a far larger part of your brain is dedicated to the functions of eyesight than to those of hearing, taste, touch, or smell. We tend to take eyesight for granted, yet when vision problems develop, most of us will do everything in our power to restore our eyesight to normal.

The most common forms of vision impairment are errors of refraction—the way light rays are bent inside the eye so images can be transmitted to the brain. **Nearsightedness, farsightedness,** and **astigmatism** are examples of refraction disorders. **Retinal detachment, color blindness,** and **night blindness** are systemic disorders of the eye that lead to distorted or inaccurate vision. Cataracts, conjunctivitis, glaucoma, and macular degeneration are other diseases of the eye that respond in varying degrees to medical treatment.

## CAUSES

**Nearsightedness** and **farsightedness** have to do with the way the eye brings images into focus on the back of the eyeball, where 10 layers of light-sensitive nerve tissue make up the retina. **Nearsightedness,** or myopia, which affects about 20 percent of the population, is the result of images being focused in front of the retina rather than on it *(right),* so distant objects appear blurred. A nearsighted person holds a book close to the eyes when reading and has to sit in the front of the classroom or movie theater to see clearly. The condition runs in families and affects men and women equally, usually appearing in childhood and stabilizing in the twenties.

**Farsightedness,** or hyperopia, is the opposite of nearsightedness: The lens of the eye focuses images slightly behind the retina, making nearby objects appear blurry. Children often overcome mild farsightedness through a natural process called accommodation: As the eye grows, the eye muscles contract, bringing the focal point forward onto the retina. With age, the eye's natural ability to accommodate tends to diminish.

**Astigmatism,** often associated with near- or farsightedness, occurs when the eye lacks a sin-

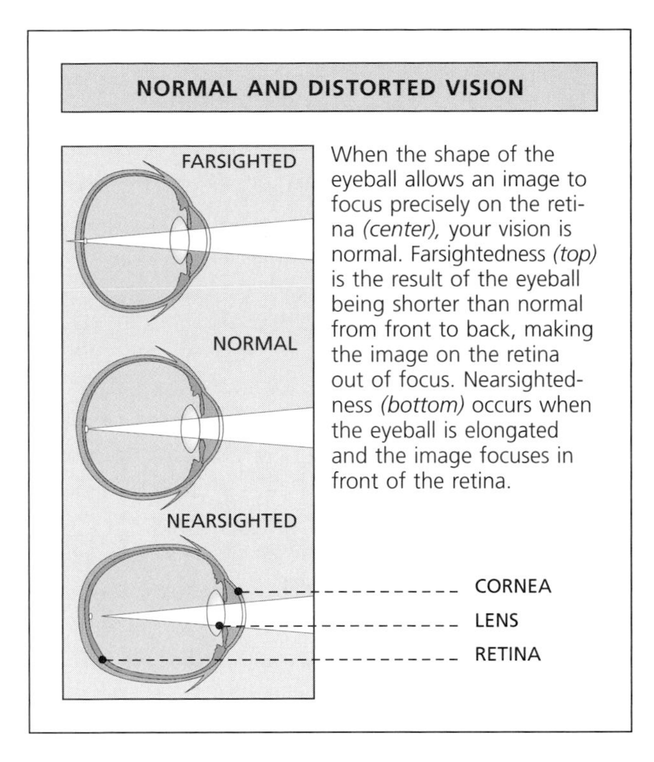

When the shape of the eyeball allows an image to focus precisely on the retina *(center)*, your vision is normal. Farsightedness *(top)* is the result of the eyeball being shorter than normal from front to back, making the image on the retina out of focus. Nearsightedness *(bottom)* occurs when the eyeball is elongated and the image focuses in front of the retina.

gle point of focus. The condition is a result of an uneven curvature of the cornea or, in some cases, an abnormality in the lens. People with astigmatism have a random, inconsistent vision pattern, in which some objects appear clear and others blurry. Astigmatism is usually present from birth and neither improves nor worsens over time.

**Presbyopia** is blurred vision at normal reading distance. It typically starts at about age 40 and is the reason many older people use glasses.

**Retinal detachment** occurs when a part of a retinal layer is pulled out of place, or when a hole or tear occurs. Although a detached retina is not painful, it is definitely a medical emergency. If the retina is not reattached to its source of nutrients promptly, the cells die and blindness can result. Risk factors for the condition include nearsightedness, previous eye surgery or injury, and congenital thinness of retinal tissue.

**Color blindness** is a disorder of the retina's light-sensitive cone cells, which respond to colors. Most people with color blindness see colors normally in bright light but have difficulty distinguishing reds and greens in dim light. Color blindness occurs mostly in men, afflicting 8 percent of the male population. It is extremely rare for someone to be totally color-blind—that is, able to see only shades of gray.

**Night blindness**—difficulty seeing in dim light—occurs when the retina's rod cells, which distinguish light from dark, begin to deteriorate. The precise cause is unclear, but it may be linked to a liver disorder, a vitamin-A deficiency, or a disease of the retina, such as retinitis pigmentosa, an inherited disorder.

**Eyestrain** does not affect your vision, but it accompanies some vision disorders and may bring on a headache. It is often the result of eye muscles becoming strained from holding the same focus too long. If you wear prescriptive lenses, eyestrain may be an indication that you need new glasses or a different prescription. Eye exercises or resting the eyes every 30 minutes helps relieve eyestrain, especially if you work with computers.

### DIAGNOSTIC AND TEST PROCEDURES

Annual eye examinations by your ophthalmologist are essential to monitor the health of your eyes and diagnose suspected disorders. Checking the external and internal portions of your eye and your eye's movement will reveal crossed eyes or other forms of strabismus *(see Eye Problems).*

A Snellen test employs letters of decreasing size to determine the sharpness of your vision and to detect nearsightedness, farsightedness, and astigmatism. An ophthalmologist will examine the cornea using a slitlamp microscope to detect signs of clouding in the lens of the eye, known as a cataract. Examinations with an ophthalmoscope can reveal abnormalities of the retina, macula, and optic nerve.

## TREATMENT

If routine testing indicates that your vision is impaired, conventional treatment calls for wearing corrective glasses or contact lenses, practicing sensible eye care, and, in some cases, having corrective surgery. Almost 60 percent of the population wears corrective lenses, and that number in-

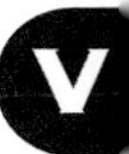

creases dramatically after the age of 65. A far smaller percentage ever need surgery for vision disorders, but those who do benefit from sophisticated, highly successful procedures.

### CONVENTIONAL TREATMENT

Conventional treatment for disorders such as **nearsightedness, farsightedness**, and **astigmatism** depends primarily on corrective prescription lenses. Disorders such as cataracts, macular degeneration, and **retinal detachment** require surgical treatment.

To treat **nearsightedness** your ophthalmologist will usually prescribe lenses to focus visual images correctly on the retina. Normally you have a choice between wearing conventional eyeglasses and contact lenses. As an alternative to corrective lenses, or in severe cases, surgical techniques are used to treat nearsightedness. Radial keratotomy is a surgical procedure in which tiny, spokelike incisions are made in the cornea, flattening the center and focusing images correctly on the retina. Each eye is examined and operated on individually, and success is relatively good. More than three-quarters of those who have had the surgery report corrected or partially corrected vision. The procedure has potential complications, however: Vision may be erratic, the cornea may become infected, and there is some risk of the cornea's rupturing.

Excimer laser treatment may offer results similar to those of radial keratotomy. The laser beam removes microscopic amounts of tissue from the center of the cornea. This effectively flattens the cornea so that light rays focus correctly on the retina.

If **farsightedness** has not accommodated naturally and the disorder persists into adulthood, glasses or contact lenses can be prescribed, but they usually are not necessary until age 40 or older. People typically seek treatment for farsightedness when they begin to complain of eyestrain, especially at the end of the day.

For **astigmatism**, the accepted prescription is a lens that will correct or neutralize the effect of the uneven cornea. You will normally have a choice between glasses and contact lenses.

Some cases of **retinal detachment** can be corrected with laser surgery, which has a high rate of success. If the peeling or tearing of the retina is extensive, additional corrective surgery may be necessary.

### ALTERNATIVE CHOICES

Alternative remedies rely on correcting mineral and vitamin deficiencies that may contribute to vision problems and on relieving the strain of overworked eyes. They can complement medical remedies prescribed by an ophthalmologist to treat your particular vision disorder.

#### ACUPRESSURE

Traditional Chinese relaxation therapy calls on the natural healing powers of your body to soothe overworked eyes, to ease headaches, and to relieve eyestrain from reading or working at a computer for extended periods.

If you are **nearsighted** or **farsighted**, or suffer from **astigmatism,** try the exercises Chinese children use to start the school day:

- Place both thumbs against the upper eye socket next to the bridge of your nose and knead vigorously.
- Pinch the bridge of your nose with your thumb and forefinger, then squeeze repeatedly.
- Using both forefingers, press and knead the bone under your eyes next to your nose.
- Place your forefingers on your temples at the side of your head behind your eyes and knead.

#### HERBAL THERAPIES

A daily 200-mg dose of bilberry *(Vaccinium myrtillus)* is reported to be useful for improving microcirculation, the flow of blood in the vessels of the eye, particularly for people with **night blindness** and **nearsightedness**.

#### HOMEOPATHY

If you develop **eyestrain** and your eyes are sore after a period of close work, the recommended over-the-counter remedy is Ruta in 12x potency, three or four times a day for two days.

#### NUTRITION AND DIET

To help strengthen the retina, people with **night blindness** can take up to 25,000 IU of vitamin A in fish liver oil daily. Zinc, which is found in high concentrations in oysters, may be helpful for night blindness. It is said to aid in adaptation to darkness and to strengthen the retina. Selenium, magnesium, and vitamin C supplements are antioxidants reported to prevent deterioration of the retina, especially in diabetics.

### AT-HOME REMEDIES

When your eyes feel tired or overworked, take time to rest and reinvigorate them. Lie down in a dark room or sit quietly with your eyes covered. To soothe sore eyes and refresh puffy, red eyelids, try this old-fashioned remedy: Put a thick slice of fresh cucumber over each closed eyelid and relax for 15 to 30 minutes.

For itchy or irritated eyes, try a refreshing herbal eyewash. Steep 2 or 3 tsp of chamomile *(Matricaria recutita)* flowers or 1 tsp of dried eyebright *(Euphrasia officinalis)* in a pint of boiling water. Allow the brew to cool and strain out the residue. Put ½ tsp in an eyecup and rinse each eye several times a day.

## PREVENTION

Resting your eyes when they are overworked is the first line of defense against vision problems. Eye exercises and a well-balanced, nutritious diet will help your eyes remain healthy and your vision acute.

Maintenance of your healthy eyesight depends on getting sufficient vitamin A, which plays a key role in the eye's ability to adjust to different degrees of light. To help prevent or postpone vision disorders, you should cut your consumption of refined sugar. If you smoke, stop. Do everything possible to stay away from tobacco smoke, exhaust fumes, and other kinds of polluted air. Finally, do not let yourself get overtired. When your body is rested, your circulation improves and your eyes get the supply of oxygenated blood they need.

### COMMON MYTHS ABOUT YOUR EYES

*Contrary to popular belief, the following activities may temporarily strain your eyes, but they will not impair your vision:*

- *reading in poor light.*
- *reading without your glasses.*
- *wearing the wrong glasses.*
- *working at a computer for long periods of time.*
- *sitting close to a television screen or computer monitor.*

#### EYE EXERCISES TO RELIEVE EYESTRAIN

- When using a computer or doing concentrated activity such as sewing or reading, rest your eyes for 5 minutes at 30-minute intervals. Look away from your work, close your eyes, or simply stare off into space.
- Blink regularly. This action helps prevent evaporation of the tear film that protects the cornea. Blinking also breaks the continuous focus when you have been reading or looking at a computer screen, increasing the amount of concentrated activity you can perform.
- If you are driving for long stretches, alternately focus on the dashboard and a faraway object. Changing the focus periodically will relax your eye muscles and prevent eyestrain.
- Palm your eyes. Sit comfortably, breathe deeply, and cover your eyes with the palms of your hands.
- Breathe deeply for several minutes. Roll your head around with a circular motion while stretching your neck and shoulders, then turn your head from side to side and up and down, repeating several times.
- While yawning, stretch and maneuver the muscles of your face to relieve tension. ■

# VITILIGO

## SYMPTOMS

- White patches of skin are often located symmetrically on both sides of the body; borders of the irregularly shaped spots may be raised.
- Patches can appear at any time, though their appearance is often stress related.
- Patches are most common in exposed areas such as the face, neck, and hands but can emerge anywhere.
- Hair may gray and the whites of the eyes may change color.

## CALL YOUR DOCTOR IF:

- the depigmentation is severe enough to affect your self-esteem and social activities; there are many treatments available that can offset the effects of vitiligo.

As many as two million people in the United States have this disease, which results in white patches on the skin. Sometimes the patches appear symmetrically; for example, you may have almost identical patterns on your right and left index fingers.

The first signs of pigment loss often appear before you reach age 20, and there may be cycles of rapid loss of color followed by little or no change. The dormancy period can last for years.

The progression of the disease varies. One patient might develop a few spots at first and then nothing more happens for years, while another might lose all skin pigmentation in six months. Emotional or physical stress can be contributing factors.

Vitiligo itself does not endanger your health, but it is sometimes associated with thyroid problems, pernicious anemia, Addison's disease (decreased adrenal gland function), and alopecia areata (patches of hair loss). For most patients, however, the greatest risk is loss of self-esteem.

## CAUSES

Doctors don't know what causes vitiligo, though the disease does tend to run in families; up to a third of all patients have a relative who also suffers from the condition. Chemical agents such as phenol (often used as a disinfectant) and catechol (used in dyeing and tanning), as well as emotional and physical stress, may precipitate the onset of vitiligo.

The underlying problem is that cells called melanocytes cease producing melanin, which gives skin its color. There are three prominent theories on why this happens in vitiligo patients: Abnormal nerve cells might injure nearby pigment cells; the body might be destroying its own tissue (an autoimmune response) because it perceives the pigment cells as foreign; or pigment-producing cells might self-destruct (autotoxic response), leaving a toxic residue that destroys new pigment cells. Whatever the cause, the problem is never life-threatening and rarely even a health risk.

## TREATMENT

Most treatments for vitiligo involve drawing more pigmented cells to the skin's surface. A therapy known as psoralen ultraviolet A (PUVA), which combines an oral drug and ultraviolet light, has proved particularly effective, especially for patients in advanced stages of the disease.

Alternative medicine has little to offer for vitiligo patients, since the only way to influence the progression of the disease is to alter the body's production of melanin or to transplant healthier cells to the affected areas. Certain relaxation techniques, however, may prove helpful if you find that stress triggers episodes of depigmentation.

### CONVENTIONAL MEDICINE

There are two basic approaches to treating vitiligo: trying to restore normal pigment, or depigmenting the rest of the skin—which makes the skin very pale but uniform in color. For mild forms of the disease doctors usually start with topical corticosteroids, which have a good record of restoring small patches. In instances where vitiligo has affected more than 20 percent of the body's surface, PUVA treatments are commonly prescribed. At least half of all vitiligo patients regain pigment in most areas with these treatments.

Researchers continue to hunt for alternatives to PUVA therapy because of its many side effects, including liver damage, cataracts and other eye problems, a phototoxic reaction that causes skin blistering, and nausea. Khellin, derived from the roots of the *Ammi visnaga* plant, has proved to be an effective substitute. It does not induce phototoxicity, though at high doses it can cause nausea, dizziness, insomnia, and an increase in liver enzyme levels.

If vitiligo has created patches on more than half of your skin, you might consider having the remaining color removed—a process known as depigmentation. Before you take this step, however, consider that it can take months to years to complete and is irreversible. The drug of choice, a combination of monobenzone and hydroquinone, destroys melanocytes. Potential side effects include contact dermatitis, severe itching, abnormally dry skin, pigment deposits in the cornea, and graying hair.

**RECOGNIZING VITILIGO**

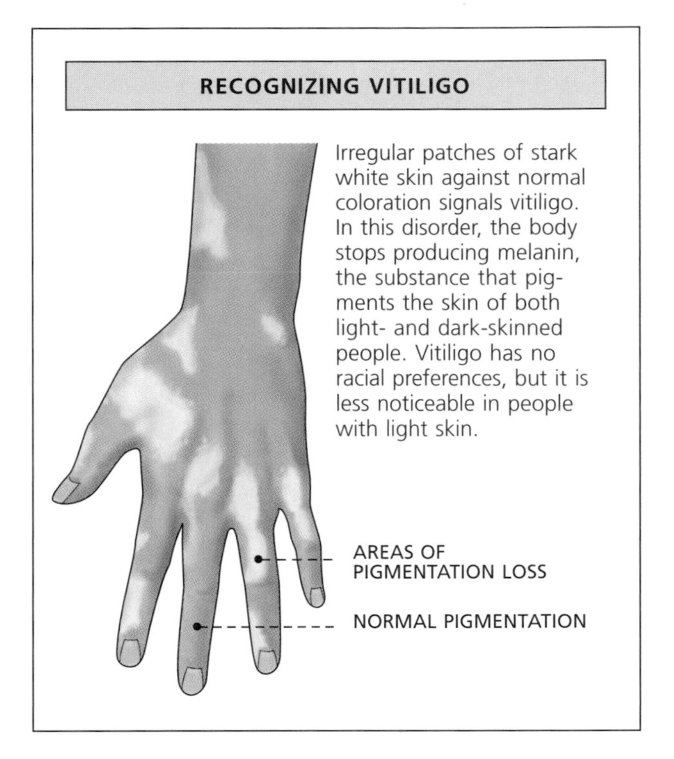


Irregular patches of stark white skin against normal coloration signals vitiligo. In this disorder, the body stops producing melanin, the substance that pigments the skin of both light- and dark-skinned people. Vitiligo has no racial preferences, but it is less noticeable in people with light skin.

### ALTERNATIVE CHOICES

**Homeopathic** therapy is probably the best alternative for vitiligo patients who want to avoid potent conventional medicines. Consult a professional about a homeopathic treatment plan.

To reduce the stress that can aggravate vitiligo, try **mind/body** relaxation techniques such as **guided imagery, yoga,** or **hypnotherapy.**

### AT-HOME REMEDIES

To properly treat vitiligo you must see a doctor. One step you can take at home that might help is to expose patches of affected skin to the sun (while protecting healthy skin with a sunscreen). The ultraviolet radiation from the sun may promote repigmentation. ■

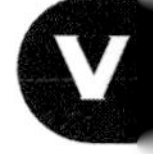

# VOMITING

*Read down this column to find your symptoms. Then read across.*

| SYMPTOMS | AILMENT/PROBLEM |
| --- | --- |
| For other conditions that may involve vomiting, see also Nausea. | |
| ◆ vomiting that appears to be brought on by a specific situation, such as a long car trip or a stressful encounter. | ◆ Motion sickness; anxiety |
| ◆ small amounts of vomiting; burning chest pain (heartburn); difficulty swallowing; shortness of breath. | ◆ Hiatal hernia |
| ◆ vomiting, headache, nausea; symptoms may be worse with exposure to bright light. | ◆ Migraine headache; possibly meningitis |
| ◆ vomiting preceded by intense dizziness, to the extent that everything around you appears to spin; possibly, ringing in your ears. | ◆ Inner ear disorder; possibly Ménière's disease |
| ◆ diarrhea, vomiting, nausea, and fever lasting 48 hours or less, sometimes after you eat rich, spicy, or possibly spoiled foods, drink an excessive amount of alcohol, or ingest a drug you have never taken before. | ◆ Gastroenteritis (also called stomach flu or intestinal flu) |
| ◆ vomiting accompanied by fever, lower abdominal pain, and frequent, malodorous, and/or painful urination. | ◆ Kidney infection |
| ◆ recurrent vomiting accompanied by yellowish skin and/or whites of eyes. | ◆ Jaundice |

| WHAT TO DO | OTHER INFO |
| --- | --- |
| ◆ For motion sickness, ask your doctor about preventive treatment such as antinausea drugs that you can take before you travel. For anxiety, find a relaxation technique—such as yoga—that you're comfortable with and will practice regularly. See also Stress. | ◆ Ginger *(Zingiber officinale)* capsules may alleviate motion sickness, as may acupressure. |
| ◆ See your doctor for an accurate diagnosis. Over-the-counter antacids are often the first line of defense against heartburn; avoiding stomach irritants such as alcohol, tobacco, and caffeine can also help. | |
| ◆ If you suspect meningitis, **call 911 or your emergency number now.** Migraines may respond to various analgesics (over-the-counter and prescription varieties). | ◆ While meningitis requires emergency medical treatment, symptoms of migraine headache may be relieved by a variety of alternative choices. Herbalists often recommend taking a daily 125-mg capsule of feverfew *(Chrysanthemum parthenium)* to prevent migraines. |
| ◆See your doctor. You may need antibiotics to clear up an ear infection. | |
| ◆ Rest, drink plenty of fluids, and eat bland foods. You may need an antibiotic if your stomach bug is the result of a bacterial infection. | ◆ Take care not to let vomiting persist, or your body will lose important fluids and become dehydrated. To prevent dehydration, drink room-temperature beverages such as water, fruit juice, or soda that has been allowed to go flat. |
| ◆ Call your doctor today. You may need prescription antibiotics to treat the infection. | ◆ If you are prone to kidney infections, drinking cranberry juice daily may keep them at bay. Cranberry capsules are also available. |
| ◆ Call your doctor. There are many possible causes of jaundice, and some are serious. | ◆ If your skin is yellow but the whites of your eyes are still white, you likely have carotenemia, not jaundice. Carotenemia is a harmless effect of high levels of the pigment carotene in the body and can be brought on by a diet rich in leafy green vegetables, carrots, and oranges. |

| SYMPTOMS | AILMENT/PROBLEM |
|---|---|
| ◆ vomiting accompanied by severe pain in or around one eye. | ◆ Glaucoma |
| ◆ vomiting, fever, headache, nausea; unusual sleepiness and/or confusion; possibly, staggered walk. | ◆ Meningitis; encephalitis (inflammation of the brain, usually caused by a virus transmitted by mosquitoes); Reye's syndrome (a neurological disorder typically seen in children, which may occur after aspirin has been given for an infection or chickenpox) |
| ◆ nausea and vomiting; whitish bowel movements; dark urine. | ◆ Hepatitis |
| ◆ intense, recurrent abdominal pain that is not relieved by vomiting; loss of appetite. | ◆ Appendicitis; stomach ulcer; possibly stomach cancer |
| ◆ vomit that smells like feces, accompanied by constipation. | ◆ Intestinal obstruction (the intestines are blocked); possibly, colorectal cancer |
| ◆ headache, vomiting, drowsiness, confusion and/or aberrant behavior. | ◆ Possibly, brain cancer or an aneurysm |
| ◆ severe headache that occurs several hours or days after a head injury; nausea and possibly vomiting; drowsiness, confusion; dilation of one or both pupils. | ◆ Concussion (neurological problems caused by head trauma); severe cases may also include bleeding within the skull |
| ◆ vomit containing blood or material that looks like coffee grounds. | ◆ Internal bleeding, possibly from a stomach ulcer, stomach cancer, or throat cancer |
| ◆ You are—or may be—in the first three months of pregnancy, and have vomited on several days of the past week or more. | ◆ Normal effects (sometimes called morning sickness, though it can occur any time of day) often felt during the first three months of pregnancy |

| WHAT TO DO | OTHER INFO |
| --- | --- |
| ◆ Call your doctor today. Depending on the type of glaucoma, you may need beta-adrenergic blockers to reduce eye pressure or surgery to help the eye drain fluid. | ◆ Blindness may occur in as little as three to five days with some types of glaucoma. Early, fast treatment is essential. |
| ◆ **Call 911 or your emergency number now.** Each of these illnesses is serious; Reye's syndrome in particular escalates quickly and can be fatal. | ◆ To avoid Reye's syndrome, never give aspirin to a child with fever; use acetaminophen instead. |
| ◆ **Call 911 or your emergency number now.** You may need emergency care. | ◆ Improved nutrition and a specific diet may help in recovery. |
| ◆ **Call your doctor now.** An accurate diagnosis is essential. Appendicitis requires immediate surgery. | ◆ In the United States, 1 in 15 people gets appendicitis. It is most common between ages 10 and 30. |
| ◆ **Call 911 or your emergency number now.** Intestinal obstruction can be fatal within hours if left untreated. Successful treatment of colorectal cancer depends on an early and accurate diagnosis. | ◆ Scar tissue from a previous surgery is the most frequent cause of intestinal obstruction. |
| ◆ **Call 911 or your emergency number now;** these are serious conditions that may require immediate surgery. | |
| ◆ **Call 911 or your emergency number now.** Although a mild concussion may not require medical treatment, there is no way to tell if bleeding is occurring. Bleeding within the skull is a medical emergency. | ◆ Prevent head trauma whenever you can by using seat belts in vehicles and wearing helmets for sports such as bicycling, in-line skating, and ice skating. |
| ◆ **Call 911 or your emergency number now.** Internal bleeding calls for prompt intervention, as well as a follow-up evaluation to determine its cause. | |
| ◆ Try not to let your stomach become empty, which seems to make morning sickness worse. Eat soda crackers or other breads frequently to prevent nausea or to calm existing nausea. See Pregnancy Problems. | ◆ Vitamin $B_6$ may help combat morning sickness, but consult with your doctor before trying any supplements, medications, or therapies. |

# WARTS

## SYMPTOMS

- Common warts are small, hard, rough lumps that are round and elevated; they usually appear on hands and fingers and may be flesh-colored, white, pink, or granulated.
- Digitate warts are horny and finger-like, with pea-shaped bases; they appear on the scalp or near the hairline.
- Filiform warts are thin and thread-like; they commonly appear on the face and neck.
- Flat warts appear in groups of up to several hundred, usually on the face, neck, chest, knees, hands, wrists, or forearms; they are slightly raised and have smooth, flat, or rounded tops.
- Periungual warts are rough, irregular, and elevated; they appear at the edges of fingernails and toenails and may extend under the nails, causing pain.

See also Genital Warts and Plantar Warts and the Visual Diagnostic Guide.

## CALL YOUR DOCTOR IF:

- over-the-counter remedies don't work.
- you are a woman and develop genital warts, which in rare cases may indicate cervical cancer.
- you are older than 45 and discover what looks like a wart; it may instead be a symptom of a more serious skin condition, such as skin cancer.
- warts multiply and spread, causing embarrassment or discomfort.
- you notice a change in a wart's color or size; this could indicate skin cancer.

After acne, warts are the most common dermatological complaint. Three out of four people will develop a wart (verruca vulgaris) at some time in their lives. Warts are slightly contagious, and you can spread them to other parts of your body by touching them or shaving around infected areas. Children and young adults are more prone to getting warts because their defense mechanisms may not be fully developed, but it is possible to get a wart at any age.

## CAUSES

Warts are caused by the human papilloma virus (HPV), which enters the skin through a cut or scratch and causes cells to multiply rapidly. Usually, warts spread through direct contact, but it is possible to pick up the virus in moist environments, such as showers and locker rooms.

### DIAGNOSTIC AND TEST PROCEDURES

In most cases you don't need to undergo tests for other conditions if you develop a wart. But if you're over 45, your doctor may want to examine the growth, possibly after removing it, to ensure that it is benign.

## TREATMENT

Nearly every doctor says that the best treatment for warts is no treatment at all. Most people develop an immune response that causes warts to go away by themselves. One-fifth of all warts disappear within six months, and two-thirds are gone within two years. However, if your wart doesn't disappear, or if it's unsightly or uncomfortable, you can try self-treatment or seek help from your doctor.

### CONVENTIONAL MEDICINE

If you decide to treat your own wart, your first-choice remedy should be an over-the-counter medication in liquid, gel, pad, or ointment form. Most of these contain salicylic acid, the main constituent of aspirin, which softens abnormal skin cells and dissolves them.

First, soak the wart in warm water for five minutes to help the medication penetrate the skin. Then gently rub off dead skin cells with a washcloth or pumice stone. Before applying the medicine, coat the area around the wart with petroleum jelly to keep the medicine away from healthy or sensitive skin.

If over-the-counter treatment fails, your doctor can remove a wart by:

- freezing it with liquid nitrogen.
- burning it off with electricity or a laser.
- excising it (a minor surgical procedure).
- dissolving it by wrapping it in a plaster patch impregnated with salicylic acid.

Any of these treatments can cause scarring, so instead you may want to ask your doctor about a prescription patch that clears up warts by delivering a continuous dose of medication.

## ALTERNATIVE CHOICES

### CHINESE HERBS

A doctor of Chinese medicine may place a slice of ginger *(Zingiber officinale)* root on top of the wart and cover it with smoldering mugwort *(Artemisia).* The burning herb enables the ginger to release its antiviral constituents. This process is called indirect moxibustion.

### HERBAL THERAPIES

Several herbs contain chemicals thought to fight viruses and help treat skin conditions. Herbalists recommend applying the sticky juices of dandelion *(Taraxacum officinale),* milkweed *(Asclepias syriaca),* and celandine *(Chelidonium majus).* An ointment of thuja *(Thuja occidentalis)* applied four or five times a day may also help.

### HOMEOPATHY

Homeopathic medicines for warts include Causticum, Nitric acid, and Antimonium crudum.

### NUTRITION AND DIET

To strengthen your immune system, eat dark green and yellow vegetables, which contain vitamin A, as well as onions, garlic, Brussels sprouts, cabbage, and broccoli, which contain sulfur. Supplements to help fight off warts include beta carotene, L-cysteine, zinc, and vitamins B complex, C, and E.

## AT-HOME REMEDIES

There are countless folk cures for warts. One that may have some validity is rubbing the wart with a slice of raw potato or the inner side of a banana skin; both contain chemicals that may dissolve the wart. You might also try any of the following applications:

- vitamins A and E, which are generally good for skin conditions.
- a paste of crushed vitamin C tablets and water.
- over-the-counter medicines or a paste of crushed aspirin; both contain wart-dissolving salicylic acid.
- aloe *(Aloe barbadensis),* dandelion, or milkweed juices.
- cotton soaked in fresh pineapple juice, which contains a dissolving enzyme.

# PREVENTION

Practice good hygiene, and eat balanced meals high in vitamins A, C, and E to boost your immune system. Avoid stress, which can compromise your immunity, and learn to relax.

**CAUTION!**

**Be sure your growth is a wart. It could be any of several benign skin growths, such as a mole or a corn or callus, but there is also a chance it could be a form of skin cancer. Warts are usually pale, skin-colored growths with a rough surface. If your growth doesn't look like this, play it safe and see a doctor. Also check with your doctor if a wart's appearance changes.** ■

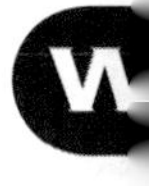

# WHEEZING

## SYMPTOMS

- a whistling sound and labored breathing, particularly when exhaling; sometimes accompanied by a mild feeling of tightening in the chest.

## CALL YOUR DOCTOR IF:

- wheezing is accompanied by a fever of 101°F or above. You may have an upper-respiratory infection such as acute bronchitis.
- breathing is so difficult that you feel that you are suffocating. This is either a sign of a severe asthma episode or an allergic reaction *(see Allergies)*; **get emergency medical help immediately.**
- you wheeze most days and cough up greenish or gray phlegm. You may have chronic bronchitis or emphysema.
- you begin wheezing suddenly and cough up frothy pink or white phlegm. This may be a sign of heart disease; **get emergency medical help immediately.**

Many people with respiratory allergies know that bouts of wheezing almost always come with the arrival of hay fever season. Mild wheezing may also accompany respiratory infections such as acute bronchitis or emphysema. But the characteristic whistling sound of wheezing is the primary symptom of the chronic respiratory disease asthma.

A variety of conventional and alternative remedies can alleviate wheezing. However, you should be regularly monitored by a conventional doctor if you have asthma, severe allergies, chronic bronchitis, or emphysema.

## CAUSES

The whistling sound that characterizes wheezing occurs when you attempt to breathe deeply through bronchial passages that are constricted or excreting excess mucus due to allergy, infection, or other irritation. With your lungs' airways partially blocked, your bronchial muscles may tighten because of increasing anxiety. This makes the wheezing worse, because it is more difficult for you to exhale completely.

In some people, wheezing is the result of asthma or allergic reactions to pollen, chemicals, pet dander, dust, foods, or insect stings. People with acute bronchitis also produce excess mucus in the respiratory tract, which can cause the lungs' passageways to become blocked. People with these respiratory diseases may also be more vulnerable to developing allergies. Wheezing may also be caused by cystic fibrosis or obstruction from a foreign body.

### DIAGNOSTIC AND TEST PROCEDURES

To determine the cause of your wheezing, your physician will ask you questions to determine if you have allergies. For example, if you have no history of lung disease and you always wheeze after eating a certain food or at a certain time of year, your doctor may suspect that you have a

YOGA

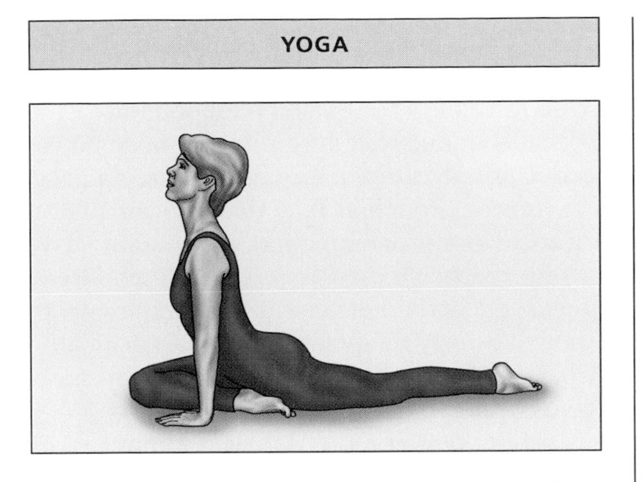

The **Pigeon** may enhance breathing. From a kneeling position, slide your left leg straight behind you. Take a deep breath and stretch up through your torso while arching your back slightly. Hold the position for 20 or 30 seconds, breathing deeply. Exhale and relax. Repeat with the other leg.

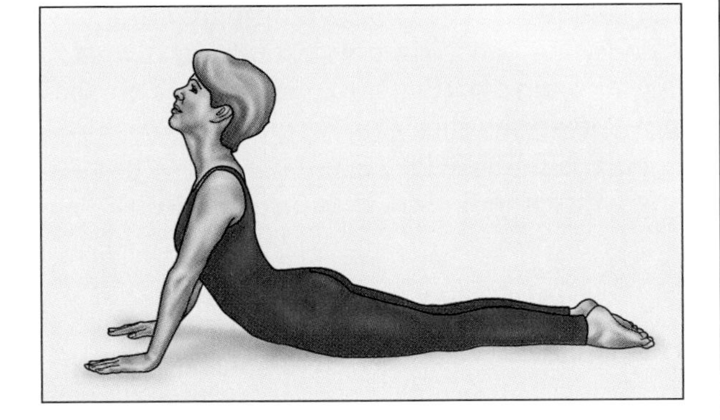

To ease wheezing spasms, try the **Cobra.** Place both forearms on the floor, elbows directly under your shoulders. Inhale and push your chest upward, straightening your arms while pressing your pelvis against the ground *(above).* Hold for 15 seconds, breathing deeply, then slowly relax.

food or respiratory allergy. There are a variety of tests your doctor may use to determine the exact nature of your allergy, including skin tests and blood tests. Your doctor may also administer a pulmonary function test to evaluate the volume of air moving through your bronchial passages. If your wheezing appears related to chronic bronchitis or emphysema, your doctor may also want to take x-rays.

## TREATMENT

You must see a conventional medical doctor to determine the cause of your wheezing and receive treatment for it. Alternative therapies, however, can help ease discomfort.

### CONVENTIONAL MEDICINE

If your wheezing is caused by asthma, your doctor will probably prescribe bronchodilators, drugs that help dilate the constricted airways. If you have allergies, your doctor will almost certainly prescribe antihistamines, drugs that counteract the allergy-producing chemicals in your body. If you have acute bronchitis, your doctor will probably prescribe an antibiotic to clear up your respiratory infection; generally, any mild wheezing that accompanies acute bronchitis disappears when the infection does. In cases of chronic bronchitis or emphysema, your doctor may prescribe an expectorant, to clear excess mucus, or a bronchodilator. In emergencies, when wheezing is so severe that it is difficult or impossible for you to breathe, a medical team may administer a shot of epinephrine to open clogged respiratory passages.

### ALTERNATIVE CHOICES

Many alternative therapies for asthma may be effective for wheezing. See Asthma for specific suggestions, including **Chinese medicine, reflexology,** and **herbal therapies.** But remember: If you have asthma, serious allergies, chronic bronchitis, or emphysema, you need to be monitored regularly by a conventional physician.

#### YOGA

Several postures may help relieve wheezing by teaching you how to control your breathing and release stress. Particularly effective positions include the Pigeon and the Cobra. See the illustrations at left. ■

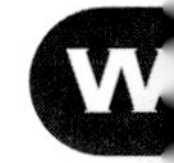

# WHOOPING COUGH

## SYMPTOMS

- in the early stage, a runny nose, a persistent cough, and sometimes a low-grade fever.
- after 7 to 14 days, severe spasms of coughing, in which each cough is followed by a high-pitched whooping sound as the person forces air over a swollen larynx (voice box). Young babies are often too weak to make the whooping sound.
- sometimes, vomiting after coughing episodes.
- particularly in infants under two months, interrupted breathing (apnea), during which the infant's lips may turn blue from lack of oxygen.

## CALL YOUR DOCTOR IF:

- your child has not been vaccinated against whooping cough and has recently been exposed to the illness.
- you suspect your child has whooping cough, especially if the child has a cold and cough that have lasted a week or more.
- your child's lips turn blue and your child experiences periods of breathing poorly, an indication of severe respiratory distress. **Seek emergency medical care immediately.**
- your child still seems unwell with a persistent cough and fever after the whooping cough spells have cleared up; the child may have developed a secondary respiratory infection, such as pneumonia or bronchitis.

Whooping cough, a highly contagious respiratory infection, is considered one of the most serious of traditional childhood diseases. Most states require children to be vaccinated against it. If untreated, it can cause lung damage and recurrent bronchial infections; in infants, it can lead to brain damage and even death. It is most often associated with very young children, but teenagers and adults can also become infected, though usually much less seriously. Fortunately, it has become uncommon in the U.S. because of the widespread immunization of children.

The first symptoms—usually a runny nose, dry cough, and mild fever—begin about 7 to 10 days after exposure. After another week, the characteristic cough may develop: violent spasms of coughing followed by a high-pitched whooping sound, though in babies this sound is often muted. The person may cough up copious amounts of thick saliva, and vomiting is common. This coughing phase usually lasts up to 6 weeks; during this time patients are susceptible to secondary infections that can be quite serious. The last phase is a recovery period of up to a month, during which the patient regains strength.

## CAUSES

Whooping cough is caused by the *Bordetella pertussis* bacterium. It is spread by airborne droplets from a cough or sneeze or through contact with contaminated sheets or clothing.

## TREATMENT

Whooping cough requires prompt medical treatment; delay can lead to serious complications, particularly in children.

### CONVENTIONAL MEDICINE

A pediatrician will probably prescribe erythromycin, an antibiotic that can be effective in reducing the length and severity of the infection, especially if started in the first 10 days of illness. Codeine may be prescribed to relieve coughing.

In severe cases or if your child is under a year old, hospitalization may be required to prevent dehydration and to permit quick administration of oxygen should the patient have difficulty breathing.

## ALTERNATIVE CHOICES

Alternative therapies, which are primarily aimed at relieving the cough, should be used only in conjunction with conventional medicine.

### ACUPRESSURE

To relieve a severe cough, try pressing Bladder points 43, 12, or 13. See pages 22–23 for information on point locations.

### HERBAL THERAPIES

For cough relief, try wild black cherry *(Prunus serotina)* bark syrup, a favorite remedy with children. Other herbs that might help relieve the cough include sundew *(Drosera rotundifolia),* thyme *(Thymus vulgaris), (Lactuca canadensis).* Consult a medical herbalist for dosages.

### HOMEOPATHY

Homeopathic remedies can help supplement conventional care. See a trained practitioner, whose remedies may include Carbo vegetabilis, Drosera, or Coccus cacti.

### OSTEOPATHY

Manipulation of the spinal segments of the chest and ribs may encourage lymphatic drainage and reduce the severity of the cough.

## AT-HOME CARE

- To help ease coughing spasms, have your child sit up and lean forward. Keep a bowl nearby to catch any phlegm that may be coughed up.
- If your child is vomiting, try feeding him immediately afterward, when it may be easier to keep food down.
- Increase liquids to offset dehydration and to thin mucus.
- To aid your child's breathing, use a cool-mist humidifier. Direct the mist away from your child and change any clothes or bedding that becomes damp. Use a humidifier with a humidistat, which keeps the air from becoming too humid, and make sure both the water and the humidifier stay clean to prevent mold and other germs from growing.
- Keep your child away from cigarette smoke, which can aggravate respiratory distress.

**CAUTION!**

**If your child is producing a lot of mucus, don't give him cough suppressants. Such medications will prevent him from effectively expelling mucus from a blocked airway.**

## PREVENTION

The DPT (diphtheria, pertussis, and tetanus) vaccine is given in five doses between the ages of two months and six years. The vaccine has been shown to be 90 percent effective when the child receives all five doses; however, it does not provide permanent immunity. Five years after the final dose, a previously immunized child is no longer protected. Reimmunization is not recommended, however, because the vaccine can trigger severe side effects in older children and adults. Because some family members may no longer be immune to the illness, doctors often recommend that others in the family take a 10-day preventive course of erythromycin when a child comes down with whooping cough.

Minor reactions to the DPT vaccine—mild fever, fretfulness, and drowsiness—are common. But if your child develops a very high fever, persistent crying, or convulsions, he may be having a severe reaction to the vaccine. **Seek emergency medical care immediately.** Fortunately, such reactions are very rare. Most medical experts believe that the risks of whooping cough far exceed the risks of the vaccine. ■

## SYMPTOMS

- Severe anal itching especially at night, restlessness, and difficulty sleeping may indicate **pinworms.**
- Itching on the soles of your feet suggests **hookworms;** in some cases this may be accompanied by a rash, coughing bloody sputum, and fever, followed by loss of appetite, diarrhea, palpitations, anemia, and fatigue.
- Nausea, diarrhea, abdominal pain, dizziness, changes in appetite, and fatigue indicate a **large tapeworm**—probably originating in beef, pork, or fish.
- Loss of appetite and weight, irritability, diarrhea, abdominal pain, and vomiting are symptoms of **small tapeworms**—originating in a rodent or dog.
- Diarrhea and cramping that last up to a week, followed by fever, muscle pain, conjunctivitis, and facial swelling around the eyes are signs of **trichinosis.**
- Wheezing, coughing, or other breathing difficulties, followed by vomiting, stomach pain, and bloating, suggest **ascariasis.**
- Small red lesions that may itch—followed by coughing, wheezing, or bronchitis; diarrhea; abdominal pain; and flatulence—are signs of **threadworms.**

## CALL YOUR DOCTOR IF:

- you experience any combination of the listed symptoms; you need a medical diagnosis for the possibility of worms.

Parasitic **roundworms** and **tapeworms** that infest humans come from unsanitary living conditions and poor food preparation. They range in size from half-inch pinworms to tapeworms more than 30 feet long. Of the roundworms, **pinworms** and **ascarids** (the worms that cause **ascariasis**) are the most common parasites affecting children in the United States. **Trichinosis** is a disease caused by a microscopic roundworm; if not treated, the worm larvae can cause muscle damage and cardiac or neurological complications. **Hookworms** are roundworms that live on blood, glucose, and oxygen they suck from the intestinal wall, often causing anemia. Like **hookworms, threadworms** can spread to the lungs and cause chronic coughing; both types often infest people sharing living quarters, as in prisons or mental institutions.

The several types of **tapeworms** that infest humans are generally not harmful unless they penetrate the intestinal wall and move to another part of the body. Any worm infestation can lead to respiratory or cardiovascular complications, but most are easily treated and cause no lasting harm.

## CAUSES

Most **roundworms** share a similar life cycle inside the body, but their methods of infestation differ. **Pinworms** live in people's lower intestinal tracts. The female worm leaves the anus to deposit eggs in the anal area at night. This produces an irritating itch that—when scratched—transfers the eggs to the host's fingers; the eggs can thus spread by touch through an entire household. If inadvertently eaten, the eggs hatch in the intestines and the cycle continues. The roundworm that causes **ascariasis** can enter the body in unwashed or raw food contaminated with the worm's eggs; it may also be picked up from soil that contains the eggs. **Hookworms** and **threadworms** enter the body in contaminated drinking water or through bare feet. The larvae migrate to the small intestine, where they may live for several years, taking nutrients from the intestinal walls. Their eggs are excreted in feces; if the infested feces contaminate soil, the cycle is repeated. You can contract the roundworm that causes **trichinosis** by eating raw or undercooked pork or game, which may contain living worm larvae encased in cysts. After digestive juices dissolve the cysts, the larvae circulate through the blood and the lymphatic system before digging into muscle and forming a cyst with new larvae.

**Tapeworms** also enter the body in raw or undercooked beef, fish, or pork. In rare cases, children may swallow tapeworm-infested fleas or lice that live on vermin or household pets.

### DIAGNOSTIC AND TEST PROCEDURES

A physician may diagnose **pinworms** by using a piece of sticky tape to pick up any eggs that may be around the anal area; the tape is then checked under a microscope. The worm itself is sometimes visible in stool samples or around the anus. **Roundworms, hookworms, threadworms,** and **tapeworms** can be diagnosed from stool samples as well, and sometimes tapeworm segments are found in bedding or clothes. To diagnose **trichinosis**, a physician will test samples of blood or muscle tissue.

## TREATMENT

### CONVENTIONAL MEDICINE

Most worms respond to medicines specific to the type of worm. **Hookworms** and **threadworms** are treated with pyrantel or mebendazole. Doctors usually treat **pinworms** with three oral doses of mebendazole, two weeks apart. Since the eggs can spread, everyone in the household must be treated. Washing all bed linens and clothing is essential to eradicate all pinworm eggs. You can relieve itching in the anal area with petroleum jelly.

Most cases of **trichinosis** are mild and do not need medication; if symptoms are severe, the medicine of choice is mebendazole. Trichinosis that spreads to the respiratory, cardiovascular, or central nervous system is rare and is treated with corticosteroids to fight inflammation.

After you have completed a course of treatment, have your doctor repeat the diagnostic tests to make sure the worms are gone. If not, another course of treatment may be necessary. **Tapeworms** may not clear your system for up to five months.

### ALTERNATIVE CHOICES

Once you have seen a doctor for an accurate diagnosis, alternative treatments can be used to flush worms from your system.

#### HERBAL THERAPIES

Check with a licensed herbalist about using these herbs, since they can be toxic:

- For **pinworms** and **roundworms**, steep 1 or 2 tsp wormwood *(Artemisia absinthium)* in a cup of boiling water for 10 to 15 minutes; drink three times daily. Over-the-counter tinctures of wormwood and black walnut *(Juglans nigra)* are also recommended; follow dosages on the labels.
- For **roundworms** and **threadworms,** steep 1 tsp dried tansy *(Tanacetum vulgare)* or 2 tsp dried balmony *(Chelone glabra)* in a cup of boiling water for 10 to 15 minutes; drink three times daily. Avoid tansy if you are pregnant.

#### NUTRITION AND DIET

Pineapple, papaya juice, and pumpkin seeds are all said to be tough on worms. Try over-the-counter grapefruit-seed extract to flush worms out of your intestines; follow dosage directions on the label.

## PREVENTION

- Make sure children always wash their hands after going to the bathroom and before eating.
- Keep fingernails short to reduce the chances of picking up **pinworm** eggs underneath them.
- Have all your four-legged pets checked and treated for worms in the spring and fall.
- Avoid **trichinosis** by thoroughly cooking pork.
- Wash thoroughly in hot, soapy water tools and utensils that come in contact with raw meat.
- Always wear shoes in areas where **hookworms** and **threadworms** may live in the soil, particularly in the southeastern U.S. ■

# YEAST INFECTIONS

## SYMPTOMS

- painless white patches in your mouth or throat that may come off when you eat or brush your teeth; this indicates **oral thrush,** most common in infants, the elderly, and AIDS patients.
- white patches in the mouth and throat, sometimes associated with painful swallowing; these are symptomatic of **esophageal thrush,** a potential complication of AIDS.
- peeling skin on the hands, especially between the fingers, and swollen nail folds above the cuticle; possibly painful, red, and containing pus.
- itchy or burning shiny, pink rash with a scaly or blistered edge in the folds of the skin. This indicates **intertrigo.**
- in women, vaginal itching and irritation; redness and swelling of the vulva; unusually thick, white discharge; and pain during intercourse. These are signs of a **vaginal yeast infection,** also known as **moniliasis.**
- in men, red patches and blisters at the end of the penis and around the foreskin, possibly accompanied by severe itching and pain. These are symptoms of **balanitis.**

## CALL YOUR DOCTOR IF:

- you have any of the symptoms for the first time; you need a professional evaluation before beginning treatment.
- the infection does not respond to treatment or recurs; you may have a more serious disorder such as diabetes or an HIV infection.

Yeast, or fungal, infection—sometimes called **candidiasis**—takes many forms. Yeast infections often develop where a moist environment encourages fungal growth, especially on the webs of fingers and toes, nails, genitals, and folds of skin. *(See Athlete's Foot.)* **Oral thrush** is a painless, often recurrent infection of the mouth and throat; it is common in babies, young children, and the elderly, but can affect all ages. **Moniliasis** is a painful vaginal yeast infection experienced by many women, most commonly during pregnancy or treatment with antibiotics. *(See Vaginal Problems.)* **Balanitis** is a less common but equally irritating infection of the penis. *(See Penile Pain.)* **Systemic yeast infections** can occur in cases of diabetes, AIDS, and other ailments or drug treatments that suppress the immune system.

## CAUSES

*Candida albicans* is a fungal organism, or yeast, that thrives in your mouth, gastrointestinal tract, and skin; your body produces bacterial flora that keeps it in check. When fungal growth exceeds the body's ability to control it, yeast infection develops. This can happen when you are weakened by illness or upset by stress. Modern antibiotics that treat many ailments can actually kill the bacteria that otherwise control fungal outbreaks.

Yeast infections are common among dishwashers and people whose hands are often in water, in children who suck their thumbs or fingers, and in people whose clothing retains body moisture. The diaper rash called **candidal dermatitis** is caused by yeast growth in the folds of a baby's skin. Diabetics are especially prone to yeast infections because they have high levels of sugar in their blood and urine and a low resistance to infection—conditions that encourage yeast growth. In rare cases the candida fungus may invade the bloodstream through an intravenous (IV) tube or urinary catheter. If the infection travels to the kidneys, lungs, brain, or other organs, it can cause serious systemic complications, but these develop only in people who are seriously ill or who have other health problems that weaken the immune system, such as drug addiction or diabetes.

### DIAGNOSTIC AND TEST PROCEDURES

To diagnose **oral thrush,** a doctor will examine the white patches and may take a sample for testing. To check for **vaginal yeast infection,** a doctor may take a vaginal wet smear. If your physician thinks you have a **systemic yeast infection,** a blood, stool, or tissue sample will be tested for the fungus.

## TREATMENT

Treatment will depend on your specific condition but will focus on counteracting the growth of the yeast organism that causes the infection.

### CONVENTIONAL MEDICINE

Your doctor will probably treat **oral thrush** with an antifungal medication such as clotrimazole or ketoconazole. Babies with oral thrush are typically given nystatin with a dropper. Infections of the skin or nails can be treated with topical applications of clotrimazole. For **vaginal yeast infection,** an over-the-counter intravaginal cream containing miconazole or clotrimazole is typically suggested. If over-the-counter medications are not effective, your doctor may prescribe a cream with terconazole or an oral antifungal drug containing fluconazole. If your doctor determines that you have a **systemic yeast infection,** you may get intravenous doses of amphotericin or flucytosine.

### ALTERNATIVE CHOICES

Alternative remedies can strengthen the immune system to resist yeast infections, and can treat specific yeast infections and prevent recurrence.

#### HERBAL THERAPIES

For healing yeast infections on your skin, apply full-strength tea tree oil (*Melaleuca* spp.) two to three times daily; a slight burning sensation is normal, but discontinue if the treatment is painful. An over-the-counter salve containing calendula *(Calendula officinalis)* is good for rashes in children over two years of age.

### CHRONIC YEAST INFECTION

*Although the diagnosis is not universally accepted, some doctors recognize a condition called chronic candidiasis, or chronic yeast infection, that may affect the gastrointestinal, nervous, endocrine, and immune systems. Treatment focuses on eliminating predisposing factors, such as prescription or over-the-counter drugs, foods with high refined-sugar or yeast content, high-carbohydrate vegetables, and milk products. Your doctor may also test you for underlying conditions, such as diabetes or thyroid problems.*

*An herbal remedy for chronic yeast infection is tea brewed from 1 to 2 grams of dried root of barberry (Berberis vulgaris) or goldenseal (Hydrastis canadensis) in a cup of boiling water, taken three times a day. With your doctor's approval, you may want to try taking daily supplements of 45 mg iron, 45 mg zinc, and 200 mcg selenium (avoid higher doses of selenium).*

#### HOMEOPATHY

Numerous homeopathic remedies are used to treat yeast infections; ask a licensed homeopath about which one best suits your symptoms.

## PREVENTION

- If work keeps your hands in water for long periods, wear rubber gloves. When you're done, wash your hands and apply a mild prescription or over-the-counter antifungal cream.
- Wear cotton or silk underclothes, which, unlike nylon and other synthetics, allow excess moisture to evaporate. Wash and dry your underclothes thoroughly; change them often. ■

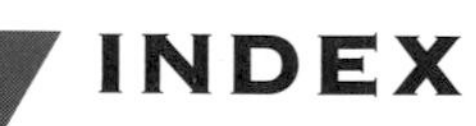

# INDEX

*Page numbers in italics refer to illustrations or illustrated text.*

## A

# C

# D

# E



# F

# G



# H

# I

## J



## K



## L



## M

# N

## Q



## R

# V



# W



# Y



# Z

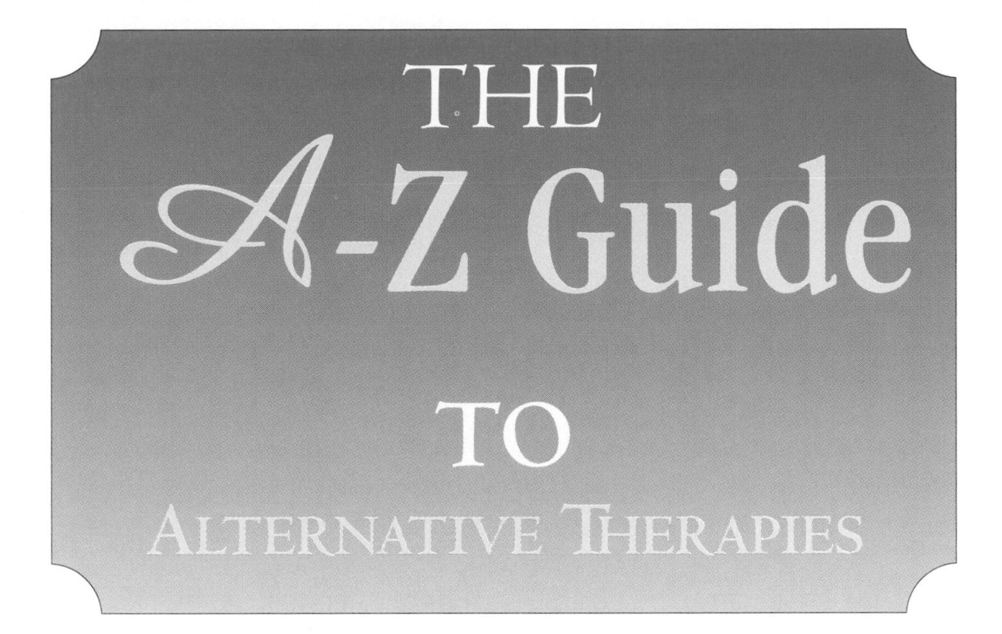


BY THE EDITORS OF TIME-LIFE BOOKS
ALEXANDRIA, VIRGINIA

# Consultants

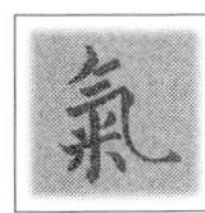

**ZOË BRENNER**
LAc, Dipl Ac and Dipl Ch (NCCA), FNAAOM
*has practiced acupuncture since 1977 and Chinese herbal medicine since 1984. She teaches Oriental medicine and the history and philosophy of Chinese medicine at the Traditional Acupuncture Institute in Columbia, Maryland, and lectures in other schools around the United States.*

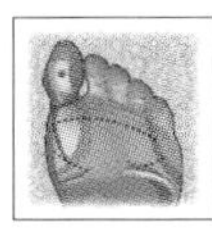

**DWIGHT C. BYERS**
*began teaching with his aunt, Eunice Ingham, who pioneered and developed the original Ingham method of reflexology. Byers now serves as president of the International Institute of Reflexology in St. Petersburg, Florida, which offers seminars worldwide.*

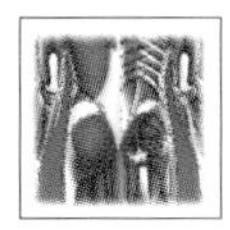

**DEBORAH CAPLAN,** MA, PT
*is a licensed physical therapist and a certified teacher of the Alexander technique. She studied with F. M. Alexander and is a founding member of the American Center for the Alexander Technique, Inc. The author of Back Trouble, she specializes in teaching the Alexander technique to people with back problems.*

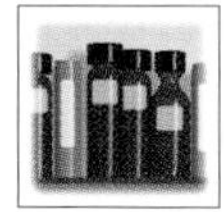

**JOHN G. COLLINS,** ND, DHANP
*teaches dermatology and homeopathy at the National College of Naturopathic Medicine in Portland, Oregon. He also has a private practice in Gresham, Oregon.*

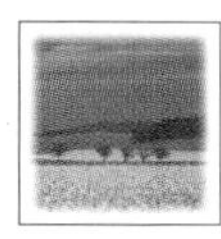

**KYLE H. CRONIN,** ND
*specializes in women's healthcare in her medical practice in Phoenix. Dr. Cronin is also cofounder of Southwest College of Naturopathic Medicine and Health Sciences, where she is dean of Curricular Development.*

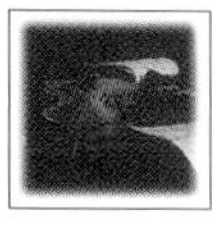

**BARBARA CROWE,** RMT-BC
*teaches music therapy at Arizona State University, Tempe. She frequently gives presentations on music therapy and sound healing and is writing a book on the theory of music therapy. She is past president of the National Association for Music Therapy.*

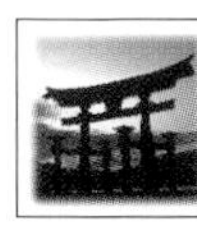

**PALI C. DELEVITT,** PhD
*consults on alternative therapies at the cancer center of the University of Virginia, where she also teaches in the School of Medicine. Dr. Delevitt has consulted on curriculum development for the medical schools of Columbia University, Emory University, and Indiana University.*

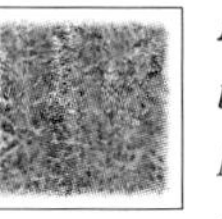

**ADRIANE FUGH-BERMAN,** MD
*is chair of the National Women's Health Network, a science-based advocacy group. An expert on herbs and nutritional medicine, she has lectured internationally on diverse alternative medicine issues and formerly directed field investigations for the National Institutes of Health Office of Alternative Medicine.*

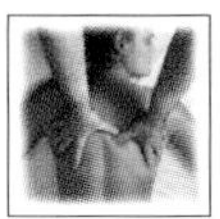

**ELLIOT GREENE,** MA
*is past president of the American Massage Therapy Association and currently maintains a private practice in Silver Spring, Maryland. Certified in therapeutic massage by the National Certification Board for Therapeutic Massage and Bodywork, he has spent more than 24 years in the field. He was formerly on the board of directors of the National Wellness Coalition.*

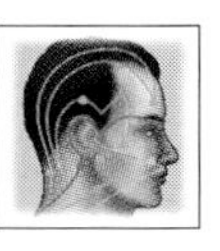

**GARY KAPLAN,** DO
*is a family physician and a specialist in chronic pain medicine. He is president of the Medical Acupuncture Research Foundation and serves on the clinical faculty of Georgetown University Medical School. Dr. Kaplan is director of the Kaplan Clinic in Arlington, Virginia, where he is in private practice.*

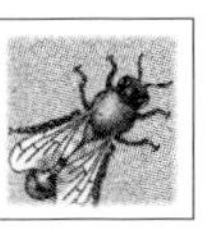

**CHRISTOPHER M. KIM,** MD
*is past president of the American Apitherapy Society, an organization that informs the public on the therapeutic uses of bee venom and other bee products. A pain-medicine specialist, Dr. Kim is medical director of the Monmouth Pain Institute in Red Bank, New Jersey, and president of the International Pain Institute.*

# Consultants

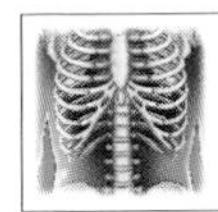

**DANA J. LAWRENCE,** DC, FICC
*has been a faculty member at the National College of Chiropractic in Lombard, Illinois, for more than 17 years. He is the director of the college's Department of Publication and Editorial Review, and editor of its Journal of Manipulative and Physiological Therapeutics.*

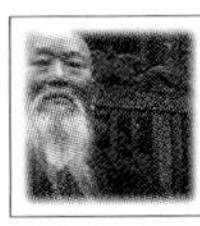

**JEFFREY MIGDOW,** MD
*has been practicing holistic medicine for 17 years. In his medical practice, Dr. Migdow counsels patients on lifestyle and recommends a wide variety of homeopathic, nutritional, and other therapies. He is also a director of yoga-teacher training at the Kripalu Center for Yoga and Health in Lenox, Massachusetts. He began his yoga training more than 20 years ago and has been teaching yoga for 10 years.*

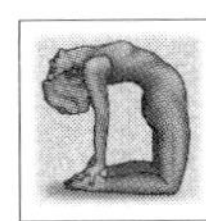

**DONALD G. MURPHY,** PhD
*is a basic scientist who retired from the National Institutes of Health after a career in biomedical research and research administration. He is a martial arts master instructor with experience in aikido, jujitsu, judo, tae kwon do, qigong, and t'ai chi. Dr. Murphy provides experiential training in life force (bioenergy, chi, ki) and is an adjunct faculty member at the Uniformed Services University of the Health Sciences in Bethesda, Maryland.*

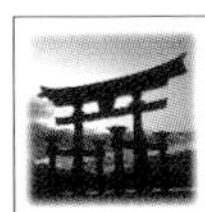

**CHRISTINA PUCHALSKI,** MD, OCDS
*utilizes her patients' spiritual background in her work as an internist and primary care physician at the George Washington University Hospital in Washington, D.C. Dr. Puchalski was instrumental in creating and integrating a course on spirituality and medicine into the curriculum at George Washington University Medical School.*

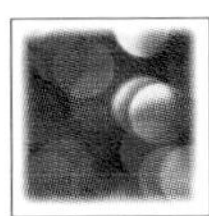

**BEVERLY RUBIK,** PhD
*is founding director of the Institute for Frontier Science in Philadelphia. Her interests in alternative medicine include light therapy, bioelectromagnetic therapy, spiritual healing, acupuncture, and homeopathy.*

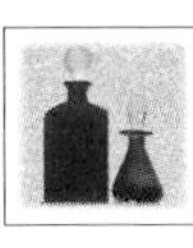

**KURT SCHNAUBELT,** PhD
*founded and directs the Pacific Institute of Aromatherapy in San Rafael, California. Drawing on his background in chemistry, Dr. Schnaubelt has written numerous articles and books on scientifically based aromatherapy.*

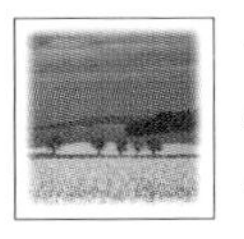

**J. JAMISON STARBUCK,** JD, ND
*practices family medicine in Missoula, Montana. A former practicing attorney, she is past president of the American Association of Naturopathic Physicians and a member of the Homeopathic Academy of Naturopathic Physicians.*

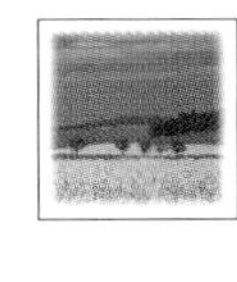

**MICHAEL A. TANSEY,** PhD
*is a pioneer researcher and authority on biofeedback, EEG neurofeedback, and the Instrumental Cartography of Consciousness. He is past president of the Society for the Study of Neuronal Regulation.*

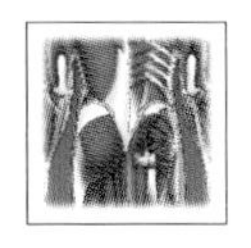

**DICK W. THOM,** DDS, ND
*teaches clinical and physical diagnosis at the National College of Naturopathic Medicine in Portland, Oregon. He is also a clinic supervisor at the Portland Naturopathic Clinic and maintains a general family practice at Natural Choices Health Clinic in Beaverton, Oregon.*

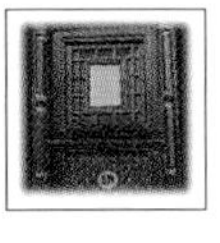

**ROBERT C. WARD,** DO, FAAO
*teaches osteopathic manipulative medicine and family medicine at Michigan State University's College of Osteopathic Medicine. He was in private family practice for 14 years prior to teaching.*

**KENNETH G. ZYSK,** PhD
*researches Ayurvedic medicine as the project director of the Indic Traditions of Healthcare at Columbia University. Dr. Zysk also teaches in the Department of Near Eastern Languages and Literature at New York University, and in the Department of Religion at Columbia University. He is senior editor of a series of books on Indian and Tibetan medicine for the University of California Press.*

# Contents

# Contents

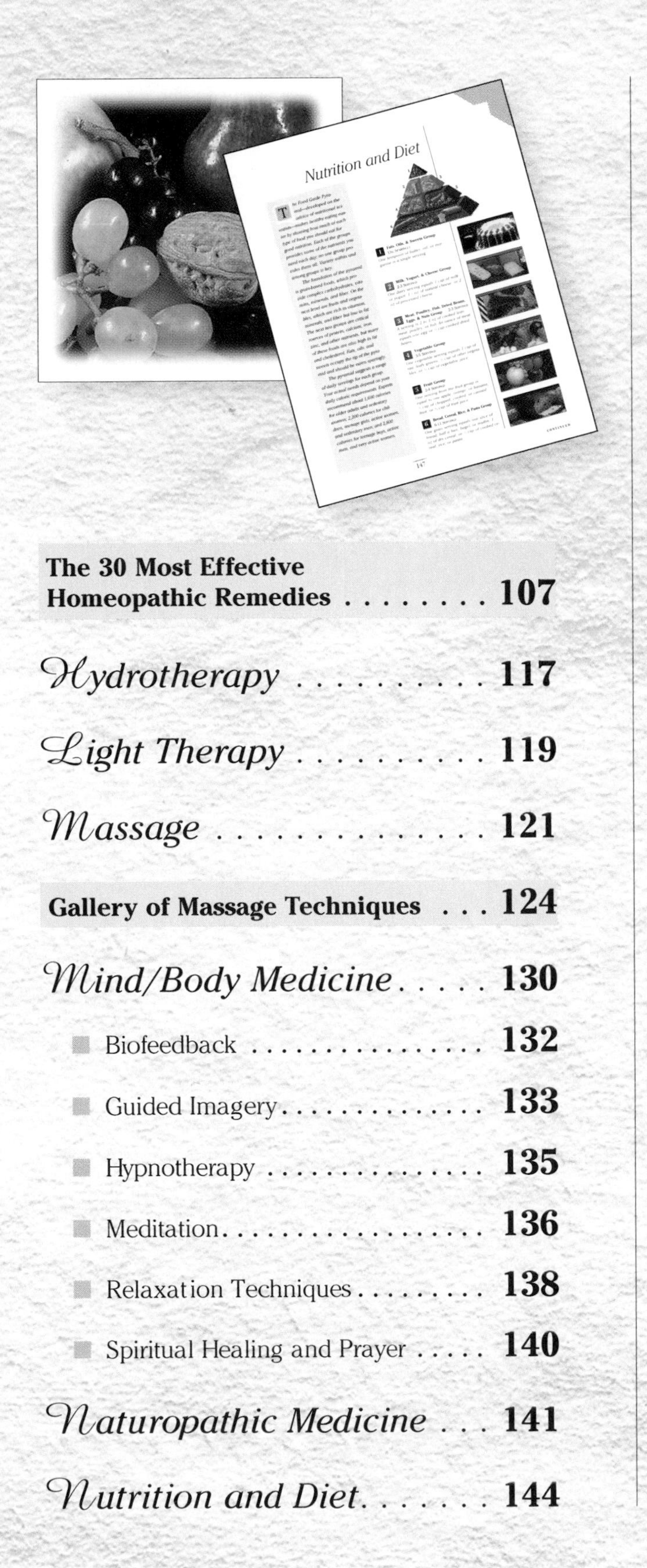
Nutrition and Diet



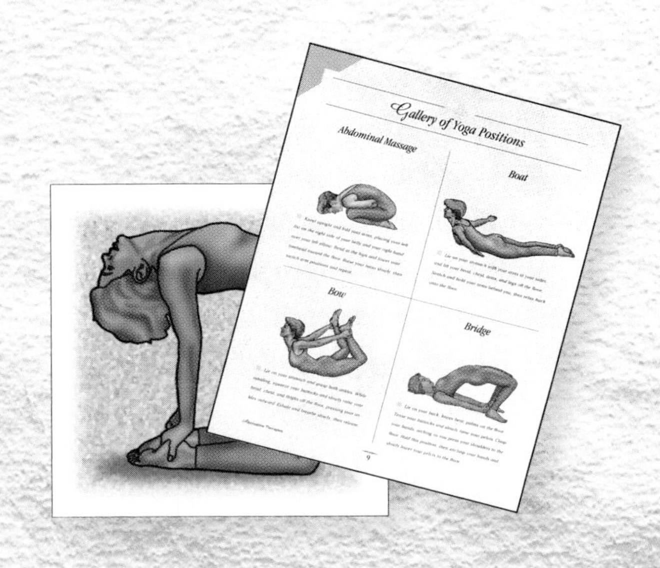
Gallery of Yoga Positions

Abdominal Massage

Boat

Bow

Bridge

CONTINUED

# Introduction

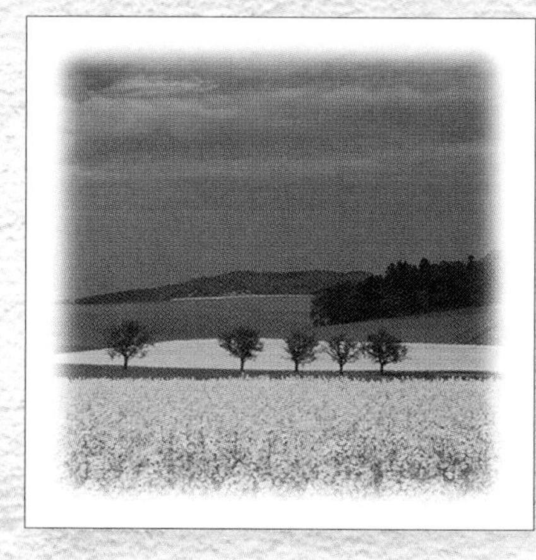

*In my work as a physician—and as a practitioner of alternative medicine—I am constantly reminded of the importance of keeping an open mind when it comes to finding what's best for my patients. Years of experience have shown me that no single approach to healthcare has all the answers; the search for healing solutions often requires a willingness to look beyond one remedy or system of treatment. At the same time, I also feel a deep responsibility to be selective—to recognize important distinctions among the vast array of treatment options available. Because the same therapy can affect different patients in different ways, an approach that works for one person may do nothing for another. My job, then, is not just to seek out which remedies are available or safe, but to prescribe the course of treatment that best suits the patient's condition and lifestyle. I've discovered, though, that I can't do this job alone. Whatever the therapy, patients respond dramatically better to treatment when they take an active, confident role in their own healthcare.*

*More than ever before, taking such an active role in your own health requires a good working knowledge of alternative medicine—practical knowledge that this book is expressly intended to give you. While conventional physicians generally view health as the absence of disease, alternative practitioners think of it as a balancing of body, mind, and spirit. Central to alternative medicine is the principle of holism, or the idea that all aspects of a person are interrelated; disharmony in one aspect upsets the balance and stresses the body, eventually leading to illness.*

*Alternative practitioners use a number of methods to bolster the body's own defenses and restore balance to help overcome disease. Among these therapies are ancient healing systems that were ignored by Western society but are now being rediscovered for their powerful therapeutic ability.*

*The Alternative Advisor offers an in-depth look at the wide variety of healing approaches—some dating to the dawn of civilization—that are used to treat ailments ranging in severity from the common cold to skin cancer. This section of the book addresses the pros and cons of particular therapies, explaining their origins, who can benefit from them, and specifically how they are used both to treat ailments and to help maintain wellness.*

*Besides the variety and scope of its treatment options, what I find particularly impressive about The Alternative Advisor is its pervading sense of responsibility—its honest recognition that alternative methods are not always sufficient on their own, and that in some cases the best medicine is so-called conventional treatment. In other words, when conventional medications or treatments such as surgery are necessary, this book does not hesitate to say so. The authors and editors take great pride in presenting an objective, reasoned look at alternative medicine. I share that pride and sense of responsibility, and I know that my fellow consultants do as well. After all, the health of our patients depends on it.*

*Alternative medicine has flowered in the past few decades as more and more people seek to avoid the drugs and surgery of conventional healthcare—or at the very least supplement them with other approaches. Already, thousands of medical doctors (including myself) have incorporated alternative therapies into their practices. Health insurance companies now cover certain alternative methods, including acupuncture, which has been used in China for millennia but was practically unknown in this country until 20 years ago. Indeed, the face of healthcare is changing, moving toward a more open-minded view of nonconventional remedies—some new, some long forgotten. Ironic as it sounds, it looks as though the future of medicine may well lie in these healing traditions of the past. Knowing more about them—and having practical advice about how to use them at your fingertips—may be one of the best things you can do for your health.*

***—Jeffrey Migdow, MD***

*Former Medical Director, Kripalu Center for Yoga and Health*

# A-Z Guide to Alternative Therapies

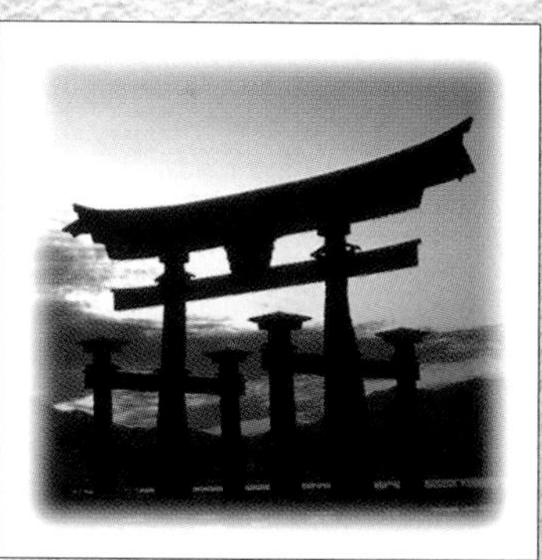

*In this section, 24 alternative therapies are arranged by name in alphabetical order. Most are listed individually, but in some cases a few similar or related techniques are grouped together under a single umbrella heading. Bodywork, for instance, is a general category for various therapies that involve bodily manipulation or techniques for improving posture and movement. Examples include Hellerwork and Reiki. (Note: Massage and chiropractic, though generally considered to be bodywork techniques, are listed separately.) Therapies that rely on the healing power of the mind—biofeedback, guided imagery, and hypnotherapy, to name a few—are discussed under the group heading Mind/Body Medicine. If you're not sure where to look for a particular therapy, you can find it easily in the index.*

*Each entry offers a comprehensive, "big picture" look at a given therapy as well as a close examination of its various elements. An introduction sets the stage, defining the technique and explaining its working principles. Next comes a brief review of the technique's historical origins, identifying the key players and explaining how their methods evolved over the decades or millennia into the therapy as practiced today.*

*Under "What It's Good For," you'll find general information about how this therapy acts on the body to improve health. Specific disorders commonly treated with this method are listed as "Target Ailments," each of which is the subject of a full entry elsewhere in the book (see Common Ailments, beginning on page 194). "Preparations/Techniques" delves into the nuts and bolts of the therapy; here you'll learn such things as how healing substances are prepared and administered, and what techniques or equipment is used. Under "Visiting a Professional," you'll find out what you can expect when visiting a practitioner's office. Because wellness is a big part of alternative medicine, most entries describe how a given therapy helps promote and maintain lasting good health. "What the Critics Say" attempts to characterize—and occasionally rebut—criticisms that have been leveled against this form of therapy. A special "Licensed & Insured?" box explains the licensing requirements for practitioners and whether their services are covered by health insurance, and another box labeled "For More Info" lists addresses and phone numbers of organizations you can contact to learn more about the topic.*

*Besides the alphabetized list of therapies, this first section of The Alternative Advisor also features 10 illustrated galleries that give practical, in-depth information about selected remedies and therapeutic techniques. The acupressure, t'ai chi, and yoga galleries, for example, show exactly how and where to apply healing pressure to the body or how to perform certain positions for relaxation and good health. Another gallery provides step-by-step instruction in therapeutic massage, while others explore such health-related topics as vitamins and minerals, herbs, essential oils, and homeopathic remedies.*

## How to Choose a Practitioner

*When searching for an alternative practitioner, you may want to begin with a recommendation from a conventional doctor. Illness-related self-help groups and books on alternative healing can also be good sources for names. You may find that family and friends can provide valuable opinions based on their experience with particular practitioners. In your search, don't hesitate to act on personal considerations such as a preference for a male or female practitioner, or an older or younger one. If you have beliefs or philosophies that play a major role in your healthcare, be sure that you choose a provider who will respect your views.*

*You should fully investigate any alternative practitioner's background and experience and be aware of any licensing requirements in your state or district. Be extremely suspicious of anyone who expresses hostility or derision toward mainstream medicine or makes grandiose claims for a cure. A conscientious practitioner understands that every therapy has its limitations. Get explicit information about the treatment you will receive, and remember that you are in charge of the entire treatment process. Above all, trust your own instincts and judgment.* ■

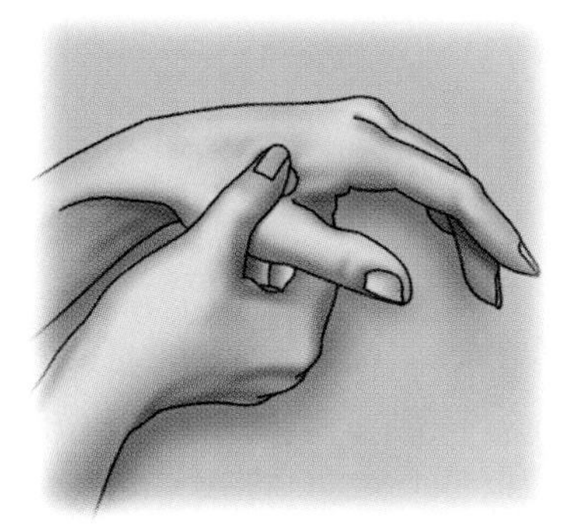

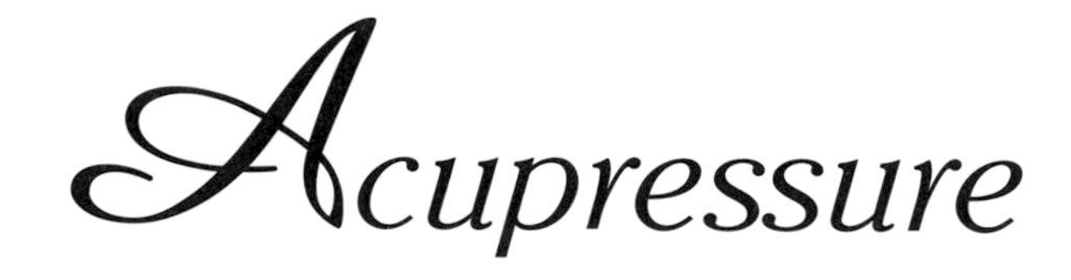

# Acupressure

### Target Ailments

- Allergies
- Arthritis
- Asthma
- Athletic Injuries
- Back Problems
- Chronic Fatigue Syndrome
- Common Cold
- Constipation
- Diarrhea
- Earache
- Headache
- Immune Problems
- Indigestion
- Insomnia
- Motion Sickness
- Nausea
- Pain, Chronic
- TMJ Syndrome
- Toothache

*See Common Ailments, beginning on page 194.*

*An integral part of the traditional practice of Chinese medicine (pages 57-60), acupressure has become increasingly popular and accepted in the West. Its simple, noninvasive techniques have shown beneficial effects for a wide array of health problems—even if the theory behind it remains questionable to many conventional medical practitioners.*

*Like acupuncture (pages 32-33), acupressure is based on the concept of chi (sometimes spelled "qi"), defined in Chinese medicine as an essential life force that flows through the body, circulating through invisible passageways called meridians (see the illustrations on pages 34-35). The movement, or flow, of chi is said to vary with the mental, physical, and spiritual changes of daily living. According to this theory, when chi flows freely and evenly, harmony and good health are possible; however, if chi circulation is stagnant, overstimulated, or unbalanced, illness is likely.*

*The invisible meridians carrying chi are said to reside within the body's interior. However, there are specific places on the skin, called acupoints, where chi may be accessed and guided using deep, focused finger pressure. By improving chi circulation, practitioners encourage the harmonious equilibrium of mind and body believed to be essential for physical and spiritual health. And once this internal harmony is achieved, they claim, the body is able to invoke its self-healing capabilities.*

## *Origins*

The various therapeutic techniques of Chinese medicine, including acupressure, are among the most ancient healing approaches in the world, dating back some 5,000 years. Acupressure itself probably originated as a combination of acupuncture and massage.

## *What It's Good For*

Acupressure techniques address hundreds of ailments. In addition to those listed at left, studies have shown that acupressure can hasten recuperation from stroke and surgery. And at some hospitals, elastic acupressure wristbands (designed to relieve motion sickness) are used to reduce the

> **LICENSED & INSURED?**
>
> *No. Although acupuncturists are licensed, acupressurists are not. Acupressure is often viewed by insurance companies as massage; as such, it may or may not be covered. Contact your insurance provider for more-specific information.*

# Acupressure

anesthesia-induced nausea that often follows surgery. Acupressure can also be valuable during pregnancy, as it may relieve morning sickness, indigestion, and backache; alleviate the pain of childbirth; and enhance recuperation. But be sure to read the caution at right.

### *Preparations/Techniques*

Acupressure can be performed by a trained specialist or by patients in their own homes. A specialist can provide comprehensive treatment, which involves the redirecting of chi around the meridians; the American Association of Oriental Medicine can help you locate a good practitioner. To try acupressure yourself for local, symptomatic relief, first identify which acupoints you will use. This may be a single point, or several points in a specific order *(see the Gallery of Acupressure Techniques, pages 18-31)*. Locate the first acupoint with your fingertips, then press lightly with one finger. Gradually increase the pressure until you are comfortably pressing as firmly as you can. Hold this pressure steadily until you begin to feel a very faint, even pulse at the acupoint. (This usually takes three to 10 minutes, or longer for severe problems.) When you're ready to release, reduce the pressure from the acupoint very slowly. You may occasionally feel some discomfort, but if the pressure is actually painful, ease up. There is no "correct" amount of pressure that you should strive for; everyone's needs are different, and the amount required at one acupoint will vary from that needed at another.

For best results, apply pressure to the same acupoints on both sides of the body; when working with a series of acupoints, complete the set on one side of the body before continuing to the other side. In some forms of acupressure, such as shiatsu, pressure is applied sequentially, from one end of the meridian to the other. To work on hard-to-reach spots (such as your back), either ask a partner for help, or place a tennis or golf ball on the floor and then lie on top of it.

### *Wellness*

Beyond its many potential healing effects, acupressure may also be beneficial in maintaining overall good health. Acupressure releases tension in muscle fibers, promoting the movement of blood and nutrients to the tissues. Many people report acupressure induces peaceful rejuvenation and clarity of thought, as well as improved athletic performance.

### *What the Critics Say*

Because no one is certain just how acupressure works, its critics typically claim that it is simply not effective, offering the placebo effect to explain its success. Studies testing the placebo effect do not support this criticism, however. ■

### CAUTION

**If you have a serious illness, ask your doctor before using acupressure. Never press on an open wound, swollen or inflamed skin, bruises, varicose veins, or a lump. Avoid sites of recent surgery and sites of a suspected bone injury. If you have atherosclerosis, avoid direct pressure on the carotid arteries. If you are pregnant, avoid pressure to the lower abdomen, and don't use points Spleen 6 or Large Intestine 4 (some believe these points can induce miscarriage).**

### FOR MORE INFO

Following is a list of organizations you can contact to learn more about acupressure:

**American Association of Oriental Medicine**
433 Front Street
Catasauqua, PA 18032
(610) 433-2448
fax: (610) 264-2768
e-mail: AAOM1@aol.com

**National Certification Commission for Acupuncture and Oriental Medicine**
PO Box 97075
Washington, DC 20090-7075
(202) 232-1404
fax: (202) 462-6157

# Gallery of Acupressure Techniques

## Bladder 10

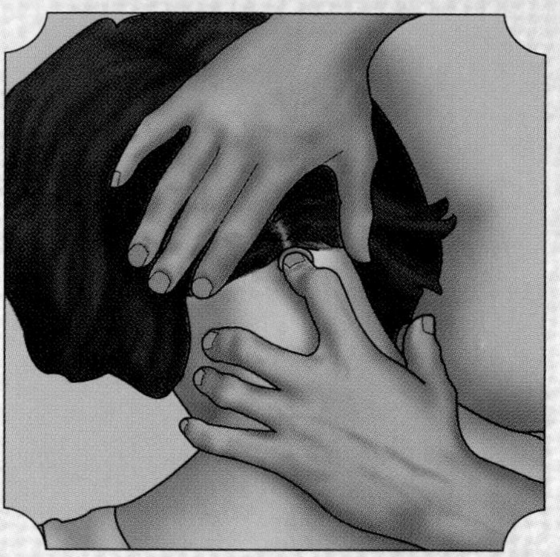

Locate the ropy muscles one-half inch below the base of the skull. Press inward using the thumb or a finger.

## Bladder 13

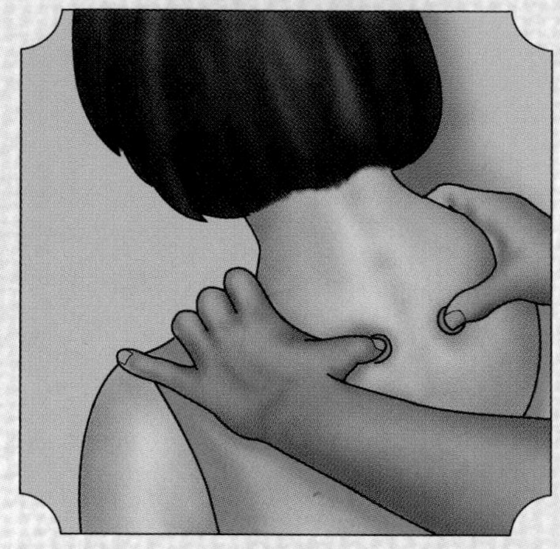

Use your thumbs or fingers to press into the muscles one-half inch outward from either side of the spine and one finger width below the upper tip of the shoulder blade.

## Bladder 23

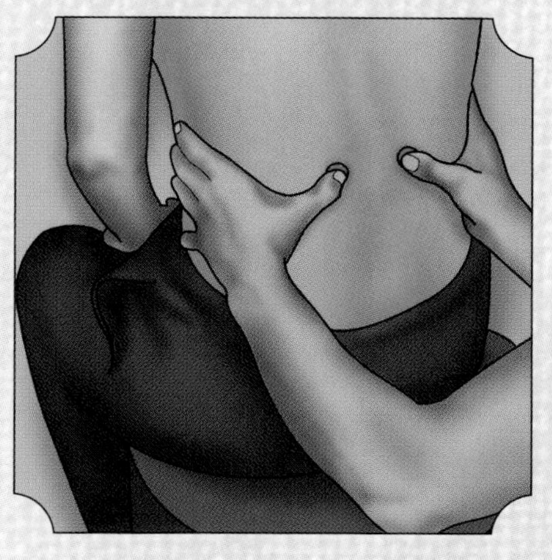

This point site is level with the space between the second and third lumbar vertebrae. Find BL 23 by aligning your thumbs or fingers about an inch outward from either side of the spine, just behind the navel, then press inward.

## Bladder 25

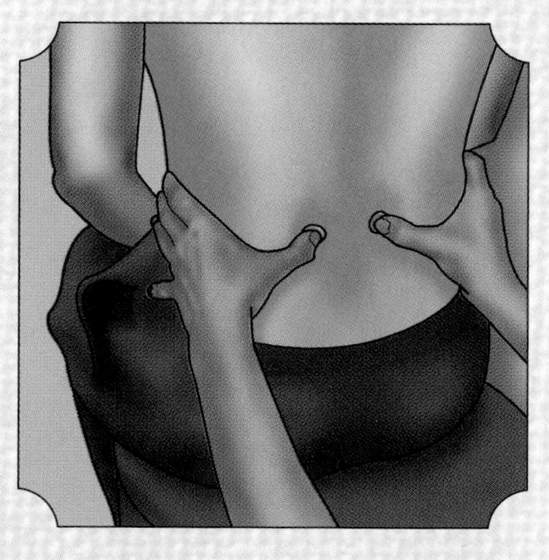

With your thumbs or fingers, press into the muscles about an inch outward from either side of the spine, about midway between BL 23 (left) and the bottom of the spine. The point is level with the fourth and fifth lumbar vertebrae.

# Gallery of Acupressure Techniques

## Bladder 32

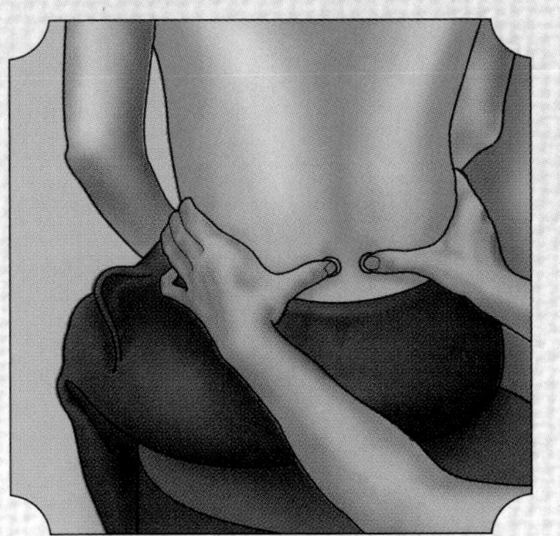

At the base of the spine, directly above the tailbone, use your thumbs or fingers to press into the muscles one-half inch outward from either side of the spine.

## Bladder 40

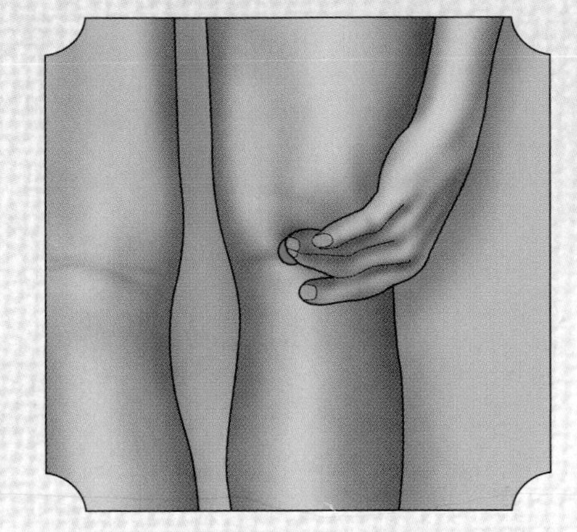

With your leg slightly bent, find the fold on the back of your knee where the knee bends. Use your middle finger to press inward on the fold, between the two tendons.

## Conception Vessel 4

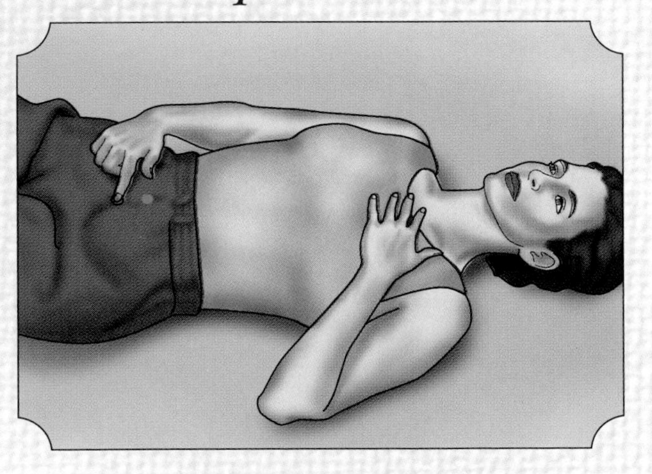

Locate this point, which lies just below CV 6 (right), by measuring four finger widths down from the navel on the midline of the abdomen. With your index finger, gradually press as deep as possible on the point site.

## Conception Vessel 6

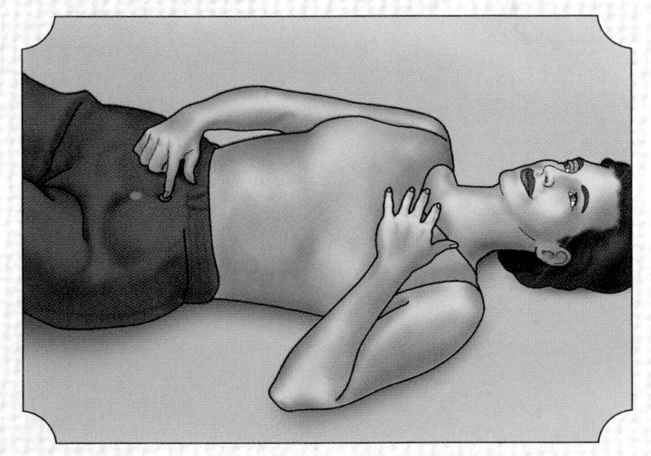

Measure three finger widths below the navel—or about one finger width up from CV 4 (left)—then press inward on this point as far as you can, using your index finger. Inhale slowly and deeply, relaxing as you exhale.



CONTINUED

# Gallery of Acupressure Techniques

## Conception Vessel 12

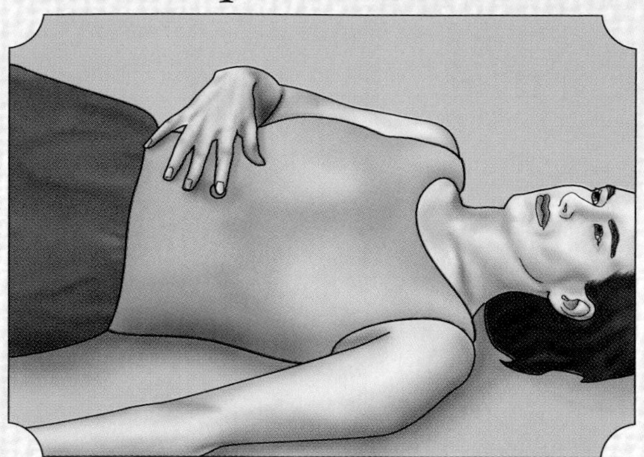

This point lies four thumb widths above the navel along the midline of the belly, about halfway between the navel and the bottom of the breastbone. Press softly inward, using your index finger.

## Conception Vessel 17

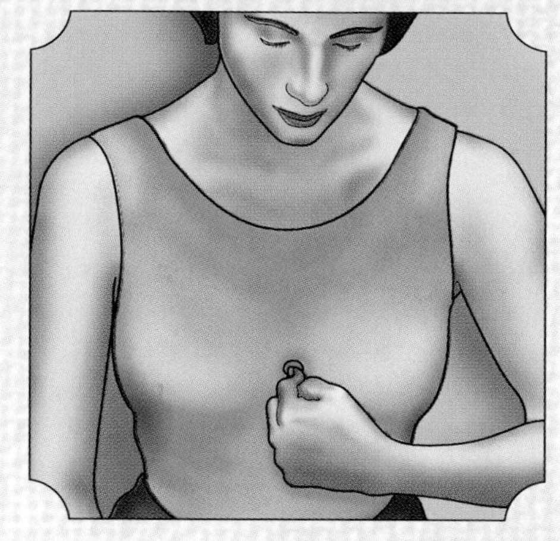

Place your index finger in the center of your chest, midway between the nipples, and press lightly.

## Conception Vessel 22

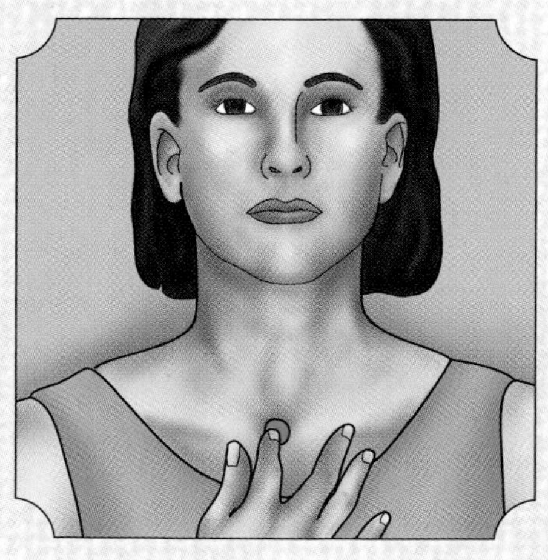

This point lies directly below the Adam's apple, midway between the collarbones in the large hollow at the base of the throat. Place the tip of your index or middle finger on the point site and press downward lightly.

## Gall Bladder 2

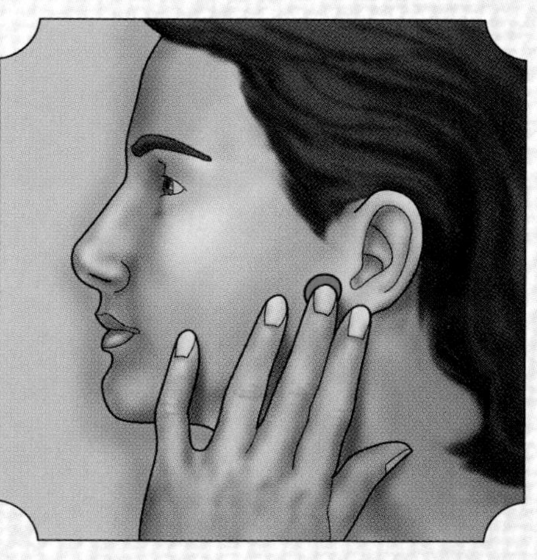

Open your mouth and, feeling along the jawbone, locate the depression directly in front of your ears. Place the tips of your middle fingers about one-half inch below the base of the depression. Close your mouth and press steadily on the point.

# *Gallery of Acupressure Techniques*

## *Gall Bladder 20*

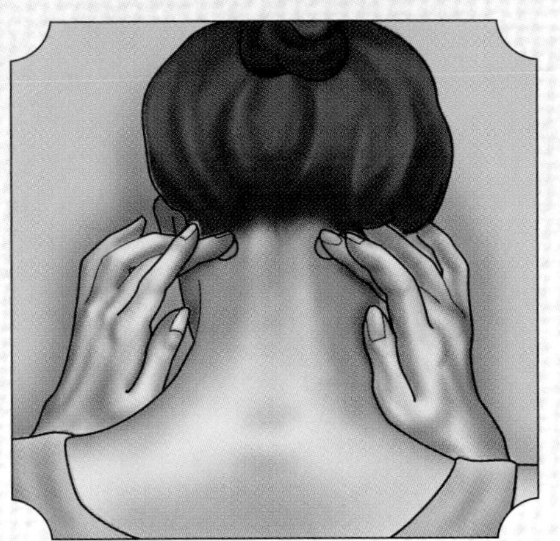

*Place the tips of your middle fingers in the hollows at the base of your skull, about two inches apart on either side of the spine. Press firmly.*

## *Gall Bladder 21*

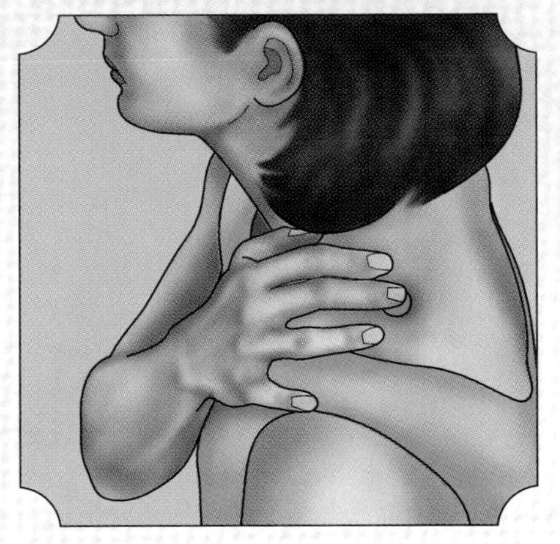

*Apply pressure with your right middle finger to the highest point on your left shoulder muscle, one or two inches out from the base of the neck. Repeat on the other side. (Use light pressure if you are pregnant.)*

## *Gall Bladder 34*

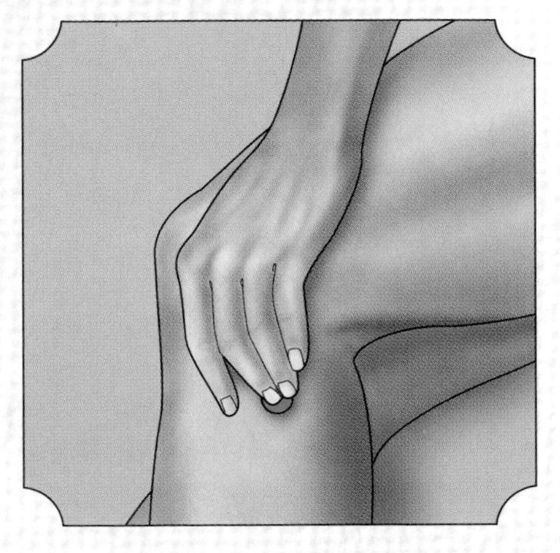

*While seated with legs bent, locate the bony indentation on your lower leg just below and to the outside of the kneecap. Apply firm pressure to the point with your finger or thumb.*

## *Gall Bladder 39*

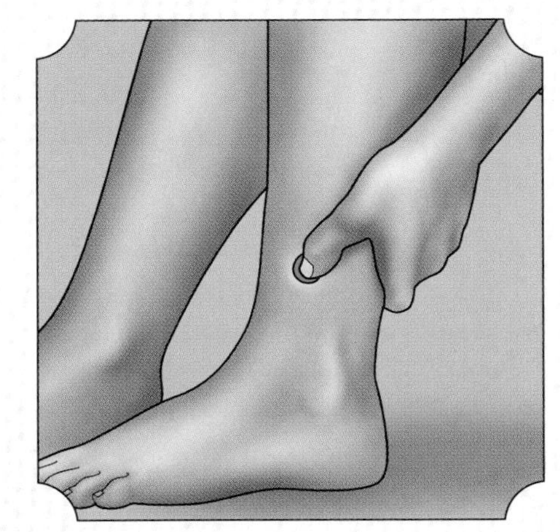

*To find this point, measure four finger widths above the outside anklebone, in front of the fibula, on the lower leg. Apply pressure with the tip of your finger or thumb.*



CONTINUED

# Gallery of Acupressure Techniques

## Governing Vessel 4

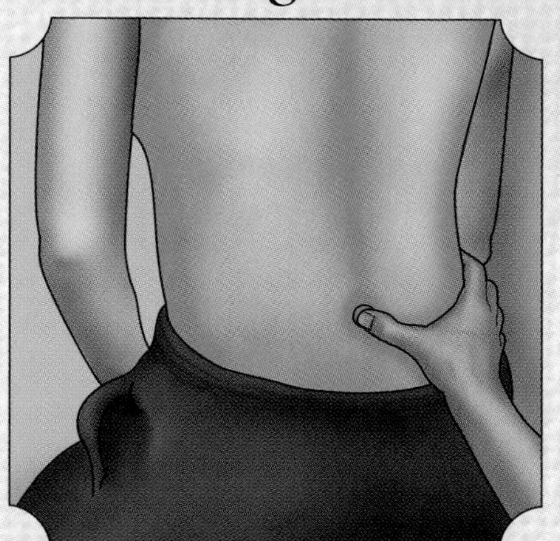

Press hard with your thumb on the midline of the spine, directly behind the navel. The point is located between the second and third lumbar vertebrae.

## Governing Vessel 14

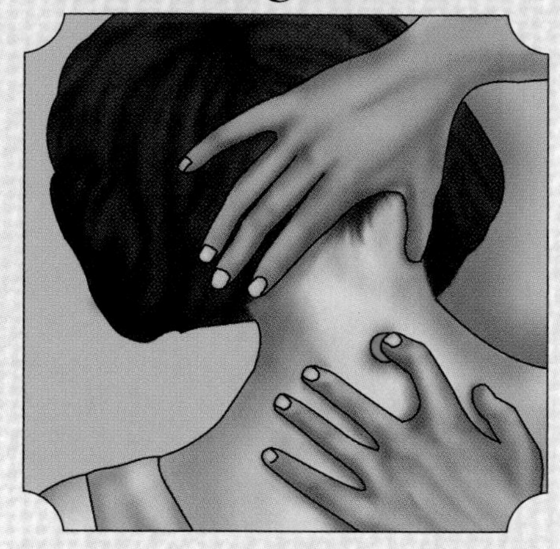

Tilt your head and locate the seventh cervical vertebra, the most prominent bone on the back of your neck. Have a helper press the thumb or index finger hard between this bone and the first thoracic vertebra below it.

## Governing Vessel 20

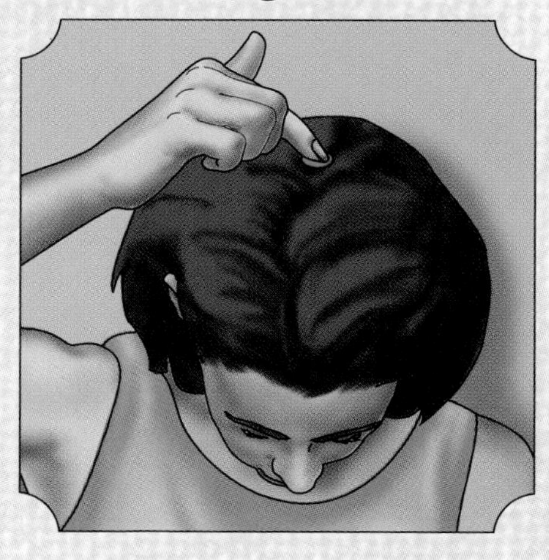

This point is located on the flat spot at the top of the head, midway along an imaginary line connecting the upper part of the ears. Apply pressure with your thumb or index finger. (Do not press this point if you have high blood pressure.)

## Governing Vessel 24.5

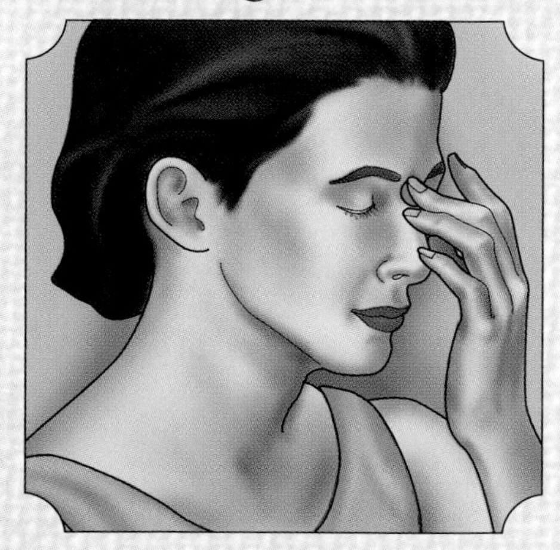

Place the tip of your middle finger at the top of the bridge of the nose, between your eyebrows. Press lightly.

# *Gallery of Acupressure Techniques*

## *Governing Vessel 25*

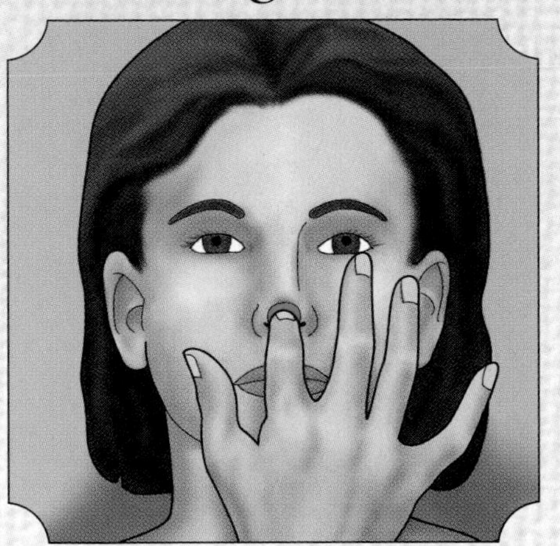

Lightly press the tip of your nose with the end of your finger.

## *Heart 3*

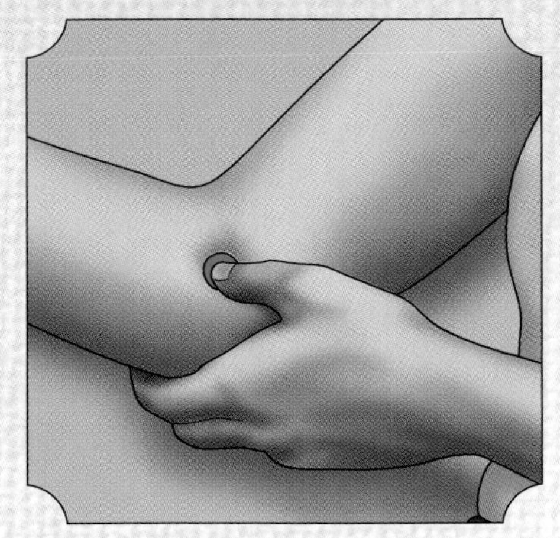

On the inside of the upper arm, use your thumb to apply pressure next to the tendon in the indentation near the inside elbow crease, in line with the little finger.

## *Heart 7*

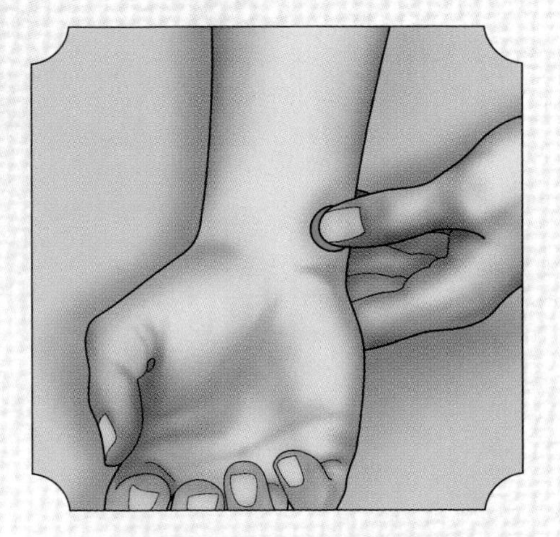

This point is located on the crease along the inside of the wrist, directly in line with the little finger. Squeeze firmly, using the thumb and index finger of your other hand.

## *Kidney 1*

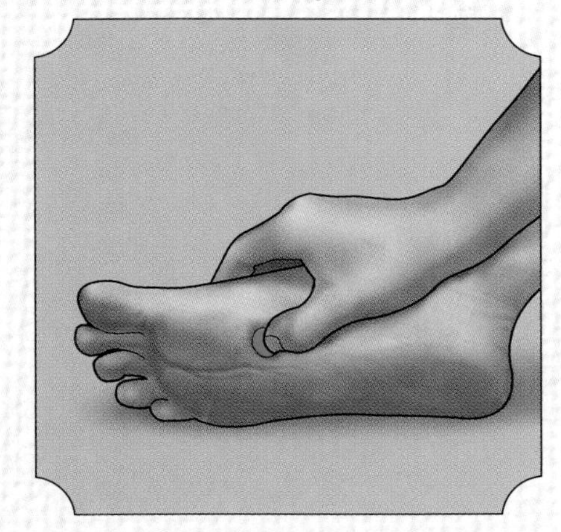

Use one or both thumbs to press just behind the ball of the foot, in the slight indentation of the back of the large pad that corresponds to the big toe. (Do not use this point if you have low blood pressure.)



CONTINUED

# Gallery of Acupressure Techniques

## Kidney 3

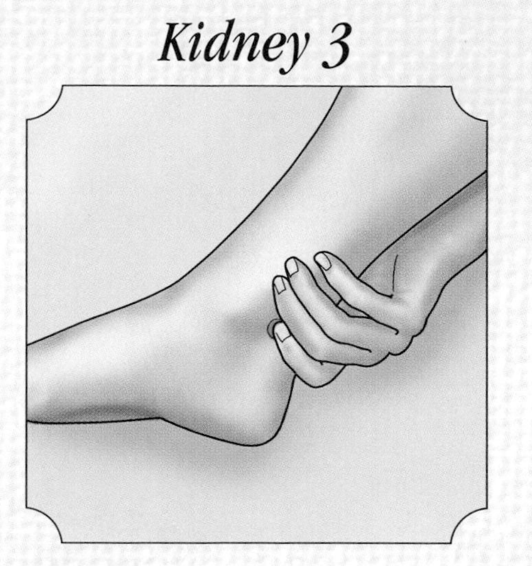

This point lies midway between the inside anklebone and the Achilles tendon at the back of the ankle. Apply pressure with your thumb or index finger. (Avoid using this point after the third month of pregnancy.)

## Large Intestine 4

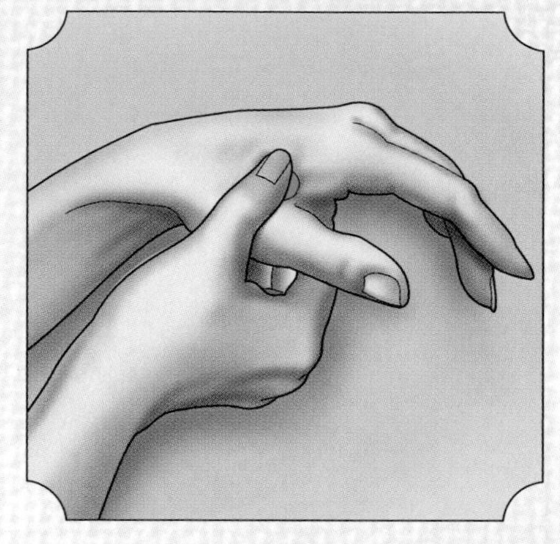

Use the thumb and index finger of your right hand to squeeze the webbing between the thumb and index finger of your left hand. Switch hands and repeat. (Do not apply pressure to this point if you are pregnant.)

## Large Intestine 10

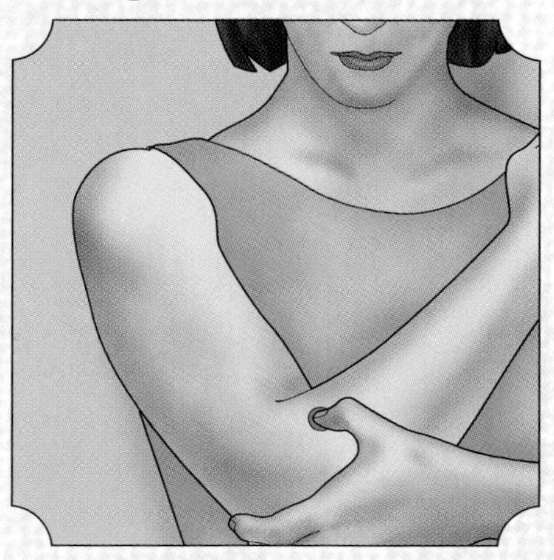

With your arm bent and your palm down, measure two thumb widths below the edge of the elbow crease. The point site lies in the groove between the muscles on the outside of the arm. Press hard with your thumb, then repeat on the other arm.

## Large Intestine 11

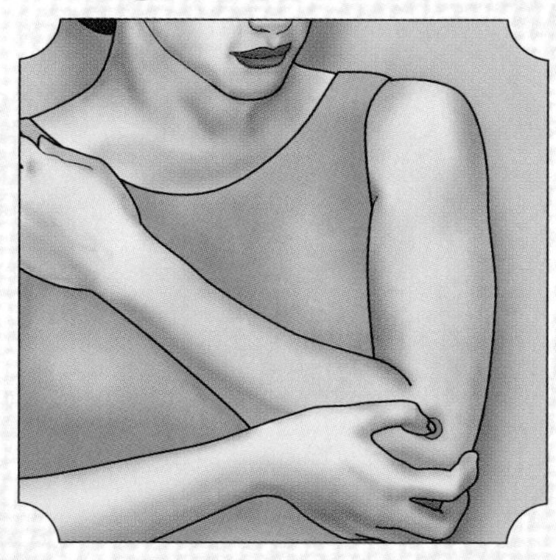

With your arm bent, use your thumb to press deeply on the outer edge of the elbow crease. Repeat on the other arm.

# Gallery of Acupressure Techniques

## Large Intestine 20

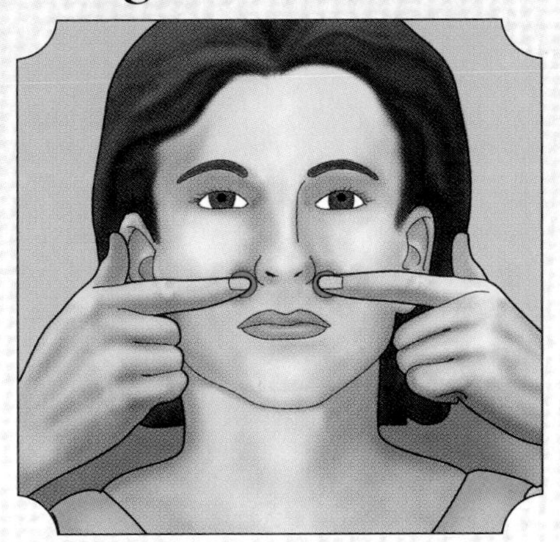

Using your index or middle fingers, press hard on the outer edge of the nostrils at the base of the nose.

## Liver 2

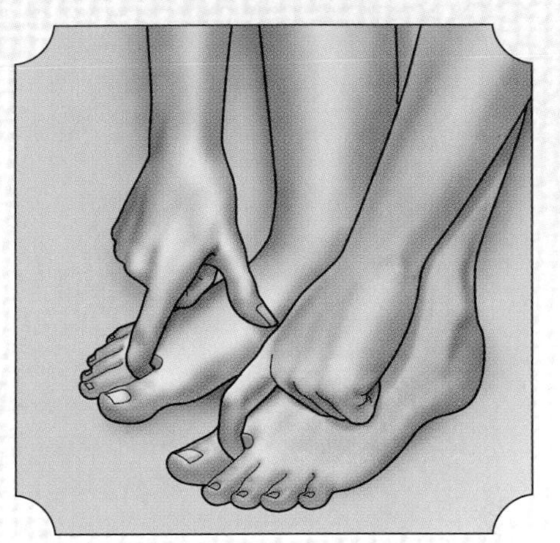

On the top of each foot, use your index finger to press into the webbing between the big toe and the second toe.

## Liver 3

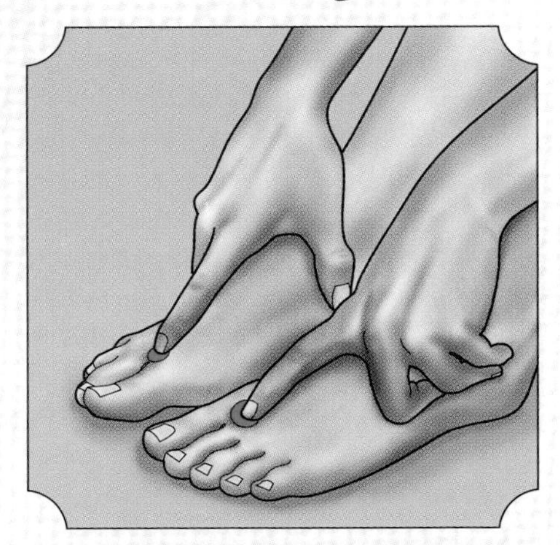

Place your index fingers next to the large knuckle of each big toe, then press into the groove on top of the foot between the big toe and the second toe.

## Liver 8

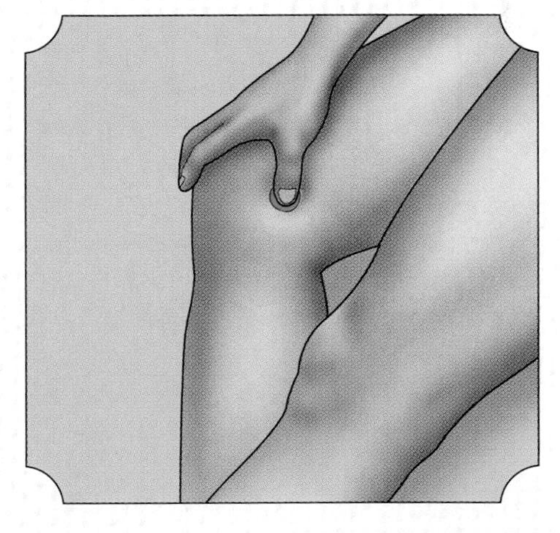

Bend the right knee and place your right thumb just above the knee crease on the inside of the leg. The point lies just below the knee joint (swing your leg a few times to help locate it). Press, then repeat on the other leg.



CONTINUED

# Gallery of Acupressure Techniques

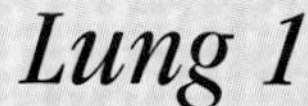

## Lung 1

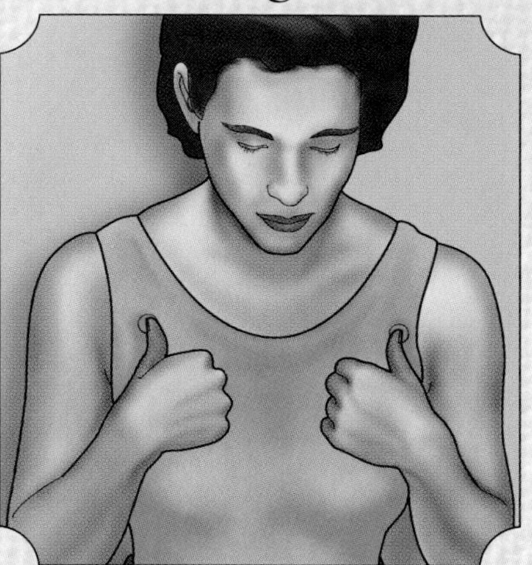

Place the thumb or index finger of each hand about one-half inch below the large hollow under the collarbone, on the outer part of the chest near the shoulder. Apply pressure gently.

## Lung 5

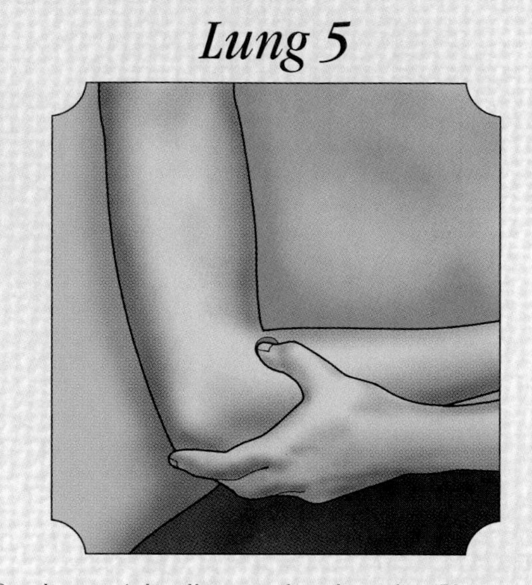

Bend your right elbow and make a fist. Place your left thumb on the outside crease (thumb side) of the elbow alongside the taut tendon and press firmly. Repeat on the other arm.

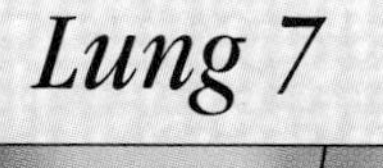

## Lung 7

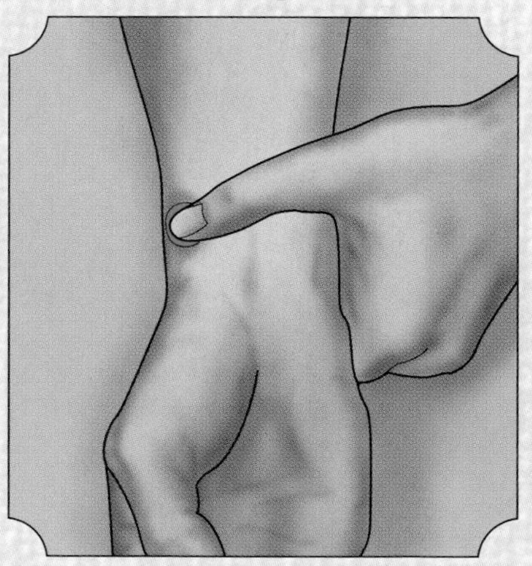

On the thumb side of the inner forearm, measure two finger widths above the crease in the wrist. Apply steady, firm pressure to the point site with your thumb, then repeat on the other arm.

## Lung 10

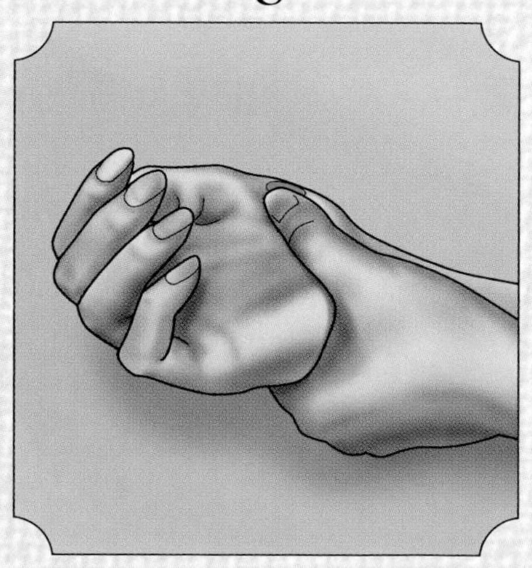

On the palm side of the hand, locate this point at the center of the pad at the base of the thumb. Apply pressure with your other thumb while taking several deep breaths.

# Gallery of Acupressure Techniques

## Pericardium 3

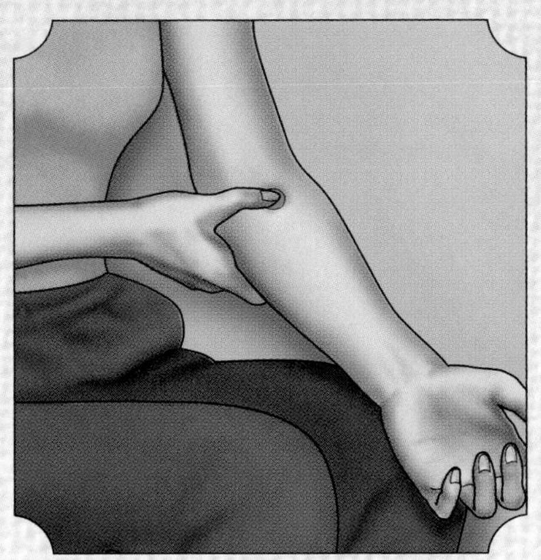

*Locate the point along the biceps tendon at the elbow crease, in a direct line with your ring finger. Use your thumb to apply firm pressure, then repeat on the other arm.*

## Pericardium 6

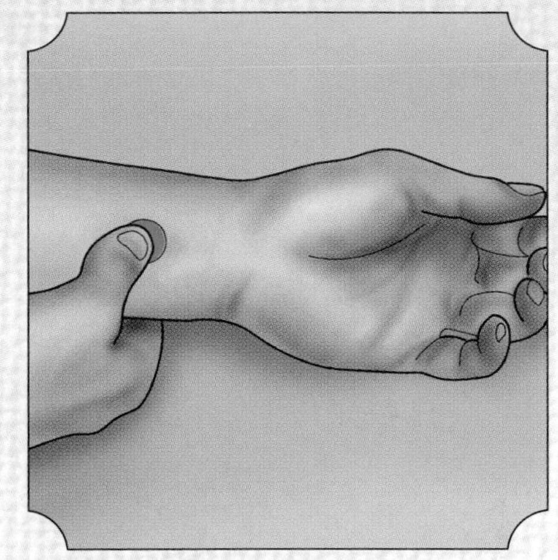

*To find this point, measure two finger widths above the center of the wrist crease on the inside of your arm. With your thumb, press between the two bones of the forearm. Repeat on the other arm.*

## Small Intestine 3

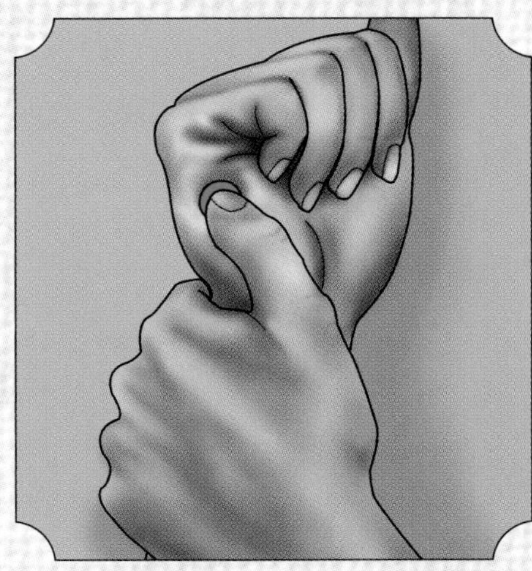

*Make a loose fist, then twist your wrist to view the side of your little finger. Using your thumb, apply pressure to the side of your palm just below the knuckle of the little finger, between the bone and muscle.*

## Small Intestine 17

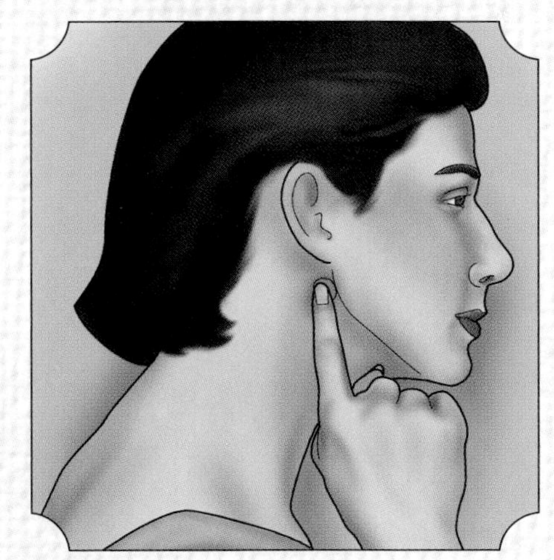

*Place your index fingers just below your earlobes, in the indentations at the back of the jawbone. Apply light pressure while breathing deeply.*



CONTINUED

# Gallery of Acupressure Techniques

## Spleen 3

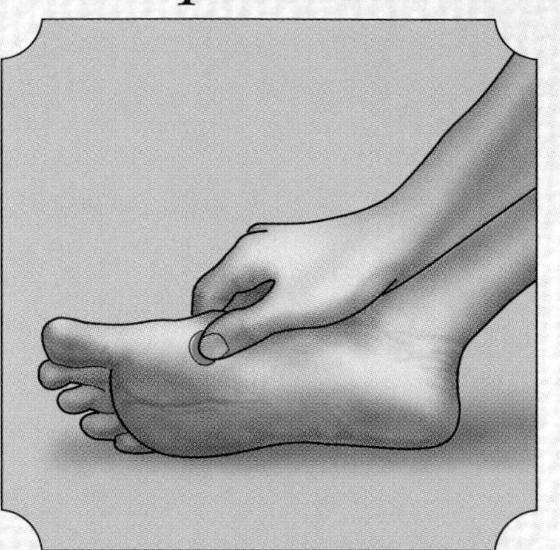

Locate the indentation on the inside of the foot, just behind the bulge made by the large joint of the big toe. Maintain steady pressure on the point site with your thumb. Repeat on the other foot.

## Spleen 4

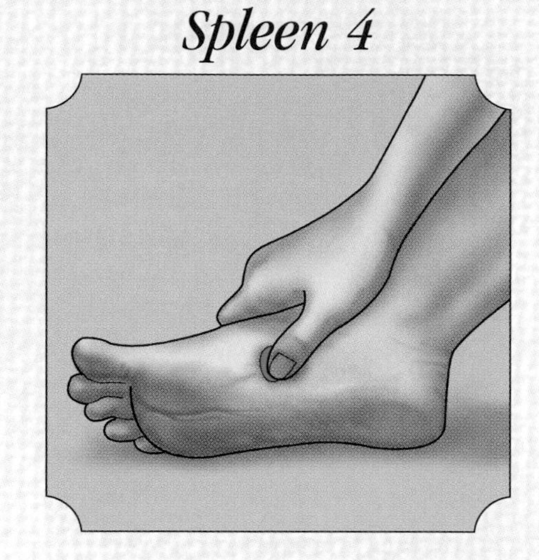

On the inside arch of your foot, measure one thumb width back from the ball of the foot. Apply pressure to this point with your thumb, and then repeat on the other foot.

## Spleen 6

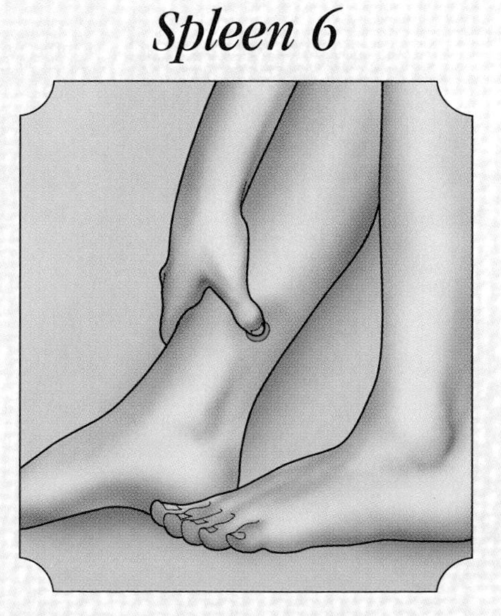

Measure four finger widths up from the top of the right inside anklebone. With your thumb, press near the edge of the shinbone. Repeat on the other leg. (Do not apply pressure to this point if you are pregnant.)

## Spleen 8

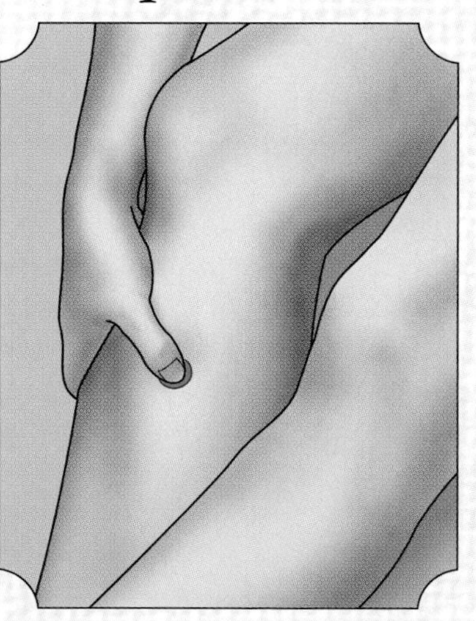

On the inside of the lower leg, locate the depression four finger widths below the knee. Press firmly between your calf muscle and your leg bone.

# Gallery of Acupressure Techniques

## Spleen 9

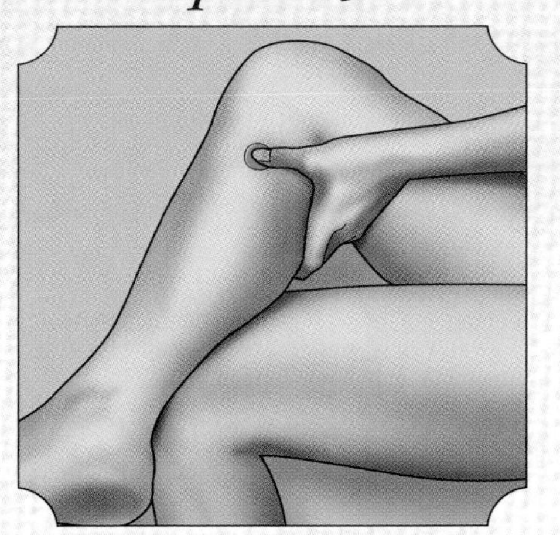

Place your thumb in the depression between the tibia and calf muscle on the inside of your leg, just below the knee joint. Press under the large bulge of the bone.

## Spleen 10

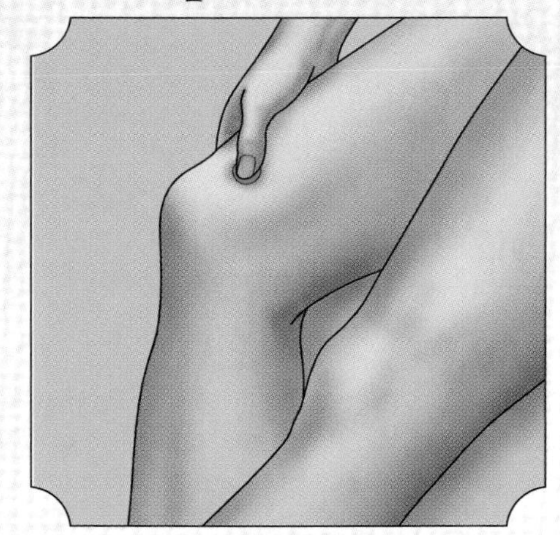

Bend your knee slightly to find this point, located two thumb widths up from the top of your knee, in line with the inner edge of the kneecap. Press on the bulge of the muscle with your thumb.

## Spleen 12

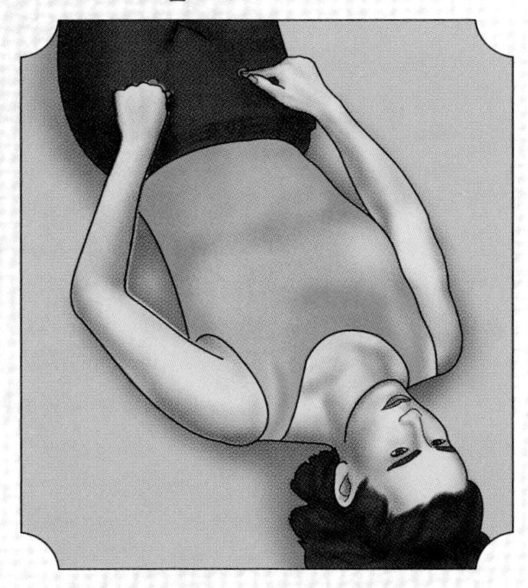

In the pelvic area, use your fingertips to press the middle of the crease where the leg joins the trunk of the body.

## Stomach 2

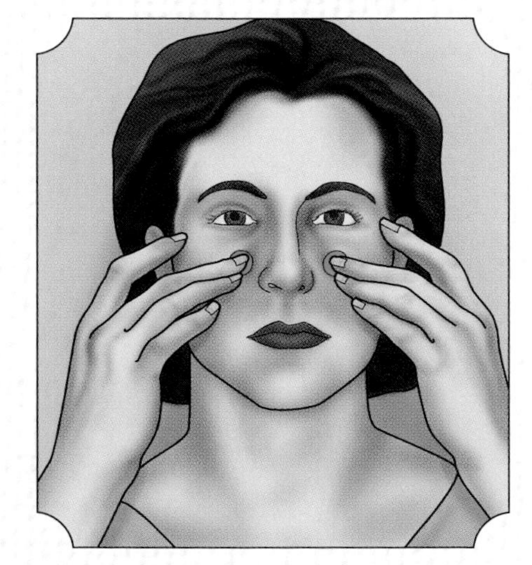

Measure one finger width below the lower ridge of the eye sockets, in line with the pupils. Press into the indentation of the cheeks.



CONTINUED

# Gallery of Acupressure Techniques

## Stomach 3

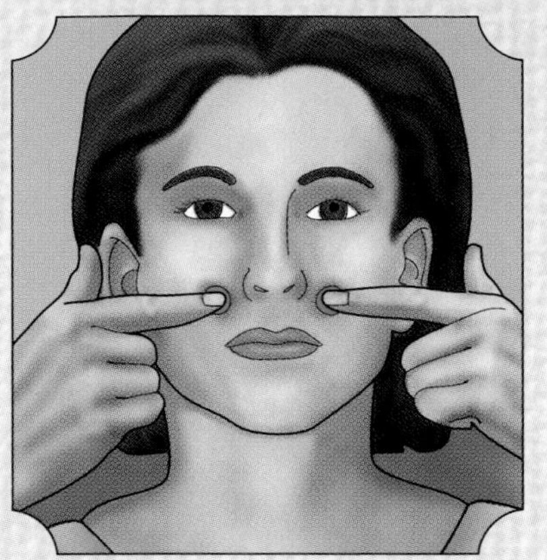

*Place your index fingers at the bottom of your cheekbones, directly under the pupils of your eyes, then press firmly.*

## Stomach 7

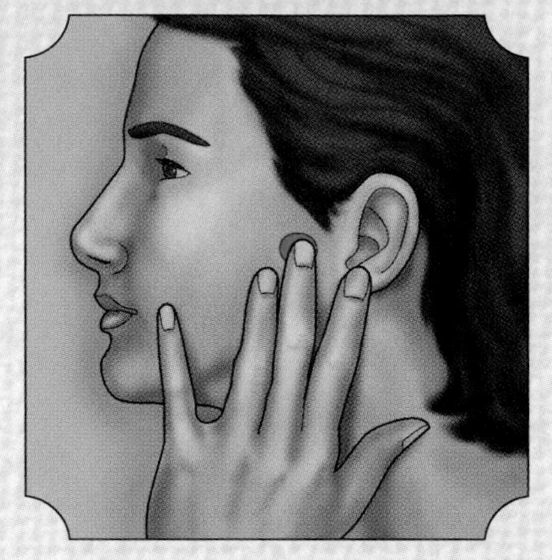

*With your middle finger, feel on either side of your jaw one thumb width in front of your ears. Press the point site in the slight indentation along the upper jaw line.*

## Stomach 25

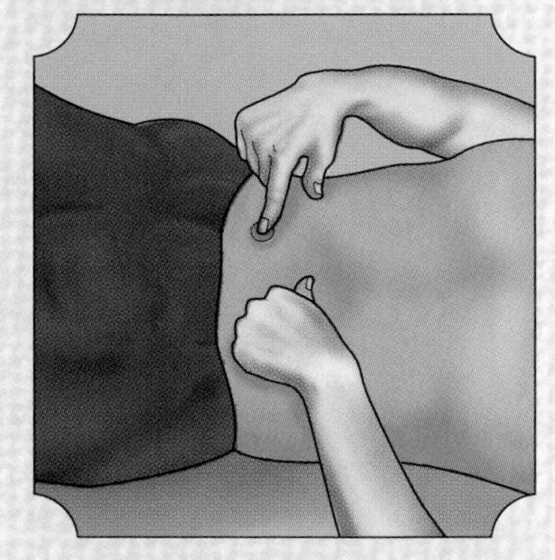

*Place the index fingers of both hands two finger widths from your navel on either side. Press down firmly and breathe deeply.*

## Stomach 36

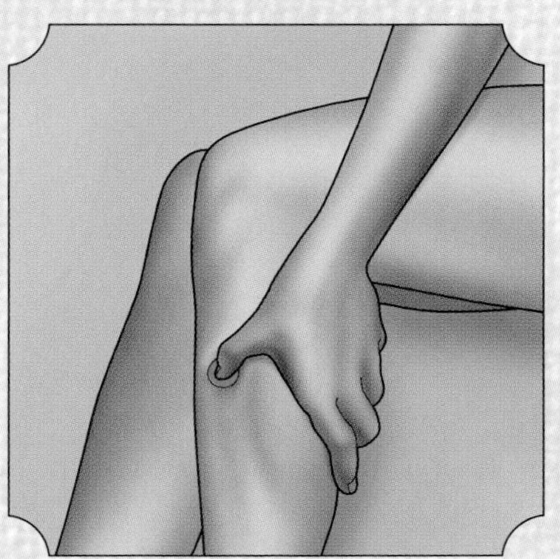

*Measure four finger widths below the kneecap just outside the shinbone (flex your foot; you should feel a muscle bulge at the point site). Press the point steadily with a finger or thumb, then repeat on the other leg.*

## Stomach 44

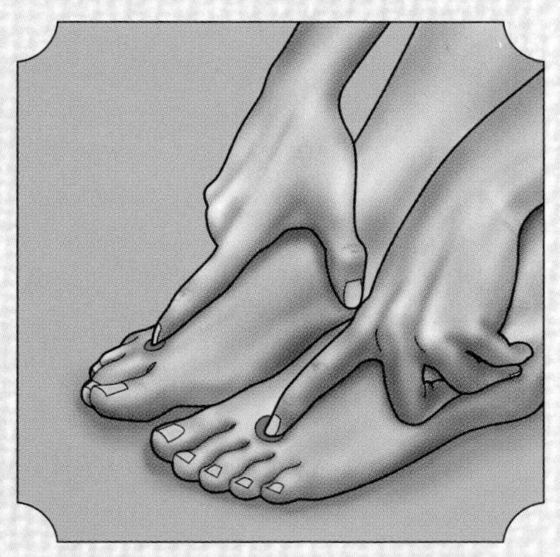

*Using your index fingers, press lightly on the webbing between the second and third toes of each foot.*

# Gallery of Acupressure Techniques

## Triple Warmer 3

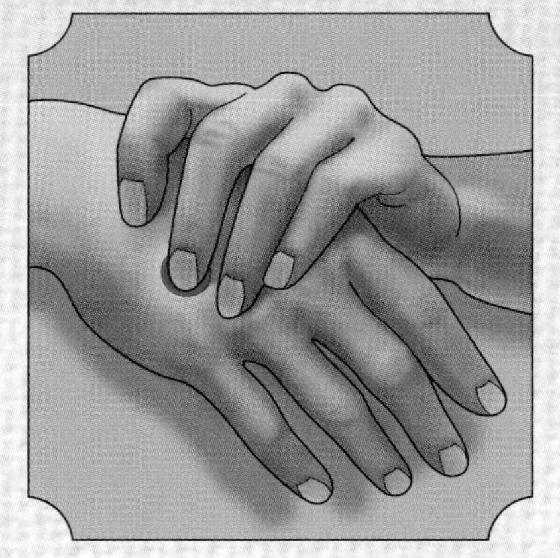

*On the back of the hand, press firmly into the furrow just below the fourth and fifth knuckles (between the ring and little fingers). Repeat on the other hand.*

## Triple Warmer 5

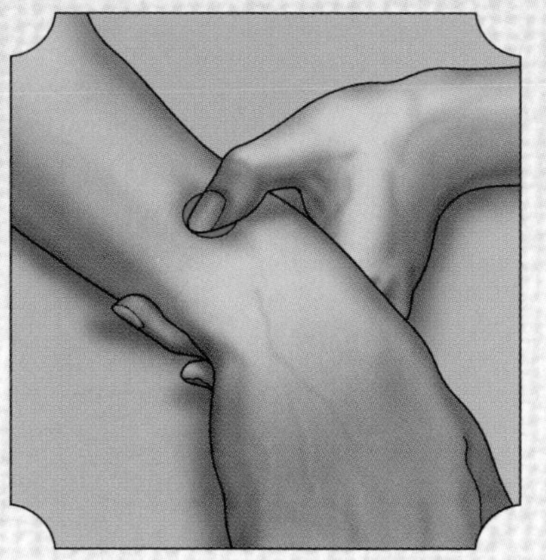

*Center your thumb on the top of your forearm, two thumb widths from the wrist joint, and press firmly. Repeat on the other arm.*

## Triple Warmer 6

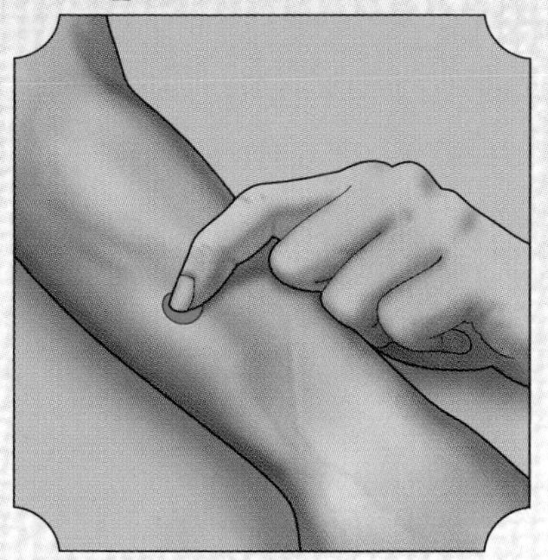

*Measure about three finger widths from the wrist on the top of the forearm, then press this point with your thumb or index finger. Repeat on the other arm.*

## Triple Warmer 17

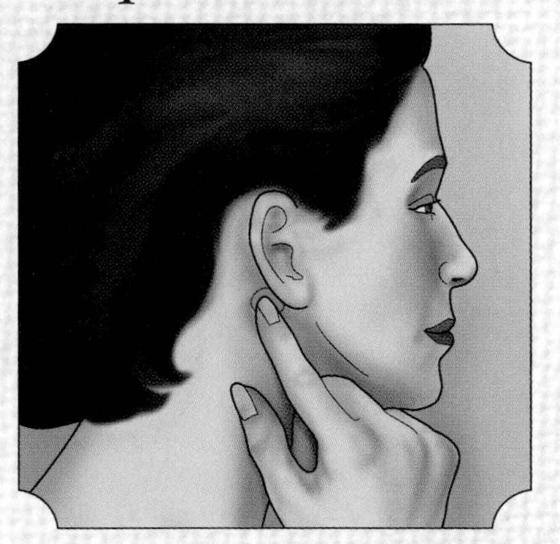

*Using the tips of your index or middle fingers, find the hollows behind the earlobes where the ears meet the jawbone. Press lightly and breathe deeply.*

## Hiccup 1

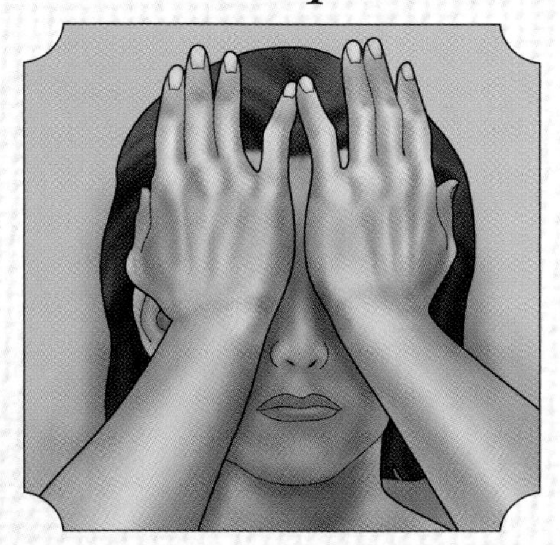

*To stop hiccups, place your palms over both eyes, with heels resting on your cheekbones. Massage gently by pressing the pads below your thumbs toward your palms, then follow instructions for Governing Vessel 25.*

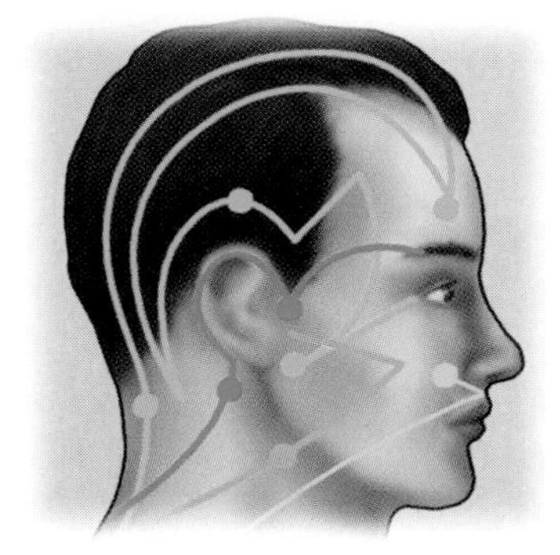

## Target Ailments

- Arthritis
- Asthma
- Athletic Injuries
- Back Problems
- Bursitis
- Chronic Fatigue Syndrome
- Common Cold
- Depression
- Earache
- Gout
- Headache
- Hemorrhoids
- Indigestion
- Insomnia
- Nausea
- Pain, Chronic
- Sinusitis
- Sore Throat
- Stress
- Tendinitis
- Toothache

*See Common Ailments, beginning on page 194.*

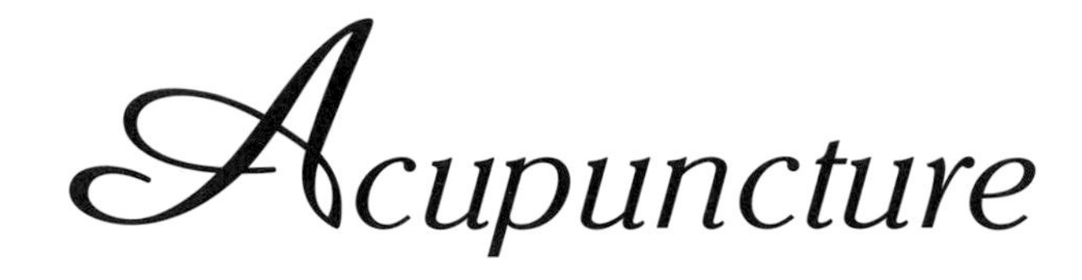

# Acupuncture

*The healing technique of acupuncture, like other therapeutic approaches in the traditional practice of Chinese medicine (pages 57-60), is founded on the principle that internal harmony is essential for good health. Fundamental to this harmony is the concept of chi (sometimes spelled "qi"), a vital energy or life force that ebbs and flows with changes in a person's mental, physical, and spiritual well-being. Chi is said to circulate through the body within 14 invisible channels called meridians (see the illustrations on pages 34-35), forming a network called the web of life. A balanced, freely flowing chi is said to generate good health, while a sluggish, blocked, or overstimulated chi is believed to cause illness. Acupuncturists strive to encourage proper chi circulation by manipulating it at "chi gateways" just below the skin; the manipulation is achieved by inserting hair-thin needles at these gateways, which are more commonly known as acupoints. The stimulation that results is said to enable a person to achieve internal harmony, a state that allows the body's self-healing mechanisms to engage.*

### *Origins*

Acupuncture has been practiced in China for about 4,500 years. Its spread to the West has been relatively slow but steady. The first real surge in popularity in the United States came in 1971, following a story by a *New York Times* journalist who had been successfully treated for pain with acupuncture during a visit to China.

### *What It's Good For*

Traditionally, acupuncturists have treated scores of different illnesses, as indicated by the list at left, which represents only a sampling of them. Although acupuncture's primary use in the United States has been to alleviate pain, its therapeutic applications have been gradually expanding. Today,

**LICENSED & INSURED?**

**YES!** *Currently 33 states and the District of Columbia have set standards for acupuncturists. Choose a practitioner who is a physician or who is board-certified in acupuncture by the National Certification Commission for Acupuncture and Oriental Medicine. For help finding a certified acupuncturist in your area, contact the American Association of Oriental Medicine.*

*In 1996 the FDA classified acupuncture needles as a type of medical device. This indirectly boosts acupuncture's credibility and increases the likelihood that your insurance provider will pay for your acupuncture treatments. Coverage varies tremendously. Your provider's claims office is your best information source.*

acupuncture is employed in treating addictions, controlling weight, and enhancing recuperation following surgery or stroke.

### Visiting a Professional

In order to properly evaluate your needs, during a first visit an acupuncturist will observe you closely, check your pulse, look at your tongue, and ask many questions about your health and your lifestyle. These are customary diagnostic routines employed by practitioners of all forms of Chinese medicine.

After this evaluation, the therapy itself can begin. Typically, the acupuncturist inserts acupuncture needles into the skin at the appropriate acupoints, then twirls them and, possibly, applies a gentle electric current (which is believed to enhance effectiveness). The needles may penetrate as little as a fraction of an inch (on the fingertips, for example) or as much as three or four inches (where a thick layer of fat or muscle exists). The procedure usually causes little pain, although patients often feel numbness where the needles are inserted, and perhaps a bit of tingling.

In addition to—or sometimes instead of—inserting needles, acupuncturists may opt for a treatment called moxibustion. This consists of applying heat directly above acupuncture points by means of small bundles of smoldering herbs, usually mugwort leaf. The practitioner may also employ acupressure *(pages 16-17).*

### Wellness

Because acupuncture's ultimate goal is to maximize the body's own healing abilities, it is little surprise that acupuncture treatments are considered helpful in maintaining as well as restoring health. Indeed, acupuncturists are trained to recognize so-called disharmonies early, often before they develop into full-blown disease.

### What the Critics Say

Although the American Medical Association does not officially sanction acupuncture, more than 2,000 of the United States' 12,000 acupuncturists are MDs. But many physicians find it hard to accept acupuncture's invisible energy-path theory of effectiveness. The "placebo effect" is most often cited as the reason acupuncture works—an argument that has not, however, held up to scientific testing. Some say that the pain of inserting acupuncture needles distracts the patient from his or her original pain, but this would not account for acupuncture's reputed success in treating other, painless ailments; also, properly inserted needles are not usually painful.

Research indicates that acupuncture stimulates the body to release its own natural painkillers (endorphins and enkephalins), as well as an anti-inflammatory agent (cortisol). Whether enough of these natural chemicals are released to account for acupuncture's apparent success has yet to be determined. ■

#### CAUTION

**While acupuncture can help one manage the pain of labor and delivery, it is generally not recommended for other purposes during pregnancy because it may stimulate uterine contractions and could induce labor.**

#### FOR MORE INFO

Following is a list of organizations you can contact to learn more about acupuncture:

**National Acupuncture and Oriental Medicine Alliance**
14637 Starr Road, SE
Olalla, WA 98359
(206) 851-6896
fax: (206) 851-6883

**American Association of Oriental Medicine**
433 Front Street
Catasauqua, PA 18032
(610) 433-2448
fax: (610) 264-2768
e-mail AAOM1@aol.com

**American Academy of Medical Acupuncture**
5820 Wilshire Blvd, Suite 500
Los Angeles, CA 90036
(800) 521-2262
fax: (213) 937-0959
e-mail: KCKD71F@prodigy.com

**National Certification Commission for Acupuncture and Oriental Medicine**
PO Box 97075
Washington, DC 20090-7075
(202) 232-1404
fax: (202) 462-6157



CONTINUED

# Acupuncture CONTINUED

## Meridians and Acupoints

*Chinese medicine teaches that energy flowing through invisible channels in the body called meridians may be manipulated by pressure (acupressure), the insertion of fine needles (acupuncture), or warmth (moxibustion) to treat disease and improve health. Meridians and related acupoints are listed below. For more information, see the Gallery of Acupressure Techniques, pages 18-31.*

● Bladder
**1** BL 1
**2** BL 2
**3** BL 7
**4** BL 10
**5** BL 13
**6** BL 23
**7** BL 25
**8** BL 27
**9** BL 28
**10** BL 29
**11** BL 30
**12** BL 31
**13** BL 32
**14** BL 33
**15** BL 34
**16** BL 40
**17** BL 57
**18** BL 58
**19** BL 60

● Conception Vessel
**20** CV 4
**21** CV 6
**22** CV 12
**23** CV 17
**24** CV 22

● Gall Bladder
**25** GB 2
**26** GB 8
**27** GB 14
**28** GB 20
**29** GB 21
**30** GB 30
**31** GB 34
**32** GB 39
**33** GB 40
**34** GB 41

● Governing Vessel
**35** GV 4
**36** GV 14
**37** GV 16
**38** GV 20
**39** GV 24.5
**40** GV 25
**41** GV 26

● Heart
**42** HE 3
**43** HE 7

● Kidney
**44** KI 1
**45** KI 2
**46** KI 3
**47** KI 5
**48** KI 6
**49** KI 7
**50** KI 27

● Large Intestine
**51** LI 4
**52** LI 10
**53** LI 11
**54** LI 15
**55** LI 20

● Liver
**56** LV 2
**57** LV 3
**58** LV 8

● Lung
**59** LU 1
**60** LU 5
**61** LU 6
**62** LU 7
**63** LU 9
**64** LU 10

● Pericardium
**65** PE 3
**66** PE 6
**67** PE 7

● Small Intestine
**68** SI 3
**69** SI 4
**70** SI 5
**71** SI 8
**72** SI 10
**73** SI 11
**74** SI 17

● Spleen
**75** SP 3
**76** SP 4
**77** SP 6
**78** SP 8
**79** SP 9
**80** SP 10
**81** SP 12
**82** SP 16

● Stomach
**83** ST 2
**84** ST 3
**85** ST 6
**86** ST 7
**87** ST 16
**88** ST 18
**89** ST 25
**90** ST 35
**91** ST 36
**92** ST 40
**93** ST 44

● Triple Warmer
**94** TW 3
**95** TW 4
**96** TW 5
**97** TW 15
**98** TW 17
**99** TW 21

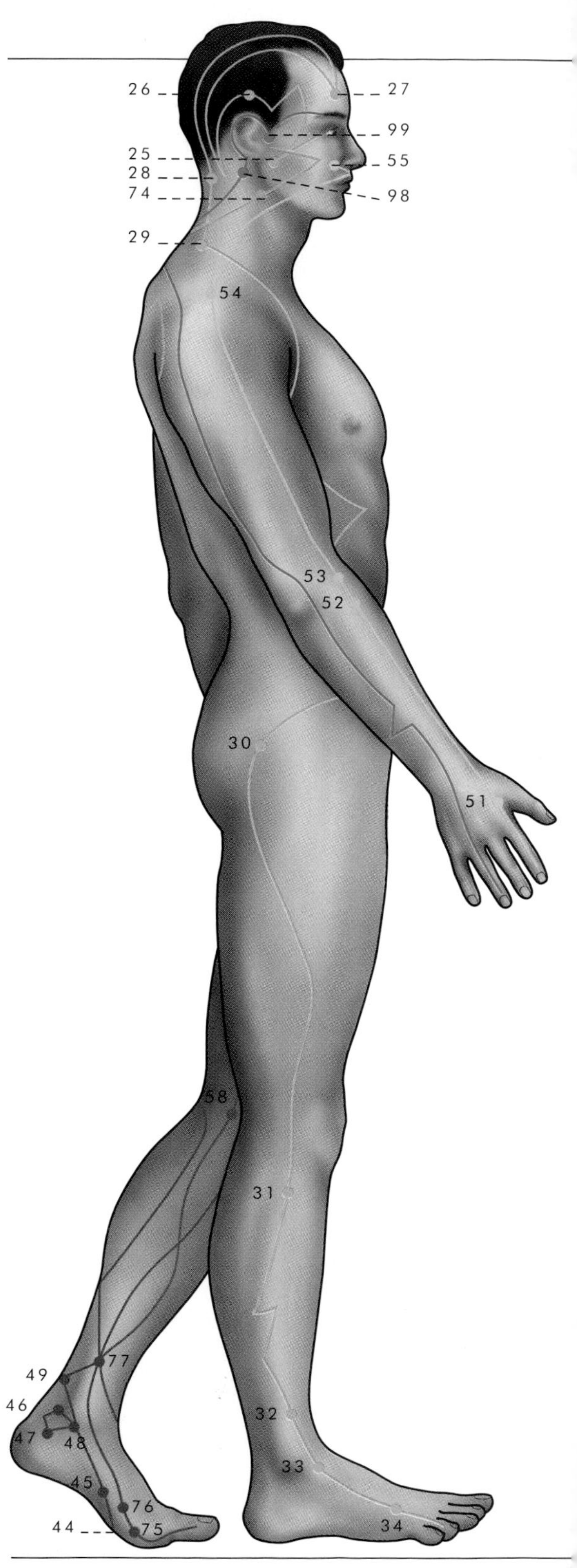

# Acupuncture

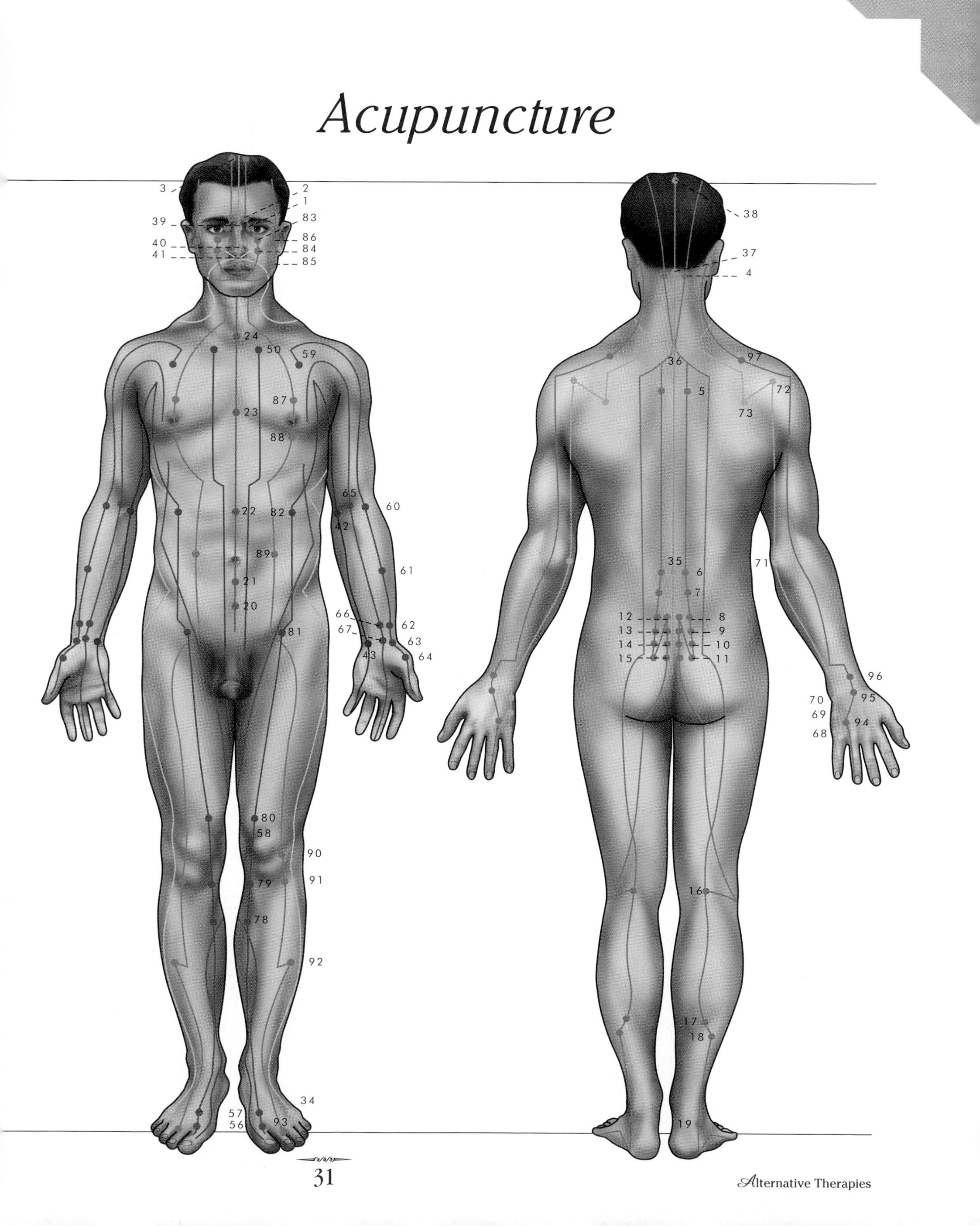

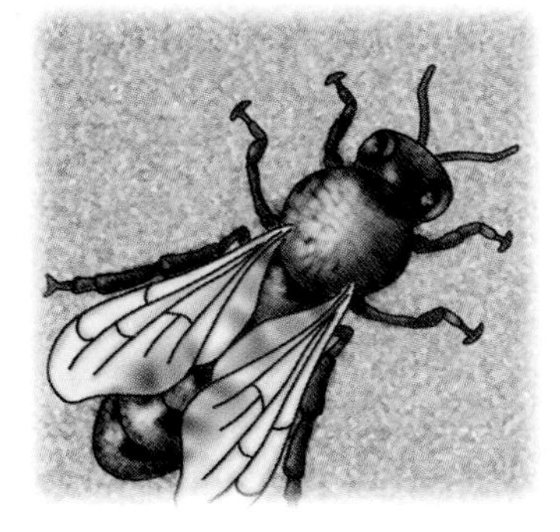

**Target Ailments**

**For Bee Venom Therapy:**

- Arthritis
- Bursitis
- Headache
- Menopause
- Multiple Sclerosis
- Premenstrual Syndrome
- Tendinitis

*See Common Ailments, beginning on page 194.*

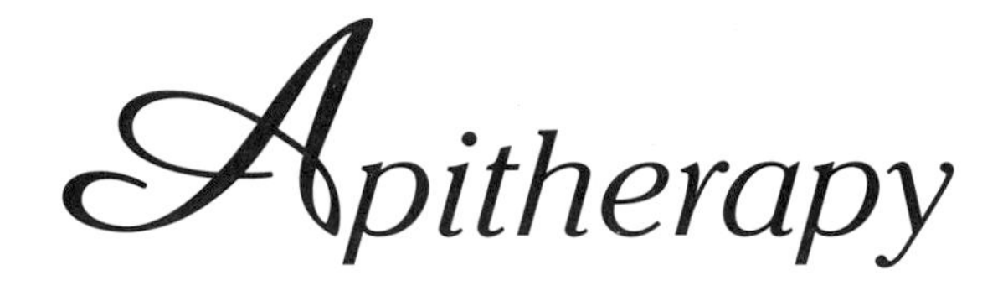

# Apitherapy

*Apitherapy is the therapeutic use of any of the products of the honeybee. Honey itself, for example, has been shown to have antiseptic and antibacterial properties, as does a substance known as propolis, which is made by bees from tree resin and is used to cement the hive together. Bee pollen has high concentrations of vitamins and minerals and so is sometimes incorporated into nutritional therapy, while royal jelly—a potent food made specially for the queen bee—is reputed to have energizing effects and to stimulate hormone production.*

*Perhaps most surprising and controversial are reports of success in the use of honeybee venom—administered either by injection or directly by stinging—to reduce symptoms such as pain and inflammation in chronic illnesses.*

## Bee Venom Therapy

Although by definition a poison, bee venom contains among its active ingredients the peptide melittin, a potent anti-inflammatory agent. Inside the body, melittin stimulates the adrenal glands to produce cortisol, a natural steroid with powerful healing properties and none of the complications of synthetic steroids. When venom is introduced into tissues that are already inflamed by disease, the area becomes further inflamed in reaction to the venom, but at the same time the body's anti-inflammatory agents are called into action; as they work to shrink the swelling caused by the venom, these agents are also thought to help reduce the inflammation resulting from the original condition.

## Origins

Apitherapy dates back to the ancient civilizations of Greece and China. Bee stings were used by the Greek physicians Hippocrates and Galen, and apitherapy is mentioned in both the Bible and the Koran. Phillip Terc, an Austrian physician, initiated the modern study of intentional bee stings with his 1888 work entitled "Report about a Peculiar Connection between the Beestings and Rheumatism." Medical and lay practitioners today number in the thousands.

**LICENSED & INSURED?**

*Bee venom therapy does not require a licensed practitioner. But when a physician administers the treatment (using either live bees or a hypodermic needle), the procedure may be covered by medical insurance as part of an office visit. Although bee venom presently is approved by the U.S. Food and Drug Administration only as a desensitizing agent, some physicians have won approval to use it as an "investigational new drug."*

# Apitherapy

## What It's Good For

Raw (unheated, unfiltered) honey can be used topically as a wound or burn dressing. Bee pollen is a potent dietary supplement and may also be helpful in treating seasonal allergies. The germ-fighting properties of propolis make it effective for treating sore throat, colds, and flu. Royal jelly, long a staple of folk medicines and also sometimes used in cosmetics, has been used to treat vascular diseases and illnesses that cause weakness or tiredness.

Venom therapy may help reduce pain and swelling in osteoarthritis, rheumatoid arthritis, and other inflammatory and degenerative diseases. It is also used to treat various autoimmune diseases. Because of anecdotal reports of significant symptom reduction in multiple sclerosis, venom therapy is being used extensively by patients with that disease, and research is under way to document the therapy's effects. Additionally, venom therapy may help alleviate migraine headaches.

## Preparations/Techniques

Most honeybee products are available in commercial preparations and are either applied topically or taken internally by mouth. Bee venom is delivered at specific sites related to the illness or at acupuncture points, and is administered either through a hypodermic needle or directly by the bee in the form of stings. Some physicians perform the treatment—a must in the case of injection—but the therapy is also sometimes administered by beekeepers, patients themselves, or a partner.

When the stinging method is used, a supply of bees is kept in a jar containing honey; each bee is removed with tweezers and held over the specified area of the body until it stings. The stinger is removed after three to five minutes. The number and frequency of stings depend on the patient and the specific problem.

Injections cost more than stinging, and it is not known whether the processing of the venom reduces its healing effect. On the other hand, bee stings are extremely painful, and the amount of venom cannot be standardized. A less painful method, used infrequently in the United States, involves removing the stinger from the bee and applying it to the skin.

## What the Critics Say

Because most of the evidence for the efficacy of bee venom therapy consists of anecdotes rather than double-blind studies, many Western physicians remain skeptical. Some say multiple sclerosis naturally waxes and wanes and that the benefits reported may be due to either natural remission or the placebo effect. Critics have pointed to occurrences of localized infection and scarring, which result from leaving the stinger in for too long. ■

### CAUTION

**Bee venom can cause a serious and potentially fatal allergic reaction, including severe respiratory distress and shock. Before beginning treatment, you should be allergy-tested; also, be sure an emergency bee sting allergy kit containing epinephrine is on hand during treatment. You should not be concerned about minor swelling and itching caused by the venom; this is a desirable inflammatory response necessary to the healing process.**

### FOR MORE INFO

Following is a list of organizations you can contact to learn more about apitherapy:

**The American Apitherapy Society**
PO Box 54
Hartland Four Corners, VT 05049
(802) 436-2708
fax: (802) 436-2827

**The Multiple Sclerosis Association of America**
706 Haddonfield Road
Cherry Hill, NJ 08002
(800) 833-4672
(609) 488-4500

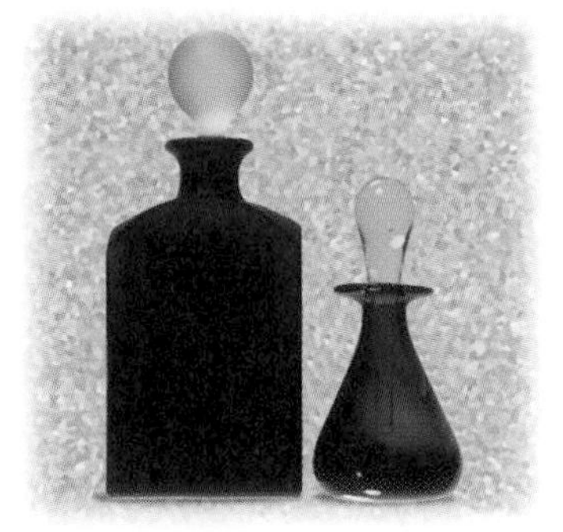

## Target Ailments

- Bladder Infections
- Bronchitis
- Common Cold
- Conjunctivitis
- Depression
- Flu
- Gas and Gas Pains
- Immune Problems
- Indigestion
- Insomnia
- Laryngitis
- Menopause
- Motion Sickness
- Muscle Cramps
- Nausea
- Sexually Transmitted Diseases
- Stress
- Tendinitis
- Tonsillitis
- Yeast Infections

*See Common Ailments, beginning on page 194.*

# Aromatherapy

*Aromatherapy is the therapeutic use of essential oils—concentrated, fragrant extracts of plants—to promote relaxation and help relieve various symptoms. Suppliers of aromatherapy oils extract them from specific parts of plants—the roots, bark, stalks, flowers, leaves, or fruit—by two methods: Distillation uses successive evaporation and condensation to pull the oils from the plants; cold-pressing squeezes rinds or peels through a machine to press out the oils. Users then administer the oils in several ways, generally by applying them to the skin or inhaling their scents.*

*Some practitioners believe the oils have both physical and ethereal (spiritual) qualities and effects. They assert that the oils work on the emotions because the nerves involved in the sense of smell are directly linked to the brain's limbic system, which governs emotion, and that the active components of the oils give them specific therapeutic value, with antiseptic, antibacterial, and antiviral effects common to many of them.*

### *Origins*

Ancient people used aromatic substances for medicinal, cosmetic, and religious purposes. In the 10th century, the Arab doctor Avicenna described methods of distilling plants, although there is evidence that what came to be known as aromatherapy may have been known even in ancient times.

French chemist René-Maurice Gattefossé, who worked in a perfume factory, inaugurated the modern scientific use of essential oils in the 1920s and coined the term *aromatherapy.* After burning his hand in a chemical explosion, he quickly healed it without infection or scarring by applying lavender oil, which happened to be nearby. Gattefossé went on to classify the oils and their properties.

Aromatherapy gained widespread popularity in the United Kingdom and France in the 1980s, but it is less well known and researched in North America.

### *What It's Good For*

Aromatherapists believe that all the oils affect the emotions in some way and that many also work on physical ailments. They think that as well as relieving stress, some oils may improve sluggish circulation, relieve pain, reduce swelling, or cleanse the body of impurities. Others are used to

**LICENSED & INSURED?**

*Aromatherapy practitioners are not licensed in the United States today, although licensed healthcare providers may include aromatherapy as one of their techniques.*

# Aromatherapy

treat bacterial or viral infections, burns, hypertension, arrhythmias, respiratory conditions, insomnia, depression, and many other ailments.

Although patients with asthma may benefit from aromatherapy, they should use the oils only under a practitioner's supervision.

## *Preparations/Techniques*

Essential oils may be applied externally and used in massage, or incorporated into compresses and ointments. They may also be inhaled or taken internally (orally, rectally, or vaginally). Remember to follow all dilution, dosage, and treatment guidelines as well as the cautions on the chart on the following pages.

A common aromatherapy technique is to dilute the oils in a vegetable carrier oil, such as safflower or sweet almond oil, for an aromatherapy massage. You can use basic massage strokes on yourself or a partner *(see the Gallery of Massage Techniques, pages 124-129)* to encourage relaxation or relieve specific problems. If you are prone to allergic reactions, test the oils first by putting a drop of oil on the inside of your elbow and waiting 24 hours for any reaction. During the massage, the skin absorbs the oil at the same time that the user inhales it.

Another way to use the oils is in an aromatic warm bath, which adds the therapeutic qualities of water to those of the oils. You may also apply hot or cold compresses, creams, or lotions made from the oils directly to the skin. For respiratory conditions, insomnia, depression, or stress, try breathing in the aromas using a steam inhaler or a fan-assisted apparatus. Remember to close your eyes when inhaling.

Buy oils from a reputable company and don't shop by price alone, because adulteration with chemicals and cheaper herbs is common. Consult a qualified health practitioner before taking oils internally. Some oils, such as thuja, wormwood, mugwort leaf, tansy, hyssop, sage, and eucalyptus, should never be taken internally.

## *Wellness*

Essential oils are often incorporated into wellness programs because they are easy and pleasant to use. Aromatherapists believe that regular use can reestablish balance and harmony within the body as well as soothe the mind and emotions.

## *What the Critics Say*

Critics from conventional medicine point to the general lack of research in the field and to unscientific pronouncements of its proponents, such as references to ethereal effects and to the so-called subtle parts of the plants. Critics with a holistic viewpoint have faulted aromatherapy because the whole plant is not used. They note that chemical changes occur after a flower is cut that may adversely affect the therapeutic value of a given type of plant. ■

### CAUTION

**Because the oils used in aromatherapy are available over the counter, some people may assume that they are all safe. However, they can have potentially serious side effects, including neurotoxicity and inducement of abortion, as well as skin reactions, allergies, and liver damage. Overexposure to oils by inhalation can produce headache and fatigue. It's best to have a health-care professional supervise you when you use oils.**

### FOR MORE INFO

Following is a list of organizations you can contact to learn more about aromatherapy:

**National Association for Holistic Aromatherapy**
PO Box 17622
Boulder, CO 80308-7622
(800) 566-6735

**Pacific Institute of Aromatherapy**
PO Box 6723
San Rafael, CA 94903
(415) 479-9121
fax: (415) 479-0119



CONTINUED

# The 15 Most Effective Essential Oils

| Name | Parts Used | Properties | Target Ailments |
|---|---|---|---|
| ***Bay laurel*** *Native to the Mediterranean, this hardy evergreen shrub or tree has dark green leaves and black berries. Its oil is greenish yellow and has a powerful spicy scent.* | BERRIES<br>DRIED LEAVES<br>YOUNG TWIGS | An overall strengthener; can be an antiseptic, diuretic, or sedative, and may help to expel gas and clear the lungs. | ■ **Bay laurel** helps in digestive problems and appetite loss, relieves chronic bronchitis, colds, flu, and tonsillitis, and treats scabies and lice. It also aids in rheumatic aches and pains and reduces swollen lymph nodes. CAUTION: Use in moderation. Avoid if pregnant. |
| ***Clary sage*** *This southern European plant has small blue or white flowers and large, hairy leaves. The oil is colorless or pale yellow-green and is used extensively in foods and drinks.* | FLOWERING TOPS<br>LEAVES | A powerful, quick-acting relaxant; has warming effects; eases inflammation; anticonvulsive and antiseptic. | ■ **Clary sage** soothes anxiety and stress, relieves menstrual and menopausal symptoms, and treats burns and eczema. CAUTION: Avoid during pregnancy or if you have high blood pressure. Do not drink alcohol while using. |
| ***Eucalyptus globulus*** *This native Australian evergreen is cultivated in several areas, including the state of California. The oil ranges from clear to yellow and has a penetrating smell.* | LEAVES<br>TWIGS | Strongly antiseptic; antibacterial; expectorant; has stimulating, astringent, and analgesic actions. | ■ **Eucalyptus globulus** reduces fever; fights colds, flu, sinusitis, and cough; helps relieve the symptoms of bronchitis; and is helpful in skin conditions such as boils and pimples. CAUTION: Do not take internally. |
| ***Everlasting*** *This strongly scented herb, with multi-branched stem and bright flowers, is native to the Mediterranean region and grows wild in the Pacific Northwest.* | FLOWERS<br>FLOWERING TOPS | Anti-inflammatory and painkilling properties; prevents internal hemorrhage and swelling after injury. | ■ **Everlasting** is effective in skin conditions such as scarring, sunburn, and wounds. It relieves congestion of the liver or spleen, helps in bronchitis and flu, and is used to treat tendinitis, arthritic pain, and muscle aches, sprains, and strains. |
| ***German chamomile*** *Native to Europe and Asia, this widely cultivated aromatic herb has feathery leaves and white flowers, and produces an inky blue strong-scented oil.* | FLOWERS | Anti-inflammatory, sedative, and painkilling properties; also antiallergic and antiseptic. | ■ **German chamomile** alleviates digestive upsets, menstrual and menopausal problems, inflamed skin, burns, acne, boils, sunburn, and cuts. It aids in arthritis and muscular pain, and helps to relieve symptoms of hay fever and bronchitis. |
| ***Lavender*** *Native to the Mediterranean, this evergreen shrub is now grown worldwide. You may release its familiar aroma by rubbing a flower or leaf between the fingers. The oil is clear or yellow-green.* | FLOWERING TOPS | Known for its calming, soothing, and balancing effects; also has analgesic and antiseptic properties. | ■ **Lavender** relieves headache, depression, insomnia, stress, muscular aches and sprains, menstrual pain, and nausea. It also soothes skin conditions such as cuts, wounds, insect bites, burns, and athlete's foot. |
| ***Lemon-scented eucalyptus*** *This tall evergreen, sometimes called a gum tree, is native to Australia. Its colorless or pale yellow oil has long been used for sachets in linen closets.* | LEAVES<br>TWIGS | Sedative, anti-inflammatory, antiseptic, and deodorant action; can kill bacteria, viruses, and fungi. | ■ **Lemon-scented eucalyptus** soothes mosquito bites and skin irritations. It also helps athlete's foot and herpes sores and relieves muscle tension and stress. CAUTION: Do not take internally. |

# Aromatherapy

| Name | Parts Used | Properties | Target Ailments |
|---|---|---|---|
| ***Niaouli***<br>*Principally from Australia, this evergreen has a spongy bark and white flowers. The yellow or greenish oil has a camphorous odor and is found in health aids such as toothpaste.* | LEAVES<br>YOUNG TWIGS | Antiseptic, analgesic, and antiallergic properties, as well as tissue-stimulating action helpful for healing. | ■ **Niaouli** combats allergies, bronchitis, colds, and flu; cleans minor wounds and burns; aids in acne, boils, and insect bites; and helps relieve muscle aches and pains as well as toothache. It may also be used to treat bladder infection. |
| ***Palmarosa***<br>*Native to India and Pakistan, this wild tropical grass has a long stem and aromatic leaves. The oil is pale yellow or olive in color, with a sweet floral scent.* | FLOWERS<br>LEAVES | Antiviral, antibacterial, and antiseptic properties, as well as an overall strengthening effect. | ■ **Palmarosa** is diluted with almond oil to treat skin conditions such as cuts and wounds, acne, dermatitis, cold sores, and scars. It also relieves symptoms of flu, fights intestinal and other infections, and is helpful in stress-related conditions. |
| ***Peppermint***<br>*This perennial herb native to Europe and western Asia is cultivated around the world. Its oil is colorless, pale yellow, or green and is a popular flavoring agent.* | FLOWERING TOPS<br>LEAVES | Produces a warming effect (after an initial cooling action) and can relieve pain; also stimulates the liver. | ■ **Peppermint** relieves indigestion, nausea, and headache. It is helpful for neuralgia and muscle pain, and can aid in bronchitis, sinusitis, and motion sickness.<br>CAUTION: Use in moderation. Do not give to children under 30 months of age. |
| ***Rosemary***<br>*This Mediterranean evergreen shrub has silvery green leaves and pale blue flowers. The oil is colorless to pale yellow-green; its scent is minty in oils of good quality.* | FLOWERING TOPS<br>LEAVES | A stimulant that invigorates the whole body and helps eliminate toxins; antiseptic and diuretic properties. | ■ **Rosemary** is effective for indigestion, gas, and liver problems. It fights bronchitis and flu, reduces fluid retention, and helps treat depression.<br>CAUTION: Avoid during pregnancy or if you have epilepsy or high blood pressure. |
| ***Tarragon***<br>*This bushy perennial plant native to Asia and Europe has narrow green leaves and small flowers. The colorless oil has an aroma similar to anise and is a popular food seasoning.* | LEAVES | Antispasmodic, diuretic, and mild laxative properties; stimulant. | ■ **Tarragon** helps with menstrual and menopausal symptoms and with digestive ailments such as gas, indigestion, hiccups, and loss of appetite. It can aid in stress-related problems and in overcoming shock.<br>CAUTION: Avoid during pregnancy. |
| ***Tea tree***<br>*Native to New South Wales, Australia, the tea tree or shrub has small, narrow leaves and yellow or purple flowers. Its tart oil ranges from colorless to pale yellow-green.* | LEAVES<br>TWIGS | Antiseptic action against bacteria, fungi, and viruses; soothing to the skin and mucous membranes. | ■ **Tea tree** fights colds, flu, tonsillitis, bronchitis, and sinusitis, and can treat skin ailments such as abscesses, acne, and burns. It also helps clear vaginal thrush, vaginitis, and bladder infections, and helps control *Candida* infection. |
| ***Thyme***<br>*This evergreen shrub native to the Mediterranean area has gray-green leaves and clusters of purple or white flowers. The oil's natural color varies from red- or orange-brown to yellow.* | FLOWERING TOPS<br>LEAVES | Strongly stimulating, antiseptic, and antibacterial properties; also has antispasmodic and digestive actions. | ■ **Thyme** helps in laryngitis and coughs and fights skin, bladder, and other infections. It relieves joint pain, treats diarrhea and gas, and can help to expel intestinal worms.<br>CAUTION: Avoid during pregnancy or if you have high blood pressure. |
| ***Ylang-ylang***<br>*Native to the Philippines, ylang-ylang is a tall tropical tree with large, fragrant flowers. The clear or yellow oil, used in perfumes and soaps, has a sweet, spicy aroma.* | FRESH FLOWERS | Both stimulant and sedative properties; also can regulate heart action. | ■ **Ylang-ylang** helps with acne and oily skin and aids in depression, insomnia, impotence, and other stress-related disorders. It can be a backup therapy for high blood pressure.<br>CAUTION: Overuse can cause headache or nausea. |

## Target Ailments

- Allergies
- Angina
- Arthritis
- Cancer
- Cholesterol Problems
- Chronic Fatigue Syndrome
- Common Cold
- Constipation
- Depression
- Diabetes
- Diarrhea
- Flu
- Gas and Gas Pains
- Headache
- Heartburn
- High Blood Pressure
- Immune Problems
- Insomnia
- Irritable Bowel Syndrome
- Premenstrual Syndrome

*See Common Ailments, beginning on page 194.*

# Ayurvedic Medicine

*Ayurvedic medicine is a system of diagnosis and treatment that has been practiced in India for more than 2,500 years. The term "ayurveda" comes from the Sanskrit roots āyuh, which means longevity, and veda, meaning knowledge. Ayurvedic theory holds that the human body represents the entire universe in microcosmic form, and that we come to know how we function as organisms only by observing and understanding the world around us. The key to health is maintaining a balance between the microcosmic body and the macrocosmic world, a relationship that is expressed in the concept of three physiological principles called doshas. The role of the Ayurvedic physician is to restore and maintain, through different types of therapies, diet, lifestyle, and natural medicines, the balance of the three doshas that is appropriate for a given individual.*

### The Three Doshas

According to Ayurvedic theory, every person contains some amount of the universe's five basic elements: earth, air, fire, water, and ether (or space). To describe and understand the combination of these elements that makes up each unique individual—and thereby to gain insights into aspects of personality as well as of physiology—Ayurvedic healers rely on the concept of *doshas.*

Doshas are general categories; each dosha consists of one or more of the universe's five basic elements. Ayurvedic practitioners recognize three main types of dosha: *vata, pitta,* and *kapha.* Together these are called the *tridosha.*

Vata, "wind," is a combination of ether (space) and air. As such, vata is associated with lightness and dispersion, and this concept encompasses both the movement of fluids and cells through the body and the flow of thoughts through the mind. According to Ayurvedic principles, people who are strongly influenced by vata are said to be active and often restless. Creative people often have a strong vata component in their makeup.

Pitta, "bile," is composed of fire (some descriptions also mention wa-

**LICENSED & INSURED?**

*No. There is currently no licensing board for Ayurvedic practitioners and no recognized form of certification, though the need for some form of regulation is growing as Ayurveda increases in popularity. Insurance providers are generally reluctant to pay for Ayurvedic therapies, although your expenses may be covered if your treatment is performed by a licensed physician. Ask your insurance provider's claims representative for information about your coverage.*

ter). The key to this dosha is the concept of transformation—apparent in such physical processes as the digestion of food to produce energy. Pitta is said to be the controlling force behind all of the body's metabolic activities. Persons primarily influenced by pitta are thought to be doers, in the sense of being quick to change things as needs arise. They also may be extremely competitive or aggressive.

Kapha, "phlegm," is made up of earth and water elements. Structure is integral to kapha, as this dosha is said to provide the body's physical strength, stability, and wound-healing abilities. A predominantly kapha person might be relatively heavy and muscular, and would be likely to be characterized as having a stable, tranquil personality.

### *Doshic Balance*

A given individual's natural constitution—known in Ayurvedic medicine as that person's *prakriti*—is a unique balance of the three doshas. Each person's prakriti is said to be present at the moment of conception. While every prakriti contains a certain amount of vata, pitta, and kapha, one dosha usually predominates. According to Ayurveda, your prakriti not only describes your constitution but also regulates your physical, emotional, and mental processes. By living a lifestyle that conforms to your specific prakriti, you can achieve optimum health. If, however, in the course of your daily life you subject yourself to overeating, stress, inadequate or excessive sleep, or other similar conditions, you can excite one or more of the doshas, causing a disruption of your doshic balance (and therefore your prakriti), which is virtually guaranteed to lead to illness.

Ayurvedic practitioners advocate diets and lifestyles that reinforce the doshic balance, and encourage close vigilance (through body and mind-awareness techniques such as meditation) to identify imbalances. When an imbalance is detected and confirmed by an Ayurvedic practitioner, immediate corrective measures are prescribed using Ayurvedic therapies and remedies.

### *Origins*

Historical evidence suggests that the medical system we now call Ayurveda began in India around the sixth century BC, coinciding roughly with the lifetime of the Buddha (although some scholars contend that it began much earlier). According to tradition, holy men, or *rishis,* gathered together in a hermitage high in the Himalayas to compile the healing wisdom they had attained via divine inspiration. Their medical knowledge was then transmitted to the people as part of the sacred Hindu scriptures known as the Vedas. The rishis intended that Ayurveda would maximize wellness of the body and the mind, and that this would create an unencumbered path to a person's spiritual fulfillment.

CAUTION

**Some Ayurvedic preparations contain harmful substances such as lead, mercury, and arsenic. Although these substances may be described as "inactivated" and therefore safe, their safety has not been proved: Avoid all preparations containing even minute amounts of heavy metals or dangerous chemicals. Ayurvedic medicine is a comprehensive system of healthcare; however, it is not always appropriate for treating serious injuries or problems that require surgery.**



CONTINUED

# Ayurvedic Medicine CONTINUED

Through the centuries, Ayurvedic philosophy has spread worldwide. In the last few hundred years, foreign influence in India has overshadowed much traditional knowledge, including Ayurveda. The last 35 years or so, however, have witnessed a powerful resurgence in interest, among both practitioners and patients. In India today, Ayurveda is a popular—though not exclusive—choice for 80 percent of the population; conventional Western-style allopathic medicine, homeopathy, Arabic Unani medicine, and Siddha medicine, in the south, are also commonly practiced.

Ayurveda is steadily growing in popularity in the United States, where two types of Ayurvedic medicine coexist: traditional Ayurveda and Maharishi Ayur-Veda. Traditional Ayurveda is based on the ancient textbooks of the master physicians Caraka, Sushruta, and Vagbhata. Many traditional practitioners have been trained in India's Ayurveda colleges. They practice largely on their own in the United States, as there is currently no unifying professional organization.

Maharishi Ayur-Veda is a modern effort by Maharishi Mahesh Yogi (the Indian teacher who introduced transcendental meditation to the United States in the 1960s) to blend traditional Ayurvedic medicine with transcendental meditation. Maharishi Ayur-Veda practitioners are trained in North America, and this is the more popular type of Ayurvedic medicine in the United States. (Maharishi Ayur-Veda is also the name of a company that sells Ayurvedic products and services.)

## What It's Good For

While its primary focus is preventive, Ayurveda also encompasses healing remedies for hundreds of ailments. Practitioners especially recommend Ayurvedic therapies for the relief of chronic, metabolic, and stress-related problems. Numerous studies are under way to determine if Ayurvedic remedies may inhibit breast cancer; increase mobility and reduce the pain of arthritis; allay chemotherapy's side effects; hasten recuperation following conventional surgery; decrease serum cholesterol; alleviate symptoms of Parkinson's disease; reduce insulin dependence for diabetics; and assist in recovery from heroin addiction.

## Two Forms of Treatment

Ayurvedic practitioners use many preparations and techniques, including hatha-yoga *(see Yoga, pages 182-183),* sounds, scents, foods, spices, colors, minerals, medicines, and gems. These can be separated into two basic types of Ayurvedic treatment: constitutional and therapeutic.

Constitutional treatments encompass adjustments in lifestyle and the taking of preparations that are believed to enhance and preserve good health. These preventive measures might include engaging in *pranayama,* or breathing exercises; readjusting your sleeping and eating schedules to correspond with your prakriti;

performing Ayurvedic massage (called *abhyanga*) to reestablish your energy flow, or *prana;* or taking regular herbal supplements called *rasayanas* to cleanse your body and harmonize your prakriti. The principal form of constitutional treatment is known as *panchakarma,* and it can last anywhere from three days to three weeks. It is an intensive and individualized five-step cleansing process that incorporates a special diet and various massages, herbal treatments, and evacuation procedures, all with the goal of purifying the body and the mind.

Therapeutic treatments are specific healing regimens. According to Ayurvedic theory, all disease originates in the gastrointestinal tract, and is ultimately caused by decreased enzyme activity and poor digestion. Improperly digested foods are said to form a sludgelike substance called *ama* that blocks the body's digestive and energy channels. Practitioners use therapeutic treatments (called *anamaya*) to fight disease by ridding the body of ama and reestablishing a balanced prakriti. These treatments might include medicinal remedies (selected from some 8,000 herbal, mineral, fruit, and vegetable preparations used in Ayurvedic practice); cleansing procedures such as therapeutic vomiting (inducing vomiting to expel toxins) or herbal enemas; and bloodletting, which is believed to detoxify the blood.

Dietary change is by far the most common form of constitutional and therapeutic treatment. Certain foods are credited with the ability to strengthen or weaken the doshas, and practitioners often suggest specific diets to help reestablish a patient's prakriti.

OF SPECIAL INTEREST

### Healing Elements

*Using medicinal herbs and prescribing nutritional changes are not the only healing techniques espoused by Ayurvedic practitioners. Colors, aromas, gems, and stones are also believed to activate the body's healing potential. When worn or held close to the body, certain stones and gems are said to release their healing energy and engage the body's own energy centers. Aromas are said to help soothe the mind—a belief shared by practitioners of aromatherapy (pages 38-39)—and to pacify disturbed doshas. The seven colors of the rainbow are believed to be related to the tridosha, and therefore to be helpful in balancing the prakriti. To take advantage of color therapy, practitioners may advise patients to drink water from a glass wrapped in colored paper. The color's power is said to infuse the water and be transported to the person who drinks it.*

## *Visiting a Professional*

Ayurveda dictates that every person is responsible for his or her own health. This is not to negate the value of the practitioner-patient relationship, however. Although Ayurvedic preparations are available to everyone, it is difficult (if not impossible) to identify




CONTINUED

what you need without a practitioner's help. And when illness strikes, a practitioner's advice is essential.

Expect your first visit with your *vaidya,* or Ayurvedic doctor, to last 45 to 90 minutes. In determining your unique tridosha and prakriti, he or she will ask many questions about your emotional, spiritual, and physical health, your diet, and your lifestyle. You may also be asked to complete a written questionnaire that delves further into your physical and spiritual health.

Your vaidya will check your pulse to help establish your prakriti and determine your overall condition; rates, intensities, and rhythms of an individual's pulse are believed to indicate specific physical, mental, and metabolic conditions. The practitioner will observe you closely, paying particular attention to the condition of your tongue, skin, lips, eyes, and nails. Some practitioners also rely on laboratory analysis of blood, urine, and stools to help in diagnosing your prakriti.

After determining your constitution, your vaidya will use an integrative approach to consider your specific physical, emotional, mental, and spiritual needs, and recommend treatments to harmonize your lifestyle with your prakriti.

### *Wellness*

Preventive medicine is the central tenet of Ayurvedic healing. According to Ayurveda, health is achieved and maintained by first identifying a person's prakriti and then assigning the proper constitutional or therapeutic remedies to maintain his or her doshic balance. Practitioners encourage their patients to stay in close contact, so that therapies and regimens may be adjusted as needed.

### *What the Critics Say*

Ayurveda's use of nonstandard techniques of diagnosis and treatment and its reliance on organic medicines tend to make conventional Western physicians and scientists uneasy. But not all conventional physicians oppose Ayurveda. Some doctors have received introductory Ayurvedic training and use Ayurveda to complement their conventional-style practices. As Ayurveda's popularity continues to increase within the general population of the United States, this trend is likely to continue.

Some criticism of Ayurveda is directed specifically toward the Maharishi Ayur-Veda system. Detractors allege that the promoters of Maharishi Ayur-Veda may be more interested in selling medicine than in healing. Some insist that descriptions of Maharishi Ayur-Veda's power and potential have been wildly exaggerated. Others question whether Maharishi Ayur-Veda represents authentic Ayurvedic science. Still, Maharishi Ayur-Veda is the most popular form of Ayurvedic medicine in the United States. Both traditional Ayurveda and Maharishi Ayur-Veda therapies are currently being investigated in scientific laboratories around the world. ■

**FOR MORE INFO**

Following is a list of organizations you can contact to learn more about Ayurvedic medicine:

**Ayurvedic Institute**
11311 Menaul NE, Suite A
Albuquerque, NM 87112
(505) 291-9698

**Indic Traditions of Healthcare**
**Dharam Hinduja Indic Research Center Columbia University**
Mail Code 3367
1102 International Affairs Building
New York, NY 10027
(212) 854-5300
fax: (212) 854-2802
e-mail: dhirc@columbia.edu

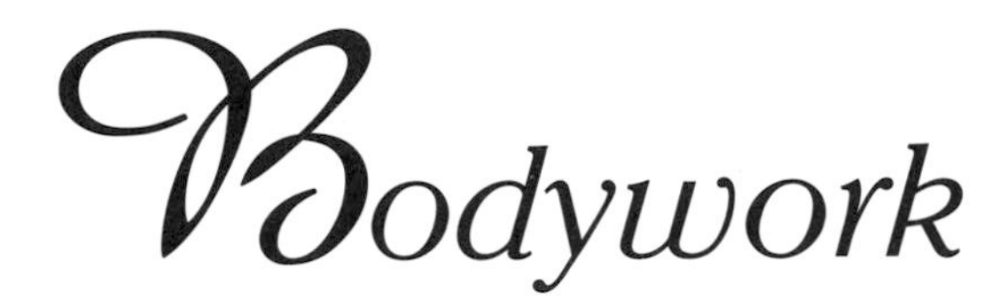

# Bodywork

*Bodywork is an umbrella term for the many techniques that promote relaxation and treat ailments (especially those of the musculoskeletal system) through lessons in proper movement and posture, exercise, massage, and various other forms of bodily manipulation. These techniques can be divided into three broad categories—massage, movement awareness and structural realignment, and energy balancing—although the majority include more than one of these elements. Most take a holistic view of health and emphasize treatment of the mind as well as of the body. Skeptics point out, however, that therapeutic claims made for these techniques are usually based on anecdotal observation rather than on controlled scientific studies.*

*Some of the many bodywork techniques are explored in detail below and on the following pages. Massage, which is generally considered a form of bodywork, is described separately on pages 121-123.*

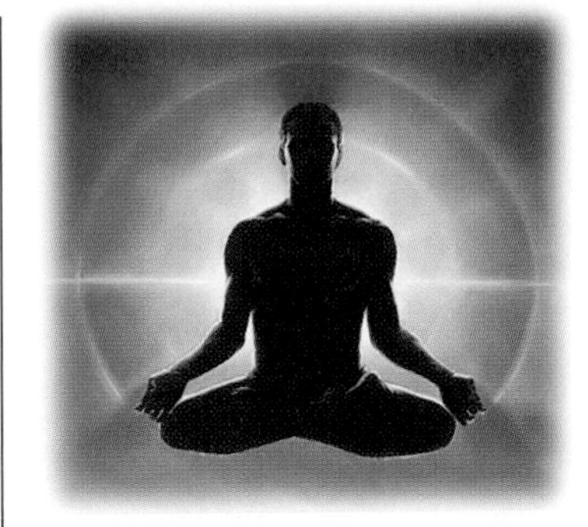

## Alexander Technique

*This form of bodywork was developed in the late 1800s by an Australian Shakespearean actor named Frederick Matthias Alexander, whose voice often became hoarse during performances, jeopardizing his career. When the rest and medication prescribed by his physician failed to provide a reliable cure, Alexander decided to find out for himself the cause of his vocal problem. Using a mirror, he studied the way he spoke and concluded that he was unconsciously tensing his body in a way that was interfering with the correct relationship between his head, neck, and back—and that this tension was affecting his voice. In the course of finding a way to correct this damaging habit, Alexander developed the muscle-releasing and postural technique that bears his name. Although he cured his propensity to hoarseness and returned to the stage, Alexander eventually left acting—and Australia—to teach his technique to others in England and America.*

*What It's Good For* • The Alexander technique teaches people how to release painful muscle tension, improve posture, and move with greater ease. Old, damaging habits of sitting, moving, and speaking are replaced with new, more efficient ones. People who practice the technique find it reduces stress and fatigue.

### Target Ailments

- Arthritis
- Athletic Injuries
- Back Problems
- Bursitis
- Pain, Chronic
- Tendinitis

*See Common Ailments, beginning on page 194.*



CONTINUED

# Bodywork CONTINUED

Because it improves postural habits, the technique can also help relieve back, knee, and other pain caused by the improper use of muscles; it is especially helpful for disk problems and sciatica. The technique has also been effective in relieving the discomfort associated with arthritis, bursitis, and other conditions involving muscles and joints.

*Preparations/Techniques* • The Alexander technique is traditionally taught in one-on-one lessons, although some instructors also offer group classes. Basic to the technique is learning how to release your neck muscles so that your head can balance freely on top of your neck. This, in turn, allows your back to lengthen, eliminating compression in the spine.

During a lesson, the teacher will analyze the way you sit, stand, walk, and bend. He or she will then use verbal instructions and gentle touch to guide you into releasing muscle tension, improving posture, and moving with more freedom. You will learn to apply this improved use of your body to everyday tasks, from sitting in a chair to carrying packages to talking on the phone. The Alexander technique does not involve exercises. However, you will learn to apply it to any sport or exercise program you do on a regular basis. Advocates believe this will help you avoid injury and also increase the benefit you receive from your regular exercise program.

Lessons in the Alexander technique generally last 30 to 45 minutes. Wear loose, nonrestrictive clothing. Your instructor will work with you while you are lying on a table and also while you are moving about.

*Wellness* • Practitioners of this technique believe it promotes wellness by helping people learn how to move within their physical environment in a relaxed and efficient manner that promotes healthy mental and physical functioning.

*What the Critics Say*
Although correcting poor posture has been known to help prevent back and neck pain, the specific therapeutic benefits of the Alexander technique have not been demonstrated in controlled scientific studies. One study has shown that the technique can be beneficial to healthy adults by enabling them to breathe more efficiently, but it involved only a small number of participants.

LICENSED & INSURED?

*Practitioners must complete a three-year, 1,600-hour instructional program at an approved school to obtain a certification to practice the Alexander technique. Some insurance companies will cover a portion of the cost of Alexander technique therapy if you first get a referral from your physician.*

CAUTION

**You should avoid bodywork that involves massage if you have an open wound, a bone fracture or dislocation, an infectious disease, a contagious skin condition, severe varicose veins, or any heart problem. Some health professionals are concerned that the deep massage associated with some of these techniques may cause existing cancer cells to metastasize, or spread, in the body. If you have cancer, you may want to ask your bodywork practitioner to consult with your oncologist before undergoing one of these techniques.**

FOR MORE INFO

Contact the following organization to learn more about the Alexander technique:

**North American Society of Teachers of the Alexander Technique**
(800) 473-0620
e-mail: nastat@ix.netcom.com

# Bodywork

## Aston-Patterning

*This type of bodywork was developed in the 1970s by a California dancer named Judith Aston. A decade earlier, two separate car accidents had left her with a disabling back injury. At a doctor's suggestion, Aston went to see Ida Rolf, whose unique form of deep massage and postural retraining known as Rolfing (page 54) helped Aston regain full body movement. Aston began working with Rolf to develop a movement maintenance program that would help people sustain structural changes brought about by Rolfing. She eventually broke away from Rolfing to develop and teach her own form of bodywork.*

*What It's Good For* • Practitioners claim it can help relieve acute or chronic pain such as that caused by poor posture or muscle tension. They also believe it can improve balance, increase strength and endurance, and relieve fatigue. The goal is to help people find more comfortable and efficient ways to work, play, and rest.

*Preparations/Techniques* • Aston-Patterning is generally taught in one-on-one sessions with a trained practitioner. Each session can last from one to two hours and may include any or all of the following components: movement education, or neurokinetics, which involves learning how to decrease body tension and move more efficiently; three types of bodywork that release tensions held in different body structures; ergonomic training, which teaches how to modify home and work environments in ways that encourage good posture and efficient movement; and fitness training, which helps to stretch, loosen, and tone muscles throughout the body.

*Wellness* • Like most alternative therapies, Aston-Patterning focuses on promoting health and well-being—goals it seeks to achieve by improving how the body moves and functions.

*What the Critics Say*
Critics note that Aston-Patterning's therapeutic effectiveness has not been demonstrated in controlled studies.

**LICENSED & INSURED?**

*Practitioners must complete several one- to two-week training sessions over a period of three years to obtain a certification to practice. Some insurance companies will cover part of the cost of Aston-Patterning treatment if you first get a referral from your physician.*

### Target Ailments

- Athletic Injuries
- Back Problems
- Stress

*See Common Ailments, beginning on page 194.*

**FOR MORE INFO**
Contact the following organization to learn more about Aston-Patterning:

**The Aston Training Center**
PO Box 3568
Incline Village, NV 89450
(702) 831-8228



CONTINUED

# Bodywork CONTINUED

## Feldenkrais Method

*This bodywork technique was developed by Moshe Feldenkrais, a Russian-born Israeli physicist who became interested in the physics of body movement during the 1940s, after experiencing a disabling knee injury. He drew on the earlier work of Frederick Matthias Alexander (pages 47-48)—as well as on his own intense study of anatomy, biochemistry, neurophysiology, and other sciences related to human movement—to create this system for improving posture, movement, and breathing.*

*What It's Good For* • Feldenkrais practitioners claim the method can help people with chronic musculoskeletal problems, such as back or knee pain. They also report success helping people overcome some of the physical limitations brought on by an injury or by a chronic medical condition, such as cerebral palsy or multiple sclerosis. Other benefits cited include improved digestion, more restful sleep, greater mental alertness, increased energy, and reduced stress.

*Preparations/Techniques* • The Feldenkrais method teaches how to recognize and then break improper habits of movement. You can learn the technique through a group class or one-on-one lessons. In group classes a practitioner verbally guides students through a sequence of movements designed to teach how to relax and abandon habitual patterns of movement that reveal unconscious tension. Private lessons provide similar guidance, although here the practitioner also uses slow, gentle touch to help you feel exactly where and how your body is tensing and moving incorrectly. Both types of sessions last about 45 minutes to an hour. You'll also learn exercises to practice at home.

*Wellness* • Feldenkrais practitioners believe that by helping people release unnecessary muscle tension and move in a freer and more graceful way, injuries and stress-related illness can be prevented.

*What the Critics Say*
The small amount of objective research that has been done on the therapeutic benefits of the Feldenkrais method has been inconclusive.

**LICENSED & INSURED?**

*Practitioners must complete 800 hours of instruction over a period of three to four years to obtain a certification to practice. Insurance companies usually do not cover the cost of Feldenkrais treatments.*

### Target Ailments

- Back Problems
- Insomnia
- Multiple Sclerosis
- Pain, Chronic
- Stress

*See Common Ailments, beginning on page 194.*

**FOR MORE INFO**

Contact the following organization to learn more about the Feldenkrais method:

**The Feldenkrais Guild**
524 SW Ellsworth Street
PO Box 489
Albany, OR 97321
(800) 775-2118

# Bodywork

## Hellerwork

*Hellerwork was developed by Joseph Heller, a former aerospace engineer who began studying with Ida Rolf in the early 1970s. At the time, Rolfing (page 54) did not include movement education, which Heller thought essential for helping people break old, destructive movement patterns. Nor did it include an exploration of the psychological dynamics behind such habits, which Heller believed was also necessary to root out tension. So in 1978 Heller founded his own method, which includes deep massage, movement education, and therapeutic discussion.*

*What It's Good For* • Hellerwork is based on the premise that a misaligned body limits movement and flexibility, leading to fatigue, physical deterioration, and premature aging. By realigning the body, Hellerwork is thought to release chronic tension and increase flexibility, which in turn reduces stress, increases energy, and creates an overall feeling of youthfulness.

*Preparations/Techniques* • The Hellerwork program consists of eleven 90-minute private sessions, each with a theme, such as "reaching out," and concentrating on a different part of the body. Each session begins with a deep connective-tissue massage to reduce body tension and realign the musculoskeletal system. Movement lessons follow on how to sit, stand, bend, and walk with more fluidity and balance. The practitioner will also ask about emotional patterns that may have led to physical tension. You may be asked, for example, about how easy or difficult it is for you to be assertive or to reach out to others. The therapy, however, does not require you to answer any questions that you find too painful or uncomfortable.

*Wellness* • Practitioners believe Hellerwork promotes wellness by breaking the muscular rigidity caused by unconscious habits, so people can better align themselves with gravity and move with more ease and energy.

*What the Critics Say*

The therapeutic benefits of this technique have not been demonstrated in controlled studies.

**LICENSED & INSURED?**

*Practitioners must complete 1,250 hours of study and training with certified Hellerwork trainers to obtain a certification to practice. Some insurance companies will cover part of the cost of Hellerwork treatments, especially if performed by a physical therapist, as long as you first get a referral from your physician.*

### Target Ailments

- Athletic Injuries
- Back Problems
- Carpal Tunnel Syndrome
- Stress

*See Common Ailments, beginning on page 194.*

**FOR MORE INFO**

Contact the following organization to learn more about Hellerwork:

**Hellerwork International**
406 Berry Street
Mount Shasta, CA 96067
(800) 392-3900; (916) 926-2500
e-mail: hwork@snowcrest.net



CONTINUED

# Bodyword CONTINUED

## Target Ailments

- Arthritis
- Athletic Injuries
- Back Problems
- Carpal Tunnel Syndrome
- Headache
- Menstrual Problems
- Multiple Sclerosis
- TMJ Syndrome

*See Common Ailments, beginning on page 194.*

## Myotherapy

*The term "myotherapy" is used here to refer specifically to the technique known formally as Bonnie Prudden Myotherapy. It is an offshoot of trigger point injection therapy, a medical treatment developed in the 1940s that involved injecting saline and the drug procaine directly into painful muscles, or "trigger points," to get them to relax. In 1976 physical fitness pioneer Bonnie Prudden discovered that the injections were unnecessary, as simple manual pressure on the trigger points could produce similar results. This finding led to the development of her form of myotherapy—a deep-pressure massage used to reduce tension and pain originating in specific points in the muscle layers of the body.*

*What It's Good For* • Practitioners claim this therapy is beneficial for a variety of muscle-related conditions, including back, shoulder, and neck pain; headaches; repetitive motion injuries; menstrual cramps; sports injuries; and TMJ syndrome. They say it can also help relieve pain associated with such diseases as arthritis, multiple sclerosis, and lupus. Practitioners emphasize, however, that myotherapy does not cure disease, but rather helps relieve pain and ease recovery.

*Preparations/Techniques* • Sessions last about an hour. The therapist will ask questions about your sports activities, occupation, injuries, and illnesses, and will test your muscles' strength and flexibility. Then, using fingers, knuckles, and elbows, the therapist will apply pressure to trigger points—those areas in your muscles that the therapist believes are responsible for your pain. Treatment is followed by passive stretching of affected muscles. You will be given corrective exercises to do at home to help keep your muscles free of spasms and pain.

*Wellness* • Myotherapists believe that by reducing pain and helping to restore the body's full range of motion, they can improve an individual's overall health and sense of well-being.

*What the Critics Say*
Critics point out that massaging trigger points is not unique to this therapy alone.

**LICENSED & INSURED?**

*Practitioners must complete a 1,300-hour training program at the Bonnie Prudden School for Physical Fitness and Myotherapy to obtain a certification to practice. Some insurance companies will cover part of the cost of treatments if you first get a referral from your physician.*

**FOR MORE INFO**

Contact the following organization to learn more about myotherapy:

**Bonnie Prudden Pain Erasure**
7800 East Speedway Boulevard
Tucson, AZ 85710
(520) 529-3979
(800) 221-4634

# Bodywork

## Reiki

*Reiki (pronounced ray-key) practitioners claim this ancient form of healing originated in Tibet thousands of years ago and was rediscovered in the mid-1800s by Mikao Usui, an educator at a Christian seminary in Kyoto, Japan. According to Reiki tradition, Usui spent 21 days fasting on a sacred mountain outside Kyoto, where he experienced a vision that revealed how the universal life energy described in ancient Sanskrit writings could be activated through a hands-on approach to healing. Usui named this healing method Reiki, after the healing aspect of the energy.*

*What It's Good For* • Reiki is used to treat a wide variety of conditions, from minor ailments such as heartburn to chronic diseases such as arthritis.

*Preparations/Techniques* • Only a trained practitioner may administer Reiki. During a healing session, the practitioner will gently lay his or her hands over the chakras, or energy centers, of your body to enable healing energy to flow more fully into your body. Treatments last from 30 to 60 minutes and are usually carried out in four sessions over four successive days. For some conditions, people receive treatments once a week for one or two months. You will be instructed to drink substantial quantities of water and herb tea during the treatment period to help cleanse your body of toxins. You may be told to avoid stimulants, such as coffee and white sugar, which can interfere with the cleansing process.

*Wellness* • Reiki practitioners believe the body becomes ill when the universal life energy is out of balance. Thus, by bringing balance and harmony to the body, Reiki enables the body and the mind to heal and remain healthy.

*What the Critics Say*
Evidence of Reiki's benefits is mainly anecdotal; very few controlled studies of it have been done. Because Reiki is often used to treat illnesses, critics worry that seriously ill patients will not receive the conventional medical care they need. Competent Reiki practitioners, however, do not discourage their patients from receiving such care.

**LICENSED & INSURED?**

*First- and second-degree Reiki practitioners are certified by their training organization. Becoming a master Reiki therapist requires a long apprenticeship with another master. Insurance companies usually do not cover the cost of Reiki treatments.*

### Target Ailments

- Arthritis
- Athletic Injuries
- Chronic Fatigue Syndrome
- Heartburn
- Indigestion
- Insomnia
- Irritable Bowel Syndrome
- Pain, Chronic
- Stress

*See Common Ailments, beginning on page 194.*

**FOR MORE INFO**
Following is a list of organizations you can contact to learn more about Reiki:

**The Reiki Alliance**
PO Box 41
Cataldo, ID 83810-1041
(208) 682-3535

**Reiki Outreach International**
PO Box 609
Fair Oaks, CA 95628
(916) 863-1500
fax: (916) 863-6464

**The Reiki Center of Los Angeles**
16161 Ventura Blvd., Suite 802
Encino, CA 91436
(818) 981-9100
e-mail: joyce@Reiki-Center.Org



CONTINUED

# Bodywork CONTINUED

## Rolfing

*This form of bodywork was developed in the 1940s and 1950s by Ida Rolf, a biochemist who wanted to improve the health of her friends and family and cure her own spinal curvature problem. After much study she decided that many physical and mental problems are caused by the body being out of alignment with gravity. She felt that by deeply massaging the fascia—the connective tissue enclosing muscles—most bodies could be brought back into alignment. This deep massage was called structural integration, but it became better known by its trademarked name, Rolfing.*

*What It's Good For* • Rolfing is said to ease chronic pain and stiffness, especially that caused by poor posture. Many athletes, dancers, musicians, and others seeking to improve physical performance in their professions and daily activities say they have been helped by Rolfing. Rolfers also claim the technique can help ease anxiety caused by chronic stress.

*Preparations/Techniques* • Rolfing is usually applied in 10 one-hour sessions. In each session, a specific area is massaged, or "manipulated." Rolfers use their fingers, knuckles, and elbows during the sometimes painful manipulations. The intent is to loosen adhesions in the fascia and bring the head, shoulders, thorax, pelvis, and legs into improved alignment with gravity. In a separate program, patients are instructed on how to move their body in more efficient ways.

*Wellness* • Rolfers believe that stretching and lengthening the fascia, and thus bringing the body into proper alignment with gravity, helps keep the body in a state that is free of stress.

*What the Critics Say*
Critics point out that no large, controlled studies of Rolfing have been carried out. One study of 10 cerebral palsy patients had mixed results. Critics are also concerned that some Rolfers use the technique to treat depression and other psychological disorders but are not qualified to do so.

**LICENSED & INSURED?**

*Rolfing practitioners must complete a two- to three-year training program at the Rolf Institute and 400 additional hours of classwork to obtain a certification to practice. Some insurance companies will cover part of the cost of Rolfing treatments if you first get a referral from your physician.*

### Target Ailments

- Athletic Injuries
- Back Problems
- Carpal Tunnel Syndrome
- Stress

*See Common Ailments, beginning on page 194.*

**FOR MORE INFO**
Contact the following organization to learn more about Rolfing:

**The Rolf Institute**
205 Canyon Boulevard
Boulder, CO 80306
(800) 530-8875
e-mail: Rolf Inst@aol.com

# Bodywork

## Therapeutic Touch

*During the 1970s Dolores Krieger, a nursing professor at New York University, brought together a variety of ancient "hands-on" healing practices into a modern technique she called therapeutic touch. Like many of its older predecessors, therapeutic touch is based on the premise that disease reflects a blockage in the flow of energy that surrounds and permeates the body. Krieger devised a four-step process by which a therapeutic touch practitioner could detect and free these blockages, thus healing the body.*

*What It's Good For* • Therapeutic touch practitioners claim it can be used to ease a variety of ailments, including arthritis, chronic back pain, headaches, constipation, and colic in babies. Practitioners also report it can help wounds and broken bones to heal faster and can reduce fevers. Therapeutic touch is frequently used to reduce stress and anxiety. It has been used in some hospitals, for example, to relax people before and after surgery and to alleviate pain.

*Preparations/Techniques* • Despite its name, therapeutic touch does not involve actual physical contact. Each session begins with the practitioner assuming a relaxed, meditative state. The practitioner then moves his or her hands in slow, rhythmic motions two to six inches above the patient in an effort to detect blockages in the body's energy field that may be causing or contributing to illness. When perceiving a blockage, the practitioner "unruffles" the field with a downward sweep of the hands. After this, the practitioner transfers energy to the patient via what is called noncontact touch. Sessions last about 20 minutes. Once you become proficient in the technique, you can practice it on yourself and on others.

*Wellness* • Therapeutic touch is most commonly used to relieve pain and other symptoms of illness, but some practitioners also use the technique to help prevent the body from becoming ill in the first place.

*What the Critics Say*
Although conceding that the technique may comfort some patients, critics of therapeutic touch say that its healing value has not been demonstrated in well-designed, controlled scientific studies.

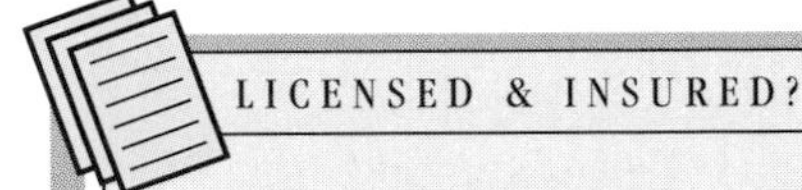

LICENSED & INSURED?

*Therapeutic touch practitioners are neither licensed nor certified. Insurance companies occasionally cover the cost of treatments.*

### Target Ailments

- Arthritis
- Back Problems
- Bronchitis
- Bursitis
- Cancer
- Circulatory Problems
- Constipation
- Endometriosis
- Headache
- Heart Problems
- High Blood Pressure
- Immune Problems
- Menopause
- Menstrual Problems
- Pain, Chronic
- Stress

*See Common Ailments, beginning on page 194.*

**FOR MORE INFO**

Contact the following organization to learn more about therapeutic touch:

**Nurse Healers Professional Associates**
1211 Locust Street
Philadelphia, PA 19107
(215) 545-8079



CONTINUED

# Bodywork CONTINUED

## Trager Psychophysical Integration (Trager Approach)

*This type of bodywork was first developed in the 1920s by a young Miami boxer named Milton Trager, who was told by relatives and friends that he had an uncanny knack for massaging away their aches and pains. He eventually gave up boxing to become a physical therapist and later a physician, and over the next seven decades treated thousands of patients with his unique and gentle form of massage. In the 1970s Trager began teaching his technique to others, who now offer it in the United States and other countries to people seeking relief from chronic pain and other ailments.*

*What It's Good For* • The Trager approach is used in the treatment of all kinds of chronic pain, including back pain, headaches, muscle spasms, and TMJ syndrome. A few small studies have shown it to be beneficial for some people with severe neuromuscular problems produced by injury or with such diseases as multiple sclerosis or muscular dystrophy.

*Preparations/Techniques* • Sessions last 60 to 90 minutes. The patient lies or sits on a table while the practitioner applies gentle touch and rhythmic rocking and shaking movements to the body to relax and loosen joints and muscles. Practitioners work in a meditative state called hook-up, which enables them to better sense minute responses of the patient's body. Patients are also taught a series of exercises to practice at home. Called mentastics, they are intended to help identify and correct chronic tension patterns that affect posture and movement.

*Wellness* • Trager practitioners believe that this form of movement reeducation brings people into a relaxed and physically graceful state that enhances wellness and helps make the body more resistant to injury and illness.

*What the Critics Say*
Because large, controlled studies involving the Trager approach to bodywork have never been conducted, its ability to help people suffering from chronic pain or other ailments cannot be stated with any degree of certainty.

**LICENSED & INSURED?**

*Trager practitioners must complete more than 200 hours of training at the Trager Institute to obtain a certification to practice. Some insurance companies will cover part of the cost of Trager treatments if you first get a referral from your physician.*

### Target Ailments

- Back Problems
- Headache
- Multiple Sclerosis
- Pain, Chronic
- TMJ Syndrome

*See Common Ailments, beginning on page 194.*

**FOR MORE INFO**

Contact the following organization to learn more about the Trager approach:

**The Trager Institute**
21 Locust Avenue
Mill Valley, CA 94941-2806
(415) 388-2688
e-mail: Trager D@aol.com

# Chinese Medicine

*Chinese medicine is an ancient system of healthcare that uses a variety of techniques—including acupuncture (pages 32-33), acupressure (pages 16-17), herbal therapy (pages 70-73), qigong (pages 165-166), and massage (pages 121-123)—to treat disorders by restoring the balance of vital energies in the body.*

*Unlike Western medicine, which tends to focus on specific parts of the body immediately affected by disease or injury, Chinese medicine takes a more global, holistic approach to healthcare, fashioning remedies to treat the entire body rather than just its component parts. Practitioners of Chinese medicine think of the human body not as a bundle of cells, bones, and tissues but rather as a complex system of interrelated processes—an ecosystem unto itself, constantly influenced by the push and pull of opposing forces within it. These physicians regard the human being as both a part of nature and a separate entity, complete and self-contained. It is, they believe, a microcosm of the grand cosmic order, moved by the same rhythms and cycles that shape the natural world. At the core of Chinese medicine is the belief that disease is the result of disturbances in the flow of a bodily energy called chi or qi (pronounced "chee") or a lack of balance in the complementary states of yin (characterized by darkness and quiet) and yang (characterized by light and activity).*

## Chi and the Dynamics of Yin and Yang

Defined in early Chinese writings as "basic stuff," chi is thought to be the force that animates life and enlivens all activity. Powerful yet invisible, chi cannot be isolated, measured, or quantified; it is known not through direct observation but through its observable effects. Just as blood courses through the vessels of the circulatory system, chi flows through the body primarily by way of invisible channels called meridians. Practitioners of Chinese medicine believe that maintaining the proper movement of chi through these meridians is essential to good health.

Wellness also requires preserving a delicate balance, or equilibrium, between the contrasting states of yin and yang. Translated literally, the Chinese character for *yin* depicts the shady side of the mountain, *yang* the sunny side; together they symbolize the dual nature of all things. According to Chinese theory, yin and yang coexist harmoniously in the body. Polar opposites, they represent alternate phases in the natural cycle, contradicting and at the same time complementing one another. In a healthy body, the darkness and inactivity of yin are perfectly counterbalanced by the

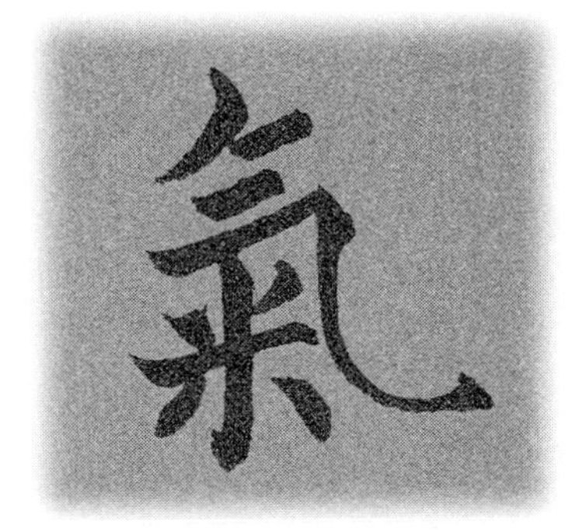


### Target Ailments

- Allergies
- Arthritis
- Asthma
- Bursitis
- Common Cold
- Constipation
- Depression
- Diarrhea
- Earache
- Flu
- Headache
- Hemorrhoids
- High Blood Pressure
- Insomnia
- Menstrual Problems
- Nausea
- Pain, Chronic
- Sore Throat
- Stomach Ulcers
- Stress
- Vaginal Problems

*See Common Ailments, beginning on page 194.*



CONTINUED

lightness and activity of yang. Just as day melts into night and night into day, the body fluctuates cyclically between yin and yang. Any deviation from this orderly course causes a yin-yang disharmony, resulting in disease.

## Origins

Rooted in the philosophies of Taoism, Buddhism, and Confucianism, Chinese medicine has been practiced in China for more than 2,500 years, although the underlying principles of herbal therapy and acupuncture are even older. According to legend, the philosophical and practical groundwork of Chinese herbal medicine was laid by Emperor Shen Nung, the "Divine Farmer" who became fascinated with the apparent healing properties of certain plants. He spent years testing the efficacy of these herbs, and his observations led him to develop a theory involving nature's "opposing principles." In the centuries that followed, Chinese thinkers refined and elaborated on these principles, which came to be called yin and yang. The philosophy grew and flourished in China and from there spread throughout much of eastern Asia. It arrived with Chinese immigrants in the United States in the mid-1800s but remained relatively unknown among Americans until just a few decades ago.

## What It's Good For

Chinese medicine is used to treat a full spectrum of conditions. In recent years these methods have been subjected to increasingly rigorous study in China and elsewhere. Evidence indicates that, although some may not perform as claimed, a number of these remedies do seem to work. For example, acupuncture has been shown to be effective in the treatment of nausea, asthma, and migraines. In other studies, researchers have found that the management of chronic pain and drug addiction is more successful when acupuncture is included in a comprehensive treatment plan.

## Preparations/Techniques

Chinese medicine recognizes more than 6,000 healing substances, although only a few hundred are in practical use today. Following a sophisticated classification system, herbs are grouped according to four basic properties, or "essences"—hot, cold, warm, and cool. In general, practitioners choose plants for their ability to restore balance in individuals whose conditions are said to show signs of excessive heat or cold. For example, a hot herb such as cinnamon bark might be recommended for a condition described as cold; the cool herb chrysanthemum flower might be prescribed for a condition characterized as warm.

Herbs are further categorized according to their "flavor"—pungent, sour, sweet, bitter, or salty. An herb's taste indicates its action in the body, particularly on the movement and direction of chi. Each flavor is said to have a strong influence on a certain major organ system: Pungent herbs are associated with the lungs, sour with the liver, sweet with the spleen or pancreas, bitter with the heart, salty with the kidneys. It is important to note that the Chinese notion of body organs is much broader than the Western. The Chinese term for *heart,* for instance, encompasses not only the physical organ itself but also the general order and clarity of the mind.

Because many Chinese herbs work best when taken with others, practitioners almost always prescribe herbs in combination, occasionally blending as many as 15 in a single preparation. Some plants are used to disperse chi that has become stagnant or misdirected. Others help summon scattered reserves of chi, while still others provide nourishment or rid the body of noxious substances.

Herbs are prepared in a variety of ways. Many are cooked and made into soup or tea. In some cases the raw plants are ground into a powder, then combined with honey or some other binding agent and pressed into a pill. A number of herbs are cooked and processed into a powder and are then either mixed with warm water and swallowed or taken as capsules. Some herbs are made into pastes that are applied to the skin, while others are extracted in alcohol and used as tinctures. Mixing herbs is an extremely tricky business. Certain Chinese herbs can be poisonous in large amounts, so you should always check with a qualified practitioner for the proper dosages.

Before prescribing any type of treatment, a practitioner performs an evaluation of the patient's overall physical and mental makeup, or "individual conformation." According to Chinese theory, a single symptom by itself is meaningless; it acquires significance only in terms of how it relates to a host of other signs. The evaluation consists of four basic techniques, or stages: looking, listening and smelling (in Chinese, these are expressed by the same word), asking, and touching.

An experienced practitioner can gather a great deal of information by observing the patient's general appearance, posture, facial color, and behavior. For more detailed information, the physician looks for more specific signs, such as the alertness of the eyes and the color of the skin and nails. Crucial to the diagnosis is a careful evaluation

**LICENSED & INSURED?**

*In the United States, practitioners of Chinese medicine usually operate under the title of "licensed" or "certified" acupuncturist. Many conventional doctors have incorporated acupuncture into their practices, and some states allow chiropractic and naturopathic physicians to use the technique.*

*Few insurance providers reimburse patients for the cost of herbal treatments. But a number of companies do cover acupuncture, in some cases only if performed by a conventional medical doctor. In early 1996, the FDA removed a label classifying acupuncture needles as experimental devices, possibly clearing the way for broader insurance coverage.*



CONTINUED

# Chinese Medicine CONTINUED

of the patient's tongue, which is considered to be an excellent barometer of disharmonies in the body. To trained eyes, the shape, movement, color, texture, and moistness of the tongue—even its coating—speak volumes about the patient's condition. A red, dry tongue, for example, suggests the presence of heat; a purple tongue may indicate stagnant chi. During their examinations, practitioners take pulse readings at three points on each wrist; each point is believed to reveal conditions in different parts of the body. They also look for clues in bodily secretions, the sound of the voice, and any unusual odors emanating from the patient's body.

## *Chinese Medicine and Wellness*

Preventing disease and preserving the conditions of good health are among the fundamental aims of Chinese medicine. More than a system of after-the-fact healing techniques, it is a philosophy of life grounded on the assumption that illness is much easier to prevent than to cure. Besides providing treatment to overcome disease, practitioners strive to arm the body against conditions that bring about ill health. Historically, Chinese medical professionals have rejected the notion of quick cures, insisting that disease is caused by deep-rooted imbalances that must be treated continuously over time. (In ancient China, doctors were paid only if their patients stayed healthy.) Herbal therapy, in particular, is often prescribed to be used on a regular basis to correct small energy imbalances before they can erupt into major problems. Many Chinese herbs can be taken or eaten daily as a preventive measure in much the same way as vitamins or nutritional supplements.

## *What the Critics Say*

Many of those raised in the tradition of Western medicine dismiss Chinese medicine as so much superstition and hocus-pocus—a vague, primitive, and quasi-religious set of beliefs founded not on the principles of hard science and logical reasoning but on irrational faith and mysticism. They refute claims that Chinese medicine is appropriate for all ailments, and they attribute any positive results to other causes or to simple good luck. Nonetheless, recent studies have shown that Chinese medical techniques can be effective. Acupuncture, in particular, has proved to be especially beneficial in chronic pain management, stroke rehabilitation, drug addiction, and nausea relief. Inserting needles in the skin evidently releases endorphins and other chemicals that serve as the body's natural painkillers, although how acupuncture provides long-term pain management is unclear.

Barriers are gradually falling, and now certain medical practices of the East are starting to gain formal acceptance in cultures of the West. In one sign of this newfound recognition, the World Health Organization of the United Nations lists about 50 diseases for which it considers acupuncture an appropriate treatment. ■

**FOR MORE INFO**

Following is a list of organizations you can contact to learn more about Chinese medicine:

**American Academy of Medical Acupuncture**
5820 Wilshire Blvd., Suite 500
Los Angeles, CA 90036
(800) 521-2262
fax: (213) 937-0959
e-mail: KCKD71@prodigy.com

**Council of Colleges of Acupuncture and Oriental Medicine**
1010 Wayne Avenue, Suite 1270
Silver Spring, MD 20910
(301) 608-9175
fax: (301) 608-9576

**National Acupuncture Detoxification Association**
(addictive and mental disorders)
PO Box 1927
Vancouver, WA 98668-1927
phone and fax: (360) 260-8620
e-mail: NADAclear@aol.com

**National Acupuncture and Oriental Medicine Alliance**
14637 Starr Road, SE
Olalla, WA 98359
(206) 851-6896
fax: (206) 851-6883

**National Certification Commission for Acupuncture and Oriental Medicine**
PO Box 97075
Washington, DC 20090-7075
(202) 232-1404
fax: (202) 462-6157

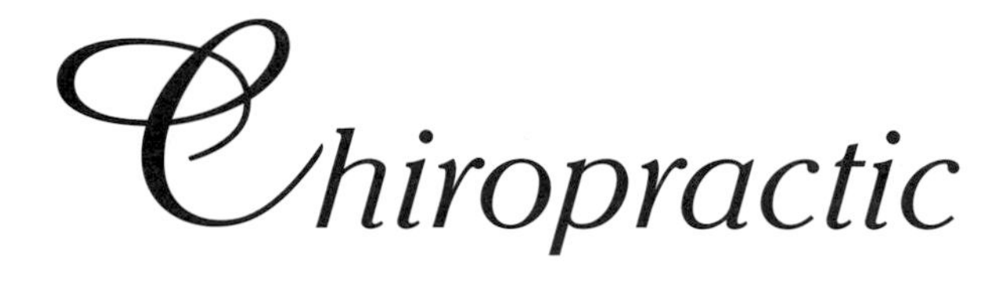

# Chiropractic

*Chiropractic is based on the concept that the human body has an innate self-healing ability and seeks homeostasis, or balance. According to general chiropractic theory, the nervous system plays an important role in maintaining homeostasis—and hence health. But "subluxations" (misalignments of bones within joints) or "fixations" (abnormalities of motion) are said to interfere with the flow of nervous impulses and diminish the body's ability to stay healthy. Through manipulation of the bones and their associated muscles and joints, particularly the spine, chiropractors work to correct these misalignments, thereby improving the function of the neuromusculoskeletal system and restoring homeostasis. The term chiropractic is derived from the Greek words "cheir" (hand) and "practikos" (done by).*

*Today, chiropractors are divided into two major camps. On one side are the straights—traditional chiropractors who adhere to the philosophy that subluxations are at the root of disease and that manipulation is the best treatment. On the other side are the mixers, so named because their approach represents a mix of traditional and progressive techniques.*

*Although chiropractic is often considered alternative medicine, it is gaining wider acceptance, in part because of recent clinical studies showing these methods to be effective in treating problems such as acute lower back pain and headache.*

## Origins

Chiropractic originated in 1895, when Daniel David Palmer, a magnetic healer who practiced laying on of hands in Davenport, Iowa, cured a janitor's deafness by pushing on a malpositioned vertebra in the man's back. To Palmer, this was proof that misalignments in the spine could impair health and that realigning the spine enhanced health by restoring the flow of nerve impulses throughout the body.

Two years later Palmer founded the first chiropractic school, and it was here, under the management of his son, that the schism currently dividing

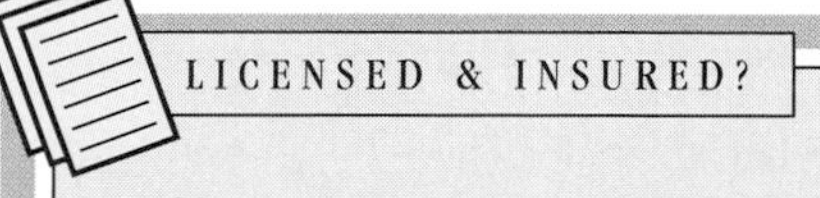

LICENSED & INSURED?

**YES!** *The services of chiropractors are covered by Medicare and, in many states, by Medicaid and most major private insurance plans. Chiropractic is taught in special five-year colleges and licensed in all 50 states according to standards established by the Council of Chiropractic Education and the Federation of Chiropractic Licensing Boards.*

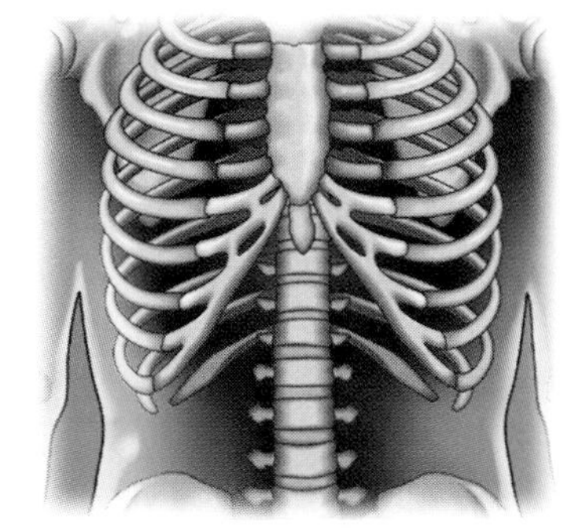

### Target Ailments

- Arthritis
- Asthma
- Back Problems
- Bursitis
- Carpal Tunnel Syndrome
- Chronic Fatigue Syndrome
- Earache
- Headache
- High Blood Pressure
- Menstrual Problems
- Muscle Cramps
- Neuralgia
- Pain, Chronic
- Premenstrual Syndrome
- Sprains and Strains
- Tendinitis
- TMJ Syndrome

*See Common Ailments, beginning on page 194.*



CONTINUED

the profession began to form. Dissatisfied with the Palmers' teachings—particularly their claims about the role of subluxations in disease—a faculty member named John Howard broke away to start his own chiropractic college (now the National College of Chiropractic) and, using Palmer's theories, to develop a program that was more firmly grounded in rational thought and solid scientific evidence. Within a decade, a number of other chiropractic schools had emerged. Practitioners who allied themselves with the Palmers became known as the straights; those who departed from the original concept were dubbed the mixers.

The straight-mixer split began a debate within the chiropractic community over the scope of its techniques and the profession's relationship with conventional medicine. While the straights concentrate almost exclusively on manipulation, the mixers employ manipulation along with a broad range of other therapeutic methods, including massage, physical therapy, and nutritional therapy.

### CAUTION

**Some people use chiropractors as their primary-care gatekeepers. But it's important to keep in mind that not all chiropractors are trained to diagnose all medical conditions, and delays in receiving the proper care can have serious consequences.**

**Chiropractic manipulation can cause severe damage if fractures or tumors are present, and in rare cases manipulation of the cervical spine (neck) can damage blood vessels in the brain, leading to stroke. However, before chiropractors begin treatment, they should carefully screen patients to determine the risk of these and other complications.**

## *What It's Good For*

Straight chiropractors believe that chiropractic manipulation can provide relief from every type of ailment, from asthma to impotence. The mixers, on the other hand, maintain that chiropractic is appropriate only for certain conditions and is particularly effective in the treatment of acute lower back pain, musculoskeletal problems, headache, and neck pain.

- **Back pain:** Studies show that spinal manipulation can relieve acute lower back pain, the most common reason that people make their first visit to a chiropractor.
- **Neck pain:** Chiropractic adjustment can often help correct painful misalignments in the neck, including those caused by whiplash injury.
- **Headache:** Spinal manipulation has been shown to decrease the frequency and intensity of migraine and tension headaches.
- **Other conditions:** Scientific studies and anecdotal evidence suggest that chiropractic can be beneficial in the treatment of otitis media, digestive problems, dysmenorrhea, hypertension, disk problems, scoliosis, sprains and some sports injuries, frozen shoulder, tennis elbow, carpal tunnel syndrome, abnormal jaw function, respiratory problems, enuresis, and arthritis in the wrist, hand, or hip.

## *Visiting a Professional*

Your first visit to a chiropractor usually begins with a general evaluation and case history: While noting your posture and gait, the practitioner will ask you about the problem and how it began, and about your medical history and lifestyle.

For the actual examination, you will be asked to wear a hospital gown. The chiropractor will palpate, or feel, your vertebrae to detect misplacement of bones or muscle weakness, and may perform a reflex test to check nerve function. You will then be instructed to bend forward, backward, and sideways while the chiropractor palpates your vertebrae and joints to determine their range of motion. The doctor may also take x-rays in order to discover any joint problems that could be worsened by manipulation.

Next, the doctor will make a diagnosis and determine a treatment plan, which may begin right away or on your second visit. In chiropractic treatment the practitioner adjusts your joints using a small controlled thrust that moves the joint slightly beyond its restricted range of motion; before making the adjustment, however, the doctor may massage the area around the joint in order to loosen tight muscles and ligaments.

If the chiropractor is adjusting your spine, you will need to lie on a padded table on your stomach or side. For an adjustment of your neck, you will be asked to sit upright. (While adjustments are being made, you may hear the joints crack just as your knuckles do when they crack.) The treatments are painless, and many patients feel improvement within nine to 12 sessions.

## *Wellness*

Unless you have a musculoskeletal problem, chiropractic may not fit into your long-term wellness plan: Some chiropractors insist that manipulation should be used to treat only specific problems, and that manipulating a healthy spine or joint accomplishes nothing. Others, however, argue that periodic chiropractic adjustments should be part of a preventive health maintenance program.

## *What the Critics Say*

- Some medical doctors maintain that misaligned vertebrae—the chiropractor's clue to health problems—are common, often harmless, and do not require treatment.
- Critics charge that frequent visits to a chiropractor are useless, whether as a preventive measure or to treat a specific condition such as back pain—which, they say, usually clears up on its own.
- Those critical of chiropractic often point out that quadriplegics can have healthy internal organs despite their extensive nerve damage. This fact, they maintain, disproves the assertion that a sound nervous system is the key to overall health.
- A number of critics argue that chiropractors should restrict their practice to treating back pain, since there is insufficient evidence to show that manipulation provides relief from any other condition. ■

**FOR MORE INFO**

Following is a list of organizations you can contact to learn more about chiropractic medicine:

**American Chiropractic Association**
1701 Clarendon Boulevard
Arlington, VA 22209
(703) 276-8800
fax: (703) 243-2593
e-mail: amerchiro@aol.com
(advocates mixer principles)

**International Chiropractors Association**
1110 North Glebe Road, Suite 1000
Arlington, VA 22201
(703) 528-5000
(advocates straight principles)

**World Federation of Chiropractic**
78 Glencairn Avenue
Toronto, Ontario M4R1M8
(416) 484-9978
fax: (416) 484-9665

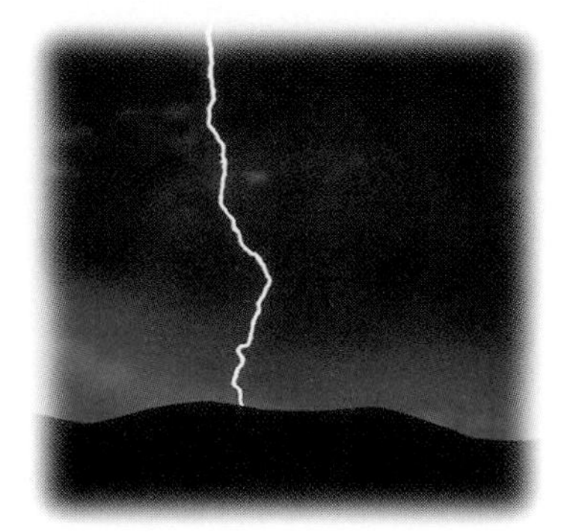

**Target Ailments**

- Headache
- Irritable Bowel Syndrome
- Pain, Chronic
- Premenstrual Syndrome
- Stress

*See Common Ailments, beginning on page 194.*

# Energy Medicine

*Energy medicine, also known as energy therapy or biofield therapeutics, is based on the premise that the human body is composed of various energy fields and that people fall ill when the energy in those fields becomes blocked, out of balance, or otherwise disturbed. Energy therapists attempt to restore health by first detecting and then removing the blockages.*

*Some energy therapists use special devices to diagnose and treat disturbed energy fields; others rely on various methods of healing touch, such as therapeutic touch (page 55), Reiki (page 53), and polarity therapy (described below).*

## The Vital Flow of Energy

Many ancient healing methods view health and sickness in terms of energy flow. Traditional Chinese medicine *(pages 57-60),* for example, posits illness as being the result of disturbances in a type of energy called *chi.* The Japanese healing technique of shiatsu *(page 17)* attempts to correct imbalances in an energy force called *ki.* And Ayurvedic medicine *(pages 42-46),* a form of healing practiced for thousands of years in India, uses body postures, breathing exercises, and meditative techniques to stimulate the flow of a variety of body energies.

Modern energy therapy has borrowed elements from these traditional approaches. The points and meridians (or energy "pathways") described in acupuncture *(pages 32-35),* for example, are often used as treatment sites by energy therapists. But some modern energy therapies have identified unique patterns of energy flow. Polarity therapy, for example, cites five currents of energy within the body, with specific points along the currents said to hold either positive or negative charges; to balance the body's energy flow, polarity therapists place their hands on points with opposite charges, creating a current.

## Origins

The earliest reference to energy healing can be found in Chinese medical texts written 2,500 to 5,000 years ago. Hippocrates also described the healing powers of "the force that flows from many people's hands." In the late 1700s, an Austrian physician named Franz Mesmer popularized the technique of laying on of hands in Europe and America with his "magnetic

**LICENSED & INSURED?**

*No. Energy therapists do not have to be licensed, although organizations for specific therapies do offer certification after completion of various training requirements.*

# Energy Medicine

healing" treatments. The technique gained renewed popularity during the 1970s when Dolores Krieger, a nursing professor at New York University, began teaching a hands-on healing method she called therapeutic touch.

## *What It's Good For*

Energy therapy is used for a variety of conditions. As a group, the techniques are reported to be most effective for healing wounds, reducing pain, and relieving anxiety. Some practitioners of energy therapy have also reported consistent success treating PMS, migraine, irritable bowel syndrome, eating disorders, and posttraumatic stress disorder. Energy therapy is also used to help people overcome addictions, and to ease the pain and anxiety of pregnancy, childbirth, and surgical treatment.

## *Preparations/Techniques*

Energy therapists use a variety of techniques to balance and release the body's flow of energy. Most involve the practitioner's placing his or her hands either directly on or very near the patient's body. The hands do not always touch the body because energy fields are said to extend outward from the body for several inches.

Practitioners first attempt to detect subtle clues, such as changes in body temperature or sensations of "electricity" or "magnetism," that indicate where your body's energy needs to be unblocked or rebalanced. Some practitioners diagnose with measuring instruments known as electroacupuncture biofeedback machines, which are said to measure electrical energy disturbances at acupuncture points.

In general, there are two views about how energy therapy heals. One is that the practitioner directs or modifies the patient's energy field in a way that facilitates healing. The other is that the source of the healing comes not from the practitioner directly, but from a universal energy field or higher spiritual power. Some practitioners meditate or pray before starting a treatment; others go into a deep meditative state during it. Some also practice mental healing—a technique in which the practitioner actively focuses his or her intention on becoming a vehicle for healing the patient.

## *Wellness*

Practitioners believe that these techniques free the body's flow of energy, thus relieving stress, increasing vitality, and contributing to overall wellness.

## *What the Critics Say*

Critics point out that energy therapy has not undergone rigorous scientific study; indeed, the very existence of bodily energy fields is widely considered unproved. In addition, most reports of energy medicine's success in healing have been anecdotal, and some critics hold that positive results are due to the placebo effect. ■

**FOR MORE INFO**

Following is a list of organizations you can contact to learn more about energy medicine:

**American Polarity Therapy Association**
2888 Bluff Street, Suite 149
Boulder, CO 80301
(303) 545-2080
fax: (303) 545-2161

**International Society for the Study of Subtle Energies and Energy Medicine**
356 Goldco Circle
Golden, CO 80403-1347
(303) 278-2228
e-mail: 74040.1273@compuserve.com

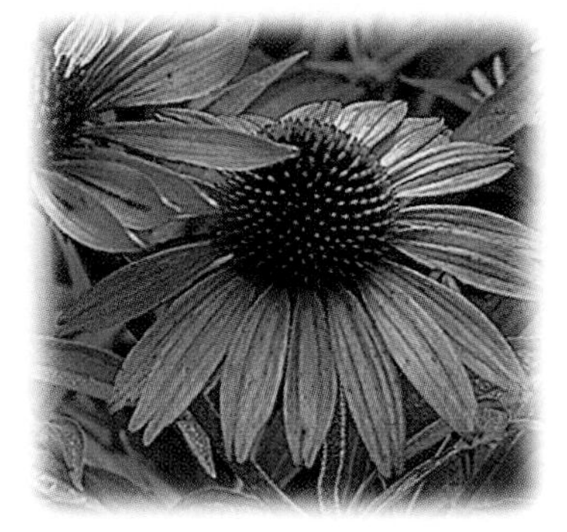

### Target Ailments

- Athletic Injuries
- Back Problems
- Chronic Fatigue Syndrome
- Depression
- Headache
- Immune Problems
- Insomnia
- Pain, Chronic
- Premenstrual Syndrome
- Stress

*See Common Ailments, beginning on page 194.*

# Flower Remedies

*Flower remedies, also called flower essences, are specially prepared liquid concentrates made by soaking flowers in pure spring water. The concentrates are diluted and sipped to treat various emotional and physical disorders. The fundamental theory behind flower-essence therapy is that physical ailments and disease, as well as psychological problems, arise from emotional disturbances; diagnosis and treatment thus involve an evaluation of personality, state of mind, and emotional makeup.*

*Like homeopathic remedies (pages 104-106), flower essences are diluted to such a degree that they do not work on a biochemical level. Practitioners say they contain specific aspects of the plants' energy, which affect the energy field of the person taking them. In this way, the flower remedies are believed to help people work with and integrate their emotions; a typical treatment might, for example, aim to develop in a fearful person the courage to face his or her fear.*

## *Origins*

Although healing with flowers goes back to ancient times, the specific use of flower concentrates to treat emotions and attitudes was developed in the 1930s by the English bacteriologist and homeopathic physician Edward Bach. After careful observation of his patients, Bach concluded not only that links existed between certain personality traits and certain illnesses but also that people with similar personalities reacted to their illnesses similarly. He searched for natural agents that would deal with the emotional precursors to disease and eventually discovered the flower essences, whose specific qualities he determined through intuition and experimentation on himself.

Today, many companies produce versions of flower essences. Among the major, well-established lines are the original 38 English essences of Dr. Bach, available from several different sources; North American flower essences, a group of over 100 remedies sometimes called California remedies; and a series of Rose essences, some of which are designated as addressing specific functions of the body.

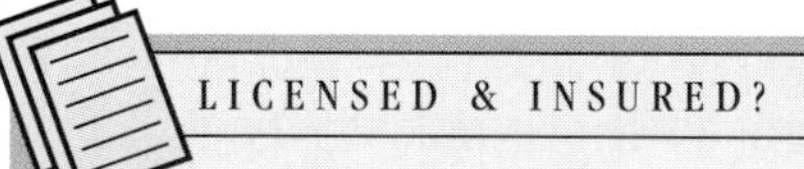

LICENSED & INSURED?

*There is no licensing of practitioners, but licensed healthcare providers might use flower essences as part of a treatment that may be covered by insurance. Depending on the manufacturer, some flower essences are sold as dietary supplements. Others are enrolled in the official homeopathic pharmacopoeia and classified as homeopathic medicines.*

# Flower Remedies

## What It's Good For

Proponents say flower remedies are helpful for numerous physical ailments and emotional states. Each of Bach's original 38 remedies corresponds to a negative mood or state of mind. The 38 are divided into seven groups of emotions: fear, uncertainty, insufficient interest in present circumstances, loneliness, oversensitivity to influences and ideas, despondency and despair, and overconcern for the welfare of others. Within each of the seven groups are subcategories of the emotion, each with a specific remedy. For example, subcategories under fear include terror, fear of an unknown cause, and fear for other people.

The group of English remedies includes a combination formula of five of the 38 essences that is said to be beneficial for a variety of problems, such as physical injury, shock, pain, or severe emotional upset. Among the brand names for this combination are Rescue Remedy, Five Flower Formula, and Calming Essence.

## Preparations/Techniques

The remedies, usually obtained in liquid concentrate form (called the stock) and preserved in alcohol or vinegar, may be bought at health food stores and some pharmacies, by mail order, or through a practitioner. Preparation of the essences is a complex process that takes into account a variety of factors, including the plants' environment and the climatic conditions at the time of collection and concentration.

You can match your own emotions and state of mind with those listed in the chart on pages 68-69 to choose one or more remedies (up to six at a time) for yourself or your children. To administer, place 2 to 4 drops of the stock under your tongue four times daily or place several drops in a large glass of water and sip a few times a day. Flower essences may also be used topically or added to baths.

## Visiting a Professional

If you are unfamiliar with these remedies, it may be helpful to seek out a practitioner at first. The practitioner is likely to choose your remedies by observing you and asking you questions, and possibly by evaluating the results of certain physical tests.

## What the Critics Say

Critics point out that claims of effectiveness are based on intuition rather than science and therefore are unsubstantiated. Some say any reported positive effects are due to the placebo effect; however, proponents point to benefits experienced by animals and children, who presumably would not be susceptible to the placebo effect. Proponents also claim there is no evidence of side effects, ill effects following a wrong diagnosis, or harmful interactions with any other medicines. ■

### CAUTION

**Some practitioners say that the essences may bring unresolved emotional issues to the surface for consideration, which may be psychologically unsettling, yet beneficial in the long run.**

**People who are sensitive to the alcohol in some remedies can dilute the remedy or use a few drops on the wrist or lips rather than ingesting.**

### FOR MORE INFO

Contact the following organizations to learn more about flower essences:

**Flower Essence Society**
PO Box 459
Nevada City, CA 95959
(800) 736-9222; (916) 265-9163
(North American and English essences)

**Perelandra Ltd.**
PO Box 3603
Warrenton, VA 20188
(540) 937-2153
fax: (540) 937-3360
(Rose essences)

**Nelson Bach USA Ltd.**
Wilmington Technology Park
100 Research Drive
Wilmington, MA 01887
(800) 334-0843
(the official Bach flower Essences)

**Ellon USA, Inc.**
644 Merrick Road
Lynbrook, NY 11563
(800) 423-2256
(English essences)



CONTINUED

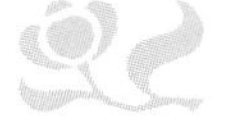

## 39 Essential Flower Remedies

*This chart lists the 38 Bach essences plus the combination formula Rescue Remedy. Each entry describes—in language typically used by practitioners—the mental and emotional states for which that remedy is said to be beneficial. Up to six Bach remedies may be taken at a time. The illustrations show four common herbs from which additional essences—beyond Bach's originals—have been developed.*

**Agrimony**
Proclivity to conceal worry and deny pain, restlessness, distressed by arguments and confrontation.

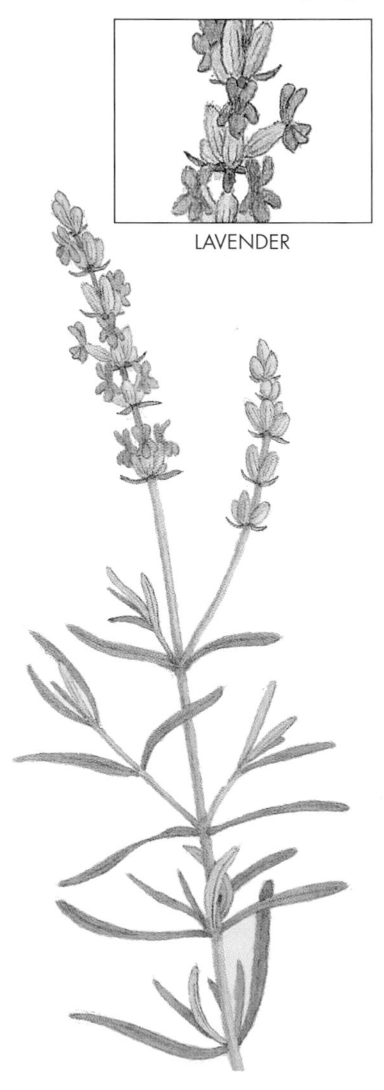

LAVENDER

**Aspen**
Unexplained anxiety, apprehension, fears of unknown origin, tending to have nightmares.

**Beech**
Intolerant, critical, dissatisfied, negative, unwilling to make allowances.

**Centaury**
Weak-willed, submissive, easily influenced or imposed upon, difficulty saying no.

**Cerato**
Distrust of self and own ability, overdependent on the advice of others.

**Cherry Plum**
Desperation, fear of emotional breakdown, uncontrolled and irrational thoughts.

**Chestnut Bud**
Failure to learn from experience, lack of observation, repeating mistakes.

**Chicory**
Possessiveness, self-love, self-pity, controlling, demanding, attention-seeking.

**Clematis**
Indifference, daydreaming, inattention, absorbed in own thoughts, impractical.

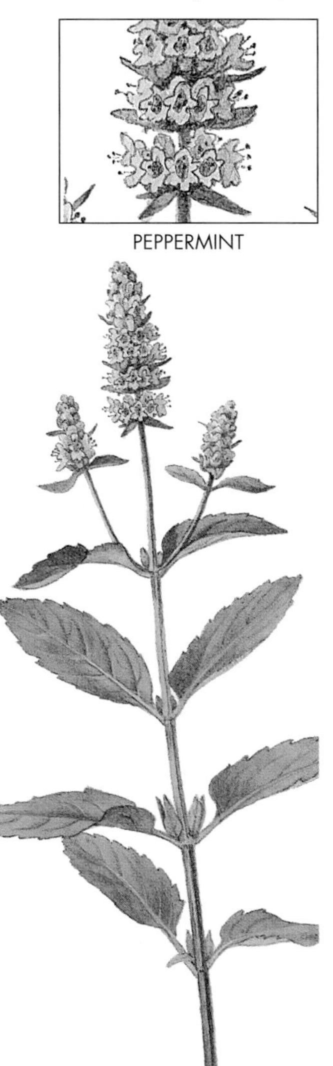

PEPPERMINT

**Crab Apple**
Self-disgust, shame, feeling of uncleanness.

**Elm**
Occasional feelings of inadequacy, being overwhelmed by responsibility.

**Gentian**
Doubt, depression, discouragement after setback, skepticism, negativity.

**Gorse**
Hopelessness, despair, resignation, loss of will, pessimism, defeatism.

**Heather**
Self-centered, talking incessantly about oneself, obsessed with own problems.

**Holly**
Hatred, envy, jealousy, suspicion, strong negativity, feeling cut off from love.

**Honeysuckle**
Nostalgia, homesickness, living in the past, regretful, loss of interest in the present.

**Hornbeam**
Fatigue, feeling of

# Flower Remedies

being burdened, temporary mental and physical exhaustion, procrastination.

**Impatiens**
Impatience, irritability, intolerance, impulsivity, nervous tension, overexertion.

**Larch**
Lack of confidence, despondency, self-censorship, feelings of inferiority.

**Mimulus**
Fear or anxiety of known things, timidity, shyness, nervousness.

**Mustard**
Deep depression of unknown cause, sadness that comes and goes unexpectedly.

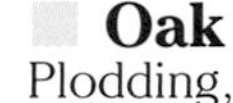

SAGE

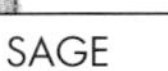

**Oak**
Plodding, uncomplaining, inflexible, overachieving, obstinate.

**Olive**
Complete exhaustion, depletion after illness or long-term stress.

**Pine**
Self-reproach, guilt, self-blame, inability to accept self, apologetic.

**Red Chestnut**
Excessive fear or anxiety for loved ones, anticipation of trouble.

**Rock Rose**
Sudden alarm, terror, panic, hysteria, nightmares, feelings of horror.

**Rock Water**
Self-repression, self-denial, self-martyrdom, perfectionism, obsessiveness.

**Scleranthus**
Uncertainty, indecision, hesitancy, confusion, wavering, lack of mental clarity.

**Star-of-Bethlehem**
Grief, distress, past or present trauma such as that sustained from bad news, accident, or fright.

**RESCUE REMEDY**
**Star-of-Bethlehem, Rock Rose, Impatiens, Cherry Plum, Clematis**
Trauma, terror, panic, stress, desperation, disorientation.

**Sweet Chestnut**
Extreme mental anguish, utter dejection, hopelessness, despair.

**Vervain**
Overenthusiastic, tendency to impose will, argumentative, fanatical, overbearing.

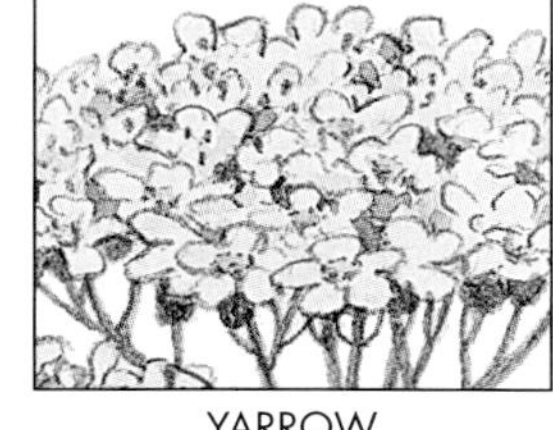

YARROW

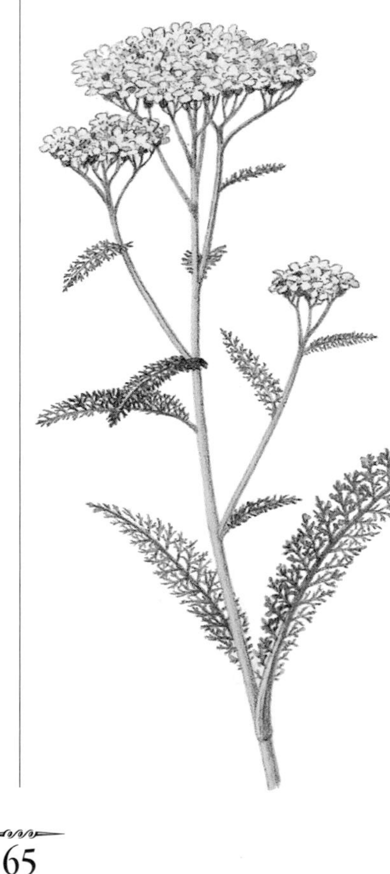

**Vine**
Dominating others, tyrannical, ambitious, arrogant, inflexible, ruthless.

**Walnut**
Difficulty in adjusting to transition or change, including relocation, a new job, divorce, menopause, or puberty.

**Water Violet**
Pride, aloofness, self-reliance, noninterfering, enjoys being alone.

**White Chestnut**
Persistent unwanted thoughts, internal arguments, worry, preoccupation.

**Wild Oat**
Dissatisfaction due to uncertainty regarding career, lack of direction or commitment.

**Wild Rose**
Resignation, apathy, surrender, failure to make effort, lack of hope.

**Willow**
Resentment, bitterness, grumbling, self-pity, blaming others, dissatisfaction, victim role.

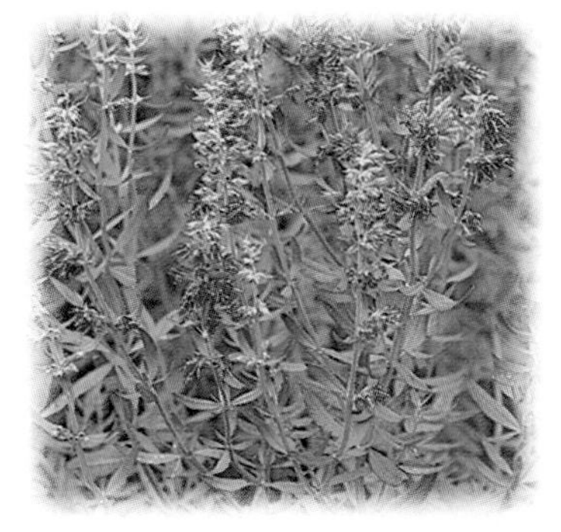

## Target Ailments

**Herbs are used for ailments affecting all body systems.**

- Cardiovascular System
- Digestive System
- Immune System
- Musculoskeletal System
- Nervous System
- Reproductive System
- Respiratory System
- Skin
- Urinary System

*See Common Ailments, beginning on page 194.*

# Herbal Therapies

*Herbal medicines are prepared from a wide variety of plant materials—frequently the leaves, stems, roots, and bark, but also the flowers, fruits, twigs, seeds, and exudates (material that oozes out, such as sap). They generally contain several biologically active ingredients and are used primarily for treating chronic or mild conditions, although on occasion they are employed as complementary or supportive therapy for acute and severe diseases.*

*Across the spectrum of alternative medicine, the use of herbs is varied: Western herbology, Chinese medicine, and Ayurvedic medicine differ in the way practitioners diagnose diseases and prescribe herbal remedies. Naturopathic physicians may use herbs from any of these systems.*

### Western Herbs

Medicinal plants in the group known as Western herbs bear English as well as Latin names and are categorized in several ways. Normalizers, or tonics, have a gentle, healing effect on the body. Another type, called effectors, have powerful actions and are used to treat illnesses. Herbs are also frequently grouped into more than 20 categories according to how they affect the body. Some of these categories are familiar—anti-inflammatories, diuretics, laxatives. Other, less well known classes include diaphoretics (herbs that promote perspiration and therefore the elimination of waste products through the skin) and nervines (herbs that act to strengthen the nervous system).

In many cases, herbs are also grouped according to the body systems they affect. The cardiovascular system, for example, responds well to herbs that strengthen blood vessels; these herbs include ginkgo, buckwheat, and linden. The digestive system, on the other hand, benefits from the relaxing effects of chamomile. Individual herbs can act on a body system in different ways. For instance, the sedative valerian, the cardiotonic herb hawthorn, and the herb St.-John's-wort, which has an antidepressant effect, invoke distinct responses from the nervous system.

> **LICENSED & INSURED?**
>
> *Naturopaths and acupuncturists are licensed on a state-by-state basis, and in some states their services are covered by medical insurance. However, Ayurvedic physicians and clinical or medical herbalists are not licensed, and insurance companies usually do not provide coverage for their services.*

### Traditional Chinese Herbs

Another group of herbs, used by practitioners of Chinese medicine, are

# Herbal Therapies

part of a larger system of healing that attempts to help the body correct energy imbalances *(see Chinese Medicine, pages 57-60).* Chinese herbs are classified according to certain active characteristics (such as heating, cooling, moisturizing, or drying) and are prescribed according to how they influence the various organ systems. Practitioners of Chinese medicine also recognize five herb "tastes"—sweet, sour, salty, pungent, and bitter—each of which is associated with a particular physiological action. Chinese herbal prescriptions usually contain several herbs, perhaps as many as a dozen. These combinations are chosen not only for their effect on specific diseases but also for their ability to balance potential side effects and direct the therapy to a certain area of the body.

## Origins

People have used plants for medicine since before recorded history, and all known cultures have long histories of folk medicine that include the use of herbs. Physical evidence of the existence of herbal remedies was found in the burial site of a Neanderthal man who lived more than 60,000 years ago.

Early observations of the characteristics of herbs and the way certain plants affected animals and humans were amassed in collections called pharmacopoeias or materia medicas. Many traditional herbalists believed that a healing energy inherent in the plants, and not the chemical constituents alone, accounted for the beneficial effects—a theory that is being explored by some contemporary practitioners.

Ancient cultures such as those of Greece and Rome developed well-defined herbal pharmacopoeias, and some herbal knowledge came to Europe from the Middle East during the Crusades. In the United States, herbs were used for many years to prevent various ailments and treat minor emergencies. In fact, American physicians relied on herbal preparations as primary medicines through the 1930s.

During the latter part of the 20th century, the use of plant remedies declined with advancements in medical technology and developments in the production of new pharmaceuticals. A 1992 report on alternative medicine prepared for the National Institutes of Health expressed concern that our knowledge of herbs—as medicinal plants and as unique species—may soon be lost. Recently, however, interest in herbal therapy has increased dramatically, partly in response to the growing perception that medicinal drugs are expensive, may cause side effects or allergic reactions, and are not capable of curing every disease.

## What It's Good For

Herbal therapy offers remedies for virtually every ailment affecting all body systems. For a list of specific herbs and some of their medicinal uses, see The 75 Most Effective Herbs, on pages 74-103.

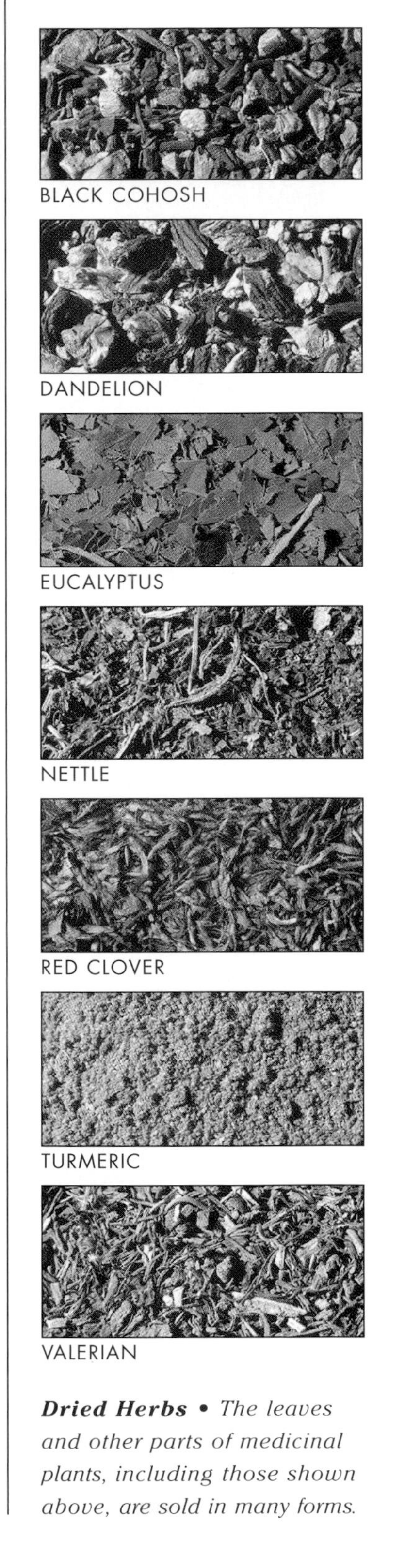


***Dried Herbs*** • *The leaves and other parts of medicinal plants, including those shown above, are sold in many forms.*



CONTINUED

# Herbal Therapies CONTINUED

CAUTION

**Use herbs with caution at all times. Be especially careful if you have allergies, are sensitive to drugs, are taking drugs for a chronic illness, or are older than 65 or younger than 12. To help minimize any adverse reactions, start with the lowest appropriate dose. Be aware that some herbs are toxic if taken incorrectly; comfrey, for example, can cause liver damage if taken in excessive amounts for too long a time.**

## *Preparations/Techniques*

Herbs are available in various forms at health food stores and pharmacies, and many can be ordered by mail. Although Chinese herbs can usually be bought at Asian food stores, these products are more likely to be dispensed by practitioners, who are familiar with the combination formulas. Many practitioners of Chinese medicine also dispense Western herbs.

Herbal remedies can be prepared at home in a variety of ways, using either fresh or dried ingredients. Herbal teas, or infusions, can be steeped to varying strengths. Roots, bark, or other plant parts can be simmered into strong solutions called decoctions. Honey or sugar can be added to infusions and decoctions to make syrups. You can also buy many herbal remedies over the counter in the form of pills, capsules, or powders, or in more concentrated liquid forms called extracts and tinctures. Certain herbs can be applied topically as creams or ointments, soaked into cloths and used as compresses, or applied directly to the skin as poultices.

## *Visiting a Professional*

Because some herbs can be toxic or carcinogenic, all medicinal plants should be used only under the guidance of a healthcare practitioner who is familiar with herbal medicine. The major professional herbalists in the U.S. include naturopathic physicians specializing in botanical medicine, acupuncturists trained in Chinese herbal medicine, Ayurvedic doctors, and trained medical or clinical herbalists.

Practitioners select a plant or formula that is appropriate for the patient rather than for just the complaint alone. Typically, the herbalist will take your personal and family history and may either perform a physical examination or request the results of a recent exam. He or she may evaluate any personal, social, or lifestyle factors that affect your health, then make recommendations regarding diet, exercise, or other lifestyle modifications. The practitioner will then suggest one or more remedies deemed appropriate for your condition. The exact form and dosage will depend on the strength of the herb, the effects desired, your age, and your constitution. In the case of Chinese medicine, the choice of herbs is based on a diagnostic system that evaluates specific individual characteristics, including the pulse rate and the appearance of the tongue *(see Chinese Medicine, pages 57-60).*

## *Wellness*

Herbs can be of great value when used in a program of self-care and preventive medicine. But because they vary in strength from gentle remedies that can be eaten like food to potential lethal poisons, medicinal plants should always be used under the supervision of a professional. A practitioner can advise which of the milder "tonic" herbs, such as dandelion and nettle, are safe and appropriate for your condition. A number of culinary herbs—including thyme and rosemary, which act as digestive stimulants and antiseptics—may also be used in a preventive health program.

## What the Critics Say

Those suspicious of herbal therapy often point to the widespread availability of what they consider inaccurate or deceptive information about herbs. Although herbs cannot legally be labeled as to their efficacy in fighting diseases, advocacy literature—some of it carrying extreme claims of therapeutic effectiveness—may be sold alongside herbs on store shelves. Sometimes dangerous herbs are recommended, and in other cases herbs are said to be imbued with magical or mystical properties. Such claims draw fire from critics either because they are unscientific or because they leave the erroneous impression that potentially dangerous plants are harmless.

Herbal therapy also is criticized because medicinal plants have not been tested for efficacy according to rigid pharmaceutical standards. However, these tests are very expensive. Because herbs are natural products and cannot be patented, any company paying for such testing would likely never recover its losses. Furthermore, there's continuing debate over whether such testing should be performed on the entire herb or only on its active ingredients. Some remedies depend on the actions of several components (or several herbs) working together. Another problem is that sometimes an herb's active ingredients are not known.

Proponents of herbal therapy point out that the pharmaceutical industry grew out of herbal treatment and that plant extracts are still used to make drugs. For example, digitalis, used to treat heart disease, comes from the foxglove, and morphine comes from the opium poppy. About 25 percent of today's prescription drugs are at least partially derived from plants. ■

OF SPECIAL INTEREST

### Using Herbs Safely

*Purchasing herbs is generally safer than harvesting your own plants. Many herbalists also advise against collecting your own herbs from the wild. Plants have natural variations that can be misleading, and the consequences of a mistake can be severe: A number of people have died from ingesting toxic wild plants believed to be benign substances. Because all forms of herbs lose potency over time, you should look for a source that provides the freshest possible product.*

*If you consistently develop nausea, diarrhea, or headache within two hours of taking an herb, discontinue its use immediately. Call your practitioner if the symptoms are prolonged. Women who are pregnant or breastfeeding are advised not to take medicinal amounts of herbs without first consulting a healthcare professional.*

### FOR MORE INFO

Following is a list of organizations you can contact to learn more about herbal therapy:

**The American Herbalist Guild**
PO Box 746555
Arvada, CO 80006
(303) 423-8800

**Herb Research Foundation**
1007 Pearl Street, Suite 200
Boulder, CO 80302
(303) 449-2265

**National Acupuncture and Oriental Medicine Alliance**
14637 Starr Road, SE
Olalla, WA 98359
(206) 851-6896

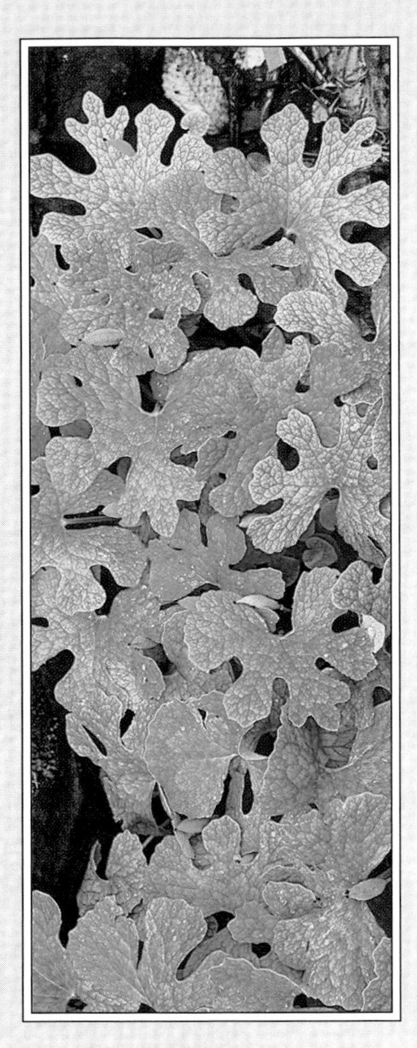

**Bloodroot**

## Aloe

*Aloe barbadensis*

*The translucent gel obtained from the inner leaves of this tropical herb works externally to relieve minor burns, skin irritations, and infections; taken internally, it provides relief from stomach disorders. Among its ingredients are several that reduce inflammation. Aloe gel is also used as a beauty aid and moisturizer because it contains polysaccharides, which act as emollients.*

**TARGET AILMENTS**

**Take internally for** digestive disorders, gastritis, stomach ulcers.

**Apply externally for** minor burns, infected wounds, insect bites, irritated skin or eyes, bruises, chickenpox, sunburn, poison ivy, acne.

**PREPARATIONS**

**Over the counter:** Aloe is available as powder, fluidextract, powdered capsules, or bottled gel.

**At home:**

Eyewash: Dissolve ½ tsp powdered aloe gel in 1 cup water. Add 1 tsp boric acid to accelerate the healing process. Pour through a coffee filter before applying to the eyes.

Bath: Add 1 to 2 cups gel to a warm bath to relieve sunburn or skin lesions.

Combinations: Use aloe gel externally with wheat-germ oil and safflower flower to reduce bruising.

**SIDE EFFECTS**

**Not serious:** The use of aloe may result in allergic dermatitis, intestinal cramps, or diarrhea. Try a lower dosage or stop using the product.

**SPECIAL INFORMATION**

- If you are pregnant or have a gastrointestinal illness, consult an herbalist or a licensed healthcare professional before taking aloe internally.

## Astragalus

*Astragalus membranaceus*

*The perennial plant astragalus, or milkvetch root, has sprawling stems and pale yellow blooms. Western herbalists believe that substances known as polysaccharides in this herb stimulate the immune system and generally strengthen the body, promoting tissue regeneration, speeding metabolism, and increasing energy. The herb is also used in traditional Chinese medicine.*

**TARGET AILMENTS**

**Take internally for** general weakness and fatigue, loss of appetite, spontaneous perspiration, diarrhea, blood abnormalities, chronic colds and flu, AIDS, cancer. (Take with conventional medical treatment.)

**PREPARATIONS**

**Over the counter:** Astragalus is available as prepared tea, fluidextract, capsules, and dried root.

**At home:**

Chinese: Combine 1 part honey, 4 parts dried root, and a small amount of water in a wok or skillet. Allow mixture to simmer until the water evaporates and the herbs are slightly brown.

Combinations: For spontaneous perspiration, astragalus is mixed with Asian ginseng. As an immune system stimulant, the herb is combined with siler *(Ledebouriella divaricata)*. Blood abnormalities are treated with a mix of astragalus and dong quai. Herbalists combine astragalus and atractylodes (white) for diarrhea.

Western: Boil 1 oz astragalus root in 1 cup water for 15 to 20 minutes to make a tea.

**SIDE EFFECTS**

None expected.

**SPECIAL INFORMATION**

- Pregnant women should check with their practitioners before using astragalus.

## Black Cohosh

*Cimicifuga racemosa*

*The knotty black rhizome and root of black cohosh contain substances that act like the female hormone estrogen. It is prescribed for several menstrual and menopausal conditions. The herb also acts as a sedative and is believed to promote urination, dry up discharges of fluid, aid in expelling mucus from the lungs, and relieve coughing spasms.*

### TARGET AILMENTS

**Take internally for** menstrual discomfort, menopause, PMS, headache, bleeding gums, coughs.

**Apply externally for** sciatica, neuralgia, muscle spasms, rheumatism.

### PREPARATIONS

**Over the counter:** Black cohosh is available as tincture, syrup, capsules, fluidextract, and also as dried root and rhizome.

**At home:**

Decoction: Boil ½ tsp powdered rootstock per cup of water for 30 minutes and let cool. Add lemon and honey. Take as much as a cup per day, 2 tbsp at a time.

### SIDE EFFECTS

**Not serious:** Prolonged use may irritate the uterus.

**Serious:** Overdoses or prolonged use can cause dizziness, diarrhea, nausea, vomiting, abdominal pain, headaches, joint pains, and lowered heart rate. It can contribute to abnormal blood clotting, liver problems, and breast tumors. If any symptoms develop, stop using black cohosh and call your doctor immediately.

### SPECIAL INFORMATION

WARNING: Because it can cause serious side effects, use black cohosh only under medical supervision. Do not use if you have heart problems.

❧ Do not use if you are pregnant or if you have been told not to take contraceptive pills.

## Black Walnut

*Juglans nigra*

*Native Americans used the bark of the black walnut, a tree that grows in the eastern U.S., to treat skin problems such as ringworm. They drank a tea made from the bark as a laxative, and they chewed on the bark to relieve headache pain. Today black walnut's bark, leaves, fruit rind, and liquid extracts are prescribed by herbalists for constipation, fungal and parasitic infections, and mouth sores. Black walnut is rich in tannins and contains a large amount of iodine, which makes it a good antiseptic. Also, the herb is believed to relieve toxic blood conditions. And some evidence indicates that, if used internally over a long period, the herb will help eliminate warts caused by viruses.*

### TARGET AILMENTS

**Take internally for** constipation, intestinal worms and parasites, warts, mouth sores.

**Apply externally for** ringworm, scabies, eczema, herpes, psoriasis, sores, pimples, athlete's foot, jock itch, cold sores.

### PREPARATIONS

**Over the counter:** Black walnut is available as tincture, extract, dried bark, leaves, and fruit rind.

**At home:**

Decoction: Simmer the bark in boiling water for 10 to 15 minutes. Take 1 tbsp three or four times a day.

Gargle: Use the decoction as a mouthwash or gargle to treat mouth sores.

Extract: Rub on the affected area twice a day.

Poultice: Make a poultice from the green rind of black walnut and apply to the sites of ringworm.

### SIDE EFFECTS

None expected.

## Bloodroot

*Sanguinaria canadensis*

*Named for the crimson extract made from its root, bloodroot not only looks forbidding but is potentially toxic and can cause severe side effects if ingested in excess. For this reason, herbalists prescribe the root of this perennial plant primarily as an external remedy to relieve eczema, venereal blisters, rashes, and other skin disorders. Bloodroot is a major ingredient in many mouthwashes and toothpastes because of its ability to kill the bacteria that can lead to gingivitis (gum disease) and the buildup of plaque.*

### TARGET AILMENTS

**Take internally for** gingivitis. (Use as toothpaste and mouthwash.)

**Apply externally for** fungus, athlete's foot, venereal blisters, rashes, eczema, ringworm, warts.

### PREPARATIONS

**Over the counter:** Bloodroot is available as tincture and dried root.

**At home:**

Tea: Boil 1 oz bloodroot in 1 cup water for 15 to 20 minutes. Drink three times daily.

Combinations: With horehound and elecampane to relieve congestion; with red sage and a pinch of cayenne to treat pharyngitis.

### SIDE EFFECTS

**Serious:** At high doses, internal use can cause burning in the stomach, vomiting, nausea, slowing of the heart rate, impaired vision, intense thirst, and dizziness. Stop using immediately if these symptoms develop, and consult your practitioner.

### SPECIAL INFORMATION

WARNING: Bloodroot is potentially toxic. Take it internally only under the supervision of an herbalist or licensed healthcare professional.

❧ Avoid using bloodroot internally during pregnancy.



CONTINUED

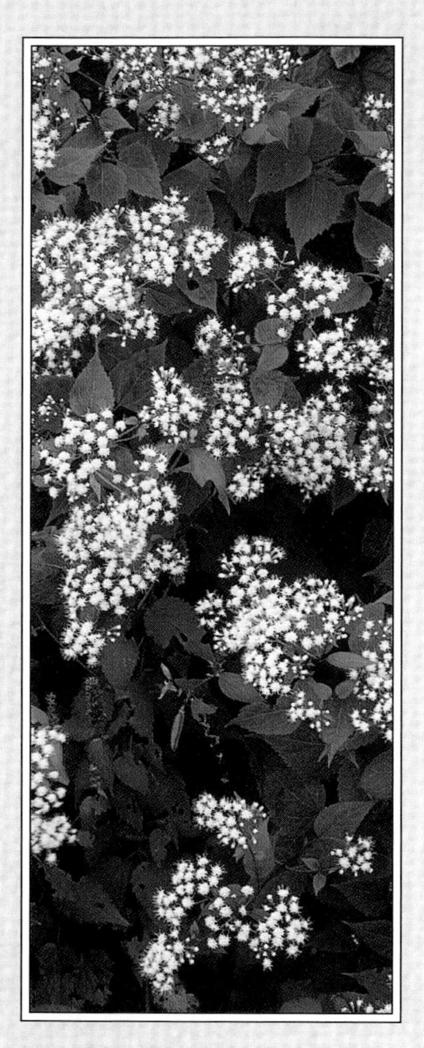

**Boneset**

## Boneset

*Eupatorium perfoliatum*

*Boneset, also called sweat plant and feverwort, was first used by Native Americans and then by the colonists to treat fever-producing illnesses. Today herbalists still recommend the herb for the aches and pains that accompany fever, especially during bouts of influenza, and to help clear mucus from the respiratory tract. It is also often used for arthritis and rheumatism.*

### TARGET AILMENTS

**Take internally for** fever, colds, flu, coughs, upper respiratory tract congestion,arthritis, and rheumatism.

### PREPARATIONS

**Over the counter:** Available in health food stores as dried leaves and flowers, and as tincture.

**At home:**

Infusion: Pour 1 cup boiling water onto 2 to 3 tsp dried herb; let steep 10 to 15 minutes. Drink as hot as possible. For fever or flu, drink a cup every half hour, up to 4 cups in 6 hours. Do not exceed 6 cups in a 24-hour period. To mask boneset's very bitter taste, mix it with an herbal tea or add honey and lemon.

### SIDE EFFECTS

**Not serious:** Large doses can cause nausea or diarrhea. Do not exceed the recommended dosage; call your doctor if you experience adverse reactions.

### SPECIAL INFORMATION

WARNING: Do not use fresh boneset. It contains a toxic chemical called tremerol that can cause vomiting, rapid breathing, and at high doses, possibly coma and death. Drying boneset removes the tremerol.

- Do not take boneset for more than two weeks at a time. If you have a history of alcoholism or liver problems, consult your herbalist before taking boneset; it is toxic to the liver.

## Bupleurum

*Bupleurum chinense*

*Bupleurum, sometimes called hare's ear or thorowax root, is often used in Chinese medicine to reduce certain types of fever and to treat irritability.*

### TARGET AILMENTS

**Take internally for** low-grade fevers; malaria; alternating chills and fever, typically accompanied by a bitter taste in the mouth, pain in the side, irritability, vomiting, or difficulty in breathing; prolapse of the uterus; vertigo combined with chest pain, and tenderness in the side or breast, often accompanied by irritability; menstrual problems; pressure in the chest, bloated abdomen, nausea, and indigestion.

### PREPARATIONS

The root is available in bulk in Chinese pharmacies, Asian markets, and some Western health food stores. Chinese pharmacies also offer mixtures containing the root.

Combinations: White peony root mixed with bupleurum is prescribed for vertigo, chest pain, and painful menstruation. Irregular menstruation, PMS, and certain kinds of depression may be treated with a blend of bupleurum and field mint. Bupleurum is often combined with bitter orange fruit to relieve pressure in the chest, abdominal pain, and irregular bowel movements, and to improve poor appetite. For information on specific dosages and additional herbal combinations, consult your Chinese medicine practitioner.

### SIDE EFFECTS

**Not serious:** Too large a dose can cause nausea.

### SPECIAL INFORMATION

- Clinical tests have indicated that the herb might be useful in treating tuberculosis, influenza, and polio.

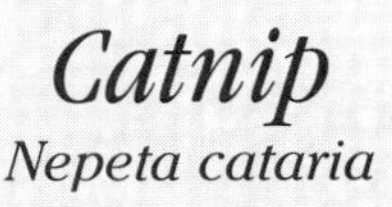

# The 75 Most Effective Herbs

## Burdock

*Arctium lappa*

*Herbalists have long prescribed burdock root for a wide range of illnesses. Today, some use it to treat urinary tract infections, arthritis, external wounds, and skin ulcers. This herb works best in conjunction with conventional medical treatment. Burdock got its name from its tenacious burrs and from "dock," the Old English word for plant.*

### TARGET AILMENTS

**Take internally for** fungal and bacterial infections; skin disorders, such as eczema and psoriasis, which cause dry, scaly skin; urinary tract infections; rheumatism; arthritis.

**Apply externally for** wounds and skin conditions.

### PREPARATIONS

**Over the counter:** Burdock is available as dried powder, slices of root, and tincture.

**At home:**

Decoction: Add 1 tsp burdock root to 3 cups water; boil for 30 minutes. Drink up to 3 cups a day to treat genital and urinary tract irritations.

Compress: Soak a clean cloth in burdock tea and place it on the skin to speed healing of wounds and skin ulcers.

Combinations: Burdock, mixed with yellow dock, red clover, or cleavers, can be taken orally for skin disorders. Consult an herbalist for more information.

### SPECIAL INFORMATION

WARNING: Because it stimulates the uterus, do not use if pregnant.

- Do not give burdock to children younger than two years of age. Older children and people over 65 should start with lower-strength doses, increasing them if needed.
- Doses higher than recommended may cause stomach discomfort.

## Calendula

*Calendula officinalis*

*The therapeutic use of calendula, whose medically active parts are its flowers, originated in ancient Egypt. One variety is the common marigold. A natural antiseptic and anti-inflammatory agent, calendula is one of the best herbs for treating wounds, skin abrasions, and infections. Taken internally, it also alleviates indigestion as well as other gastrointestinal disorders. Calendula's healing power appears to come from components known as terpenes. One of these is recognized as a sedative and for its healing effect on ulcers.*

### TARGET AILMENTS

**Take internally for** indigestion, gastric and duodenal ulcers, gallbladder problems, irregular or painful menstruation.

**Apply externally for** cuts, wounds, sores, and burns; skin rashes from measles, chickenpox, and other eruptive skin diseases; diaper rash; athlete's foot and other fungal infections.

### PREPARATIONS

**Over the counter:** Available as lotion, ointment, oil, tincture, and fresh or dried leaves and florets.

**At home:**

Rub lotions, ointments, and oils on injuries, rashes, and infections.

Poultice: Mash up the leaves, then apply directly to minor burns or scalds.

Tea: Steep 1 oz dried herb in 1 pt boiling water. For acute internal symptoms, drink two to four times a day until symptoms lessen.

Combinations: A mixture of goldenseal, calendula, and myrrh makes an antiseptic lotion.

### SPECIAL INFORMATION

- Calendula flowers can be made into an oil for external use and to ease earaches and other infections.

## Catnip

*Nepeta cataria*

*Herbalists have used the flowers and leaves of catnip, an aromatic member of the mint family, for more than 2,000 years. Today it is prescribed for easing digestion, calming nerves, and relieving muscle spasms, including menstrual cramps. Cats are strongly attracted to catnip and may become intoxicated by eating it, but the herb has no such effect on humans.*

### TARGET AILMENTS

**Take internally for** indigestion, gas, tension, difficulty in sleeping, colds, flu, bronchial congestion, fever, colic in infants, menstrual cramps.

**Apply externally for** cuts and scrapes.

### PREPARATIONS

**Over the counter:** Catnip is available in dried bulk flowers and leaves, tincture, and tea bags.

**At home:** To treat minor cuts and scrapes, press crushed catnip leaves into them before washing and bandaging them.

Tea: Pour 1 cup boiling water onto 2 tsp dried leaves and steep for 10 to 15 minutes. Drink three times a day.

Combinations: Mix with boneset, elder, yarrow, or cayenne for colds.

### SIDE EFFECTS

**Not serious:** Catnip can produce an upset stomach. If this occurs, discontinue use and call your doctor.

### SPECIAL INFORMATION

- Avoid catnip during pregnancy.
- Infants with colic can be given weak, cool infusions. For older children and people over 65, start treatment with weak preparations and increase the strength as necessary.



CONTINUED

# The 75 Most Effective Herbs

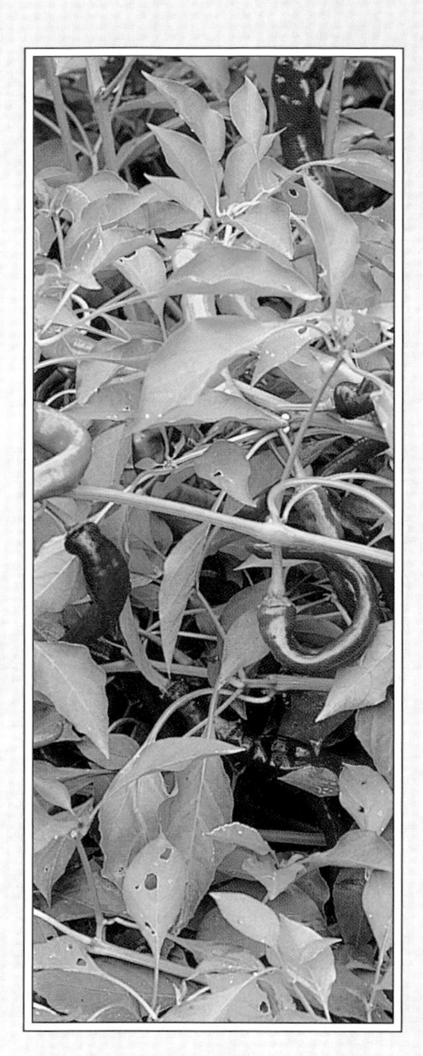

*Cayenne*

## Cayenne

*Capsicum annuum* var. *annuum*

*Regarded by herbalists as a powerful tonic, cayenne stimulates the heart and promotes blood circulation, improves digestion, and boosts energy. Like other species of hot pepper, such as tabasco, cayenne contains the natural stimulant known as capsaicin. Widely grown in Central and South America in pre-Columbian times, cayenne was carried to Spain and Europe after the early voyages of discovery.*

### TARGET AILMENTS

**Take internally for** poor circulation, indigestion, gas, physical or mental exhaustion, and lowered vitality, particularly in the elderly.

**Apply externally for** pain, including that of arthritis and diabetes, strains, sore muscles and joints, the need to stimulate blood flow or to stop external bleeding.

### PREPARATIONS

**Over the counter:** Available as powder, capsules, tincture, or oil.

**At home:**

Rub the oil on sprains, swelling, sore muscles, and joints to ease pain.

Infusion: Pour 1 cup boiling water onto ½ to 1 tsp cayenne powder and steep for 10 minutes. Mix 1 tbsp of the infusion with hot water and drink as needed.

Gargle: Combine cayenne with myrrh to treat laryngitis and to use as an antiseptic wash.

### SIDE EFFECTS

**Not serious:** In large doses, cayenne can produce vomiting, stomach pain, and a type of intoxication. Do not exceed prescribed dosages.

### SPECIAL INFORMATION

❧ Hot and spicy as a tea or tincture, cayenne can cause mild nausea at first. It's best to start with a small amount and work up gradually to the recommended dosage.

## Chamomile

*Matricaria recutita*

*Of the three types of chamomile plant, the most popular and thoroughly studied is German chamomile, used medicinally around the world for thousands of years. Modern herbalists have identified elements in the oil of the chamomile flower that appear to calm the central nervous system, relax the digestive tract, and speed healing.*

### TARGET AILMENTS

**Take internally for** stomach cramps, gas and nervous stomach, indigestion, ulcers, menstrual cramps, insomnia, colic, bladder problems. Use as a gargle for gingivitis and sore throat.

**Apply externally for** swelling and joint pain, sunburn, cuts and scrapes, teething pain, varicose veins, hemorrhoids.

### PREPARATIONS

**Over the counter:** Available as prepared tea, tincture, essential oil, and dried or fresh flowers.

**At home:**

Tea: Pour 8 oz boiling water over 2 tsp chamomile flowers and steep for 10 minutes. Drink 1 cup three or four times daily.

Fomentation: Apply three or four times daily to sore muscles; sore, swollen joints; varicose veins; and burns and skin wounds.

Herbal bath: Add no more than 2 drops essential oil of chamomile to bathwater.

### SIDE EFFECTS

None expected.

### SPECIAL INFORMATION

❧ Allergies to chamomile are rare. However, anyone allergic to other plants in the daisy family should be alert to possible allergic reactions to chamomile.

## Chaste Tree

*Vitex agnus-castus*

*Since ancient times, herbalists have used the berries of the chaste tree to manipulate the functioning of the female reproductive system. Chaste tree's natural compounds seem to aid in regulating the menstrual cycle by bringing into balance the female sex hormones, estrogen and progesterone. In addition to menstrual irregularities, chaste tree is prescribed for premenstrual syndrome and menopausal symptoms. It also aids in readjusting the body after withdrawal from long-term use of birth-control pills, in preventing miscarriage in the first three months of pregnancy, and in promoting lactation. Used by Roman matrons and medieval monks to dampen sexual ardor, chaste tree has also, paradoxically, had a reputation as an aphrodisiac.*

### TARGET AILMENTS

**Take internally for** PMS, menstrual irregularities, symptoms of menopause, prevention of miscarriage, promotion of lactation, hormone-related constipation, endometriosis, fibroid cysts in smooth muscle tissue, teenage acne.

### PREPARATIONS

**Over the counter:** Chaste tree is available as berries, powder, dried herb, capsules, and tincture.

**At home:**

Tea: Pour 1 cup boiling water onto 1 tsp ripe berries; infuse for 10 to 15 minutes. Drink three times a day.

### SPECIAL INFORMATION

- Chaste tree seems to regulate hormonal imbalances within 10 days, and relief from PMS may be noticeable by the second menstrual cycle. For optimal benefit, however, the herb should be taken for six months or longer.
- Discontinue the herb after the third month of pregnancy, since it may cause premature milk production.

## Chinese Foxglove Root

*Rehmannia glutinosa*

*The thick reddish yellow Chinese foxglove root is cooked in wine and used as a tonic. The cooked form of the root is also often used in Chinese medicine for treating disorders that are associated with aging.*

### TARGET AILMENTS

**Take internally for** lightheadedness, palpitations, blurred vision, or floaters in vision; insomnia; chronic low-grade fever and night sweats; constipation with dry, hard stools; irregular menstruation or uterine bleeding, especially after childbirth; low back pain and weak knees; weak, stiff joints; hearing loss and tinnitus; premature graying of hair.

### PREPARATIONS

The prepared root and the raw version are available from Chinese pharmacies, Asian markets, and some Western health food stores. Ask for the cooked version, which is made by soaking the root in rice wine with spices such as cardamom.

Combinations: A mixture with gelatin is prescribed for coughing and vomiting blood, nosebleeds, and uterine bleeding. The cooked root is also combined with cornus and Chinese yam to treat lightheadedness, insomnia, forgetfulness, and related symptoms. See a Chinese medicine practitioner for dosages and further herbal combinations.

### SPECIAL INFORMATION

WARNING: Those with digestive problems should use this herb carefully; the cooked herb can distend the abdomen and cause loose stools.

- Grains-of-paradise fruit is often added to preparations of Chinese foxglove root to prevent side effects such as diarrhea, nausea, and abdominal pain.

## Chinese Yam

*Dioscorea opposita*

*Chinese yam, a thick, firm root with a white cross section, is used as a tonic. Classified as neutral and sweet in traditional Chinese medicine, the herb is harvested in the winter in the mountains of Hunan and in many other Chinese provinces.*

### TARGET AILMENTS

**Take internally for** weak digestion with diarrhea and fatigue, reduced appetite, frequent urination, excessive vaginal discharge, chronic coughing and wheezing, symptoms that accompany diabetes.

### PREPARATIONS

Chinese yam is available as a fresh or dried vegetable in Chinese pharmacies, Asian food markets, and some Western health food stores. For symptoms of diabetes, slices of the fresh root are steeped in hot water to make an infusion.

Combinations: A mixture of Chinese yam, poria, and atractylodes (white) may be prescribed for loose, watery stools. Chinese yam and codonopsis root make up a preparation used to treat fatigue, general weakness, and poor appetite. Consult a Chinese medicine practitioner for information on proper dosages and other herbal combinations.

### SIDE EFFECTS

None expected.

### SPECIAL INFORMATION

- If symptoms include abdominal swelling and pain, do not use Chinese yam.

### POSSIBLE INTERACTIONS

Do not take Chinese yam with kan-sui root.



CONTINUED

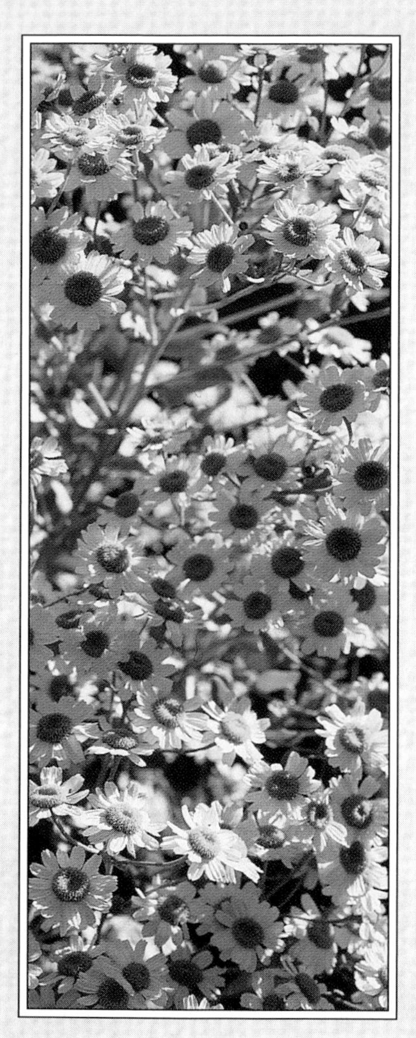

*Chamomile*

## Cinnamon Bark

*Cinnamomum cassia*

*A popular stimulant in Chinese medicine, cinnamon is usually harvested from trees after they are seven years old. Its outer bark is the common spice; the inner bark contains more oil and has stronger medicinal effects. Cinnamon bark is used to treat abdominal disorders, menstrual pain, infertility, and some forms of asthma.*

### TARGET AILMENTS

**Take internally for** lack of appetite, diarrhea, abdominal discomfort; excessive urination, impotence, and lack of sexual desire; menstrual problems and infertility; wheezing from exposure to cold.

### PREPARATIONS

Cinnamon bark is available fresh or dried at Asian food markets and pharmacies and some Western health food stores. It is normally taken in the form of powder, pill, or tincture (crushed bark mixed with alcohol).

Combinations: Used with the roots of Asian ginseng and of Chinese foxglove cooked in wine to treat palpitations of the heart and shortness of breath. Check with a Chinese medicine practitioner on dosages and other combinations.

### SIDE EFFECTS

**Serious:** Large doses can cause changes in breathing, dilation of blood vessels, and convulsions.

### SPECIAL INFORMATION

WARNING: Use this herb cautiously if you are pregnant.

WARNING: Do not use the herb when there is fever, inflammation, or hemorrhaging.

❧ In a clinical trial, an alcohol-based preparation of the bark, injected at an acupuncture point associated with the lung, seemed to help bronchial asthma.

## Coltsfoot

*Tussilago farfara*

*Coltsfoot has a long history as a cough suppressant and is still used today for that purpose and as a gentle expectorant. It is banned in Canada, but in the United States the FDA classifies it as an herb with "undefined safety." It contains an alkaloid that can seriously damage the liver, and a Japanese study found that the flower buds may be carcinogenic. Many practitioners, however, still routinely use coltsfoot on a short-term basis to treat respiratory ailments.*

### TARGET AILMENTS

**Take internally for** coughs, asthma, and emphysema.

**Apply externally for** burns, skin ulcers, inflammations, and insect bites.

### PREPARATIONS

**Over the counter:** Available in tincture, in capsules, and in bulk.

**At home:**

Tea: Pour 1 cup boiling water onto 1 to 3 tsp dried flowers or leaves and steep for 10 minutes. Drink three times a day, as hot as possible.

Compress: Soak a pad in a coltsfoot infusion for several minutes, wring out, then apply to the affected area.

Combinations: For coughs, take it with white horehound and mullein; for bronchitis, with garlic or echinacea.

### SIDE EFFECTS

**Serious:** Fever, nausea, loss of appetite, diarrhea, jaundice, or abdominal pain may result. Stop taking it and call your doctor now.

### SPECIAL INFORMATION

WARNING: Use only as prescribed by a practitioner, for short periods of time. Do not give coltsfoot to children under two, pregnant or nursing women, alcoholics, or anyone with liver disease.

## Dandelion

Taraxacum officinale

*Dandelion has a long history of medicinal use. It acts as a natural diuretic while also supplying potassium, a nutrient that is often lost through diuretic use. The plant is rich in vitamins A and C—antioxidants that are believed to help prevent cancer. The young leaves can be eaten fresh or used in herbal preparations.*

### TARGET AILMENTS

**Take internally for** poor digestion, gallbladder problems, inflammation of the liver. As a supplemental diuretic, dandelion may help relieve symptoms associated with high blood pressure, congestive heart failure, premenstrual syndrome, menstrual pain, and joint pain.

### PREPARATIONS

**Over the counter:** Available in tincture, prepared tea, capsule, and dried or fresh leaves or roots.

**At home:**

Tea: Steep 1 tbsp dried or 2 tbsp fresh leaves for each cup of boiling water for 10 minutes. Drink up to 4 cups a day.

Decoction: Simmer 1 tbsp fresh or dried root per cup of water for 15 minutes. Drink up to 4 cups a day.

Nutrition: Add fresh leaves to a salad.

### SIDE EFFECTS

**Not serious:** Allergic dermatitis, stomach upset, diarrhea, flulike symptoms, liver pain. Discontinue use and call your doctor when convenient.

### SPECIAL INFORMATION

- Consult an herbalist if you plan to use the herb longer than two or three months, or if you are pregnant, have a heart condition, or suffer from stomach discomfort.
- Use low doses for adults over 65 and children between two and 12. Do not give to children under two.

## Dong Quai

Angelica sinensis

*Also known as Chinese angelica root, dong quai is used by Chinese herbalists as a treatment for several gynecological complaints. Look for a long, moist, oily plant as the source of the root, which has brown bark and a white cross section. The herb is characterized in traditional Chinese medicine as sweet, acrid, bitter, and warm.*

### TARGET AILMENTS

**Take internally for** menstrual problems; poor blood circulation, pale complexion, possible anemia; abscesses, sores; lightheadedness, blurred vision, heart palpitations.

### PREPARATIONS

This root is available in bulk and in tablet form at health food stores and Asian markets and pharmacies. You should avoid the herb if it is dry or has a greenish brown cross section.

Combinations: Mixed with astragalus, it provides a tonic for treating fatigue. Blend it with white peony root, Chinese foxglove root cooked in wine, and cnidium root for menstrual irregularities. Dong quai is also combined with honeysuckle flowers and red peony root to form a preparation that reduces swelling and alleviates pain from abscesses and sores. Consult a Chinese practitioner for further information.

### SIDE EFFECTS

None expected if used as directed.

### SPECIAL INFORMATION

- You should not take dong quai during the early stages of pregnancy.
- Check with your Chinese medicine practitioner on the use of this herb if you have diarrhea or bloating.
- Modern acupuncturists sometimes inject the herb into acupuncture points to treat pain, especially that from neuralgia and arthritis.

## Echinacea

Echinacea spp.

*Echinacea was frequently used by Native Americans of the southwest plains in poultices, mouthwashes, and teas. Now a popular garden perennial, the plant displays purple blossoms and grows as high as five feet. Herbalists value the dried root of echinacea for its broad-based action against many types of viral and bacterial illnesses, such as colds, bronchitis, ear infections, influenza, and cystitis. Laboratory tests show that echinacea may have antibiotic effects. It seems to bolster the immune system's white blood cells in their battle against foreign microorganisms. It can also be effective as a topical medicine for eczema and other skin problems.*

### TARGET AILMENTS

**Take internally for** colds, flu, and other respiratory illnesses; mononucleosis; ear infections; blood poisoning; bladder infections.

**Apply externally for** boils, burns, abscesses, wounds, stings, hives, insect bites, eczema, and herpes.

### PREPARATIONS

**Over the counter:** Available in tea, capsule, tincture, and dried bulk form.

**At home:**

Tea: Boil 2 tsp dried root in 1 cup water and simmer for 15 minutes. Drink three times daily.

Combinations: Use echinacea with yarrow or uva ursi to treat cystitis.

### SIDE EFFECTS

None expected.

### SPECIAL INFORMATION

- Do not use echinacea continuously for more than a few weeks.
- Do not give to children younger than two; start with minimal doses for older children and older adults.
- Check with your doctor before using if you are pregnant or nursing.



CONTINUED

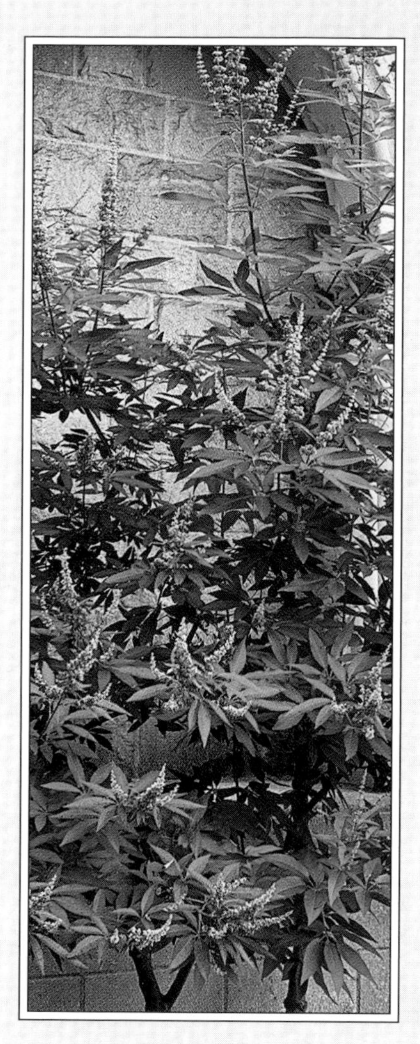

Chaste Tree

## Ephedra

*Ephedra sinica*

*Known in China as ma huang, ephedra has long been used there by healers. Its root and other parts have been used in the West as a decongestant and remedy for asthma, hay fever, and colds. Its active ingredients are central nervous system stimulants that open bronchial passages, activating the heart, increasing blood pressure, and speeding up metabolism. For this reason, herbalists warn against excessive use of the herb.*

### TARGET AILMENTS

**Take internally for** fever, respiratory ailments, hay fever, stomachache.

### PREPARATIONS

**Over the counter:** Available as fluidextract, tablets, dried bulk herb.

**At home:**

Chinese: Combine 1 part honey with 4 parts dried herb in a small amount of water. Simmer until water is gone and herbs are slightly brown.

Combinations: For fever and chills, mix with cinnamon twig; for coughing and asthma,with apricot seed; for indigestion, with licorice.

Western: Boil 1 tsp of the herb with 1 cup water for 15 to 20 minutes. Drink up to 2 cups of the tea a day.

### SIDE EFFECTS

**Serious:** Increased blood pressure or heart rate, heart palpitations. If any of these symptoms develop, discontinue use and consult your physician immediately.

### SPECIAL INFORMATION

WARNING: Because it can cause side effects—and rarely, death—consult a practitioner before taking, especially if you are on any medication. It may not be safe as a weight-loss aid.

WARNING: Do not use if you are pregnant or have heart disease, diabetes, glaucoma, or hyperthyroidism.

❧ Use mild doses for children or seniors. Do not treat children under two.

## Eyebright

*Euphrasia officinalis*

*Eyebright is an herb whose name suggests both its action and its appearance. The red spots on its white or purple flowers seem to resemble bloodshot eyes. Moreover, its dried stems, leaves, and flowers have long been used as a tonic for irritated or infected eyes. Eyebright can be applied to eyes that are itching, red, and tearing from hay fever, other allergies, or colds; it can also alleviate the symptoms of conjunctivitis. Drinking eyebright tea may help to maintain good vision and to diminish nasal congestion and coughs.*

### TARGET AILMENTS

**Apply externally for** eye irritations from allergies, colds, conjunctivitis.

**Take internally for** nasal congestion and coughs from colds, sinusitis, or allergies.

### PREPARATIONS

**Over the counter:** Available in bulk, capsules, and tincture.

**At home:**

Tea: Pour 1 cup boiling water onto 2 tsp dried eyebright and steep for 10 minutes; drink three times daily.

Compress: Boil 1 to 2 tbsp dried eyebright in 1 pt water for 10 minutes. After the water has cooled, strain it, dip a sterile cloth in it and wring it out, then put it on your eyes for 15 minutes a few times a day.

Combinations to be taken orally: For congestion, combine it with goldenrod, elder flowers, or goldenseal. For hay fever, mix it with ephedra. Consult an herbalist for dosages.

### SIDE EFFECTS

**Not serious:** Eyebright may cause a skin rash or nausea. If this occurs, lessen your dose or stop taking completely.

### SPECIAL INFORMATION

❧ Consult a practitioner before using eyebright to treat children.

## Feverfew

*Tanacetum parthenium*
(or *Chrysanthemum parthenium*)

*Feverfew is a perennial with small-blossoms that resemble daisies. In the late 1970s British researchers found feverfew leaves helpful in treating migraine headaches where other treatments had failed. They believe this relief is due to the chemical parthenolide, which blocks the release of inflammatory substances from the blood. The researchers consider these inflammatory elements to be key components in the onset of a migraine.*

**TARGET AILMENTS**

**Take internally for** migraines.

**PREPARATIONS**

**Over the counter:** Available in dry bulk, pills, capsules, and tinctures.

**At home:** Chew two fresh or frozen leaves a day for migraines. If you find the leaves too bitter, substitute capsules or pills containing 85 mg of the leaf material, but fresh leaves are best for immediate results.

Tea: Steep 2 tsp dried herb in 1 cup boiling water for 5 to 10 minutes; drink 2 to 3 cups per day.

**SIDE EFFECTS**

**Serious:** Chewing fresh or dried feverfew may cause internal mouth sores or abdominal pain. If these symptoms develop, discontinue use and notify your doctor.

**SPECIAL INFORMATION**

- Do not take if you are pregnant.
- Feverfew may interfere with the blood's clotting ability; talk to your doctor before using if you have a clotting disorder or take anticoagulant medicine.
- You may need to take feverfew daily for two to three months before it has any effect.

## Ganoderma

*Ganoderma lucidum*

*A variety of mushroom also known as ling zhi in China and as reishi in the West, ganoderma grows in mountainous regions in China. It is a rare fungus that Chinese practitioners value highly for its multiple uses. Practitioners have traditionally used it to treat psychological disturbances as well as respiratory complaints and ulcers. Ganoderma has also been prescribed to boost patients' immune systems.*

**TARGET AILMENTS**

**Take internally for** nervousness, insomnia, dizziness; asthma, allergy-related chronic bronchitis; weakened immune system; tumors; ulcers; poor blood circulation; mushroom poisoning.

**PREPARATIONS**

Ganoderma can be found in bulk at some health food stores (under the name *reishi*) and at Asian pharmacies and markets. It is also possible to obtain it in pill or tablet form, and in alcohol extracts. Consult a Chinese medicine practitioner for information on appropriate dosages. Unlike most other Chinese herbs, ganoderma is not traditionally combined with other substances.

**SIDE EFFECTS**

**Not serious:** Patients may experience dizziness, sore bones, itchy skin, increased bowel movements, hard stools, and pimplelike eruptions when they use ganoderma. Discontinue use of the herb if these symptoms develop.

**SPECIAL INFORMATION**

- The herb may be useful in conjunction with conventional medical treatment of AIDS and cancer.
- In clinical studies, ganoderma seems to have reduced blood pressure in humans and animals.

## Garlic

*Allium sativum*

*The garlic bulb has long been recognized as a medicinal remedy in Chinese and Western cultures. Garlic's active ingredient is allicin, which is also responsible for the herb's pungent smell. In China this herb is prescribed for colds and coughs and for intestinal and digestive disorders. Chinese herbalists believe garlic can be used externally as an antibiotic and antifungal treatment for skin infections. Western herbalists prescribe it for many of the same ailments as their Chinese counterparts. It is also used to reduce cholesterol and to lower blood pressure.*

**TARGET AILMENTS**

**Take internally for** colds, coughs, flu, high cholesterol, high blood pressure, atherosclerosis, digestive disorders, bladder infection, liver and gallbladder problems.

**Apply externally for** athlete's foot, ringworm, minor skin infections.

**PREPARATIONS**

**Over the counter:** Garlic is available as cloves and in tablet form.

**At home:**

Tincture: Combine 1 cup crushed cloves with 1 qt brandy. Shake daily for two weeks. Take up to 3 tbsp a day.

**SIDE EFFECTS**

**Not serious:** Allergic rash from touching or eating the herb.

**SPECIAL INFORMATION**

- Consult your practitioner before using garlic if you are pregnant.
- Garlic has a blood clot-preventing agent. If you have a blood-clotting disorder, consult an herbalist or a licensed healthcare professional.
- Garlic is thought to function as an adjunct treatment for cardiovascular disease. Consult your practitioner before using it in this capacity.



CONTINUED

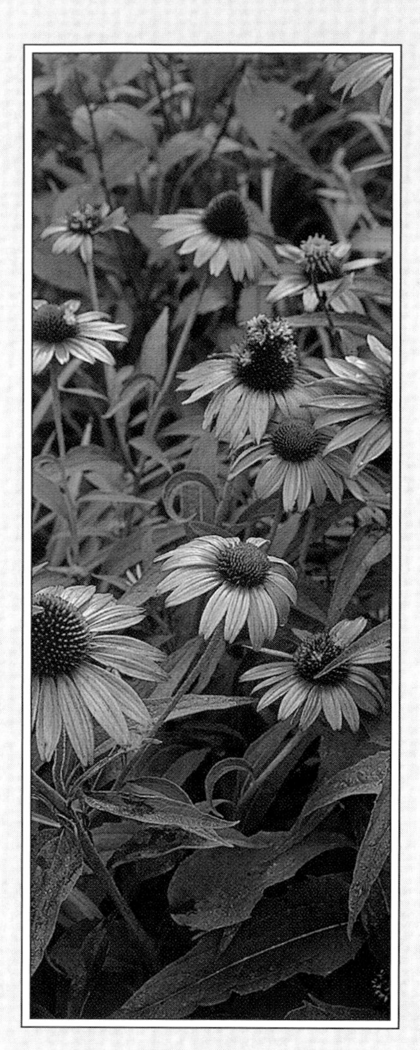

**Echinacea**

## Gentiana

*Gentiana scabra*

*Several varieties of this herb grow throughout China. Gentiana scabra, the most widely used, is a long, thick, yellow root, described as cold by Chinese herbalists. They prescribe the herb primarily for disorders of the liver and organs in the pelvic area. Gentiana tastes so bitter that Chinese herbalists use it as a standard for judging bitterness in plants.*

### TARGET AILMENTS

**Take internally for** hepatitis, jaundice, and other liver disorders; sexually transmitted diseases, vaginal discharge, inflammation of the pelvis, pain or swelling in the genital area; convulsions.

### PREPARATIONS

You can find gentiana in bulk at some health food stores and Asian pharmacies and markets. While the Chinese variety is not available in pills or tablets, the European root can be obtained in that form.

Combinations: Chinese herbalists prescribe a preparation that contains gentiana, sophora root, and plantago seeds for genital itching and vaginal discharge. A combination of gentiana with cattle gallstone and gambir is given for convulsions, especially when the symptoms appear in children. Check with your practitioner for advice on other combinations and dosages.

### SIDE EFFECTS

None expected.

### SPECIAL INFORMATION

WARNING: Chinese herbalists advise against the use of this root when diarrhea is among the symptoms.

- Gentiana is believed to have an antibiotic effect; it is also thought to be toxic to malarial parasites.

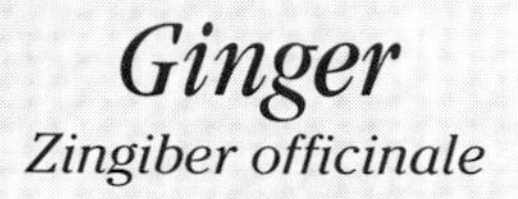

## Ginger

*Zingiber officinale*

*Ginger not only is a valued culinary seasoning but also is considered a remedy for a range of ailments. Both Chinese and Western herbalists believe it relieves motion sickness and dizziness and improves digestion. Ginger is also said to alleviate menstrual cramps. Its active constituents, gingerols, soothe the abdomen and relieve excess gas. In China, ginger, called gan-jian, is applied to first- and second-degree burns.*

### TARGET AILMENTS

Chinese: vomiting, abdominal pain, menstrual irregularity (take internally); minor burns (apply externally).

Western: motion sickness, digestive disorders, menstrual cramps, colds, flu, arthritis, high cholesterol, high blood pressure (take internally).

### PREPARATIONS

**Over the counter:** Available as fresh or dried root, liquid extract, tablets, capsules, prepared tea.

**At home:**

Chinese: Wrap fresh roots in five or six layers of rice paper. Bury under warm coals until the paper is blackened. Discard paper before use.

Rub: Treat minor burns by rubbing fresh ginger juice on the wound.

Combinations: For vomiting, ginger is mixed with pinellia root; when there is also severe abdominal pain, the herb is combined with licorice or galanga. A preparation of ginger and chamomile is used to treat menstrual irregularity.

Western: Boil 1 oz dried root in 1 cup water for 15 to 20 minutes for tea.

### SIDE EFFECTS

**Not serious:** Heartburn.

### SPECIAL INFORMATION

- Ginger may help prevent heart disease and strokes.
- If you are pregnant, consult your doctor before using.

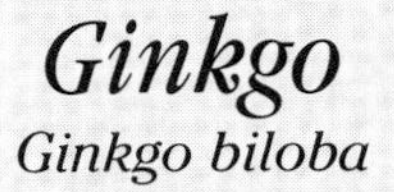

# The 75 Most Effective Herbs

## Ginkgo

*Ginkgo biloba*

*Chinese herbalists have used the fan-shaped leaves of the ginkgo tree for thousands of years to treat asthma, chilblains, and swelling. Western herbalists value it for its action against vascular diseases. It dilates blood vessels and thereby improves blood flow, especially to areas such as the lower legs and feet, as well as to the brain. Herbalists believe ginkgo can keep blood clots from forming and bronchial tubes from constricting during an asthma attack. It may also help reduce damage from macular degeneration.*

### TARGET AILMENTS

**Take internally for** vertigo; tinnitus; phlebitis; leg ulcers; cerebral atherosclerosis; diabetic vascular disease; Raynaud's syndrome; headache; depression; lack of concentration or mental and emotional fatigue in the elderly; asthma; clotting disorders, including stroke and heart attack.

### PREPARATIONS

Leaves are available in dry bulk, capsules, or tincture. You can find ginkgo biloba extract (GBE) in health food stores. Most herbalists recommend using only over-the-counter ginkgo products.

### SIDE EFFECTS

**Not serious:** Irritability, restlessness, diarrhea, nausea; check with your doctor to see if you should lower your dose or stop taking it completely.

### SPECIAL INFORMATION

WARNING: Some people cannot tolerate ginkgo even in small doses.

- Do not use if you have a bleeding disorder like hemophilia or are pregnant or nursing.
- Do not give ginkgo to children without a doctor's supervision.
- Consult a healthcare professional before using it in medicinal amounts.

## Ginseng, American

*Panax quinquefolius*

*Native Americans believed American ginseng could alleviate painful childbirths and restore energy in the elderly. American ginseng is identified by a single stalk crowned by delicate chartreuse blooms and crimson berries; its leaflets have sawlike teeth. The active ingredients of American ginseng are panaxosides, which are thought to calm the stomach and the brain and act as a mild stimulant to vital organs. American ginseng is milder than Asian ginseng and is often prescribed for people who consider Asian ginseng too potent. Both American and Asian ginseng are frequently used to treat the elderly.*

### TARGET AILMENTS

**Take internally for** depression, fatigue, stress, colds, influenza, respiratory problems, inflammation, a damaged immune system.

### PREPARATIONS

**Over the counter:** Ginseng is available as fresh or dried root, root powder, capsules, tablets, prepared tea, freeze-dried root, cured rock candy.

**At home:**

Decoction: Boil 1 oz fresh root with 1 cup water for 15 to 20 minutes. Drink up to 2 cups a day.

### SIDE EFFECTS

**Not serious:** Headache, insomnia, anxiety, breast soreness, skin rash.

**Serious:** You may experience asthma attacks, increased blood pressure, heart palpitations, or postmenopausal uterine bleeding. Discontinue use of ginseng and consult your doctor.

### SPECIAL INFORMATION

- American ginseng is considered an endangered species because of excessive harvesting.

## Ginseng, Asian

*Panax ginseng*

*Growing on the mountains of northeast China, Asian ginseng is the most potent and expensive form of ginseng. With its yellow-green flowers and red berries, it looks like American ginseng, but the stalk is longer. Its active constituents are ginsenosides, substances that strengthen the immune system and increase the body's ability to deal with fatigue and stress. Herbalists prescribe Asian ginseng root for fever, colds, coughs, and menstrual irregularities.*

### TARGET AILMENTS

**Take internally for** depression, fatigue, stress, colds, flu, respiratory problems, inflammation, a damaged immune system.

### PREPARATIONS

**Over the counter:** Ginseng is available as fresh or dried root, root powder, capsules, tablets, prepared tea, freeze-dried root, cured rock candy.

**At home:**

Decoction: Boil 1 oz fresh root with 1 cup water for 15 to 20 minutes. Drink up to 2 cups a day.

### SIDE EFFECTS

**Not serious:** Headache, insomnia, anxiety, breast soreness, or skin rash.

**Serious:** Asthma attacks, increased blood pressure, heart palpitations, or postmenopausal uterine bleeding. Stop using ginseng and consult your doctor.

### SPECIAL INFORMATION

- Use only under the direction of an herbalist or a healthcare professional if you are pregnant or have insomnia, hay fever, fibrocystic breasts, asthma, emphysema, high blood pressure, blood-clotting or heart disorders, or diabetes.



CONTINUED

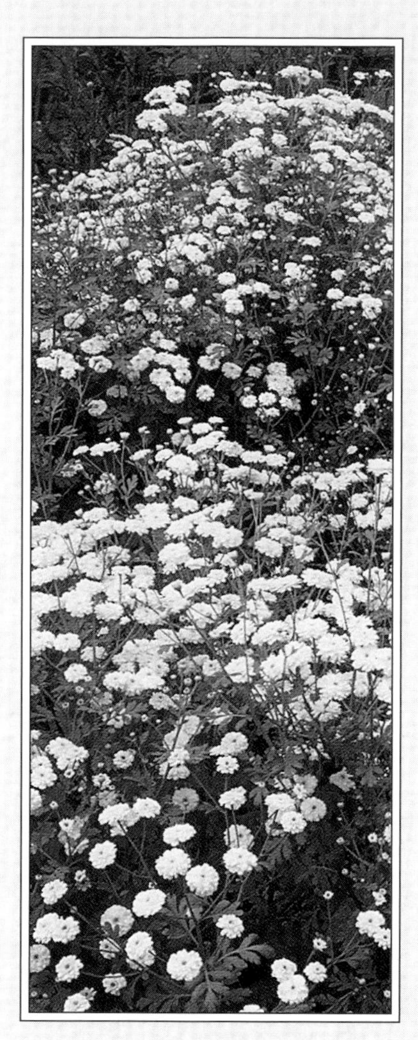

*Feverfew*

## Ginseng, Siberian

*Eleutherococcus senticosus*

*Found in the Siberian regions of Russia and China, Siberian ginseng, also called eleuthero, affects the body in a manner similar to Asian and American ginseng, although its effects are subtler and result in less-pronounced reactions. The active elements of Siberian ginseng are eleutherosides, which stimulate the immune system, increasing the body's resistance to disease, stress, and fatigue. Siberian ginseng has gained popularity as a Western herb because it does not cause the insomnia and anxiety that sometimes occur when Asian or American ginseng is used.*

### TARGET AILMENTS

**Take internally for** depression, fatigue, stress; colds, influenza, respiratory problems; inflammation, damaged immune system.

### PREPARATIONS

**Over the counter:** Ginseng is available as fresh or dried root, root powder, capsules, tablets, prepared tea, freeze-dried root, cured rock candy.

**At home:**

Decoction: Boil 1 oz fresh root with 1 cup water for 15 to 20 minutes. Drink up to 2 cups a day.

### SIDE EFFECTS

**Not serious:** Headaches, insomnia, anxiety, breast soreness, skin rashes.

**Serious:** Asthma attacks, increased blood pressure, heart palpitations, postmenopausal uterine bleeding.

### SPECIAL INFORMATION

- Siberian ginseng gained popularity in Russia when an extract was mass-produced and used in a popular colalike drink called Bodust, meaning "vigor."

## Goldenseal

*Hydrastis canadensis*

*Herbalists use the dried and powdered rhizomes and roots of the perennial goldenseal to treat several respiratory and skin infections. The herb acts as a stimulant and seems to affect the body's mucous membranes by drying up secretions, reducing inflammation, and fighting infection. Goldenseal also aids digestion and may control postpartum bleeding.*

### TARGET AILMENTS

**Take internally for** stomach problems; sore throat; infected gums, ears, and sinuses; postpartum bleeding.

**Apply externally for** eczema, ringworm, contact dermatitis, athlete's foot, impetigo.

### PREPARATIONS

**Over the counter:** Dry root is available in bulk, capsules, and tincture.

**At home:**

Tea: Pour 1 cup boiling water onto 2 tsp goldenseal; steep for 10 to 15 minutes. Drink three times daily.

Combinations: Use with meadowsweet and chamomile for stomach problems. For a skin wash, mix with distilled witch hazel; for ear infections, make drops using goldenseal and mullein. See your herbalist for exact instructions.

### SIDE EFFECTS

**Not serious:** In high doses, it can irritate the skin, mouth, and throat and cause nausea and diarrhea. If any of these develop, stop taking it.

### SPECIAL INFORMATION

- Do not take if you are pregnant.
- Do not use goldenseal without consulting a physician if you have had heart disease, diabetes, glaucoma, a stroke, or high blood pressure.
- Do not give goldenseal to children under two; for older children and older adults, start with small doses.

## Gotu Kola

*Centella asiatica*

*The gotu kola plant grows in marshy areas in many parts of the world. Its fan-shaped leaves contain the soothing agent known as asiaticoside. As a result they have been used to treat burns, skin grafts, and episiotomies. Gotu kola may also help heal outbreaks of psoriasis and may help decrease edema and promote blood circulation in the legs. It may therefore be useful in treating phlebitis.*

### TARGET AILMENTS

**Take internally for** poor circulation in the legs, edema.

**Apply externally for** burns, cuts, and other skin injuries; psoriasis. (Use a compress.)

### PREPARATIONS

**Over the counter:** Available in dry bulk, capsules, and tincture.

**At home:**

Tea: Use 1 to 2 tsp dried gotu kola per cup of boiling water; drink twice daily to improve circulation.

Compress: Soak a pad in a tea or in a tincture to help treat wounds or psoriasis. Start with a weak solution and increase the concentration of gotu kola if necessary.

### SIDE EFFECTS

**Not serious:** Gotu kola may cause a skin rash or headaches; in either case, lower your dosage or stop taking it.

### SPECIAL INFORMATION

- Do not use gotu kola if you are pregnant or nursing, or using tranquilizers or sedatives, since gotu kola may have a narcotic effect.
- Do not give gotu kola to children under two. For older children and older adults, start with low-strength doses and increase if necessary.

## Hawthorn

*Crataegus laevigata* (or *C. oxyacantha*)

*Herbalists use the flowers, fruit, and leaves of the hawthorn, a European shrub with thorny branches. They prescribe the herb as a mild heart tonic. It is thought to dilate the blood vessels, thereby facilitating the flow of blood in the arteries and lowering blood pressure. Hawthorn is also believed to increase the pumping force of the heart muscle and to eliminate arrhythmias. It may have a calming effect on the nervous system and is sometimes recommended as a remedy for insomnia.*

### TARGET AILMENTS

**Take internally** in conjunction with conventional medical treatment for high blood pressure, clogged arteries, heart palpitations, angina, inflammation of the heart muscle.

**Take internally for** insomnia and nervous conditions. Use as a gargle for sore throat.

### PREPARATIONS

Hawthorn is available as fluidextract, dried berries and leaves, capsules.

### SIDE EFFECTS

**Serious:** Taking large amounts of hawthorn may result in a dramatic drop in blood pressure, which in turn may cause you to feel faint.

### SPECIAL INFORMATION

WARNING: Use hawthorn as a heart tonic only if you have been diagnosed with angina, cardiac arrhythmias, or congestive heart failure, and only in consultation with a physician. Do not practice self-diagnosis.

- Children and pregnant or nursing women should use hawthorn only under the direction of a medical herbalist or a licensed healthcare professional.

## Horsetail

*Equisetum arvense*

*Horsetail has been valued since ancient times for its ability to stem the flow of blood, bind tissues, and increase urine production. It is rich in silica, which helps mend broken bones and form collagen, a constituent of bones and tissue. Herbalists today prescribe horsetail for wounds, urinary problems, benign prostate disorders, and the pain of rheumatism or arthritis.*

### TARGET AILMENTS

**Take internally for** bladder and kidney problems, prostatitis, ulcers; broken bones or sprains; strengthening bones and nails; joint pain.

**Apply externally for** sores and inflammation.

### PREPARATIONS

**Over the counter:** Available dried or fresh, in capsules, and in tincture.

**At home:**

Tea: Steep 2 tsp dried or 1 tbsp fresh herb per cup of boiling water for 15 minutes. Drink cold, up to 4 cups a day, 2 tbsp at a time. Apply to cuts.

Combinations: Use with hydrangea for prostate problems.

### SIDE EFFECTS

**Not serious:** Upset stomach, diarrhea, increased urination. Discontinue and call your doctor.

**Serious:** Kidney or lower back pain, or pain on urination; cardiac problems. Call your doctor now.

### SPECIAL INFORMATION

WARNING: Do not take for more than three days in a row, and follow the given dosage; extended use may cause kidney or cardiac damage.

- Use only under a doctor's care. Heart disease or high-blood-pressure patients should use with caution.
- Use mild doses for adults over 65 and children ages two to 12. Children under two and pregnant women should not use horsetail.



CONTINUED

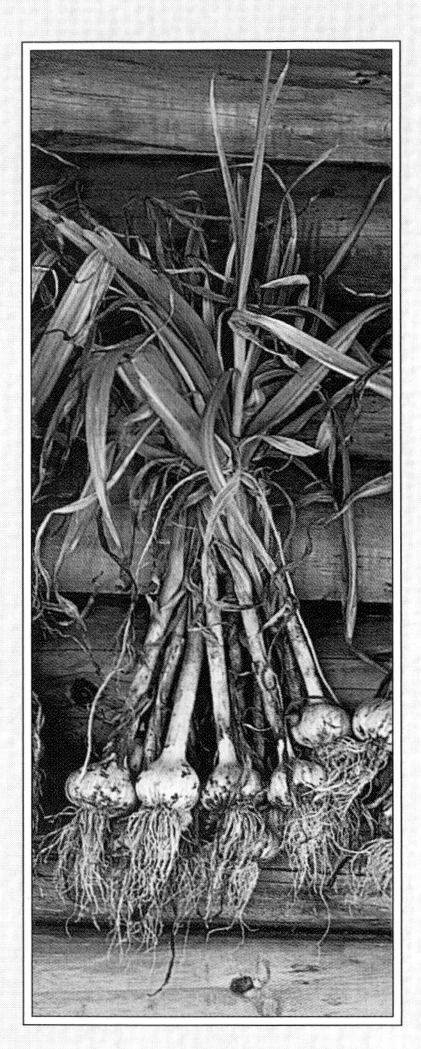

Garlic

# Hyssop

*Hyssopus officinalis*

*Hyssop, a member of the mint family, is used as an expectorant, digestive aid, sedative, and muscle relaxant. It is also used as an antiseptic; its oils may heal wounds and herpes simplex sores.*

### TARGET AILMENTS

**Take internally for** coughs, colds, bronchitis; indigestion, gas; anxiety, hysteria; petit mal seizures.

**Apply externally for** cold sores, genital herpes sores, burns, wounds, skin irritations.

### PREPARATIONS

**Over the counter:** Available dried or fresh and as tincture.

**At home:**

Tea: Steep 2 tsp dried herb per cup of boiling water for 10 to 15 minutes. Drink three times a day for cough; gargle three times a day for sore throat. Apply to burns and wounds.

Compress: Steep 1 oz dried herb in 1 pt boiling water for 15 minutes; soak clean cloth in solution and apply warm to cold sores or genital herpes sores; place on the chest to relieve congestion.

Combinations: Used with white horehound and coltsfoot for coughs and bronchitis; with boneset, elder flower, and peppermint for cold symptoms; and with sage as a gargle for sore throats.

### SIDE EFFECTS

**Not serious:** Upset stomach or diarrhea. Discontinue and call a doctor.

### SPECIAL INFORMATION

- Use hyssop only under medical supervision if you use it for more than three consecutive days.
- Do not use hyssop if pregnant; it was once used to induce abortion.
- Use low-strength preparations for adults over 65 or children between two and 12 years of age. Do not give to children under two years old.

# Juniper

*Juniperus communis*

*Juniper acts as a diuretic and thus is used to treat high blood pressure and PMS. Juniper oil is thought to have anti-inflammatory effects useful for treating arthritis and gout. Juniper teas can be taken for digestive problems.*

### TARGET AILMENTS

**Take internally for** bladder infections, cystitis, edema; digestive problems; menstrual irregularities and PMS; high blood pressure.

**Apply externally for** arthritis, gout.

### PREPARATIONS

**Over the counter:** Available in whole berries, bulk, and capsules, and as tincture.

**At home:**

Tea: Steep 1 tsp ground juniper berries in 1 cup boiling water for 10 to 20 minutes. Drink at least two times daily. Do not use for more than six weeks at a time.

### SIDE EFFECTS

**Not serious:** Individuals with hay fever may develop allergy symptoms such as nasal congestion when taking juniper. If this happens, stop taking the herb and call your doctor.

**Serious:** Juniper in high doses can irritate and damage the kidneys and urinary tract. If you develop diarrhea, intestinal pain, kidney pain, blood in the urine, purplish urine, or a faster heartbeat, stop taking juniper immediately and see your doctor as soon as possible.

### SPECIAL INFORMATION

WARNING: Because it can irritate the kidneys and urinary tract, juniper is suitable for short-term use only.

WARNING: Do not use juniper if you have or have had kidney problems.

- Pregnant women should not use juniper, because it may stimulate contraction of the uterus.

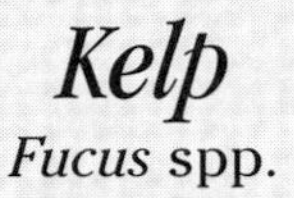

## Kelp

*Fucus* spp.

*Extracts of iodine-rich kelp, one of the many forms of seaweed, provided an effective goiter remedy for many years. Today some herbalists rely on another component of kelp's stemlike and leaflike parts, an agent known as sodium alginate. Because of its action, kelp is prescribed to aid in the treatment of heavy-metal environmental pollutants, including barium and cadmium, and to prevent the body from absorbing strontium 90, a radioactive substance created in nuclear power plants.*

*Some practitioners of alternative medicine also recommend taking kelp supplements for thyroid disorders such as mild hypothyroidism (underactive thyroid).*

### TARGET AILMENTS

**Take internally for** goiter, hypothyroidism, radiation exposure, heavy-metal environmental pollutants.

### PREPARATIONS

**Over the counter:** Available in dry bulk, capsules, and tincture.

**At home:**

Infusion: Steep 2 to 3 tsp dried or powdered kelp in 1 cup boiling water for 10 minutes; drink three times daily.

### SIDE EFFECTS

None expected.

### SPECIAL INFORMATION

WARNING: If you are already taking medication for hyperthyroidism (overactive thyroid), kelp supplements could worsen the condition.

WARNING: Do not gather your own wild kelp for use; coastal colonies may be contaminated by offshore pollutants.

WARNING: Check with your practitioner before using kelp if you have a history of thyroid problems or high blood pressure.

## Lavender

*Lavandula officinalis*

*A fragrant herb that scents clothes and helps repel moths, lavender also has medicinal properties. Herbalists prescribe lavender tea and the essential oil of lavender, both made from the plant's flowers, to treat common minor ailments such as insomnia, headache, and nausea. Anecdotal evidence suggests that lavender has a calming effect that relieves anxiety and promotes gastrointestinal relaxation. Its aroma (particularly that of L. angustifolia) is thought to stimulate mental processes and help alleviate depression, especially when it is used with other herbs. Like many aromatic essential oils, lavender oil has antiseptic qualities that may kill several types of disease-causing bacteria, and herbalists use it to treat skin ailments such as fungus, burns, wounds, and eczema.*

### TARGET AILMENTS

**Take internally for** insomnia, depression, or headache, especially when caused by stress; poor digestion, nausea, flatulence, colic.

**Apply externally for** burns, wounds, eczema, acne, candidiasis, ringworm, rheumatism.

### PREPARATIONS

**Over the counter:** Available in dried bulk, capsules, oil, and tincture.

**At home:**

Tea: Steep 1 tsp dried flowers in 1 cup boiling water for 10 minutes; drink three times daily.

Oil: To relax, use a few drops of the essential oil in a bath; rub it on your skin to ease rheumatic pains; or use a few drops in a steam inhalation for coughs, colds, and flu.

Combinations: For depression, lavender can be used with rosemary, skullcap, or kola.

### SPECIAL INFORMATION

WARNING: Do not use oil of lavender internally.

## Licorice

*Glycyrrhiza glabra*

*Licorice is one of the most commonly used medicinal herbs. Its intense sweetness masks the bitterness in any herbal mixture. Chinese and Western herbalists use licorice root as a cough suppressant and also prescribe it for digestive disorders, believing that it acts as a mild laxative and prevents stomach ulcers by forming a protective coating on the stomach wall. Practitioners think that licorice, as an external antibiotic, relieves skin irritations such as eczema and herpes sores.*

### TARGET AILMENTS

**Take internally for** cough, sore throat, colic, constipation, heartburn, stomach ulcers, arthritis, hepatitis, cirrhosis.

**Apply externally for** skin infections, eczema, herpes sores.

### PREPARATIONS

**Over the counter:** Available as dried root, liquid extract, and capsules.

**At home:**

Tea: Prepare by boiling 1 oz licorice root in 1 cup water for 15 to 20 minutes. Drink up to 2 cups daily.

Antibiotic: Sprinkle licorice powder directly on the infection or sore.

### SIDE EFFECTS

**Not serious:** Upset stomach, diarrhea, headache, edema (fluid retention), grogginess, weakness.

### SPECIAL INFORMATION

WARNING: Large amounts of licorice taken over a long period can lead to high blood pressure and edema. Consult your practitioner for advice.

- Do not use licorice root if you have edema, high blood pressure, kidney disease, or glaucoma.
- Avoid the herb if you are pregnant. It increases production of aldosterone, a hormone that regulates the salt and water balance in the body, resulting in a rise in blood pressure.

CONTINUED

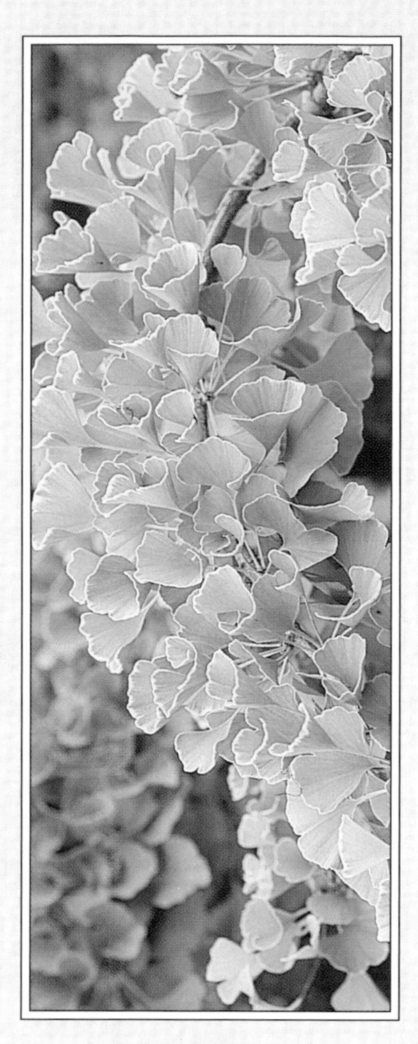

*Ginkgo*

## Lobelia

*Lobelia inflata*

*Lobelia, sometimes called Indian tobacco, is prescribed for both respiratory ailments and external conditions, but it can be extremely toxic. Because it is thought to relax overworked bronchial muscles and promote coughing, lobelia is most widely used to treat respiratory illnesses. Lobelia compresses have been used to treat skin injuries, fungus infections, and muscle strains.*

### TARGET AILMENTS

**Take internally for** pneumonia, asthma, bronchitis.

**Apply externally for** bruises, insect bites, poison ivy, fungus infections including ringworm, muscle strains.

### PREPARATIONS

**Over the counter:** Available in dried bulk, capsules, and tincture.

**At home:**

Tea: Steep ¼ to ½ tsp dried leaves in 1 cup boiling water for 10 to 15 minutes; drink three times daily.

Compress: Soak a piece of cloth in an infusion for several minutes; wring out and apply to affected area.

Combinations: For asthma, use with cayenne, skunk cabbage, and ginger.

### SIDE EFFECTS

**Serious:**

WARNING: Lobelia poisoning can cause nausea, excessive salivation, diarrhea, impaired hearing and vision, weakness, and mental confusion, and if not treated promptly can bring on respiratory failure and even death. If you develop any side effects, call your doctor at once.

### SPECIAL INFORMATION

WARNING: Use lobelia only in doses prescribed by your practitioner.

- If your practitioner prescribes lobelia for your child, monitor the child frequently for the development of any side effects.

## Lycium Fruit

*Lycium barbarum*
(or *L. chinense*)

*Similar in appearance and action, the berries of both Lycium barbarum and Lycium chinense are large, soft, and red. The fruit is sometimes known as wolfberry. In traditional Chinese medical terms, the two herbs are classified as sweet and neutral. Lycium chinense appears largely in Hebei Province, while the more common Lycium barbarum grows in a number of Chinese provinces.*

### TARGET AILMENTS

**Take internally for** night blindness, tinnitus (ringing in the ears), dizziness, and blurred vision; consumptive coughs; diabetes; sore back, knees, and legs; impotence and nocturnal emission.

### PREPARATIONS

Lycium fruit, both fresh and in the form of tablets, can be obtained from Chinese pharmacies, Asian markets, and some Western health food stores. The fruit is usually added to a dish during the last five minutes of cooking.

Combinations: When mixed with cuscuta, eucommia bark, and Chinese foxglove root cooked in wine, lycium fruit is prescribed for impotence, dizziness, and tinnitus. Practitioners also use the fruit to treat consumptive coughs, combining it with ophiopogon tuber, anemarrhena, and fritillaria.

### SPECIAL INFORMATION

- You should not take this herb if you suffer from an inflammatory ailment, weak digestion, or a tendency to become bloated.
- In a laboratory test, lycium was administered intravenously to rabbits; it seemed to reduce the blood pressure of these animals and to calm labored breathing.

## Magnolia Flower

*Magnolia liliflora*
(or *M. denudata*)

*More accurately described as magnolia buds, this herb is the unopened magnolia flower. Chinese medicine practitioners prescribe it for blocked nasal and sinus passages. The best-quality buds are green and dry; they should include none of the stems or branches. The herb is characterized in traditional Chinese medicine as acrid and warm. Growing in several Chinese provinces, magnolia is harvested in early spring, before the flowers unfold.*

**TARGET AILMENTS**

**Take internally for** nasal congestion, nasal discharge, sinus headaches, other sinus disorders.

**PREPARATIONS**

Magnolia buds are available in bulk at Chinese pharmacies, Asian markets, and some Western health food stores.

Combinations: Magnolia flowers are mixed with xanthium, angelica *(Angelica dahurica)*, and field mint to treat nasal congestion and sinus headaches, and with chrysanthemum flowers *(Chrysanthemum morifolium)* and siegesbeckia for frontal sinusitis. Consult an herbal practitioner for details of other mixtures and doses.

**SIDE EFFECTS**

**Not serious:** Because of its hairy texture, the herb can irritate the throat. Rub the herb with cotton cloth or place it in cheesecloth before mixing it into a solution. In addition, overdoses can cause dizziness and red eyes.

**SPECIAL INFORMATION**

❧ In test-tube studies, magnolia flowers seemed to inhibit the growth of several fungi on the skin.

## Marsh Mallow

*Althaea officinalis*

*For centuries people in Europe and the Middle East have eaten wild-growing marsh mallow when their crops failed. Today it is still recognized as a wilderness forage food. Herbalists use the roots, and sometimes the leaves, to treat cuts and wounds, mouth sores, stomach distress, and other ailments. And teething, irritable babies and toddlers have traditionally found comfort in sucking on a root of marsh mallow.*

*The healing substance in marsh mallow is mucilage, a spongy root material that forms a gel when mixed with water and is especially soothing to inflamed mucous membranes. One study suggests that mucilage supports the immune system's white blood cells in their fight against invading microbes. Another trial indicates that marsh mallow may help to lower blood sugar.*

**TARGET AILMENTS**

**Take internally for** sore throat, coughs, colds, flu, bronchitis, sinusitis; upset stomach, peptic ulcers, gastritis, colitis; cystitis, bladder infections, urethritis, kidney stones.

**Apply externally for** abscesses, boils, skin ulcers, scrapes, cuts, burns,other wounds; varicose veins; dental abscesses and gingivitis.

**PREPARATIONS**

**Over the counter:** Available in dried bulk, capsules, tincture.

**At home:**

Decoction: Simmer 1 to 2 tsp finely chopped or crushed root in 1 cup water for 10 to 15 minutes; drink three times daily. Use the decoction as a gargle for mouth problems.

Gel: Add just enough water to the finely chopped root to give it a gel-like consistency and use for skin problems.

**SPECIAL INFORMATION**

❧ Marsh mallow can be given in low doses to infants and children.

## Milk Thistle

*Silybum marianum*

*Milk thistle is used by herbalists to treat such liver disorders as cirrhosis and hepatitis. The active ingredient, silymarin, found in the seeds, is believed to prompt the growth of new, healthy liver cells without encouraging any malignancy that may be present. It is also thought that silymarin acts as an antioxidant, protecting the liver from damage by free radicals, harmful by-products of many bodily processes. The use of silymarin by healthy people can greatly increase the liver's content of glutathione, a key agent in detoxifying many potentially harmful substances.*

*Extracts of silymarin appear to neutralize toxins from the death cup mushroom, which can inflict lethal injury on the liver. Milk thistle also is believed to ease outbreaks of psoriasis, since these may worsen when the liver fails to neutralize certain toxins.*

**TARGET AILMENTS**

**Take internally for** liver problems; inflammation of the gallbladder duct; poisoning from ingestion of the death cup mushroom; psoriasis.

**PREPARATIONS**

**Over the counter:** Available in dried bulk, capsules, extract.

**At home:**

Tea: Steep 1 tsp freshly ground seeds in 1 cup boiling water for 10 to 15 minutes; drink three times daily. Or eat 1 tsp of freshly ground seeds. Milk thistle extract may be more effective than teas, since silymarin is only slightly water soluble. See an herbalist for more information.

**SIDE EFFECTS**

**Not serious:** Because taking milk thistle increases bile secretion, you may develop loose stools.

**SPECIAL INFORMATION**

WARNING: If you think you have a liver disorder, seek medical advice.



CONTINUED

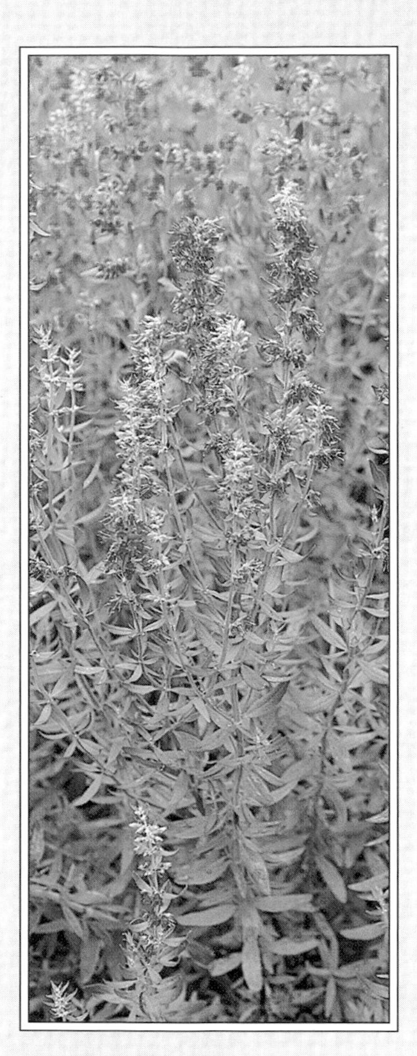

*Hyssop*

## Mugwort Leaf

*Artemisia argyi* (or *A. vulgaris*)

*Mugwort leaf is prescribed in Chinese medicine for a range of gynecological problems. In China mugwort is harvested at the end of spring or in early summer, when the leaves are growing vigorously but the flowers have not yet bloomed. The best leaves are grayish white with a thick, hairy texture. In Western tradition it is used to aid digestion and combat depression.*

### TARGET AILMENTS

**Take internally for** excessive menstrual bleeding and cramps, uterine bleeding, vaginal pain and bleeding during pregnancy, threatened miscarriage; a digestive aid; depression.

### PREPARATIONS

Leaves are available in bulk at some health food stores and Asian markets and pharmacies. The herb is also sold in pills. The dried, aged, powdered herb can be rolled in tissue paper into a cigarlike cylinder; one end is burned near the site of an injury to increase blood circulation and relieve pain. Acupuncturists sometimes use this technique instead of inserting needles.

Combinations: A mixture with gelatin is prescribed for vaginal bleeding and pain during pregnancy or for spotting between periods. Combining mugwort with dried ginger targets menstrual pain. And a preparation of mugwort leaves and kochia fruit is applied to itching lesions on the skin. For information on dosages and other preparations, check with an herbal practitioner.

### SIDE EFFECTS

None expected.

### SPECIAL INFORMATION

- A clinical trial suggests that crushed fresh leaves may eradicate warts.
- The herb seems to indicate an antibiotic effect in test-tube studies.

## Mullein

*Verbascum thapsus*

*Mullein is useful in treating diarrhea and hemorrhoids and, as an expectorant, bronchitis and coughs. The dried leaves, flowers, and roots are all used.*

### TARGET AILMENTS

**Take internally for** respiratory ailments; gastrointestinal problems such as stomach cramps, diarrhea.

**Apply externally for** external ulcers, tumors, hemorrhoids.

### PREPARATIONS

**Over the counter:** Mullein is available as tincture and as dried leaves, flowers, or roots.

**At home:**

Tea: Steep 1 to 2 tsp dried leaves, flowers, or roots per cup of boiling water for 10 or 15 minutes. Drink as many as 3 cups a day.

Compress: Soak bandages in a cooled tea made with vinegar; apply to ulcers, tumors, or hemorrhoids.

Inhalant: Boil fresh leaves in water and inhale the steam to relieve coughs and congestion.

Combinations: With elder and red clover to ease painful coughing; with gumweed for asthma; as an extract in olive oil for external ulcers, hemorrhoids, and tumors; with white horehound, coltsfoot, and lobelia for treating bronchitis.

### SIDE EFFECTS

**Not serious:** Mild stomach upset or diarrhea. Reduce dosage or discontinue; consult your doctor when convenient.

### SPECIAL INFORMATION

WARNING: If you have a history of cancer, consult your doctor before ingesting this herb; the tannin in mullein may be carcinogenic.

WARNING: Do not ingest the seeds; they are toxic.

WARNING: Do not take mullein if you are pregnant or nursing a baby.

## Myrrh

*Commiphora molmol*

*Myrrh, an oil found in the bark of certain shrubs, hardens into nuggets, called gum resin, which are powdered to make the healing herb. Myrrh fights infection by stimulating production of white blood cells and by a direct antibacterial action. It is also used as a fragrance in cosmetics and perfumes.*

### TARGET AILMENTS

**Take internally for** sinusitis, chest congestion, asthma, coughs, colds, boils; use as a mouthwash or gargle for mouth and throat infections.

**Apply externally for** wounds, abrasions (combine with witch hazel).

### PREPARATIONS

**Over the counter:** Available as tincture and as an ingredient in toothpastes, and as a powder.

**At home:**

Mouthwash: Steep 1 tsp powdered herb and 1 tsp boric acid in 1 pt boiling water. Let stand 30 minutes and strain; use when cool.

Tea: Steep 1 to 2 tsp powdered herb per cup of boiling water for 10 to 15 minutes. Drink three times a day.

### SIDE EFFECTS

**Not serious:** May cause stomach upset or diarrhea. Use a smaller amount less often or discontinue.

**Serious:** Large amounts may have a violent laxative action and may cause sweating, vomiting, kidney problems, or accelerated heartbeat. Stop using and call your doctor.

### SPECIAL INFORMATION

WARNING: Any resin tends to be hard to eliminate and can cause minor kidney damage if taken internally for extended periods. Consult your physician or herbalist before using if you are pregnant or nursing, or have kidney disease. Do not exceed recommended doses and do not give to children younger than two.

## Nettle

*Urtica dioica*

*Notorious for its stinging needles, nettle can be safely ingested when boiled or dried. Herbalists consider nettle a diuretic capable of removing toxins. Nettle has an erect stem and serrated, heart-shaped, dark green leaves.*

### TARGET AILMENTS

**Take internally for** arthritis, gout, hay fever, premenstrual syndrome, vaginal yeast infections, excessive menstrual flow, hemorrhoids, eczema, diarrhea, chronic cystitis.

**Take internally only under a doctor's supervision for** high blood pressure, congestive heart failure.

### PREPARATIONS

**Over the counter:** Nettle is available as tincture, capsules, and dried leaves and stems.

**At home:**

Tea: Steep 1 to 2 tsp dried herb in 1 cup boiling water for 10 minutes. Drink up to 2 cups a day.

Juice: Add 2 tsp juice squeezed from nettle to a vegetable or fruit drink.

Combinations: Nettle combines well with figwort and burdock to treat eczema; take orally as juice or tea.

### SIDE EFFECTS

**Not serious:** Large doses of nettle tea may cause stomach irritation, constipation, burning skin, or urinary suppression. Stop taking the herb and call your doctor.

### SPECIAL INFORMATION

WARNING: Do not use uncooked nettle; it may cause kidney damage and other symptoms of poisoning.

WARNING: Nettle is a diuretic, and it may therefore remove potassium from the body. If you use it frequently, eat foods high in potassium.

❧ Do not give nettle to children younger than two years old.

❧ To harvest, wear gloves and long pants and sleeves to avoid the sting.

## Notoginseng Root

*Panax notoginseng*

*Notoginseng root is employed in Chinese medicine to stop bleeding, reduce swelling, and alleviate pain from injuries. Unlike Western medications it seems to halt the bleeding without making the blood clot, and to stop the clotting or hematoma without causing bleeding. Practitioners of sports medicine in the West frequently use this herb as a tonic to improve stamina. The best variety, also known as pseudoginseng root (Panax pseudoginseng), is large, solid, and dark brown, with thin skin.*

### TARGET AILMENTS

**Take internally for** internal bleeding such as nosebleeds and blood in the stool and urine, coughing up blood.

**Use both internally and externally for** bleeding from injuries; swelling and pain of fractures; falls; contusions and sprains, cuts, and gunshot wounds.

### PREPARATIONS

Available in bulk from Chinese pharmacies, Asian markets, and Western health food stores, where it is sold as loose, dried roots or as tablets.

Combinations: Notoginseng can be made into a liniment for swelling and pain and is included in many injury tonics. A preparation containing notoginseng root and bletilla root is prescribed for vomiting, and for coughing up blood, nosebleeds, and blood in the urine. For information on appropriate preparations and doses, check with an herbal practitioner.

### SPECIAL INFORMATION

WARNING: Pregnant women should avoid this herb; it may cause a miscarriage under certain conditions.

❧ Notoginseng is sometimes used to treat acute attacks of Crohn's disease.



CONTINUED

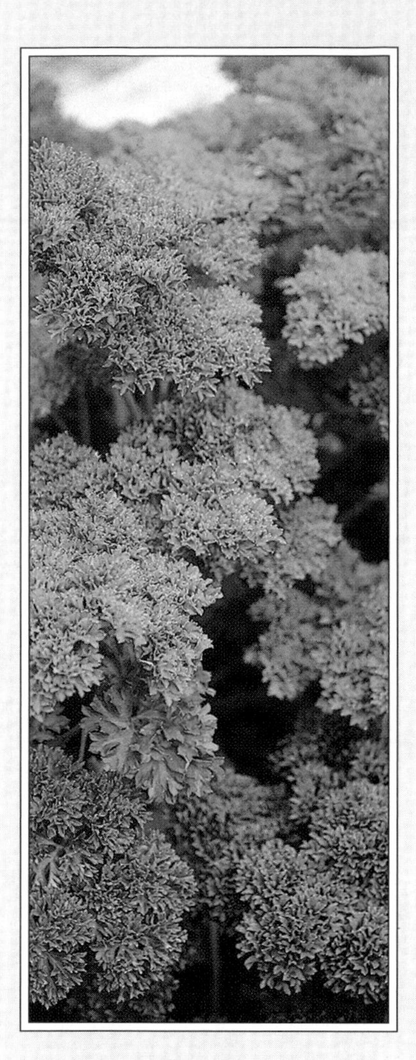

Parsley

## Parsley

*Petroselinum crispum*

*Added to salads and cooked foods or used as a garnish, the feathery leaves of parsley are a source of vitamins C and A, as well as a versatile herbal remedy. Because it eases muscle spasms and cramps, parsley is used as a digestive aid, and it is prescribed as a diuretic and mild laxative. Parsley is also considered to be an expectorant.*

### TARGET AILMENTS

**Take internally for** indigestion, congestion from coughs and colds, asthma, irregular menstruation, premenstrual syndrome, fever.

**Take internally under a doctor's supervision for** high blood pressure, congestive heart failure.

### PREPARATIONS

**Over the counter:** Available as tincture and as fresh or dried leaves, seeds, stems, and roots.

**At home:**

Tea: Steep 1 to 2 tsp dried leaves or roots per cup of boiling water for 5 to 10 minutes in a closed container. Drink up to 3 cups a day.

Nutrition and diet: Eat raw green leaves as a breath freshener.

### SIDE EFFECTS

None expected.

### SPECIAL INFORMATION

WARNING: Pregnant and nursing women should not take parsley juice or oil in medicinal doses. Eating a few sprigs served as garnish will probably not cause any harm.

WARNING: If you use this herb frequently as a medicine, you should also eat foods high in potassium, such as bananas, because diuretics deplete the body of potassium.

- Do not give medicinal doses to children younger than two years old.
- Only experienced field botanists should pick wild parsley, because of its resemblance to toxic plants.

## Passionflower

*Passiflora incarnata*

*Because of its purported calming effect on the central nervous system, herbalists use passionflower as a sedative, a digestive aid, and a pain reliever.*

### TARGET AILMENTS

**Take internally for** insomnia, anxiety, neuralgia, shingles, persistent hiccups, asthma, and to aid withdrawal from addictive disorders.

### PREPARATIONS

**Over the counter:** Available in commercial homeopathic or herbal remedies and as dried or fresh leaves, capsules, and tincture.

**At home:**

Tea: Steep 2 tsp dried herb per cup of boiling water for 15 minutes. For insomnia, drink 1 cup in the evening.

Tincture: 1 dropperful in warm water, up to four times a day, for anxiety in adults and in children weighing more than 100 pounds. For smaller children, consult a trained practitioner for dosages and give only under medical supervision.

### SIDE EFFECTS

**Not serious:** Gastric upset, diarrhea. Discontinue and call your doctor.

**Serious:** May cause sleepiness; do not take during the day if you operate heavy machinery or drive.

### SPECIAL INFORMATION

- Always use passionflower under medical supervision.
- Use only professionally prepared remedies; another species, *Passiflora caerulea,* contains cyanide.
- Do not take if you are pregnant.
- Use low-strength preparations for adults over 65 or children between two and 12 years old. Do not give to children under two years of age.

### POSSIBLE INTERACTIONS

Use caution when combining with prescription sedatives.

## Pau d'Arco

*Tabebuia impetiginosa*

*Pau d'arco is the name of both a tree and a medicinal extract from the tree's bark or heartwood. The extract is believed to be effective against bacterial, fungal, viral, and parasitic infections, and is also considered to be an anti-inflammatory agent. It is thought to destroy microorganisms by increasing the supply of oxygen to cells. For centuries before modern science isolated some 20 of its chemical ingredients, pau d'arco was used as a folk remedy. The pau d'arco tree, also called the trumpet tree, is native to Central and South America and the West Indies. It can reach a height of 125 feet.*

### TARGET AILMENTS

**Take internally for** bacterial, fungal, viral, and parasitic infections; indigestion.

### PREPARATIONS

**Over the counter:** Pau d'arco is available as capsules, tincture, and dried bark.

**At home:**

Decoction: Boil 1 tbsp bark in 2 to 3 cups water for 10 to 15 minutes. Drink 2 to 8 cups a day.

### SIDE EFFECTS

None expected.

## Peppermint

*Mentha piperita*

*Peppermint plants have stems with a purplish cast; long, serrated leaves; and a familiar minty aroma. This common, pleasant-tasting herb has been used as a remedy for indigestion since the time of the pharaohs of ancient Egypt. Menthol, the principal active ingredient, stimulates the stomach lining, thereby reducing the amount of time food spends in the stomach. It also relaxes the muscles of the digestive system.*

### TARGET AILMENTS

**Take internally for** cramps, stomach pain, gas, nausea associated with migraine headaches, morning sickness, travel sickness, insomnia, anxiety, fever, colds, flu.

**Apply externally for** itching and inflammation.

### PREPARATIONS

**Over the counter:** Available as commercial tea, tincture, and fresh or dried leaves and flowers.

**At home:**

Tea: Drink commercial brands or steep 1 to 2 heaping tsp dried herb per cup of boiling water for 10 minutes. Drink up to 3 cups a day.

Bath: Fill a cloth bag with several handfuls of dried or fresh herb and let hot water run over it.

### SIDE EFFECTS

None expected.

### SPECIAL INFORMATION

WARNING: Do not ingest pure menthol or pure peppermint; these substances are extremely toxic.

- Give only very dilute preparations to children younger than two and only under a doctor's supervision.
- Pregnant women with morning sickness should use a dilute tea rather than a more potent infusion. Peppermint should not be used by women who have a history of miscarriage.

## Polygonum

*Polygonum multiflorum* (root)

*Polygonum, which is also known as fleeceflower root and frequently called fo-ti by practitioners, is prescribed in Chinese medicine for a wide variety of disorders ranging from signs of premature aging to symptoms of malaria.*

### TARGET AILMENTS

**Take internally for** dizziness and blurred vision; insomnia; prematurely gray hair; nocturnal emission; vaginal discharge; carbuncles, sores, abscesses, scrofula, goiter, and neck lumps; constipation; sore knees and back; malaria (chronic only, not the acute stages).

### PREPARATIONS

Polygonum is available at Chinese pharmacies, Asian markets, and some Western health food stores. It can also be found in pill form.

Combinations: With lycium fruit, psorolea fruit, and cuscuta, it is prescribed for sore knees and back, dizziness, and premature aging. A preparation containing polygonum, scrophularia, and forsythia fruit is prescribed for scrofula, abscesses, and other swellings. A combination with Asian ginseng, dong quai, and tangerine peel is recommended for chronic malarial symptoms. For information on dosages and additional preparations, check with a Chinese medicine practitioner.

### SIDE EFFECTS

**Not serious:** May cause flushing of face, diarrhea, and gastric distress.

### SPECIAL INFORMATION

- The herb is not prescribed for patients with phlegm or diarrhea.

### POSSIBLE INTERACTIONS

Some traditional sources suggest that you should not take this herb with onions, chives, or garlic.



CONTINUED

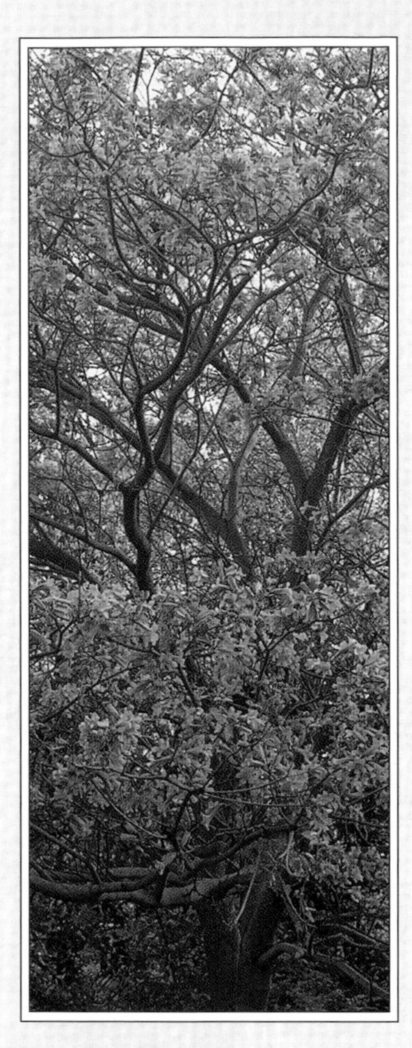

*Pau d'Arco*

## Psyllium

*Plantago psyllium*

*Psyllium, whose seeds, rich in fiber, make a safe, bulk-forming laxative, has long been used to treat constipation, diarrhea, hemorrhoids, and urinary problems. Because the herb absorbs excess fluid in the intestinal tract and increases stool volume, both diarrhea and constipation can be treated.*

### TARGET AILMENTS

**Take internally for** constipation, hemorrhoidal irritation, diarrhea.

### PREPARATIONS

**Over the counter:** Available as whole seeds, ground or powdered seeds, and in various commercial bulk-forming laxative preparations.

**At home:**

Drink: Mix 1 tsp ground seeds or powder in 1 cup cool liquid. Drink 2 to 3 cups a day.

Seeds: Take 1 tsp seeds with water at mealtimes.

### SIDE EFFECTS

**Not serious:** Psyllium can cause allergic reactions in people who have allergies to dust or grasses. Call your doctor if bothersome.

**Serious:** Severe allergic reactions are rare; if you have difficulty breathing, seek emergency help.

### SPECIAL INFORMATION

WARNING: To prevent intestinal blockage when taking psyllium as a laxative, you must drink 8 to 10 glasses of water throughout the day.

- Start using this herb gradually to allow your body to adjust to the increase in fiber.
- Do not give this herb to children younger than two years of age. Consult your pediatrician if your infant or child is constipated.
- If you are pregnant you should avoid psyllium and all laxatives, because they stimulate the lower pelvis near the uterus.

## Red Clover

*Trifolium pratense*

*The medicinal parts of this perennial are the red or purple ball-shaped flowers. Herbalists prescribe red clover for skin ailments, indigestion, and coughs. It is an anti-inflammatory agent and, as an expectorant, helps remove excess mucus from the lungs. In addition, the herb appears to act like the female hormone estrogen; it is believed to help women with menopausal symptoms.*

### TARGET AILMENTS

**Take internally for** coughs, bronchitis, whooping cough, indigestion, menopausal symptoms.

**Use internally and externally for** skin problems such as eczema and psoriasis.

### PREPARATIONS

**Over the counter:** Red clover is available in dried bulk and tincture.

**At home:**

Tea: Steep 1 to 3 tsp dried flower tops in 1 cup boiling water for 15 minutes. Drink up to 3 cups daily.

Compress: Soak a clean cloth in the infusion and apply to the skin.

### SIDE EFFECTS

**Serious:** Discontinue use if you experience stomachaches or diarrhea.

### SPECIAL INFORMATION

WARNING: Do not use red clover if you are pregnant, because of its estrogen-like behavior.

WARNING: Avoid the herb if you have estrogen-dependent cancer or a history of heart disease, stroke, or thrombophlebitis.

- If you are taking birth-control pills, consult your doctor before using red clover.
- Do not give the herb to children under two. Older children and people over 65 should start with a low dose and increase as needed.

## Red Raspberry

*Rubus idaeus*

*The berry of this biennial bush is commonly used in desserts, but herbalists value the leaves. These have high concentrations of tannin, a chemical that herbalists believe is effective in treating diarrhea, nausea, vomiting, and morning sickness in pregnancy. It is also thought that tannin, an astringent substance, helps prevent miscarriages and, during labor, checks hemorrhaging, strengthens contractions, and reduces labor pains; you should not, however, use red raspberry for this purpose at home. Red raspberry leaves are included in several herbal pregnancy formulas sold in the U.S. The herb is also used as a gargle for sore throats.*

### TARGET AILMENTS

**Take internally for** morning sickness, threatened miscarriage, problems arising during labor, diarrhea, mouth ulcers, bleeding gums.

### PREPARATIONS

**Over the counter:** Available as dried leaves or berries and as tincture.

**At home:**

Infusion: Use 1 to 2 tsp dried leaves or berries per cup of boiling water. Steep for 10 to 15 minutes. Drink cold and as desired. During pregnancy, steep ½ oz dried leaves with 1 pt boiling water for 3 to 5 minutes and drink warm, 1 pt per day. For children, dilute with more water.

### SIDE EFFECTS

**Not serious:** May cause stomach upset or diarrhea if you exceed the recommended dose.

### SPECIAL INFORMATION

- Pregnant women should take red raspberry only with the consent and under the supervision of a physician.
- Animal tests suggest that red raspberry may reduce levels of glucose (blood sugar) and hence may help in the management of diabetes.

## Rosemary

*Rosmarinus officinalis*

*Herbalists believe the leaves of rosemary stimulate the circulatory and nervous systems and serve as an antidepressant. The leaves are thought to contain antispasmodic chemicals that relax the smooth muscle lining of the digestive tract and also are used to treat muscle pain. Rosemary has antibacterial and antifungal properties.*

### TARGET AILMENTS

**Take internally for** indigestion, upper respiratory tract infections that require a decongestant, tension, muscle pain, sprains, rheumatism, neuralgia.

**Apply externally,** as an antiseptic, for skin infections.

### PREPARATIONS

**Over the counter:** Available as dried bulk, tincture, and two types of oil, one for internal use and the other for external application.

**At home:**

Tea: Use 1 tsp crushed leaves per cup of boiling water. Steep 15 minutes. To settle the stomach or clear a stuffy nose, drink 3 cups a day. For children younger than two, dilute the infusion with more water.

### SIDE EFFECTS

**Not serious:** Rosemary oil for internal use may cause mild stomach, kidney, and intestinal irritation, even in small doses. If you experience any of these discomforts, consult your physician.

**Serious:** Rosemary oil, taken internally in large amounts, can be poisonous. Keep to the prescribed dosage.

### SPECIAL INFORMATION

WARNING: Do not confuse rosemary oil for internal use with that for external use.. Never ingest the latter.

- Do not use if you are pregnant.

## Sage

*Salvia officinalis*

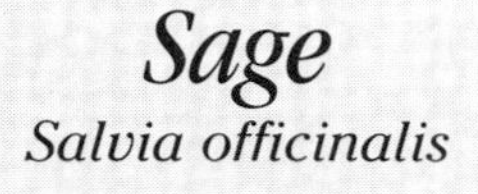

*The scientific name of sage, Salvia, derives from the Latin for "to save," which underscores the herb's early reputation as a cure-all. Modern herbalists believe sage contains an aromatic oil that reduces excessive perspiration and night sweats. Sage has antiseptic and astringent properties. It is also used to aid digestion, cleanse wounds, and stem lactation in nursing mothers.*

### TARGET AILMENTS

**Take internally for** indigestion, gas, nausea, and to stem lactation or reduce the night sweats of menopause.

**Apply externally for** bacterial infections in wounds; insect bites.

### PREPARATIONS

**Over the counter:** Available as tincture, tea, and dried or fresh leaves.

**At home:**

Tea: Steep 2 to 3 tsp leaves per cup of boiling water for 10 minutes. Drink 3 cups a day or use as a wash for infected wounds.

Compress: Soak a clean cloth in the infusion and apply to insect bites.

Fresh: Apply fresh sage leaves to minor cuts or scrapes before washing and bandaging.

### SIDE EFFECTS

**Not serious:** Drinking the tea may inflame the lips and mouth lining.

### SPECIAL INFORMATION

WARNING: Sage contains the toxic chemical thujone, which can lead to convulsions if taken in high doses. However, the heat of cooking or preparing an infusion reduces toxicity. Sage oil should not be ingested.

- Do not take if you are pregnant or nursing, or if you have epilepsy.
- Use dilute preparations for children under 12 and adults over 65.



CONTINUED

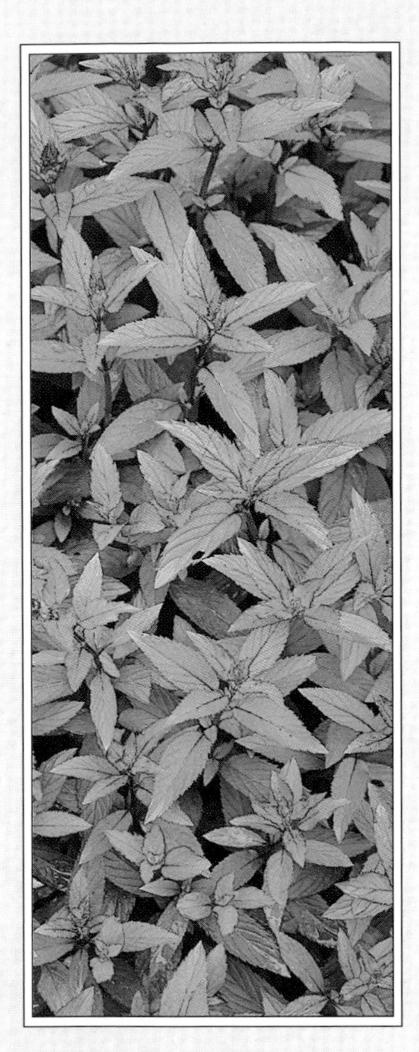

**Peppermint**

## Saw Palmetto

*Serenoa repens*

*An extract made from the berries of this shrub is used to treat and strengthen the male reproductive system. It is particularly recommended for benign prostatic hyperplasia, or enlargement of the prostate gland. Common among men over 50, the condition is thought to be caused by an accumulation of a testosterone derivative called dihydrotestosterone, which saw palmetto appears to block the production of. The herb has also been used as an expectorant, diuretic, tonic, antiseptic, sedative, and digestive aid.*

### TARGET AILMENTS

**Take internally for** benign prostatic hyperplasia; nasal congestion; asthma and bronchitis; coughs due to colds; sore throats; sinus ailments.

### PREPARATIONS

**Over the counter:** Available as fresh or dried berries and in powder or capsule form. Gel capsules are preferable to tea or tincture.

**At home:**

Infusion: Steep ½ to 1 tsp fresh berries per cup of boiling water for 10 minutes. Drink 6 oz, two or three times a day.

Decoction: Add ½ to 1 tsp dried berries to 1 cup water, bring to a boil, and simmer for 5 minutes. Drink three times daily.

Tincture: Drink 15 to 60 drops in water two or three times daily.

### SIDE EFFECTS

None expected.

### SPECIAL INFORMATION

WARNING: Do not substitute saw palmetto for medical treatment. Because the symptoms of prostate enlargement and prostate cancer are similar, men should see a doctor when they have symptoms such as urine retention, dribbling, and passage of blood in the urine.

## Skullcap

*Scutellaria baicalensis*

*Chinese herbalists prescribe the root of skullcap for a wide range of disorders.*

### TARGET AILMENTS

**Take internally for** diarrhea, dysentery; upper respiratory infections with fever; urinary tract infections, jaundice, hepatitis; tension, irritability, headache, insomnia, epileptic and other seizures; red face or eyes; coughing up or vomiting blood, nosebleeds, blood in the stool; abdominal pain and vaginal bleeding, threatened miscarriage, PMS.

### PREPARATIONS

Available in bulk from Chinese pharmacies, Asian markets, and Western health food stores. The herb can also be obtained as pills. The root is usually decocted, but it can be fried dry for use in pregnancy and to treat diarrhea and infections of the urinary tract, or cooked in wine for upper respiratory infections and redness of the face and eyes.

Combinations: A mixture with coptis is prescribed for high fever and irritability. Skullcap root mixed with anemarrhena is thought to alleviate chronic coughs. For further information on preparations and doses, consult a Chinese medicine practitioner.

### SIDE EFFECTS

None expected.

### SPECIAL INFORMATION

- Before using skullcap to treat diarrhea or the problems of pregnancy, check with a Chinese medicine practitioner.

### POSSIBLE INTERACTIONS

Some sources in traditional Chinese medicine suggest that skullcap counteracts the effects of moutan and veratrum.

## Skullcap

*Scutellaria lateriflora*

*Skullcap's leaves and blue flowers are used in many over-the-counter herbal sleep remedies. Some researchers report that skullcap calms the nervous system. Chinese medicine physicians use it to treat hepatitis. In the United States, however, skullcap is considered controversial and even useless by many medical authorities, at least partly because of its early—and unearned—reputation for curing rabies, for which it garnered the now archaic name of mad dog weed. Its current name comes from a caplike appendage on the upper lip of the flower.*

### TARGET AILMENTS

**Take internally for** nervous tension; headaches, muscle aches, and symptoms of PMS aggravated or caused by stress; insomnia; convulsions; drug or alcohol withdrawal.

### PREPARATIONS

**Over the counter:** Available as prepared tea, tincture, dried leaves, or capsules.

**At home:**

Tea: Pour 1 cup boiling water over 2 tsp dried leaves and steep for 10 to 15 minutes; drink this amount up to three times daily.

Tincture: Take ½ to 1 tsp per 8-oz glass of warm water.

### SIDE EFFECTS

**Not serious:** Stomach upset or diarrhea. Reduce intake or stop using it.

### SPECIAL INFORMATION

WARNING: Skullcap may cause drowsiness. Do not operate a car or heavy machinery after taking it.

WARNING: Taking large amounts of the tincture may cause confusion, giddiness, twitching, and possibly convulsions.

- Skullcap in medicinal amounts should be used only under professional supervision.

## Slippery Elm

*Ulmus fulva*

*The U.S. Food and Drug Administration calls slippery elm a good demulcent, or soothing agent. Herbalists recommend its use externally to ease wounds and skin problems, and internally to soothe sore throats, coughing, and diarrhea and other gastrointestinal disorders. Slippery elm's active ingredient is found in the white inner bark, whose mucilaginous cells expand into a spongy mass when mixed with water.*

### TARGET AILMENTS

**Apply externally for** wounds, cuts, abrasions.

**Take internally for** coughing, sore throats, digestive complaints.

**Use externally and internally for** gynecological problems.

### PREPARATIONS

**Over the counter:** Available in health food stores as capsules, tea, powder.

**At home:**

Poultice: For wounds that have been thoroughly cleansed with soap and water, moisten powdered bark with enough water to make a paste; apply to wound and allow to dry. This forms a natural bandage that delivers soothing agents to the wound.

Tea: Add 2 tsp powder to a cup of boiling water; simmer for 15 minutes. Drink up to 3 cups a day for throat, digestive, and gynecological problems.

Food: Mix slippery elm powder with water or milk until it has the consistency of a thin porridge.

### SPECIAL INFORMATION

- Consult your doctor if you do not improve significantly within two weeks.
- Some people may be allergic to the powdered bark; if so, discontinue use. Consult your doctor before taking larger-than-recommended doses.

## Spearmint

*Mentha spicata*

*Spearmint, used since ancient times to promote digestion, heal wounds, and relieve colds and congestion, is prescribed by herbalists today for digestive ills, colds, insomnia, and itching and inflammation. The crushed or boiled leaves release carvone, a chemical similar to but milder than the menthol found in peppermint. Many herbalists prescribe spearmint and peppermint interchangeably, although the latter is considered more potent.*

### TARGET AILMENTS

**Take internally for** upset stomach, stomach spasms, flatulence, heartburn, stomach cramps, morning sickness during pregnancy; nasal, sinus, and chest congestion; colds; headache; sore throat or mouth.

**Take internally and apply externally for** muscle pains, external infections, chapped hands.

### PREPARATIONS

**Over the counter:** Available as capsules, prepared tea, fresh or dried leaves, tincture, oil.

**At home:**

Tea: Boil 1 to 2 tsp dried herb or several fresh leaves per cup of water; steep 10 minutes. Drink up to 3 cups a day.

Tincture: Add ¼ to 1 tsp to an 8-oz glass of water and drink up to three glasses a day.

Herbal bath: Fill a cloth bag with a few handfuls of dried or fresh spearmint leaves and add to running bathwater.

### SIDE EFFECTS

None expected.

### SPECIAL INFORMATION

- Spearmint oil (carvone) may cause stomach upset if ingested. It is recommended for external use only.
- For children under two, dilute tea or tincture with water.



CONTINUED

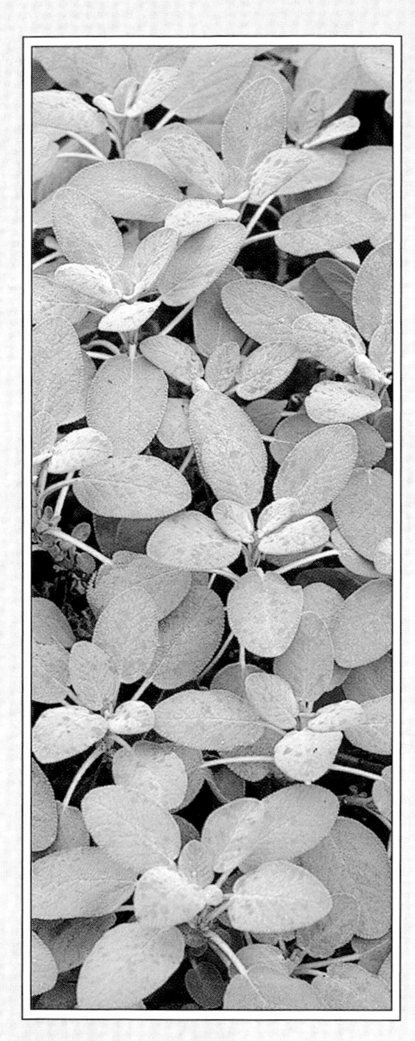

*Sage*

## St.-John's-Wort

*Hypericum perforatum*

*For centuries herbalists have used the blood red flowers of St-John's-wort to heal wounds and treat depression.*

**TARGET AILMENTS**

**Use externally for** wounds (cuts, abrasions, burns); scar tissue.

**Take internally** in consultation with an herbalist or a doctor for depression.

**PREPARATIONS**

**Over the counter:** Available as dried leaves and flowers, tincture, extract, oil, ointment, capsules, and prepared tea.

**At home:**

Tea: Add 1 to 2 tsp dried herb to 1 cup boiling water; steep for 15 minutes. Drink up to 3 cups a day.

Oil: Use a commercial preparation, or soak the flowers in almond or olive oil until the oil turns bright red.

Ointment: Use a commercial preparation, or warm the leaves in hot petroleum jelly or a mixture of beeswax and almond oil.

Fresh: Apply crushed leaves and flowers to cleansed wounds.

Tincture: Add ¼ to 1 tsp to an 8-oz glass of water and drink daily.

**SIDE EFFECTS**

**Serious:** High blood pressure, headaches, stiff neck, nausea, and vomiting. Can exacerbate sunburn in the fair-skinned.

**SPECIAL INFORMATION**

- Consult a doctor or an herbalist before using St.-John's-wort.

**POSSIBLE INTERACTIONS**

WARNING: Avoid the amino acids tryptophan and tyrosine; amphetamines; asthma inhalants; beer, coffee, wine; chocolate, fava beans, salami, smoked or pickled foods, and yogurt; cold or hay fever medicines; diet pills; narcotics; nasal decongestants.

## Tangerine Peel

*Citrus reticulata*

*Sometimes called mandarin orange peel, this herb is prescribed for digestive disorders. Practitioners of Chinese medicine believe that the peel gets better as it ages. The best samples of the fruit are thin skinned, pliable, oily, and fragrant.*

**TARGET AILMENTS**

**Take internally for** indigestion, gas; a feeling of fullness in the abdomen; nausea; loose stools; phlegm.

**PREPARATIONS**

Available at Asian food markets, Chinese pharmacies, and Western health food stores. Also available as pills.

Combinations: In a preparation with Asian ginseng, tangerine peel is used as a digestive stimulant. Chinese herbalists prescribe a mixture of tangerine peel, ripe bitter orange, and aucklandia for abdominal distention and pain. And a preparation containing tangerine peel and pinellia root is used to treat an excess of phlegm together with a stifling feeling in the chest that makes deep breathing difficult. For further information on appropriate preparations and doses, check with an herbal practitioner.

**SIDE EFFECTS**

None expected.

**SPECIAL INFORMATION**

- Do not use this herb if you have a dry cough or an excessively red tongue, or if you are spitting up blood.
- Herbalists use the red part of tangerine peel (when dried, some parts are orange and others red) to control vomiting and belching.
- Chinese practitioners also prescribe young, or green, tangerine peel for breast and side pain and for hernia pain.

## Tea Tree Oil

*Melaleuca* spp.

*The first Europeans to reach Australia made tea from the leaves of what then became known as the tea tree, which should not be confused with the common tea plant. For centuries before the Europeans arrived, native Australians were using the leaves of this tree as an antiseptic. Eventually the Europeans learned to use the leaves' volatile oil to treat cuts, abrasions, burns, insect bites, and other minor skin ailments. Modern studies show that the strong germicidal activity of tea tree oil is caused primarily by a single ingredient, terpineol. The oil, which smells like nutmeg, is extracted from the leaves by steam distillation. During World War II, tea tree oil was added to machine oils to reduce infections in the hands of workers during metal fabrication. The oils of some species of Melaleuca may irritate the skin and are not used.*

### TARGET AILMENTS

**Apply externally for** cuts, abrasions, insect bites, teenage acne, fungal infections such as athlete's foot, and other skin ailments. Use as a douche for minor vaginal infections.

### PREPARATIONS

**Over the counter:** Available as oil and also as an additive to health and beauty products such as toothpaste, soap, and shampoo. Tea tree oil is also used in flea shampoos.

**At home:**

Apply fresh leaves directly to wounds.

### SIDE EFFECTS

**Not serious:** Local skin and vaginal irritation may develop in sensitive individuals. Let your doctor know if the irritation persists.

### SPECIAL INFORMATION

- People with sensitive skin should dilute tea tree oil with a bland oil, such as vegetable oil.

## Turmeric

*Curcuma longa*

*Turmeric root, a main ingredient in Indian curries, is also used in Ayurvedic and Chinese medicine and by Western herbalists to treat a variety of ailments.*

### TARGET AILMENTS

Chinese:

**Take internally for** shoulder pain, menstrual cramps, pain after childbirth, menstrual irregularity.

**Apply externally for** infections of the skin.

Western:

**Take internally for** digestive disorders, fever, chest congestion, menstrual irregularity, arthritis pain.

**Apply externally for** pain and swelling caused by trauma.

### PREPARATIONS

**Over the counter:** Available as powdered root, capsules, liquid extract.

**At home:**

Chinese:

Combinations: Turmeric is mixed with cinnamon twig and astragalus for shoulder pain; with cinnamon bark for menstrual cramps and pain after childbirth; with dong quai for menstrual irregularity. The herb is mixed with sesame or salad oil and applied externally to swollen areas.

Western:

Decoction: Steep 1 tsp turmeric powder in 1 cup milk for 15 to 20 minutes. Drink up to 3 cups a day.

### SIDE EFFECTS

**Not serious:** Heartburn or upset stomach. Discontinue and consult your practitioner.

### SPECIAL INFORMATION

- If you are pregnant, trying to conceive or have fertility problems, or have a blood-clotting disorder, consult your practitioner before using.
- Use low-strength preparations for children, or adults over 65. Do not give to children under two.

## Usnea

*Usnea* spp.

*Usnea, or larch moss, refers to a group of lichens, plants made up of algae and fungi that grow together interdependently. Usnea is found hanging from the larch and many other trees in the Northern Hemisphere. The active ingredient, usnic acid, seems to have an antibiotic effect against the Gram-positive class of bacteria, which includes Streptococcus. It may also be effective against some fungi and protozoans. Usnea is believed to work by disrupting the cell metabolism of bacteria and other simple organisms, though it does not damage human cells. Herbalists consider it an immune system stimulant and a muscle relaxant.*

### TARGET AILMENTS

**Take internally for** colds, influenza, sore throats, respiratory infections; gastrointestinal irritations.

**Apply externally for** skin ulcers and fungal infections such as athlete's foot; use as a douche for vaginal infections and urinary tract infections such as urethritis or cystitis.

### PREPARATIONS

**Over the counter:** Available in bulk, powder, or tincture.

**At home:**

Tea: Steep 2 to 3 tsp dried lichen or 1 to 2 tsp powder in 1 cup boiling water. Take three times daily.

### SIDE EFFECTS

**Not serious:** If digestive disorders arise, reduce dosage. Call your doctor if these symptoms persist.

### SPECIAL INFORMATION

WARNING: Pregnant women should avoid using this herb because it may stimulate uterine contractions.

- Dilute tincture before ingesting; high concentrations may cause digestive problems.
- Do not use for more than three consecutive weeks.



CONTINUED

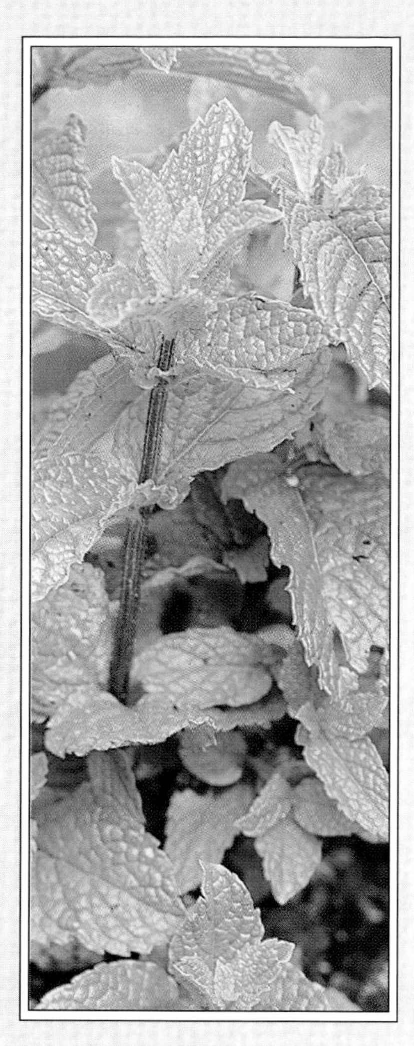

**Spearmint**

## Uva Ursi

*Arctostaphylos uva-ursi*

*Uva ursi, prescribed by herbalists for urinary problems, is also used to treat minor wounds. Its leaves contain arbutin, which is converted in the urinary tract to the antiseptic hydroquinone.*

### TARGET AILMENTS

**Take internally for** mild urinary tract infections, such as urethritis and cystitis; high blood pressure; menstrual bloating.

**Apply externally for** skin problems such as cuts and abrasions.

### PREPARATIONS

**Over the counter:** Available as dried leaves; as a tincture; and as a tea, alone or in combination with other ingredients.

**At home:**

Tea: Simmer for 5 to 10 minutes; let stand for 12 to 24 hours. To counteract the effect of the tannin content, add peppermint or chamomile. Drink 3 cups a day.

Compress: Make a tea; strain; soak a pad in the tea and apply.

### SIDE EFFECTS

**Not serious:** Taking uva ursi may produce dark green urine; this is harmless. The herb's high tannin content may cause stomach upset.

**Serious:** A 1949 study involving very high doses of hydroquinone reported tinnitus, nausea, and convulsions. Prescribed doses of the whole herb are considered safe; in case of side effects, discontinue taking until you contact your doctor.

### SPECIAL INFORMATION

- Uva ursi works only in an alkaline environment; avoid acidic foods and vitamin C when taking.
- Because hydroquinone is toxic in high doses, use uva ursi only in recommended amounts.
- Do not use if you are pregnant; it may stimulate uterine contractions.

## Valerian

*Valeriana officinalis*

*Valerian root has been used for more than a thousand years for its calming qualities, and recent research has confirmed its efficacy and safety as a mild tranquilizer and sleep aid. Valerian hastens the onset of sleep, improves sleep quality, and reduces nighttime awakenings. Unlike barbiturates or benzodiazepines, prescribed amounts leave no morning grogginess and do not interfere with the vivid dreaming sleep known as REM sleep. It is not habit forming and produces no withdrawal symptoms when discontinued.*

### TARGET AILMENTS

**Take internally for** insomnia, anxiety, nervousness, headache, intestinal pains, menstrual cramps.

### PREPARATIONS

**Over the counter:** Available dried or as capsules, tincture, and teas.

**At home:**

Tea: Steep 2 tsp dried, chopped root in 1 cup boiling water. Let stand 8 to 12 hours. Drink 1 cup before bed.

### SIDE EFFECTS

**Not serious:** A mild headache or upset stomach may develop. Reduce dosage. Tell your doctor if it persists.

**Serious:** More severe headache, restlessness, nausea, morning grogginess, or blurred vision may be caused by using too much valerian. Contact your doctor, who will probably tell you to take less or to stop using the herb.

### SPECIAL INFORMATION

- Do not take valerian with conventional tranquilizers or sedatives, because of possible additive effects.
- Paradoxically, valerian may produce excitability in some people.
- Be careful about driving until you know how the herb affects you.

## White Willow

*Salix alba*

*White willow is a source of salicin, a precursor of aspirin. Though all parts of the plant contain some salicin, the best source is the mature bark. As do other salicin-producing plants, white willow also reduces fever and inflammation. Besides salicin, willow bark contains other compounds that the body metabolizes to salicylic acid. For this reason it acts more slowly and over a longer period of time than aspirin does.*

### TARGET AILMENTS

**Take internally for** gout, minor muscle strains, menstrual cramps, headache, fever, aches and pains, pain and inflammation of arthritis.

**Apply externally for** sores, burns; pain and inflammation of arthritis.

### PREPARATIONS

**Over the counter:** Available as tea, tincture, dried bark, and capsules.

**At home:**

Tea: Steep 1 to 2 tsp powdered bark in 1 cup boiling water for 8 hours; strain. Drink up to 3 cups daily. Honey and lemon improve taste.

### SIDE EFFECTS

**Not serious:** Upset stomach, nausea, or tinnitus may result. Lower the dosage or discontinue. Call your doctor if symptoms persist.

### SPECIAL INFORMATION

WARNING: Children under 16 should not use white willow if they have a cold, flu, or other viral illness. Using salicylates may cause Reye's syndrome, a potentially fatal condition.

❧ Individuals with ulcers or other stomach problems should use white willow with caution.

### POSSIBLE INTERACTIONS

Do not mix white willow with other salicylates, such as aspirin or wintergreen oil, because of the potential for additive side effects.

## Wild Yam

*Dioscorea villosa*

*Used during the 18th and 19th centuries as a remedy for menstrual pain and complications associated with childbearing, wild yam is a perennial vine that entwines itself around fences and bushes. It is recognized by a slender reddish brown stem and drooping yellow flowers that bloom in summer. Wild yam extract, taken from the root, contains an alkaloid substance that relaxes the muscles of the entire abdominal region. Consequently, it is prescribed to alleviate menstrual cramps and to relieve the nausea and muscle tension associated with pregnancy. Wild yam also contains steroidal saponins, believed to act as anti-inflammatory agents and used to lessen the swelling of rheumatoid arthritis.*

### TARGET AILMENTS

**Take internally for** morning sickness, nausea of pregnancy, menstrual cramps, urinary tract disorders, intestinal colic, rheumatoid arthritis.

### PREPARATIONS

**Over the counter:** Available as dried root, tincture, or capsules.

**At home:**

Tea: Boil 1 oz wild yam root with 1 cup water for 15 to 20 minutes. Drink three times daily.

Combinations: For intestinal colic, wild yam is combined with calamus, chamomile, and ginger. Rheumatoid arthritis is treated with a mix of wild yam and black cohosh. Herbalists use a combination of wild yam and cramp bark for menstrual cramps.

### SPECIAL INFORMATION

❧ Herbalists sometimes prescribe wild yam for its alleged progesterone-like properties for women undergoing menopause; the effectiveness of this treatment, however, is debated. Consult a practitioner before using wild yam as a progesterone supplement.

## Yarrow

*Achillea millefolium*

*Yarrow has been used to heal wounds since ancient times. Modern investigation has revealed many chemicals in this herb that have pain-relieving and anti-inflammatory effects. The leaves, stems, and flower tops contain more than 10 active ingredients, including salicylic acid, menthol, and camphor. Two major constituents, achilletin and achilleine, are thought to help blood coagulate, while thujone (also found in chamomile) has mild sedative properties. Because yarrow may have diuretic properties, it is sometimes used to treat menstrual bloating and high blood pressure. The somewhat bitter taste of yarrow tea can be relieved by adding sweeteners. A naturalized perennial from Eurasia, yarrow is widely planted in flower and herb gardens. The herb is found growing wild in most areas of the United States.*

### TARGET AILMENTS

**Take internally for** fever, digestive disorders, menstrual cramps, anxiety, insomnia, high blood pressure.

**Apply externally for** minor wounds, bleeding. Use as a douche for vaginal irritations.

### PREPARATIONS

**Over the counter:** Available as dried herb or tea.

**At home:**

Tea: Steep 1 to 2 tsp dried herb in 1 cup boiling water for 10 to 15 minutes. Drink up to 3 cups a day.

### SIDE EFFECTS

**Not serious:** Yarrow may produce a rash or diarrhea. Stop using the herb and consult your doctor.

### SPECIAL INFORMATION

❧ If you are allergic to ragweed, you may develop a rash from ingesting yarrow.

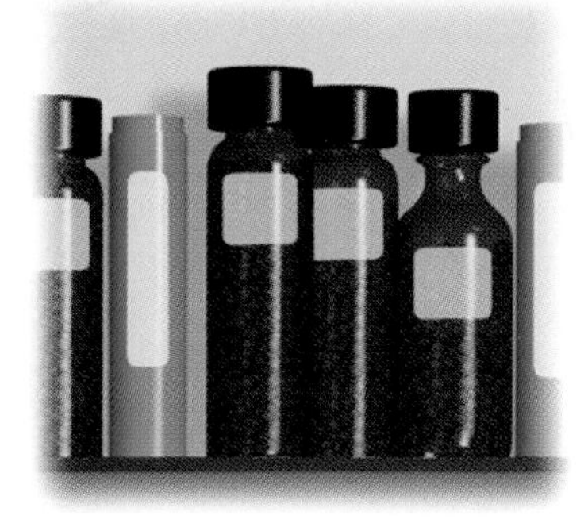

# Homeopathy

Homeopathy is a method of healing based on the idea that like cures like; that is, that substances causing specific symptoms in a healthy person can cure these symptoms in someone who is sick. Also called the law of similars, this principle gives homeopathy its name: "homeo" for similar, "pathy" for disease. The remedies are prepared from plant, mineral, and animal extracts that are highly diluted in a specific way that makes toxicity impossible and, paradoxically, increases their potential to cure.

*Homeopathic treatment, in its principles and procedures, is unlike any other system of medicinal care. Although a few conventional therapies, such as allergy desensitization and immunization, involve the use of "similars" to some degree, modern medicine relies almost exclusively on counteracting substances; laxatives, for example, are medications that work to counteract constipation.*

## Target Ailments

- Allergies
- Arthritis
- Asthma
- Athletic Injuries
- Bladder Infections
- Chronic Fatigue Syndrome
- Common Cold
- Diarrhea
- Earache
- Fever and Chills
- Flu
- Food Poisoning
- Hay Fever
- Headache
- Hemorrhoids
- Insomnia
- Menstrual Problems
- Motion Sickness
- Pneumonia
- Premenstrual Syndrome
- Sore Throat

*See Common Ailments, beginning on page 194.*

## Origins

Modern homeopathy was founded in the 1790s by a German physician named Samuel Hahnemann. Unhappy with existing medical techniques, Hahnemann experimented with small doses of substances known to cure specific diseases. Just as he had suspected, when given to healthy people these substances induced symptoms of the very diseases they were used to treat. In time, Hahnemann developed a method of preparing remedies by diluting small quantities of herbs, minerals, and animal extracts in a water-alcohol solution. The results convinced him that using increasingly smaller amounts of a substance in dilution not only eliminated unwanted side effects but actually boosted the remedy's potency. To unlock these curative powers, though, the solution had to be shaken vigorously. He called his method of preparing remedies potentizing, believing that shaking, or "succussing," the substances released their stores of vital energy.

Hahnemann was not the first to theorize that cures could be fashioned from the causes of disease. In the fifth century BC, the Greek physician Hippocrates described a system of healing by "similars"; this notion of fighting illness with like substances contrasted

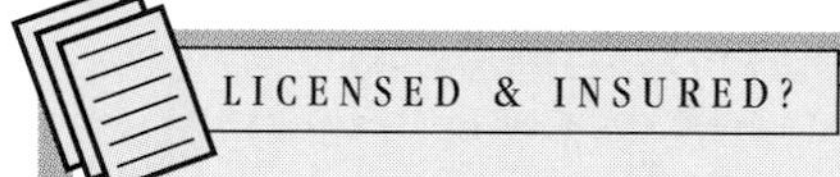

LICENSED & INSURED?

*Licensing varies from state to state for homeopathic practitioners, most of whom have prior medical training, such as a degree in medicine, osteopathy, or naturopathic medicine. The pharmaceuticals they prescribe are recognized and regulated by the FDA. Although many homeopathy products can be purchased over the counter, those offered for treating serious conditions must be dispensed under the supervision of a licensed practitioner.*

with the more orthodox practice of healing by "contraries," or antidotes. Over time, medical practitioners came to rely almost exclusively on contraries, deriving treatments from substances that reverse or work against the actions of particular diseases. Yet the principle of similars persisted in folk medicine for hundreds of years, providing the groundwork for Hahnemann's revolutionary methods.

### Testing the Remedies

Most homeopathic remedies have undergone "provings," or medical trials in which healthy individuals are given doses of undiluted or slightly diluted substances known to cause illnesses. During each test, researchers note the subjects' mental, emotional, and physical changes, which together paint a full picture of the symptoms brought on by a given substance. Responses have been recorded over the years in the materia medica, a master reference collection that gives homeopaths a basis for deciding which remedy is best suited for a patient with a particular set of symptoms.

### What It's Good For

Used for a wide range of conditions, homeopathy is especially effective for noncritical ailments and for those that do not involve severe structural damage or organ destruction. It is also appropriate for diseases for which no effective conventional treatment is available, such as viral illnesses and multiple sclerosis; for ailments that require continuous use of drugs (allergies, arthritis, and digestive problems, for example); and for behavioral and emotional disorders.

Although not every remedy has undergone conventional double-blind drug testing, clinical trials have shown a positive effect for a number of conditions, including hay fever, flu, acute childhood diarrhea, asthma, rheumatoid arthritis, and pain, as well as cardiovascular, respiratory, and gastrointestinal diseases. Further research is being conducted in the United States (under the auspices of the National Institutes of Health) and in a number of other countries.

### Preparations/Techniques

Remedies come in a variety of forms, including tablets, powders, wafers, and liquids in an alcohol base. Recently, over-the-counter combination remedies have become available for common ailments. These products, labeled according to the name of the ailment, allow self-treatment of such minor conditions as insomnia, flu, sore throat, and headache.

The specific dilution of a remedy is the ratio of active substance to inactive base. Ratios containing an *x* indicate that the remedy consists of 1 part mother tincture (concentrated extract) mixed with 9 parts alcohol base; ratios containing a *c* consist of 1 part mother tincture and 99 parts base. Further dilutions are represented

#### CAUTION

**Although homeopathic remedies are too highly diluted to cause toxicity from overdose, taking them for too long a time can cause your symptoms to worsen, and taking ones that are inappropriate for you may cause new symptoms to appear.**



CONTINUED

by a number preceding the *x* or *c*. For example, a remedy labeled 30c has first been mixed 1 part to 99; then, 1 part of the resulting mixture is diluted again with 99 parts of the base, and this process is repeated for a total of 30 times. Modern over-the-counter remedies usually have dilution ratios ranging from 1x to 30c; remedies restricted to professional use generally range from 200c to 1,000,000c.

When taking homeopathic remedies in tablet form, be careful not to touch them. Instead, pour the tablets into the bottle cap, then tip them directly onto or under your tongue. If you spill any tablets, throw them away. Practitioners recommend that the mouth be clean of flavors 15 minutes before and after taking a remedy. Avoid strong flavors and aromas—such as mint, camphor, coffee, and heavily scented perfumes—for the duration of the treatment.

### Visiting a Professional

For chronic problems, most practitioners practice "constitutional" homeopathy, which is based on the idea that the patient's constitution must be considered along with the disease itself. Acute, or short-term, conditions are usually treated with remedies specific to the illness. Typically, the practitioner takes an extensive medical history of the patient, notes the physical and psychological symptoms, then prescribes a single remedy. If this prescription does not have the desired effect, the homeopath performs another analysis and gives a second prescription. Symptom analysis is the key to success; consequently, two patients suffering from the same disorder but displaying different symptoms may receive different prescriptions.

If the correct remedy has been prescribed, healing may begin immediately or within a few days or weeks. When it does, stop taking the remedy, and start again only if your symptoms return. In some cases a prescription will cause what's known as an aggravation, or a temporary worsening of your symptoms. This is usually an indication that the remedy is going to work. Stop taking it and wait for the positive effect.

### Wellness

Homeopathic practitioners often provide constitutional treatments—regimens based on personal and family medical histories—to patients who are not sick but want to maintain or improve their general health.

### What the Critics Say

Critics argue that some homeopathic remedies are so diluted they no longer contain even a single molecule of the original healing substance. Many homeopathic remedies have been proved effective in clinical trials, but opponents attribute any therapeutic success to the placebo effect. The idea that a substance can cure by releasing energy, say skeptics, puts homeopathy in the realm of metaphysics. ■

**FOR MORE INFO**

Following is a list of organizations you can contact to learn more about homeopathy:

**National Center for Homeopathy**
801 North Fairfax Street, #306
Alexandria, VA 22314
(703) 548-7790

**International Foundation for Homeopathy**
PO Box 7
Edmonds, WA 98020
(206) 776-4147

# The 30 Most Effective Homeopathic Remedies

## Aconite • *Aconitum napellus*

Aconite grows throughout the mountainous regions of Europe, Russia, and central Asia, producing clusters of bluish violet flowers that hang from the stem like monks' cowls, giving the plant its common name, monkshood. Highly toxic, aconite was the preferred poison of the ancient Greeks. Administered in very small doses, it produces mental and physical restlessness and tissue inflammation. Homeopathic physicians prescribe *Aconite* for those patients whose symptoms resemble the effects of the poison—who seem distressed or fearful and complain of thirst and unbearable aches and pains that accompany their illnesses.

For homeopathic use, the whole plant—except the root, which is the most poisonous part—is gathered while in full bloom and pounded to a pulp. Juice is pressed from the pulp and mixed with alcohol, then diluted to nontoxic levels.

**TARGET AILMENTS**

Angina, arrhythmia, anxiety induced by sudden shock, arthritis, asthma, bronchitis, colds and flu, croup, fevers with rapid onset and chills that may be accompanied by restlessness or thirst, eye inflammations with burning pain and sensitivity to light, laryngitis, sore throat, middle ear infections, toothaches with a sensitivity to cold water.

## Allium cepa • *Allium cepa*

Cultivated worldwide, *Allium cepa,* otherwise known as red onion, has been used in folk medicine for centuries. This common garden vegetable has been applied to the skin in poultices for acne, arthritis, and congestion, and used internally to clear worms from the intestines. Modern-day herbalists find onion useful for treating conditions as varied as earaches, hemorrhoids, and high blood pressure. Homeopathic practitioners consider *Allium cepa* a remedy for conditions that are accompanied by the same symptoms as those brought on by exposure to red onions—watering eyes and a burning, runny nose.

For the homeopathic preparation, red onions are harvested in midsummer. The bulbs are pounded to a pulp and then mixed with water and alcohol through several stages of extreme dilution.

**TARGET AILMENTS**

Colds with sinus congestion that shifts from side to side in the head; coughs that cause a ripping, tearing pain in the throat; watery and inflamed eyes, hay fever; neuralgic pains; earaches.

## Apis • *Apis mellifica*

The medicinal value of *Apis,* the scientific name for the honeybee, may date back to ancient Egypt, where bees were a symbol of power, wealth, and health. Egyptian doctors revered honey over all other healing substances, and extensive methods of beekeeping were already in practice in 4000 BC. It is not the honey but the bee itself, however, that is used in homeopathic medicine.

This remedy is made from the body of the honeybee; it is used to treat those patients whose ailments are accompanied by symptoms similar to the results of a bee sting, such as redness and swelling, and also patients who express behavior considered beelike, such as restlessness or irritability. To prepare this remedy, the entire live honeybee is crushed and highly diluted by mixing it into a water-and-alcohol base.

**TARGET AILMENTS**

Bites and stings, especially those that burn, itch, or swell; conjunctivitis; edema (accumulation of fluids in body tissues) and conditions of general swelling such as hives and food allergies; headaches that include sudden, stabbing pains; red, swollen joints; mumps.



CONTINUED

# The 30 Most Effective Homeopathic Remedies

## Arnica • *Arnica montana*

Arnica, sometimes called mountain daisy, grows wild across the higher elevations of Europe, northern Asia, and parts of the United States. Mountain climbers in the Alps have traditionally chewed arnica after a long day's hike to relieve muscle aches. Homeopathic practitioners prescribe *Arnica* for bruises, sprains, strains, and other types of accidents that are sudden and may induce shock. The flowers, leaves, stem, and root of arnica are crushed to a pulp and soaked in alcohol before undergoing the homeopathic dilution process, which renders the substance nontoxic.

**TARGET AILMENTS**

Blood blisters; broken bones, sprains, strains, and other sudden injuries with swelling, tenderness, and pain where post-trauma shock is a threat; bruises; sore and swollen joints, as in rheumatism; head pain; toothache and pain from dental work; groin strain.

## Arsenicum album • *Arsenicum album*

This remedy, also called *Ars alb* by homeopathic practitioners, is an extremely dilute form of arsenic, a metallic poison derived from the chemical element of the same name. Weak preparations of arsenic have had a history of medicinal use; but slow accumulation of the element in body tissues can cause chronic poisoning, leading to gastrointestinal disorders, nausea, dehydration, and even paralysis and death. In step with the homeopathic theory that like cures like, *Ars alb* is preferred by practitioners to treat patients with various digestive complaints that are accompanied by signs of dehydration and burning pains, the same symptoms that are induced by arsenic.

In its homeopathic form, arsenic is separated from other metals like iron, cobalt, and nickel by baking at high temperatures. The extracted powder is then finely ground and weakened by mixing successively greater amounts of lactose (milk sugar) with the poison.

**TARGET AILMENTS**

Angina; anxiety disorders and panic attacks; asthma; hay fever; burns that form blisters; chronic skin problems; high fevers accompanied by chills; recurrent headaches; dry, hacking coughs; colds accompanied by excessive, watery nasal discharge and frequent sneezing; colitis, indigestion, food poisoning, Crohn's disease; influenza; insomnia; exhaustion from an illness coupled with restlessness.

## Belladonna • *Belladonna*

Belladonna, a highly toxic plant also known as deadly nightshade, grows wild across Europe, producing yellow flowers in July and dark red berries in late summer. Its name, meaning "beautiful woman" in Italian, dates from the Renaissance, when ladies of Italy dilated their pupils with belladonna eye drops for a doe-eyed appearance. Belladonna poisoning brings on a range of symptoms, including a dry mouth and hot, flushed skin, nausea, convulsive movements, and delirium. Homeopathic practitioners prescribe *Belladonna* for illnesses that are accompanied by these same symptoms. All parts of the belladonna plant are gathered for use in the homeopathic remedy. The plant is crushed and pressed, and the extracted juice is mixed with alcohol in an extremely dilute preparation.

**TARGET AILMENTS**

Common cold, flu, sore throat, painful earache, high fever with chills but with no thirst, acute inflammatory arthritis, acute bursitis, gallstones, colic, measles, mumps, acute diverticulitis, neuralgia, sunstroke, acutely inflamed varicose veins, painful toothache, painful menstrual periods, teething pains, breast-feeding complications.

## Bryonia • *Bryonia alba*

Bryonia, or wild hops, is a creeping vine commonly found along hedgerows and in forests across southern Europe. Its medicinal value was known to the Greeks, who used the root as a purgative and may have given the plant its name, derived from *bryo,* meaning "to thrust or sprout," a reference to how quickly the vine grows. Accidental ingestion of the root can cause tissue inflammation, severe vomiting, and diarrhea violent enough to cause death. Homeopathic physicians prescribe their dilute solutions of *Bryonia* for illnesses that are accompanied by similar symptoms. The homeopathic remedy is prepared from the root, which is harvested in early spring. An extract pressed from the root pulp is mixed with alcohol into an extremely dilute solution.

**TARGET AILMENTS**

Arthritis with sharp, sticking pains; backaches centered in the small of the back; bursitis; colds accompanied by chest congestion; painful coughs; sore throat with pain upon swallowing; influenza; severe headaches worsened by light, sound, or motion; dizziness; nausea, vomiting, constipation, gastritis, acute diverticulitis, stomach flu; inflammation during breast-feeding.

## Calcarea carbonica • *Calcarea carbonica*

Calcarea carbonica, or calcium carbonate, is a source of calcium, one of the most abundant natural elements in the human body. Essential to cell structure and bone strength, calcium comes from many materials, including chalk, coral, and limestone. Perhaps as a reflection of its body-building properties, *Calcarea carbonica,* also called *Calc carb,* is used by homeopathic physicians for conditions that are accompanied by symptoms of exhaustion, depression, and anxiety. Calcium carbonate prepared for homeopathic use is ground from oyster shells and used at full strength.

**TARGET AILMENTS**

Lower-back pain, broken bones, sprains, muscle cramps, constipation, chronic ear infections, eye inflammations, headaches, insomnia, eczema, allergies, teething problems, gastritis, gallstones, childhood diarrhea, menstrual problems, asthma, palpitations, arthritis.

## Cantharis • *Cantharis*

Popularly known as Spanish fly, cantharis is actually a beetle found in southern France and Spain. It produces an irritant so caustic that the skin will blister if exposed to it.

Cantharis has had a long career in medicine and has been used for all manner of disorders. In high concentrations the irritant can be toxic, prompting abdominal cramps and burning pains in the throat and stomach, vomiting of blood, diarrhea, kidney damage, convulsions, coma, and death. Homeopaths prescribe *Cantharis* for patients whose ailments are coupled with symptoms like those of cantharis poisoning.

According to homeopathic tradition, the beetles are collected at daybreak, when they are still sluggish from the cool of the night, and heated in the steam of boiling vinegar until dead. The beetles are then crushed and mixed with successively greater amounts of milk sugar, a pharmaceutical process called trituration. The resulting powder is highly dilute.

**TARGET AILMENTS**

Bladder infections or cystitis, with a constant desire to urinate accompanied by blood and pain during urination; sunburns, scalds, and blistering second-degree burns.



CONTINUED

# The 30 Most Effective Homeopathic Remedies

## Chamomilla • *Chamomilla*

*Chamomilla* is made from the flowering German chamomile plant common in Europe. The whole plant is crushed, and its juices are mixed with equal parts of alcohol, then succussed. In homeopathy *Chamomilla* is considered to work best for people who are extremely sensitive to pain, irritable, impatient, and implacable. *Chamomilla* patients sweat easily and are sensitive to wind and chills. *Chamomilla* is most often given to children who work themselves into violent temper tantrums.

**TARGET AILMENTS**

Irritability; toothaches aggravated by cold air and warm food; painful menstrual periods with severe cramping and a feeling of anger or restlessness; extremely painful earaches; teething pain, especially if the child is irritable; difficulty getting to sleep.

## Ferrum phosphoricum • *Ferrum phosphoricum*

Ferrum phosphoricum, also called ferrum phos or iron phosphate, is a mineral compound of iron and phosphorus. Both elements are present in the body independently; iron aids the exchange of oxygen in the blood, and phosphorus contributes to bone and muscle health. Ferrum phos is derived from mixing solutions of iron sulfate, phosphate, and sodium acetate. The resulting iron phosphate is ground with large quantities of lactose (milk sugar) to render it nontoxic. Homeopathic practitioners consider *Ferrum phos* good for patients who suffer from conditions accompanied by low energy and anemia.

**TARGET AILMENTS**

Tickling, hacking coughs with chest pain, headaches, fevers that begin slowly, ear infections, incontinence, rheumatic joints, early menstrual periods accompanied by headaches, anemia, fatigue, nosebleeds, sore throat, vomiting, diarrhea, palpitations.

## Gelsemium • *Gelsemium sempervirens*

Sometimes called yellow jasmine, gelsemium is not really part of the jasmine family but is related to the plants ignatia and nux vomica. A climbing vine with trumpetlike yellow flowers, it is common in the woods and coastal shoreline of the southern United States. Taken in large doses, gelsemium causes paralysis of the motor nerves, impairing physical and mental functions like vision, balance, thought, and movement; ultimately, poisoning causes convulsions and death. Homeopathic physicians prescribe dilute solutions of gelsemium for ailments that are accompanied by symptoms like those of gelsemium poisoning. In its homeopathic form *Gelsemium* is prepared from the fresh root, which is chopped, soaked in alcohol, strained, and diluted to the desired, highly dilute potencies.

**TARGET AILMENTS**

Anxiety; flu with aches, chills, and exhaustion; headache beginning in the back of the head and moving forward; measles; sore throat; fever with chills that move up and down the spine, although the patient may not feel cold.

## Hepar sulphuris • *Hepar sulphuris calcareum*

The flaky inner layer of oyster shells provides the calcium used in this homeopathic remedy, also called *Hepar sulph* and commonly known as calcium sulfide. Once an antidote for mercury poisoning, *Hepar sulphuris* is now used by homeopathic physicians to treat patients with conditions that tend to be infected, often producing pus. These disorders are accompanied by symptoms that include mental and physical hypersensitivity and an intolerance of pain and cold.

Finely ground oyster shell and sulfur are mixed together and then heated in an airtight container. The resulting powder is dissolved in hot hydrochloric acid, then combined with lactose (milk sugar) in a pharmaceutical process of dilution called trituration.

**TARGET AILMENTS**

Abscesses that are swollen and painful but have not yet opened; colds, sore throat, and earache; inflamed cuts and wounds that may be taking longer than normal to heal; aching joints; fits of coughing with chest pain, hoarseness, asthma, emphysema, croup; genital herpes; constipation.

## Hypericum • *Hypericum perforatum*

Also known as St.-John's-wort, hypericum grows in woodlands across Europe, Asia, and the United States, blooming with a profusion of yellow flowers from June to September. The flowers, if bruised, bleed a reddish juice. The dark green leaves of the plant are dotted with oil-producing pores. According to ancient healing wisdom, because hypericum seemed to resemble skin, with its pores and its simulation of bleeding on injury, it was considered ideal for all manner of flesh wounds. *(See St.-John's-wort, page 100.)* In homeopathy *Hypericum* is often prescribed for bodily injuries, among other conditions, but it is selected for the soothing effect it is said to have on injured nerves rather than for any traditional reason.

For homeopathic use the entire plant is harvested in summer, when its yellow flowers are in full bloom. It is pounded to a pulp and soaked in an alcohol solution before being weakened to the desired potencies through a vigorous dilution process.

**TARGET AILMENTS**

Backaches centered along the lower spine that may include shooting pains; bites and stings from animals and insects, especially when they have become inflamed or include nerve damage; cuts and wounds in nerve-rich parts of the body, like the fingers and lips, caused by accidents or surgery.

## Ignatia • *Ignatia amara*

The beans of this plant, sometimes called St. Ignatius bean, are in fact seeds from the fruit of a small tree native to China and the Philippines. Spanish missionaries in the Philippines were introduced to the seeds by the locals, who wore them as amulets to ward off disease. Small doses of the seed can produce mild but unpleasant symptoms of poisoning, including increased salivation, pounding headache, cramps, giddiness, twitching, and trembling; large doses can be fatal. Homeopaths may prescribe *Ignatia,* a dilute solution of the seed, for ailments that include symptoms like those associated with mild poisoning.

For the homeopathic preparation, the seeds are collected and ground to a powder, then mixed with alcohol. When the powder is saturated, the mixture is strained and diluted until it becomes a nontoxic substance.

**TARGET AILMENTS**

Anxiety; dry, tickling coughs; a sore throat that feels like there is a lump in it; painful tension headaches; indigestion; insomnia; irritable bowel syndrome; painful hemorrhoids; effects of grief, shock, or disappointment, or depression where the patient tends to sigh frequently.



CONTINUED

## Ipecac • *Ipecacuanha*

The *ipecacuanha* shrub, native to Central and South America, was named by Portuguese colonists, who called it "roadside sick-making plant" in recognition of its ability to induce vomiting. Varying dosages of its root can produce a variety of symptoms, including mild appetite stimulation, sweating, expectoration, vomiting, gastritis, inflammation of the lungs, and cardiac failure. Other health disorders can display symptoms similar to those of mild ipecac poisoning, and it is these symptoms that homeopathic practitioners hope to counteract when they prescribe *Ipecac.*

The homeopathic remedy is made from the root, the most potent part of the plant. The root is dried and then ground into a coarse powder, which is diluted either in milk sugar to be used as a dry substance or in a water-and-alcohol base. Both preparations are weakened to a nontoxic level.

**TARGET AILMENTS**

Persistent nausea, vomiting, motion sickness; menstrual problems; asthma; dry, irritating cough accompanied by wheezing; diarrhea; flu with nausea; colic; gastroenteritis.

## Kali bichromicum • *Kali bichromicum*

Kali bichromicum is often called potassium bichromate; it is a chemical compound that may be acquired from chromium iron ore or by processing potassium chromate with one of a number of strong acids. A highly corrosive substance, it is used primarily in textile dyeing, in the staining of wood, and as a component in electric batteries. It is also a very powerful poison. Homeopathic practitioners believe *Kali bichromicum* works best for conditions that are accompanied by the symptom of pain in a distinct spot, where the ache is easily located with a fingertip.

For homeopathic use this caustic chemical, also called *Kali bi,* is diluted to nontoxic levels with large amounts of milk sugar, a pharmaceutical process called trituration.

**TARGET AILMENTS**

Acute bronchitis, colds in which there is a thick mucus discharge and a heavy cough that produces pain in the chest, croup, sinusitis and resulting headaches, indigestion, pains in the joints.

## Lachesis • *Lachesis*

The South American bushmaster snake grows to a length of seven feet and kills its prey, both animal and human, by constriction or by injection of its highly poisonous venom, known as lachesis, from which this homeopathic remedy is derived. Small doses of the venom can destroy red blood cells and impair the clotting of blood. Larger amounts of lachesis poison the heart. Homeopathic practitioners believe that the conditions best treated with *Lachesis* are those accompanied by symptoms similar to the ones induced by the venom. To prepare the homeopathic remedy, venom is extracted from the snake and diluted in large quantities of lactose (milk sugar).

**TARGET AILMENTS**

Choking coughs, croup, a constricted feeling in the throat, earaches that are worse during swallowing, left-sided sore throats, indigestion, throbbing headaches, especially those that appear during menopause, insomnia, hot flashes, heart arrhythmias, hemorrhoids, sciatica.

# The 30 Most Effective Homeopathic Remedies

## Ledum • *Ledum palustre*

Ledum, sometimes called marsh tea, can be found in bogs across northern Europe, Canada, and the United States. The herb has an antiseptic smell, and its upper branches are covered with a coat of tiny brown hairs. These may have given ledum its name; in Greek, *ledos* means "woolly robe." Once used in Scandinavia for insect control, ledum has also served as a tea substitute and replaced hops in beer, although overconsumption has resulted in dizziness and a splitting headache—even before the hangover. Homeopathic practitioners consider dilute doses of *Ledum* helpful for conditions that may be accompanied by signs of infection or inflammation.

The homeopathic remedy is prepared from the whole plant, which is gathered, dried, and crushed to a powder. This is diluted to nontoxic levels in a water-and-alcohol mix.

**TARGET AILMENTS**

Animal bites or insect stings, bruises that have already discolored the skin, deep cuts or puncture wounds where there is danger of infection, gout, aching joints.

## Lycopodium • *Lycopodium clavatum*

Lycopodium, also known as club moss, grows in pastures and woodlands throughout Great Britain, northern Europe, and North America. Its spores contain a highly flammable pollen that was once used in fireworks and other pyrotechnics. Powder made from its ground-up spores has been used for internal complaints like diarrhea and dysentery since the 17th century. Homeopathic physicians use dilute doses of *Lycopodium* for complaints that are accompanied by symptoms of digestive upset, ailments that seem to develop on the right side of the body, a strong desire for sweets, anxiety, and symptoms that worsen in the early evening. To create the homeopathic remedy, pollen is extracted from the spores and diluted with milk sugar.

**TARGET AILMENTS**

Backache with stiffness and soreness in the lower back, bedwetting, colds with stuffy nose, constipation, coughs with mucus, cystitis, headache with throbbing pain, gout, indigestion accompanied by abdominal cramps, gas, heartburn, joint pain, sciatica, right-sided sore throat, eczema.

## Mercurius vivus • *Mercurius vivus*

One of the metallic chemical elements, mercury, also called quicksilver, was known in ancient Chinese and Hindu civilizations and has had a long history of medicinal use. Ingesting certain mercury compounds can cause increased perspiration and salivation; and so in ancient medicine mercury was used, along with bloodletting and purging, as a means of ridding the body of impurities. Undilute mercury is toxic, however, and severe symptoms of mercury poisoning may include nausea, inflammation of the digestive tract, and kidney failure.

Homeopathic practitioners prescribe *Merc viv,* as the homeopathic preparation of mercury is sometimes called, for conditions accompanied by symptoms of shaking, hot and cold sweats, and restlessness. *Merc viv* is made from the chemical element mercury by dilution with large quantities of milk sugar.

**TARGET AILMENTS**

Abscesses, especially dental or glandular; backache with burning, shooting pains in the lower back; chickenpox; colds with an exceptionally runny nose and pain in the nostrils; cystitis with slow urination; painful diarrhea; influenza; earache with discharge of pus; eye inflammation; indigestion; mouth ulcers; burning sore throat; toothache with increased salivation.



CONTINUED

## Natrum muriaticum • *Natrum muriaticum*

*Natrum muriaticum* is simply salt, or sodium chloride, a substance present in the natural world in quantities greater than any other except water. Essential to life and health, salt has been valued in human commerce throughout history. Roman soldiers were given a stipend, called a salarium, which they used to buy salt; from this we get the word *salary.* Homeopaths prescribe dilute solutions of *Nat mur,* as they call it, for conditions that are coupled with symptoms of extreme thirst, emotional sensitivity, and a strong desire for salt.

*Nat mur* is prepared by adding pure sodium chloride to boiling water. Once the salt has dissolved, the solution is filtered and crystallized by evaporation. The final product is diluted in water to the desired potency.

**TARGET AILMENTS**

Backaches that are relieved by firm pressure; cold sores, especially in the corners of the mouth; colds with sneezing, watery eyes, and runny nose; constipation; fevers accompanied by weakness and chills; genital herpes; eczema; anemia; hay fever; migraine headaches; menstrual irregularity; indigestion; depression caused by grief, with a desire to be alone.

## Nux vomica • *Nux vomica*

Nux vomica, also known as poison nut, is a remedy made from the seeds of an evergreen tree indigenous to parts of India, Thailand, China, and Australia. The seeds contain strychnine and have a bitter, unpleasant taste. Small doses of the seed stimulate the appetite, while somewhat larger doses decrease the appetite and cause motor dysfunction, including stiffness in the arms and legs and a staggering walk. Toxic doses can cause convulsions and death. *Nux vomica* is prescribed by homeopaths for ailments that occur from overindulgence in food, coffee, or alcohol, usually accompanied by irritability. To prepare the homeopathic remedy, poison-nut seeds are ground to a powder and then diluted with milk sugar to the desired potency.

**TARGET AILMENTS**

Colic and stomach cramps from overeating, colds with sneezing and a stuffy nose, constipation, cystitis, headache with dizziness, fevers with chills, gas and gas pains, hangovers, indigestion, insomnia, irritable bowel syndrome, nausea, menstrual cramps with a heavy flow, sinusitis, stomach flu, vomiting from overeating or eating rich foods.

## Phosphorus • *Phosphorus*

The chemical element phosphorus can be found in the cellular fluid of all living tissue. Phosphorus plays a vital role in the activity of the body's cells, most importantly in the transfer of genetic information. Many phosphorus compounds are used commercially in toothpaste, fertilizer, and laundry detergent. Phosphorus poisoning causes irritation of the mucous membranes and inflammation of tissue; over time, it can destroy bone. As a homeopathic remedy, minute doses are prescribed by practitioners for conditions accompanied by symptoms of fatigue and nervousness with a tendency to bleed easily and an unquenchable thirst for cold water. Pure phosphorus is diluted in large quantities of milk sugar to prepare the homeopathic remedy.

**TARGET AILMENTS**

Bronchitis, pneumonia, coughs with congestion and burning pains in the chest, visual problems resulting from eyestrain, gastritis, nosebleeds, indigestion accompanied by vomiting or pain, stomach ulcers, kidney infections, nasal polyps, hepatitis, anemia, hemorrhages, diarrhea, menstrual problems.

# The 30 Most Effective Homeopathic Remedies

## Pulsatilla • *Pulsatilla nigricans*

Common in the meadowlands of northern and central Europe, the pulsatilla, or windflower, contains a caustic substance, and chewing the plant may cause blisters in the mouth and throat. Homeopathic physicians often prescribe *Pulsatilla* to patients with conditions accompanied by a thick yellow or white discharge. For homeopathic use the plant is collected when in full bloom and pounded to a pulp. The pulp is steeped in an alcohol-and-water solution and then strained and diluted.

**TARGET AILMENTS**

Bedwetting, breast infections, chickenpox, coughs, headaches, eye inflammation, fever with chills, hay fever, incontinence, indigestion, aching joints that improve with movement and cold compresses, urethritis in men, late menstrual periods, otitis media, sciatica, sinusitis, varicose veins, depression.

## Rhus toxicodendron • *Rhus toxicodendron*

This vinelike shrub, also known as poison ivy, grows throughout North America and is well known for the itchy red rash its oil can cause on the skin. The medicinal history of its leaves and stalk began in the late 18th century, when it was used to treat conditions such as paralysis and rheumatism. The effects of its undilute form can range from a rash to nausea, fever, delirium, swollen glands, and ulcers in the oral cavity. For this reason homeopathic practitioners use *Rhus toxicodendron,* or *Rhus tox,* as it is also called, to treat conditions that may be accompanied by fever, restlessness, and swollen glands.

*Rhus tox* is prepared from plants gathered at night, when the oil is said to be in its most potent state. The leaves and stalks are pounded to a pulp and mixed with alcohol, then strained and diluted.

**TARGET AILMENTS**

Arthritis with stiffness that is worse in the morning and better with motion; backache with stiffness along the spine; bursitis; carpal tunnel syndrome; eye inflammation with swelling, itching, and sticky matter; genital herpes; hamstring injury; influenza with painful joints; headaches; hives that itch, sting, and intensify after scratching; joint and back pains from overexertion; impetigo; poison ivy; sprains with stiffness; toothaches.

## Ruta • *Ruta graveolens*

Native to southern Europe, ruta spread across the continent in the wake of the Romans, who valued it for its medicinal properties. *Ruta* comes from the Greek *reuo,* meaning "to set free," an allusion to its historical popularity as a cure for numerous complaints, including headaches, coughs, and croup. Through centuries of use, this small shrub, sometimes called rue or rue bitterwort, has spread to herb gardens worldwide.

In large doses, ruta has toxic properties, but homeopathic physicians prescribe minute doses to treat conditions or injuries that may be accompanied by symptoms of weakness or a bruised sensation. The plant is collected just before blossoming; it is pounded to a pulp and pressed for its juice, which is then diluted in a water-and-alcohol base.

**TARGET AILMENTS**

Carpal tunnel syndrome, eyestrain caused by overwork and accompanied by heat and pain, sciatica, groin strain, sprains with pain and a bruised sensation, tennis elbow, injuries of tendons and cartilage.



CONTINUED

## Sepia • *Sepia*

The cuttlefish is a soft-bodied mollusk with eight arms that is closely related to the squid and octopus; it propels itself by squirting jets of water from special organs in its body. When threatened, it releases spurts of dark ink called sepia that cloud the water and camouflage its retreat. Sepia has been used for artistic purposes, although its ingestion, such as when a painter licks the brush, can bring about unpleasant side effects. Homeopathic physicians prescribe *Sepia* to patients with conditions whose symptoms include apathy, moodiness, and weakness. The cuttlefish ink is collected for the homeopathic preparation and diluted with large quantities of milk sugar for final use.

**TARGET AILMENTS**

Backaches and weakness in the small of the back; violent fits of coughing; cold sores and fever blisters around the mouth; exhaustion; genital herpes; hair loss; gas; headaches with throbbing pain; sinusitis; urinary incontinence; menopausal hot flashes; menstrual cramps with intense, bearing-down pain; nausea resulting from motion sickness or during pregnancy; brown spots on the skin.

## Silica • *Silica*

Silica, also called flint, is a mineral that is present in the human body in only trace amounts but is vital to the development of bones, the flexibility of cartilage, and the health of the skin and connective tissues. Many industrial operations rely on silica, including the manufacture of concrete, paper, glass, and enamelware. Flint's medicinal use is limited to homeopathy. Minute doses are prescribed for patients with conditions accompanied by excessive sweating, weakness, and extreme sensitivity to cold. For homeopathic use silica powder is mixed with sodium carbonate through a pharmaceutical process of dry substance dilution.

**TARGET AILMENTS**

Athlete's foot, constipation, wounds that have been inflamed by foreign matter, earache with decreased hearing and a stopped-up sensation, fingernails that have white spots and split easily, headaches beginning in the back of the head and spreading forward to the eyes, abscesses, swollen glands in the neck, gum infections, hemorrhoids, breast cysts.

## Sulphur • *Sulphur*

The chemical element sulphur, or more commonly, "sulfur," is present in all living tissue. It was known to ancient societies, and in the Bible it is called brimstone. Among the various conditions to which it has been applied as a medication for some 2,000 years are skin disorders such as scabies. Commercially, sulfur is used in the production of dyes, fungicides, and gunpowder. Homeopathic physicians may prescribe dilute doses of the remedy *Sulphur* to treat conditions accompanied by irritability, intense itching, burning pains, and offensive odors. The homeopathic remedy is made from pure sulfur powder that is diluted with either milk sugar or a water-and-alcohol solution.

**TARGET AILMENTS**

Asthma that is worse at night and is accompanied by rattling mucus, cough with chest pain, morning diarrhea, eye inflammation, bursitis, headaches with burning pain, indigestion, joint pain, anal itching with redness, burning vaginal discharge, eczema with intense itching and burning.

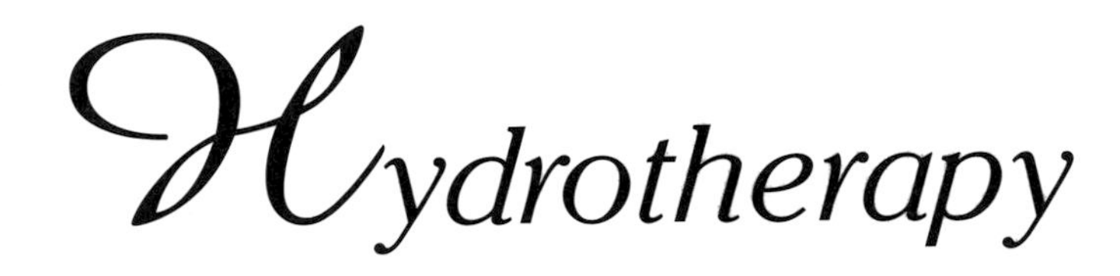

# Hydrotherapy

*Hydrotherapy, which literally means water therapy, encompasses a variety of therapeutic uses of water. As either ice, liquid, or steam, water may relieve the symptoms of numerous types of infections, acute and chronic pain, circulatory problems, and more. External hydrotherapy treatments typically involve applications of hot or cold water (or the alternation of both) to the skin. Internal treatments consist of water taken internally as a cleansing agent.*

*Treatments range from the homey footbath to sophisticated physical therapy in a hospital pool, and can include wraps, sprays, and douches, as well as the use of steam rooms, saunas, and hot and cold baths. In general, the aim is to stimulate an immune response or to detoxify the body by changing body temperature.*

## *Origins*

Using water as a source of healing is a concept as old as civilization itself. In its modern form, hydrotherapy came to the United States from Germany, where the 19th-century passion for spas and water treatments influenced such healers as the Austrian peasant Vincenz Priessnitz, the founder of hydrotherapy; and Father Sebastian Kneipp, the originator of "Kneipp's cure," which employed forms of hydrotherapy. By the turn of the century, the term "water cure" had become a catchall phrase for many forms of natural healing. Ultimately, hydrotherapy became one of the key treatments of naturopathy *(pages 141-143)*, and today, outside the home, it is practiced primarily by naturopathic doctors and physical therapists.

### *What It's Good For*

Hydrotherapy has a wide range of applications, but it is particularly useful for treating muscle and joint pain and inflammation, burns and frostbite, fevers, sinusitis, headaches, the upper respiratory tract, indigestion, pelvic pain, and stress. In pools and whirlpool baths, hydrotherapy treatment is also used to strengthen limbs after injury. Internal hydrotherapy can ease digestive problems and help detoxify the blood.

**LICENSED & INSURED?**

*Many of the techniques of hydrotherapy are practiced by licensed and insured conventional doctors, nurses, and physical therapists. For a broader-based approach to hydrotherapy as primary care, patients can visit naturopathic doctors (NDs), who practice throughout the United States and are licensed in the states of Alaska, Arizona, Connecticut, Hawaii, Maine, Montana, New Hampshire, Oregon, Utah, Vermont, and Washington. Some, but not all, insurance plans cover treatments from NDs.*

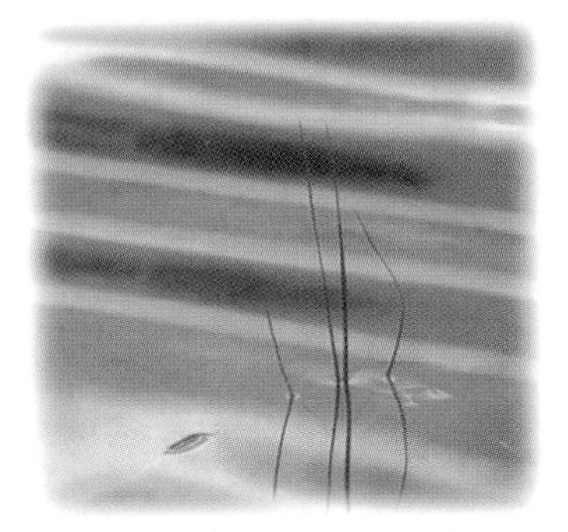

## Target Ailments

- Arthritis
- Athletic Injuries
- Bursitis
- Circulatory Problems
- Common Cold
- Fever and Chills
- Headache
- Hemorrhoids
- Indigestion
- Muscle Cramps
- Pain, Chronic
- Rashes and Skin Problems
- Sinusitis
- Stress
- Tendinitis
- Varicose Veins

*See Common Ailments, beginning on page 194.*



CONTINUED

# Hydrotherapy CONTINUED

## Preparations/Techniques

External hydrotherapy relies primarily on the effects of water temperature—hot, neutral, cold, or alternating hot and cold—to produce its effects. Hot water soothes and relaxes while stimulating the immune system. Neutral or body-temperature baths are also soothing, particularly for people with stress and insomnia. Cold water discourages inflammation and fever, while the contrast of hot and cold can improve circulation and reduce congestion.

A practitioner might recommend treatments either at a facility with the right kinds of pools and whirlpool tubs, or at home. Some treatments should take place under the watchful eye of a trained physician or therapist—hyperthermia, for example, which is a fever-inducing therapy for patients fighting viruses and infections. Paraplegics, those suffering from burns and frostbite, and anyone with diminished sensation also need to work with therapists if they are being treated in baths.

However, many of the treatments of hydrotherapy can easily be done at home. A simple example is the cold compress. For an inflamed joint or a feverish headache, take a terry cloth washcloth, wring it out in ice water, and apply it to the afflicted area. As the cloth warms up, chill it down again and repeat.

To improve immune function and for general stimulation, a hydrotherapist might suggest immediately following a hot shower with a cold one. Or if a handheld hose or sprayer is available, you can hook up the sprayer to a faucet after a hot shower and spray (or ask a friend to spray) cold water along both sides of the spine.

Hydrotherapists may also recommend adding therapeutic herbs and oils to the bath. Among them could be chamomile to soothe the skin, oatmeal for hives or sunburn, or ginger for relaxation. *(See Herbal Therapies, pages 70-73).*

## Wellness

Proponents of hydrotherapy believe that a healthy body maintains a certain internal balance. In order to keep this stability, it must constantly adjust to environmental influences such as heat, cold, food and water, and clothing. Water therapies enhance and reinforce the body's reaction to these external influences, helping it to stay well.

## What the Critics Say

Most forms of external hydrotherapy—whirlpool baths, cold compresses, and the like—are widely accepted by the medical establishment. Internal hydrotherapy, particularly the use of enemas and colonic irrigation, comes in for more criticism, however. Critics say that such methods have little scientific justification and that they can actually spread infection if not carefully applied. ■

### CAUTION

**Pregnant women, as well as those with diabetes, atherosclerosis, or a decreased sensitivity to hot and cold, should consult a doctor before using any heat therapies. When using hot water or hot packs, you should always test the temperature first to make sure it won't burn. Avoid using the microwave for heating: It can result in irregular hot and cold spots.**

### FOR MORE INFO

Following is a list of organizations you can contact to learn more about hydrotherapy:

**National College of Naturopathic Medicine**
11231 SE Market Street
Portland, OR 97216
(503) 255-4860

**Bastyr University of Natural Health Sciences**
14500 Juanita Drive, NE
Bothell, WA 98011
(206) 523-9585

**Southwest College of Naturopathic Medicine**
2140 East Broadway Road
Tempe, AZ 85251
(602) 858-9100

**Uchee Pines Lifestyle Center**
30 Uchee Pines Road, Box 75
Seale, AL 36875
Phone: (334) 855-4764

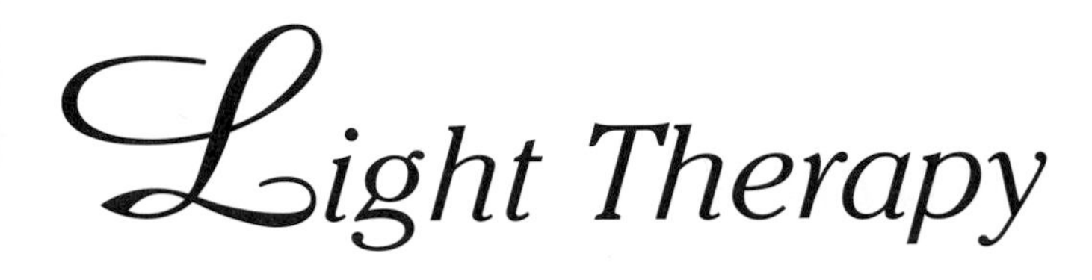

# Light Therapy

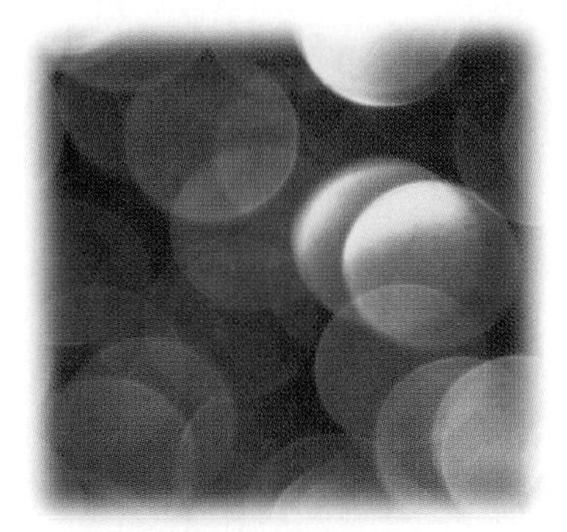

*Simply put, light therapy is the use of natural or artificial light to promote healing. Specific techniques differ primarily in the type of light involved. Full-spectrum light therapy consists of regular exposure to controlled amounts of either natural sunlight or artificial light that contains all wavelengths of light, from infrared to ultraviolet. Bright light therapy involves exposure to nonultraviolet white light in levels that match the amount of natural sunlight found outdoors shortly after sunrise or before sunset. In cold laser therapy, small beams of low-intensity laser light are applied directly to the skin. Colored light therapy focuses different colored lights on the skin.*

## *The Importance of Light*

Recent research indicates that for the body to be healthy, it must receive adequate exposure to the full and balanced spectrum of light found in natural sunlight. Adequate light is especially needed for the regulation of circadian rhythms, the daily internal pacemakers that govern a host of biological functions in humans, from hormone production to patterns of sleeping and waking. In healthy people, these rhythms run in regular cycles, reset each morning by the light of the rising sun. If the rhythms become disturbed for any reason, health problems can result.

## *Origins*

Sunlight has been used for healing throughout history. The ancient Greek physician Hippocrates prescribed sunlight for certain disorders, often sending his patients to recuperate in roofless buildings. During the Middle Ages, red light was a popular treatment for smallpox. The windows of sickrooms were covered with red curtains, and patients were wrapped in red sheets. Doctors started using bright light therapy for seasonal affective disorder and other ailments beginning in the 1980s.

## *What It's Good For*

Full-spectrum light therapy is used to treat various ailments, including high blood pressure, rashes and skin problems, depression, insomnia, PMS, migraines, jaundice in newborns, and jet lag. Bright light therapy has been shown to be highly effective in treating seasonal affective disorder (SAD), a form of depression that strikes

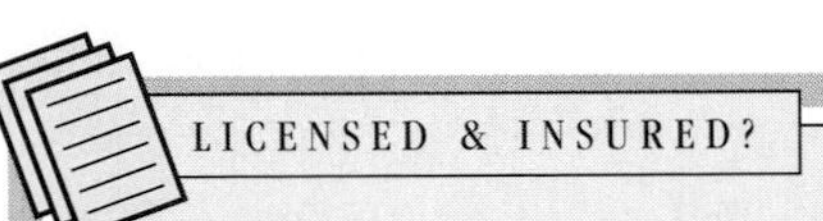

**LICENSED & INSURED?**

*Sometimes. In some states, light therapists may need a license. Insurers often reimburse for the cost of the lighting systems used to treat seasonal affective disorder and skin problems, if the lights are prescribed by a physician.*

### Target Ailments

- Arthritis
- Carpal Tunnel Syndrome
- Depression
- Headache
- High Blood Pressure
- Insomnia
- Menstrual Problems
- Pain, Chronic
- Premenstrual Syndrome
- Rashes and Skin Problems
- Seasonal Affective Disorder
- Stress
- Tendinitis

*See Common Ailments, beginning on page 194.*



CONTINUED

# Light Therapy CONTINUED

people during winter, when days are short. Bright light therapy is also used to treat bulimia, irregular menstrual cycles, and sleep disorders. Cold laser therapy is used primarily to relieve chronic pain and help heal wounds, but it is also a part of laser acupuncture, a form of acupuncture that addresses a variety of health concerns. Colored light therapy is used for depression, sleep problems, chronic pain, stress, menstrual problems, arthritis, tendinitis, sore throat, and hives and insect bites.

### *Preparations/Techniques*

Most light therapy can be self-administered, either by spending more time outdoors or by purchasing special therapeutic lights and then following the directions that come with them. Full-spectrum light therapy is accomplished indoors by installing full-spectrum lighting in place of incandescent and fluorescent lighting, which lacks the complete balanced spectrum of sunlight. Bright light therapy requires that you sit near a light box, usually for about 30 minutes, early in the morning from late fall through early spring. Cold lasers are held over the affected area of the body for specified lengths of time, generally no more than a few minutes. The treatment is then repeated once or twice a day for several days or until the condition improves. Some forms of colored light therapy also involve directing small beams of light, usually red, over the area of the body that needs healing. Another method involves bathing the body with colored light from filtered floodlights.

### *Visiting a Professional*

You may find it useful to consult a knowledgeable healthcare professional about applying some forms of light therapy to your particular health concern. Before using bright light therapy for the treatment of SAD, you should see a healthcare professional skilled in the diagnosis and treatment of that illness. Ultraviolet light therapy treatments for dermatitis, psoriasis, and other skin problems should be administered only by a professional.

### *Wellness*

People who use light therapy report that it reduces stress and relaxes and rejuvenates the body, thus contributing to an overall feeling of physical and mental well-being. Research has also shown that exposure to full-spectrum and bright light helps promote wellness by keeping the body's biological rhythms synchronized.

### *What the Critics Say*

Although the use of light therapy for the treatment of seasonal affective disorder and skin problems is widely accepted, other forms of light therapy have not undergone rigorous scientific studies. ■

## CAUTION

**If you have glaucoma, cataracts, retinal detachment, or other eye problems, check with your eye doctor before undergoing light therapy. If you have a rash and fever, obtain a professional diagnosis to rule out infections such as measles or chickenpox. Ultraviolet light therapy may cause premature aging of the skin and increase your risk of skin cancer.**

## FOR MORE INFO

Following is a list of organizations you can contact to learn more about light therapy:

**Dinshaw Health Society**
PO Box 707
Malaga, NJ 08328
(609) 692-4686
(information on color therapy)

**Institute for Frontier Science**
7711-D McCallum Street
Philadelphia, PA 19118
e-mail: 101471.1777@compuserve.com
(information on laser therapy)

**Society for Light Treatment and Biological Rhythms**
10200 West 44th Avenue, Suite 304
Wheat Ridge, CO 80033-2840
(303) 424-3697
e-mail: sltbr@resourcenter.com
(Researches light therapy for the treatment of SAD, sleep disorders, and related conditions. Send $7 for a light therapy information packet.)

# *Massage*

*Massage therapy, defined as the systematic manipulation of the soft tissues, relieves sore muscles and promotes relaxation. It is usually performed with various standard hand strokes, but sometimes pressure is applied with other parts of the body, such as the forearm, elbow, or foot.*

*The general purposes of massage are to reduce tension, improve circulation, aid in the healing of soft-tissue injuries, control pain, and promote overall well-being. Massage can gently stretch tissues, increase range of motion, and reduce some types of edema (swelling). It can also help lower blood pressure and heart rate and improve respiration. Researchers believe massage helps the brain make endorphins, chemicals that act as natural painkillers—which perhaps explains why recipients feel better and more tranquil after a massage.*

### *The Nature of Touch*

Touching is, of course, an integral part of massage, and it may play a significant role in massage's therapeutic effects. Studies have found that animals that are touched grow faster and that infants who are not touched develop more slowly, physically and psychologically, than those who are. Touch can convey the therapeutic emotions of caring and concern. Some massage therapists believe that touch can create trust and openness and help release blocked emotions.

### *Origins*

One of the earliest forms of healing, massage was mentioned in Chinese medical texts 4,000 years ago. It has been advocated in Western societies since the Greek physician Hippocrates, in the fourth century BC, referred to a technique called rubbing. In ancient Rome, Julius Caesar is said to have had himself pinched all over every day to treat his neuralgia.

At the beginning of the 19th century, a Swedish gymnastics instructor and fencing master, Pehr Henrik Ling, cured himself of an elbow ailment with percussion strokes (tapping

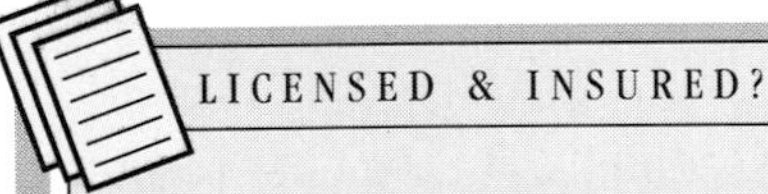

LICENSED & INSURED?

*Twenty-four states and some localities currently license massage therapy. Licensing laws are pending in additional states. Most states require 500 or more hours of education from a recognized school program as well as an examination. In 1992, the National Certification Examination in Therapeutic Massage and Bodywork was inaugurated, and states are gradually adopting it as their test. Massage is covered by some insurance companies.*

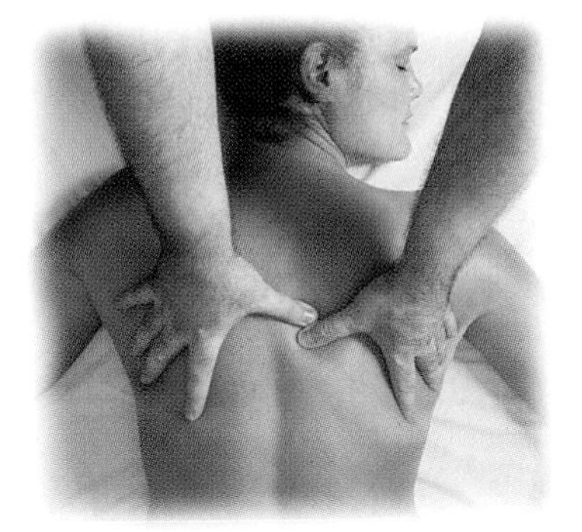

## Target Ailments

- Arthritis
- Asthma
- Athletic Injuries
- Back Problems
- Carpal Tunnel Syndrome
- Chronic Fatigue Syndrome
- Constipation
- Depression
- Headache
- Heartburn
- Immune Problems
- Insomnia
- Irritable Bowel Syndrome
- Multiple Sclerosis
- Muscle Cramps
- Neuralgia
- Pain, Chronic
- Premenstrual Syndrome
- Stomach Ulcers
- Tendinitis
- TMJ Syndrome

*See Common Ailments, beginning on page 194.*



CONTINUED

# Massage CONTINUED

movements). He subsequently developed a method of healing that became known as Swedish massage. This therapy, which was based on the then-emerging science of physiology, came to the United States in the mid-19th century. Interest dwindled, however, when healthcare in the United States took a technological turn in the early 1900s and didn't pick up again until the alternative healthcare movement gained momentum in the 1970s.

### What It's Good For

Massage is recommended for countless injuries and ailments. Well-designed studies have proved the benefits of particular methods of massage to treat pain, nausea, muscle spasm, and soft-tissue problems, as well as anxiety, depression, insomnia, and emotional stress. Massage helps premature infants gain weight and develop motor skills, and it helps elderly people relax. Researchers believe it also may improve immune system response. Many studies are under way to evaluate massage therapy further, including research on its effects in infants exposed to HIV, children with asthma, adolescents with eating disorders, adults with hypertension, and patients recovering from surgery.

Massage can also aid people who cannot use their muscles actively because of injury, illness, or paralysis. Although it cannot substitute for the normal muscular activity that rids the muscles of toxic products, massage can help the process when a person is unable to be normally active.

### Preparations/Techniques

There are approximately 100 different methods of massage therapy, about 80 of them born in the period of revival since the mid-1970s. A simple classification includes traditional European methods, contemporary Western methods, energetic manual techniques, and Oriental manual techniques.

The traditional European methods are based on longstanding Western concepts of anatomy and physiology. They use the five kinds of soft-tissue manipulation—effleurage, petrissage, friction, percussion, and vibration and jostling (the basic Swedish massage strokes)—illustrated in the Gallery of Massage Techniques that begins on page 124.

Contemporary Western methods add to the traditional techniques more recent knowledge of the effects of massage on the nervous system, posture, movement, and emotion. Also included in contemporary methods are techniques such as Rolfing and the Alexander and Feldenkrais methods *(see Bodywork, pages 47-56)* that are said to integrate the body in relationship to gravity.

Energetic and Oriental manual techniques use pressure and manipulation to assess, evaluate, and balance the energy system said to surround and infuse the

### CAUTION

**Consult a physician if you are considering massage therapy and have had an injury or a chronic illness such as heart or kidney disease. You should not use massage if you have an infection, inflammation, or cancer that could spread throughout the body or if you have a blood clot. Massage is not appropriate for some cases of edema because it can encourage more bleeding and swelling. If you have a nerve injury, you might find pressure on the skin painful. Do not use massage on your abdomen if you have high blood pressure or a peptic ulcer, and avoid massaging burned areas until they are healed.**

human body. Polarity therapy *(page 64)* and therapeutic touch *(page 55)* are energetic techniques. Oriental methods include shiatsu and acupressure *(pages 16-17)*.

## Visiting a Professional

You can find a qualified massage therapist through a physician's recommendation, a friend's advice (make sure the therapist is nationally certified or state-licensed), or by contacting one of the organizations listed below, right. On your first visit, the massage therapist should ask about your medical history and current state of health in order to tailor the therapy to your particular problems.

You will probably need to disrobe completely or partially, depending on the areas to be worked on. The therapist will position you comfortably on a massage table and provide a sheet or large towel to drape over the areas of your body that are not being massaged. During your session, pay attention to your reactions and speak up if an area is painful or tender to the touch.

## Doing It Yourself

If you are planning to practice massage with a partner, start with a few of the basic strokes and begin lightly, adding deeper strokes gradually. Wear loose clothing, remove your watch and rings, and keep your fingernails short to avoid scratching. Wash your hands thoroughly before beginning. Although shiatsu is done on the floor on a pad or futon, massage is best performed on a massage table. Keep the lighting gentle for optimum relaxation, and keep the room warm.

While massaging, keep your hands on your partner as much as possible, breaking contact gently and slowly to change areas. If your partner's muscles tighten, the pressure may be either too severe, causing discomfort, or too light, causing a tickling sensation. Do not massage directly a very tender area or the exact site of an injury. Put your body weight behind the pressure, rather than using your hands and arms alone, and keep your hands as relaxed as possible.

## Wellness

The ability of massage to reduce stress and tension, tone muscles, and enhance well-being makes it a useful part of a regular health maintenance program. Athletes often use massage to prepare muscles for strenuous activity or to recover after activity.

## What the Critics Say

Some conventional practitioners worry that ill or injured people may seek massage in place of required medical treatment; however, certified massage therapists are usually knowledgeable about the need for conventional treatment. As with any therapy, patients should be wary of any extreme or quick-cure claims. ■

### FOR MORE INFO

Following is a list of organizations you can contact to learn more about massage therapy:

**American Massage Therapy Association**
820 Davis Street, Suite 100
Evanston, IL 60201
(847) 864-0123

**National Certification Board for Therapeutic Massage and Bodywork**
8201 Greensboro Drive, Suite 300
McLean, VA 22102
(703) 610-9015

## Effleurage

*Massage of most areas of the body begins and ends with effleurage, a slow, rhythmic, gliding stroke performed with the fingertips, palms, thumbs, knuckles, or whole hand. Generally, effleurage moves from the extremities toward the heart—from wrist to shoulder, for example. An exception is the nerve stroke, which does not affect blood flow and is done in the direction opposite to a preceding series of effleurage strokes.*

*Start lightly and gradually work deeper. You may end your massage of each area with the nerve stroke, which is particularly soothing. The broad surface of the back is ideal for practicing the variations of effleurage pictured here. Keep your hands relaxed; tense, rigid hands have less sensitivity and don't feel as good to your partner.*

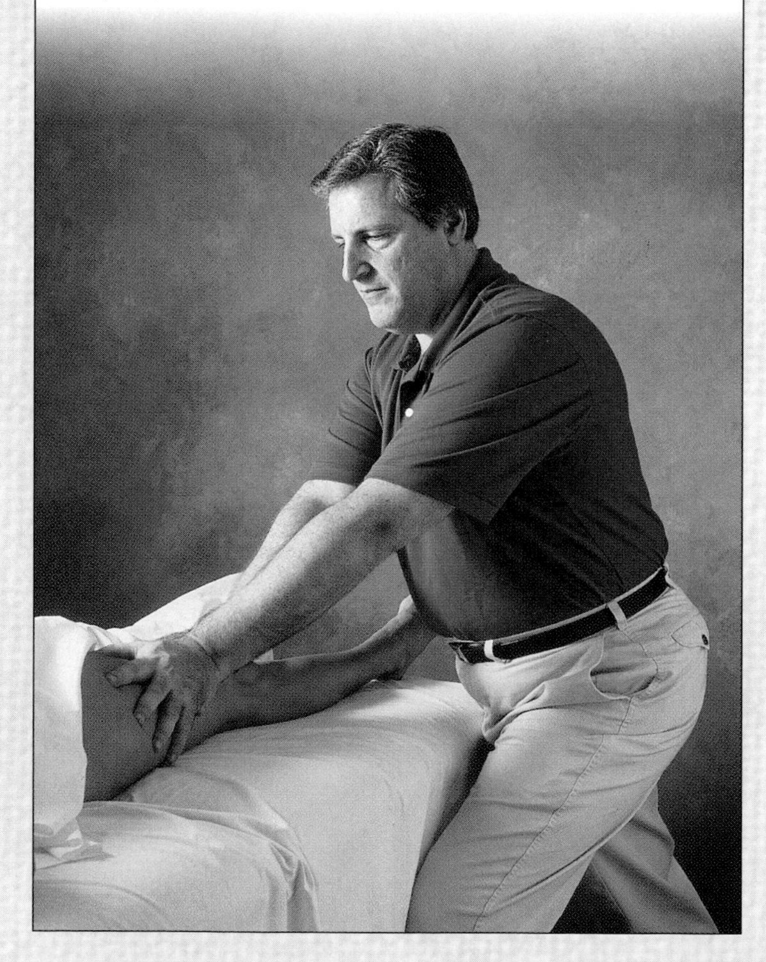

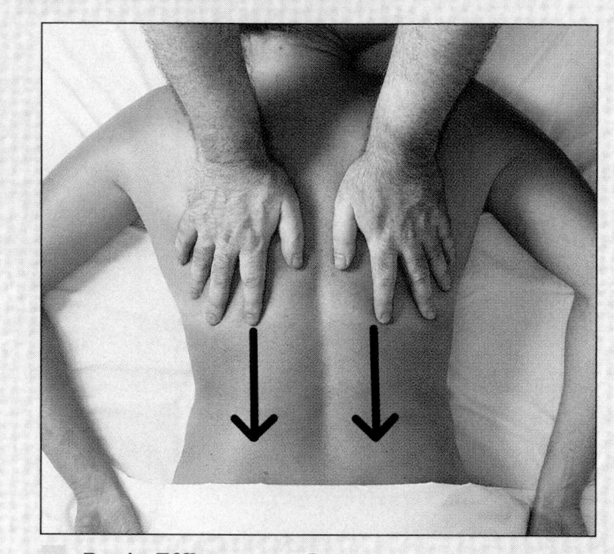

***Basic Effleurage*** • *Position your hands close together, with your thumbs an inch or two apart. Stroke downward, keeping your hands in firm and full contact with your partner's body until you reach the top of the pelvic bone.*

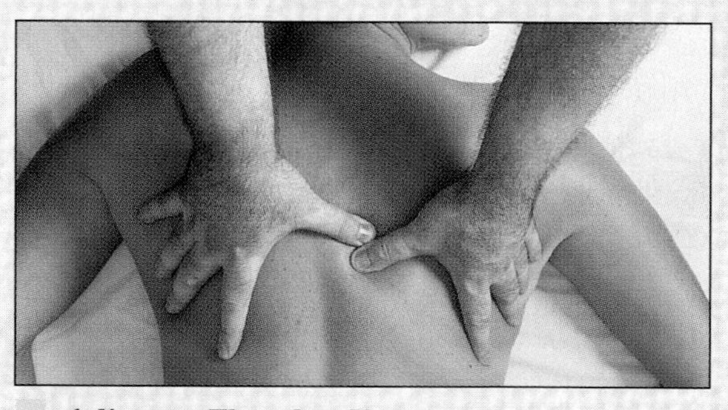

***Adjacent Thumb*** • *Place one thumb next to the other and glide down the back. Most of the pressure should be applied by your thumbs.*

***Posture*** • *Align your body properly to prevent fatigue and strain. Use the entire weight of your upper body, rather than your hands alone, for pressure; the lower body should balance and support. In general, face the direction in which your hands are moving.*

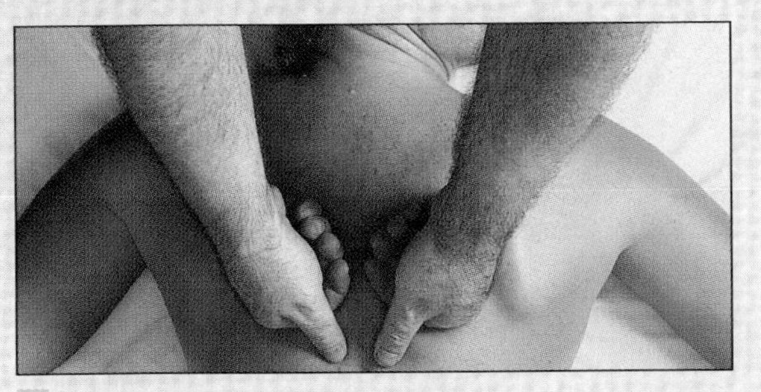

**Loose Fist** • *Work large muscles with a loose fist, making contact with the area of the fingers between the second and third joints. Glide down the back.*

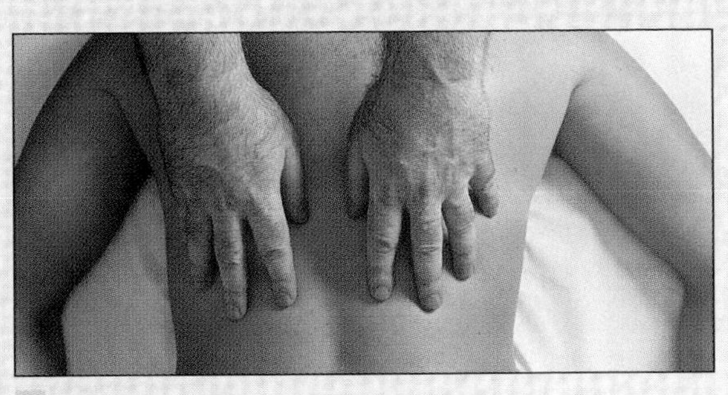

**Nerve Stroke** • *While barely touching the skin, drag your fingertips up the back, moving in the reverse direction from previous effleurage strokes.*

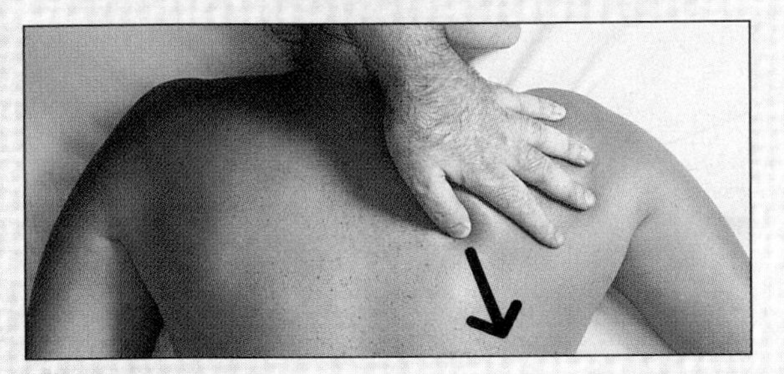

**One Thumb** • *For a deeper stroke, use one thumb to glide deeply along smaller muscles. Use a little more pressure to contact muscles that lie underneath the superficial layers of muscle.*

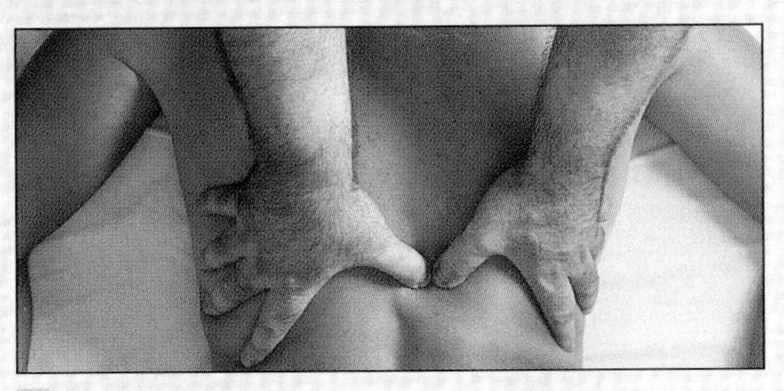

**Joined Thumb** • *Place your thumbs along the erector muscles next to the spine. Starting just below the base of the neck, slide your thumbs down, using more pressure than with previous strokes.*

## Petrissage

*A more complex technique, petrissage works specific muscle groups, usually where tissue is easily grasped. It can be performed deeply or superficially. Deep petrissage helps promote circulation and can counteract muscle tightness or degeneration. Alternately tighten and loosen your hands, fingers, or thumbs as you pick up and release muscles. Variations include rolling, heel of palm, and compression. Note the change in musculature as you go from tendons and ligaments toward the center of a muscle, which can usually withstand more pressure.*

**Hand on Hand** • *Use this stroke on the abdomen. Place the fingers of your top hand over the bottom hand for support. Ask your partner to bend her knees. Proceed clockwise in a circle, exerting even pressure.*

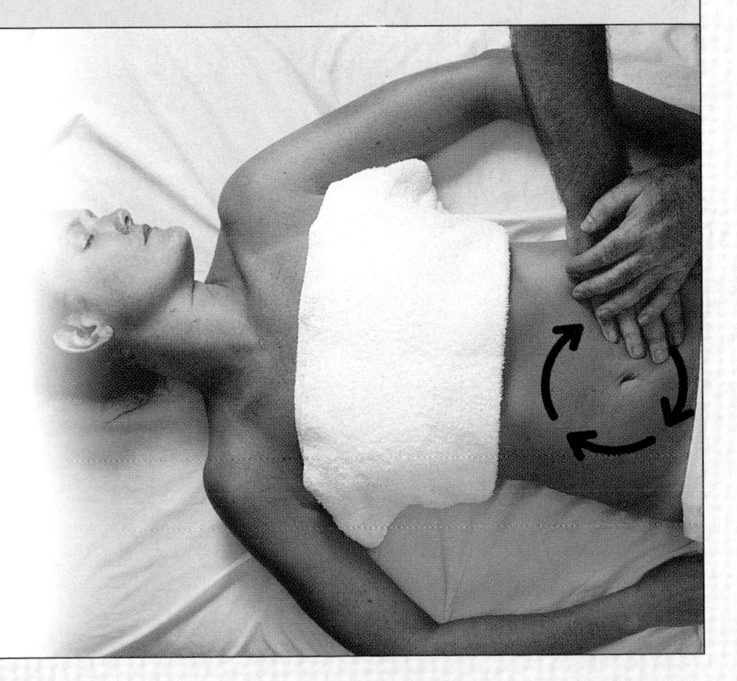



CONTINUED

# Gallery of Massage Techniques

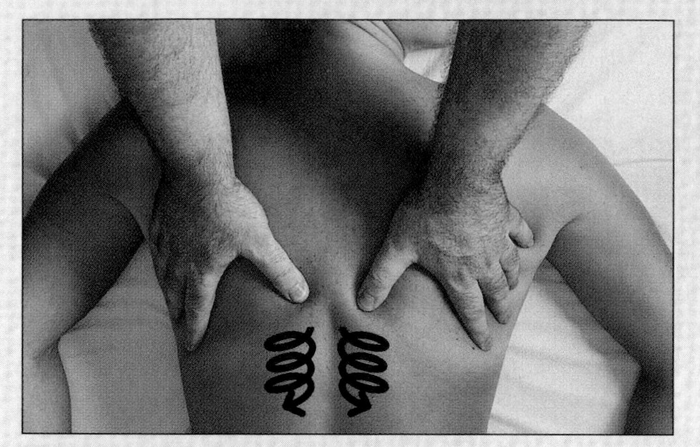

***Spiral*** • *Pressing with both thumbs while making a sweeping motion, spiral down the back, using a counterclockwise motion with the left thumb and a clockwise motion with the right thumb. Go from the base of the neck to the waist.*

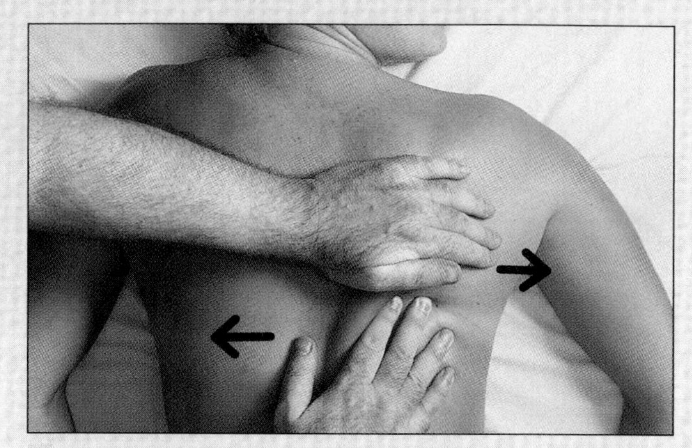

***Rolling*** • *Slide your hand firmly back and forth across your partner's back. Push with the heel of one hand, and pull/lift the skin with the fingers of the other. Note how this stroke wrings the tissues between your two hands.*

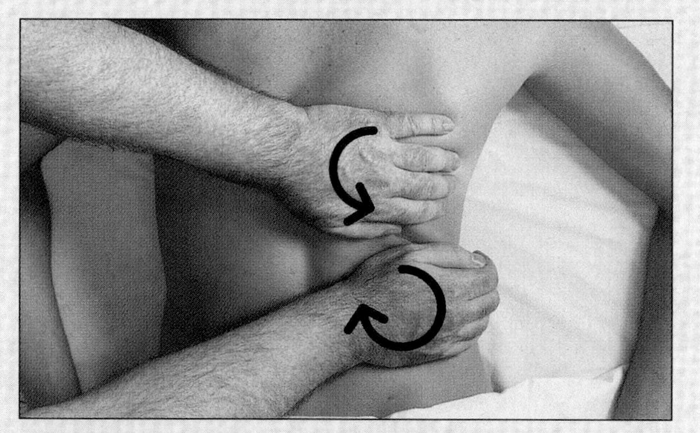

***Heel of Palm*** • *Place the heels of your palms next to your partner's spine. Alternately rotating your palms in opposite directions, push the muscle gently away from the spine as you work down the back, so the muscle is kneaded but not pinched.*

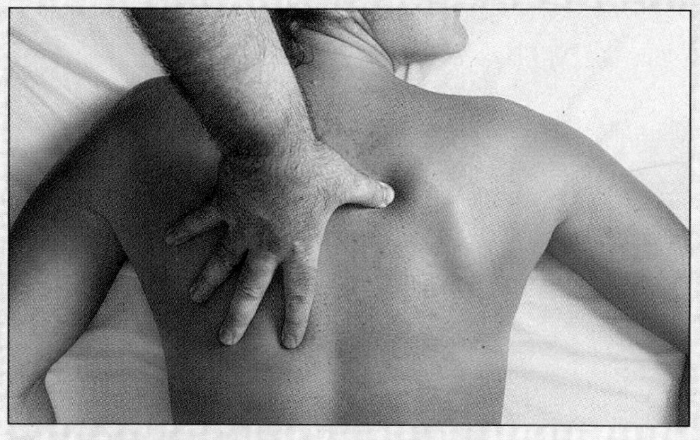

***Direct Pressure*** • *For trigger points (which feel like small marbles), for knots of muscle tension, or to execute shiatsu techniques, press with the pad of your thumb or finger straight into the tissue. Hold for five to 15 seconds or until you feel the tension release.*

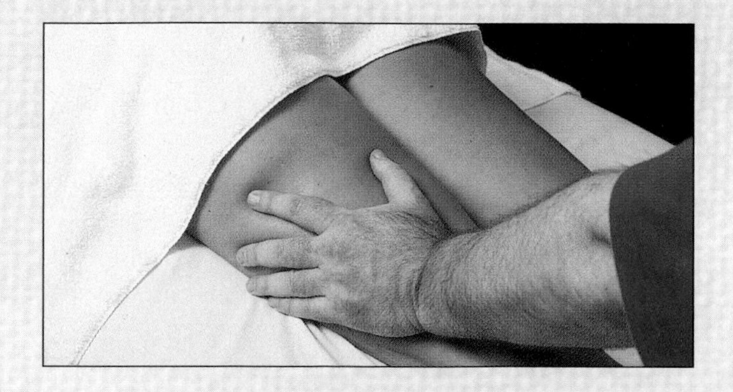

***Compression*** • *Place one palm flat with the fingers relaxed. Pump your hand up and down rhythmically, directing the pressure toward the bone underneath, then releasing the pressure. Do not use this technique on joints.*

## Friction

*Friction is often used in areas around joints. As in petrissage, you move muscle or other soft tissue away from bone. But in friction, the fingers or thumbs move over the underlying structures without sliding on the surface of the skin where the fingers or thumbs touch.*

*Because they have a relatively poor blood supply, tendons and ligaments tend to heal slowly, particularly during vigorous activities, sometimes resulting in "overuse" syndromes. Friction increases circulation and helps restore range of motion; it is a mainstay of sports massage, where it is referred to as cross-fiber stroking. Use your fingertips and thumbs to perform friction; lighten pressure if your partner experiences discomfort. Friction should not be used on an area that has been injured within the past 24 to 48 hours.*

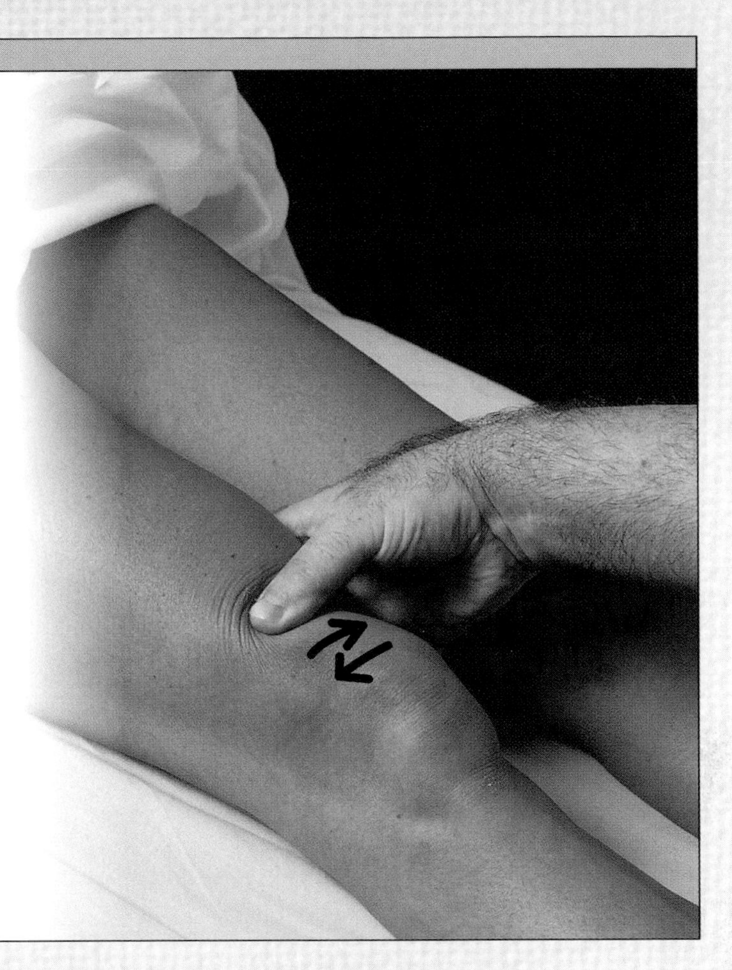

■ ***Cross-Fiber*** • *Pressing down, slide the thumb across the grain of the muscle (perpendicular to the muscle fiber) in a rhythmic motion. Keep your thumb on the same spot on the skin surface. You may feel the muscle fibers moving under your thumb.*

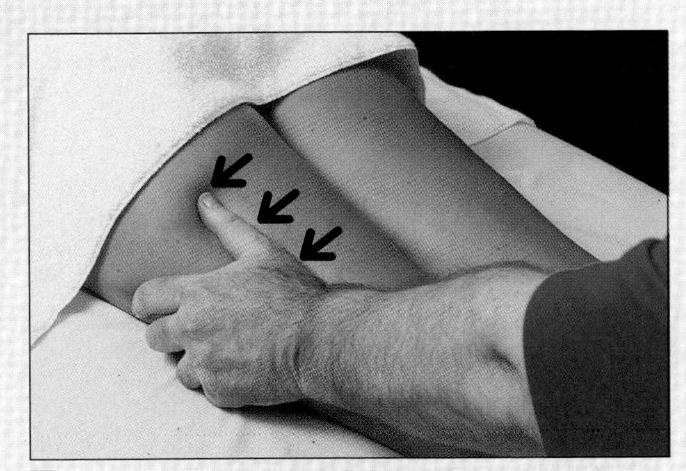

■ ***Broad Cross-Fiber Stroking*** • *Place your hand on the center of the back of the leg. While applying pressure with the outside edge of your thumb and palm, stroke across the grain of the muscle of the entire outer leg. Switch hands, and repeat on the inner portion of the leg.*

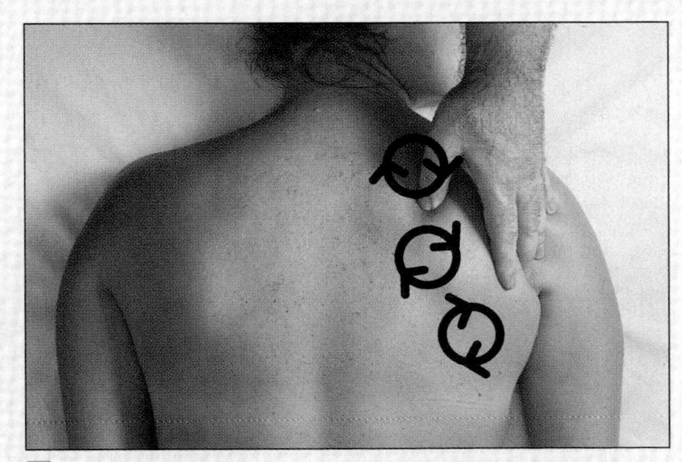

■ ***Circular Friction*** • *Locate the ropelike tissues that join the shoulder blade to the back. Using your hand for balance, place your thumb on the tissues and rotate it in small circles. Move down a bit, repeat the motion, and continue until the entire area is covered.*



CONTINUED

# Gallery of Massage Techniques

## Percussion

*Percussion strokes, also called tapotement (French for tapping), are alternate drumming hand movements performed on broad areas of the body, particularly the back. This stroke is clearly beneficial for increasing surface blood circulation, and it can help loosen phlegm and make it easier to expectorate it from the lungs.*

*When done properly, percussion is stimulating rather than painful or harsh. Keep your hands and wrists relaxed and elbows flexed. Strike the skin with alternating hands, moving rapidly over the surface you are working on. You should strike firmly but never so hard that you cause pain. Because even light percussion may cause discomfort to internal organs, do not apply it on the lower abdomen, the lower back near the kidneys, or directly on the spine.*

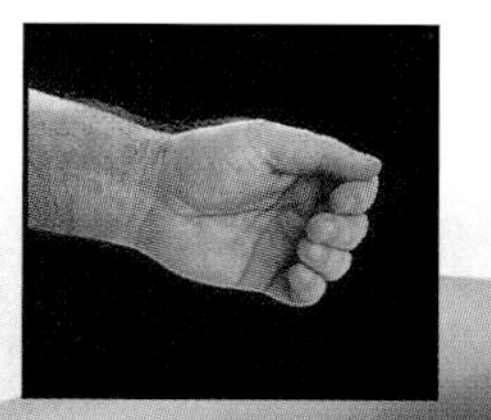

***Beating*** • *Form a loose fist (inset) and strike gently with the outside surface. Beating works best on the fleshier areas of the body, such as the back, waist, and thighs.*

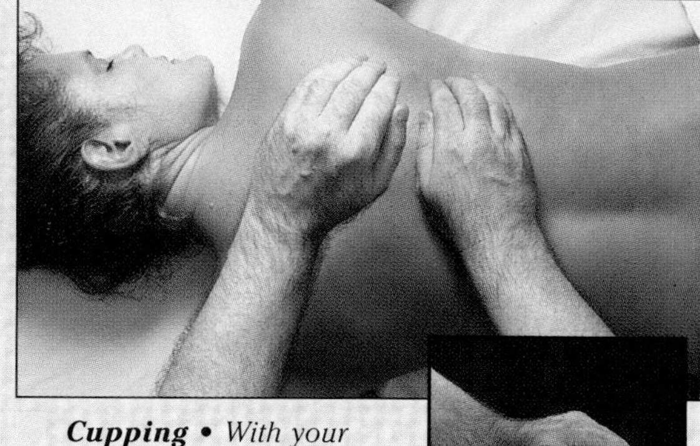

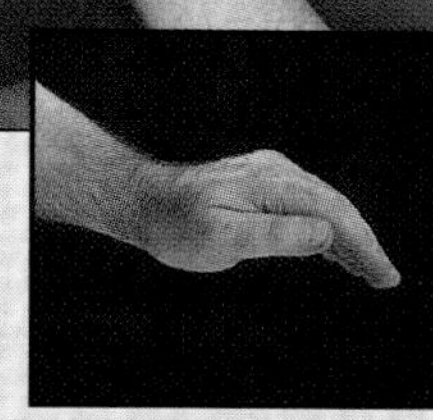

***Cupping*** • *With your hands cupped (inset), strike with your fingertips and the heels of your palms.*

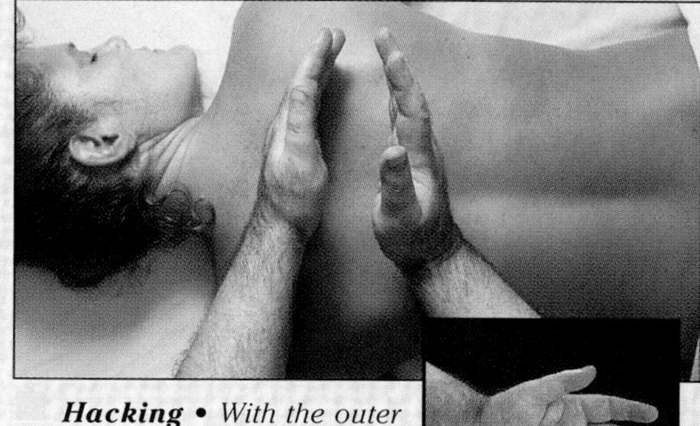

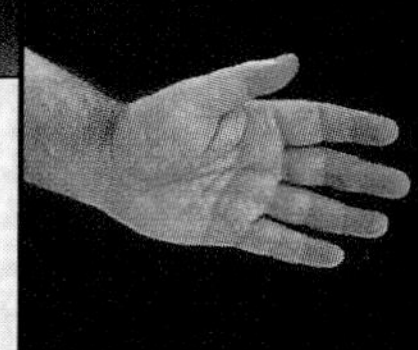

***Hacking*** • *With the outer edge of your hands, perform light, rapid chopping motions (inset) on fleshy areas like the upper shoulders. These are not hard karate chops; keep your hands relaxed with your fingers slightly separated.*

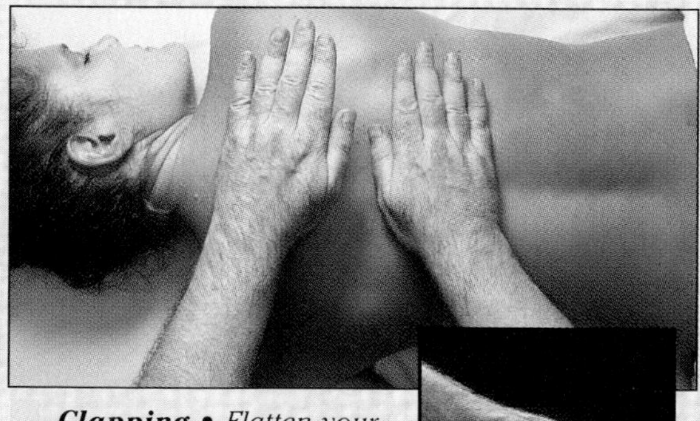

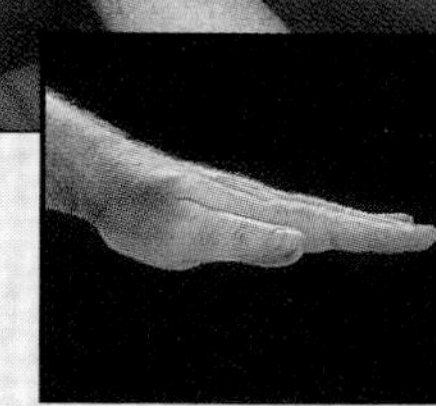

***Clapping*** • *Flatten your hand (inset); clap rapidly over fleshy areas like the upper back with the entire hand.*

# Gallery of Massage Techniques

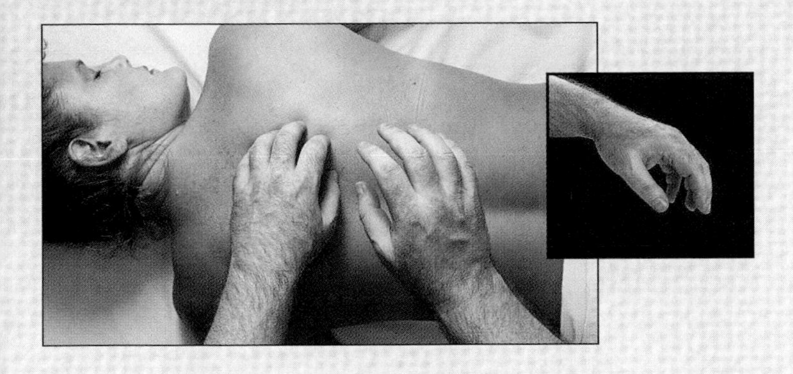

**Tapping** • *Strike with the fingertips (inset), alternating your hands quickly. Unlike other percussion strokes, tapping may be helpful on bony areas such as the shoulder blades or scalp.*

## Vibration and Jostling

*Like percussion, these techniques either stimulate or relax body tissue. The strokes are particularly effective on the limbs and fleshy areas. Vibration does not proceed in any specific direction; jostling works up and down a muscle.*

*Vibration requires a rapid contraction and relaxation of your own muscles, which sets up a vibratory wave that is transmitted to your partner through your hands. (Some professional massage therapists use mechanical vibrators for this effect.) One form of joint mobilization is a variation of vibration that uses larger motions to work the joints.*

*Jostling, which is not as strenuous, is used in sports massage, especially to treat sore muscles. If your partner's muscles tense up during massage, interrupt your sequence and relax the muscle area by jostling it for five or 10 seconds. You can insert jostling into a massage as often as you want.*

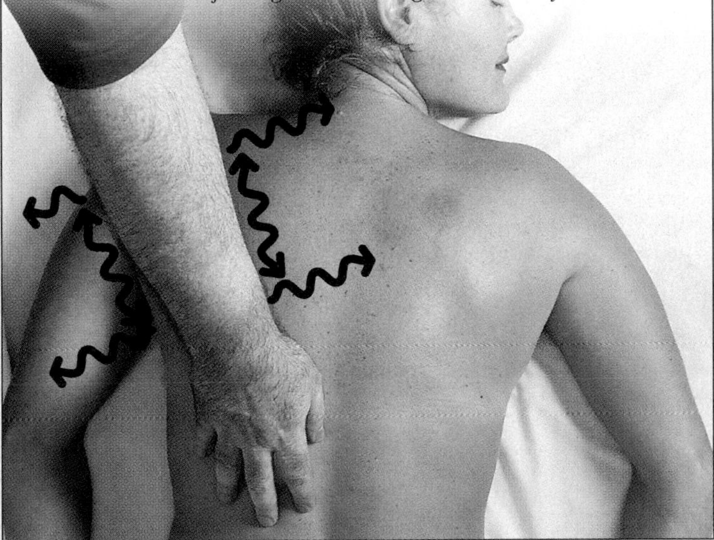

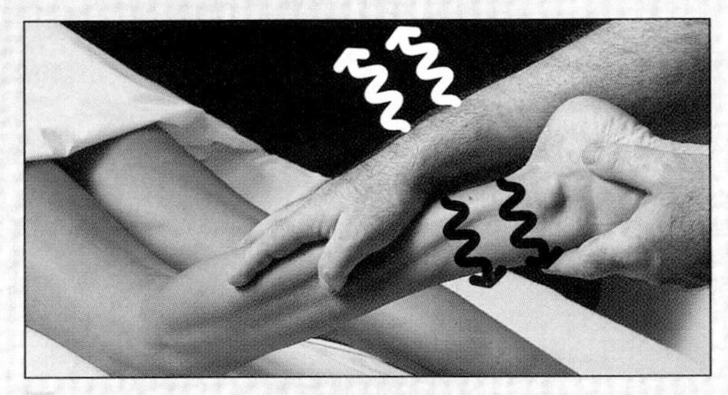

**Jostling** • *Place your hands on your partner's calf and shake back and forth, progressing along the muscle.*

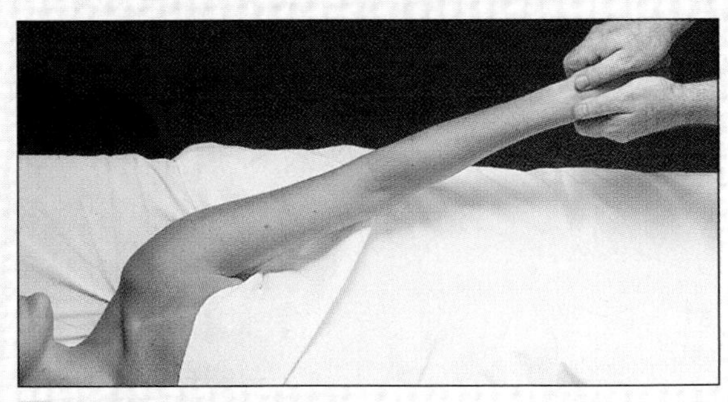

**Joint Mobilization** • *Grasp your partner's hand firmly between your hands. Move far enough away so that your partner's arm is fully extended, and shake the arm with a wavelike motion while pulling away slightly from the joint.*

**Vibration** • *With your fingertips lightly touching your partner, tense all the muscles in your arm repeatedly, creating a trembling motion (left). The vibration you create in your arm is transferred through your fingers to the area being worked on.*

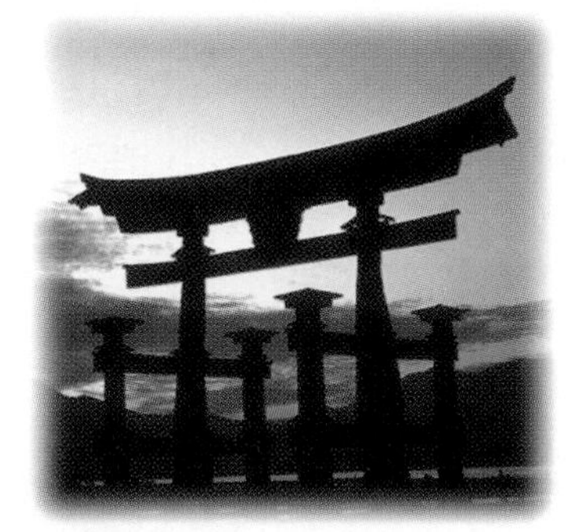

## Target Ailments

- Back Problems
- Cancer
- Chronic Fatigue Syndrome
- Depression
- Diabetes
- Headache
- Heart Problems
- High Blood Pressure
- Immune Problems
- Incontinence
- Insomnia
- Irritable Bowel Syndrome
- Menopause
- Menstrual Problems
- Pain, Chronic
- Seasonal Affective Disorder
- Stress
- TMJ Syndrome

*See Common Ailments, beginning on page 194.*

# Mind/Body Medicine

*Close your eyes and imagine holding a freshly cut, bright yellow lemon in your hand. Imagine raising it to your mouth and biting into the tart pulp. The saliva now flooding your mouth is evidence of the powerful connection between the thoughts in your mind and the physical processes of your body.*

*Western science has long viewed the mind and the body as separate entities. Using increasingly sophisticated drugs and surgical techniques, physicians have focused on the body while almost wholly ignoring the mind's role in illness and healing. Yet the mind appears to have enormous influence on the progress of disease: Studies suggest that people's opinions about the state of their own health can dramatically affect their chances of developing a serious disease later in life.*

*Mind/body medicine seeks to explore connections between the tangible body and the intangible mind, and to use these linkages to improve physical as well as mental health. The techniques are not so much treatments as they are processes that help people learn how to influence their physical reactions. A common goal among the various mind/body techniques is relaxation, an important weapon in the modern battle against stress-related disease.*

### *Stress and Relaxation*

The body reacts to stressful situations—sudden danger, for example—by releasing chemicals that produce a number of physical effects, such as an increase in heart rate, blood pressure, and muscle tension. Chronic or long-term stress can take a serious toll. It suppresses immune system activity and can lead to insomnia, anxiety, high blood pressure, depression, and possibly even cancer. Fortunately, the body has a recuperative reaction that can reverse many of the harmful effects of chronic stress: relaxation. Mind/body medicine is the quest to invoke the relaxation response and strengthen the body in pursuit of good health.

Mind/body techniques cannot replace conventional treatment, especially in the case of serious or chronic ailments, but they can be extremely useful as complementary therapies. Low in risk and cost, easy to learn, and adaptable to individual tastes, these methods can be combined and practiced in a number of ways. They can be used in conjunction with conventional or other alternative therapies to control the symptoms of disease or the side effects of certain treatments, or they can be practiced on a regular basis to promote and maintain overall health. And because they involve the active participation of the patient, mind/body techniques help foster a sense of control and self-reliance that in itself can be of significant therapeutic value.

# Mind/Body Medicine

## *The Power of the Patient*

Medical science generally has not accepted mind/body medicine, perhaps because thoughts do not lend themselves readily to scientific testing methods. However, a number of mind/body therapies—meditation, guided imagery, and prayer, for example—have been used successfully by traditional healers for hundreds of years. Even today, many physicians who do not embrace mind/body concepts acknowledge the influence the mind can have on disease. Some medical schools, in fact, teach the importance of a good bedside manner, realizing that what the patient believes about an illness—and also what the patient thinks the *doctor* believes—can change the course of the disease. The placebo effect is another familiar example of the curative power of belief: Convinced that a given medicine will bring relief, the patient actually does improve, even though the pills contain nothing but sugar.

The effectiveness of mind/body medicine depends largely on the level of patient commitment, as well as on the strength of one's belief that positive thinking can translate into better health. For these techniques to work, you must have realistic expectations and guidance from a competent, experienced therapist. Finding such a person may take some work, but the effort could pay off in long-term health benefits.

## *What the Critics Say*

Despite evidence that the mind can and does play a role in healing, a number of healthcare professionals—even some who accept the general premise—remain skeptical of mind/body techniques. Some think that the benefits are limited, that patients will become frustrated if a technique does not produce significant improvements right away, or that patients will rely solely on mind/body techniques when other types of medical care are warranted. Many conventional doctors, for example, are concerned that patients using mind/body techniques will neglect to get proper, proven treatment for serious illnesses such as cancer, heart disease, or diabetes. While mind/body methods are themselves safe and can often help people recover from disease, using them as substitutes for a doctor's care can delay necessary treatment and lead to serious problems.

Mind/body techniques also have come under attack because of possible dangers of receiving treatment from practitioners who are unlicensed or poorly qualified: For some of these therapies, practitioners are not required to pass a state examination or get special training. This, say critics, opens the way for unscrupulous practitioners to take a patient's money and offer nothing in return but false hopes. And while proponents point to numerous studies showing that thoughts and deeply held beliefs can have a tremendous effect on one's health, some skeptics argue that the claims of mind/body medicine are not supported by scientific research.



CONTINUED

## Biofeedback

*In biofeedback, sensors on the body pick up electrical signals from the muscles or brain and pass them along to a computer, which translates the pulses into images or sounds. The patient watches or listens to these processed signals and, with the help of a therapist, develops ways to affect their rate or intensity. Eventually, the patient learns to exercise conscious control over normally unconscious bodily processes, such as blood pressure and heart rate.*

*What It's Good For* • Biofeedback is used in many areas of medicine. It is especially helpful in the treatment of ailments that are caused or exacerbated by stress or anxiety, such as stress-induced hypertension and headaches. Many physical therapists use biofeedback to reeducate weak or overactive muscles, as well as to treat nerve damage and temporomandibular joint (TMJ) syndrome. Biofeedback may also be used to help reduce the frequency of epileptic seizures.

- **Headaches:** The American Medical Association sanctions biofeedback training for the treatment of certain types of headaches.
- **Raynaud's syndrome:** Thermal, or temperature regulation, biofeedback is a successful therapy for this disorder, which causes cold feet and hands due to constricted blood vessels.
- **Attention deficit disorder:** One promising new form of biofeedback aims to teach people with this disorder how to normalize brain waves associated with concentration, attention, and hyperactivity.
- **Diabetes:** Biofeedback training in relaxation techniques may help diabetics gain better metabolic control and learn to manage stress; stress can contribute to increased blood sugar levels in some people with the disease.

*Visiting a Professional*
Biofeedback is best learned with the help of a healthcare professional who has experience using its techniques to treat your condition. Learning to access and then control the body's functions usually takes at least eight to 10 visits. Consult your healthcare provider for a referral, or contact a national biofeedback society for more information.

**LICENSED & INSURED?**

*Many biofeedback therapists are licensed physicians or other healthcare professionals who have received training in these techniques. Practitioners are certified by the Biofeedback Certification Institute of America, which also sets standards. Many insurance companies reimburse patients for biofeedback training provided by a licensed healthcare provider.*

**CAUTION**

**If you use a pacemaker or other implanted electrical aid or if you have a serious heart disorder, check with your physician before using a biofeedback device that measures the output of the sweat glands. These devices use a tiny amount of electricity, and although no problems have been reported with their use, several biofeedback organizations recommend this precaution.**

**FOR MORE INFO**

Following is a list of organizations you can contact to learn more about biofeedback:

**Society for the Study of Neuronal Regulation**
4600 Post Oak Place, Suite 301
Houston, TX 77027
(713) 552-0091
fax: (713) 552-0752
e-mail: ssnr@primenet.com

**Association for Applied Psychophysiology and Biofeedback**
10200 West 44th Ave., Suite 304
Wheat Ridge, CO 80033-2840
(800) 477-8892
fax: (303) 422-8894

**Biofeedback Certification Institute of America**
10200 West 44th Ave., Suite 304
Wheat Ridge, CO 80033-2840
(303) 420-2902
fax: (303) 422-3394

# Mind/Body Medicine

## Guided Imagery

*Guided imagery is a technique that uses the mind's ability to imagine sights, sounds, movements, and other sensory experiences as a means to induce specific physical reactions in the body or to encourage changes in a patient's emotional outlook. Buddhists have used mental images to promote healing since the 13th century or earlier, and many shamanistic traditions around the world include the power of imagery. The technique can be used in many ways and can be adapted to suit different personalities; what doesn't work for one person might be the perfect therapy for another.*

*What It's Good For* • Just as lying on a warm beach, listening to the ocean waves, and feeling the warm sunshine can have a relaxing effect on your body, so can visualizing such a scene in your mind. Similarly, imagining your immune cells as a conquering army or a swarm of victorious hunters may actually boost the cells' activity and, at the same time, promote a sense of self-reliance that further improves the functioning of your immune system. Simply relaxing and allowing images to take shape in your mind may give you insight into a symptom or ailment, and perhaps even suggest ideas about how to cope with it.

Guided imagery can have a profound influence on physical as well as psychological conditions. Studies of the brain indicate that merely imagining a certain activity stimulates the same regions of the cerebral cortex as actually experiencing the activity. This suggests that guided imagery has the potential to bring about positive physiological changes in the body, allowing a patient to exercise conscious control over such vital functions as heart rate, brain-wave rhythms, and blood glucose levels.

A number of natural childbirth groups rely on a type of preparatory guided imagery called mental rehearsal, in which women imagine going through delivery before the actual event. Mental rehearsal is also frequently used by patients as a way to relieve anxiety before surgery. This sort of preview can reduce pain and side effects, and even shorten recovery time.

- **Immune problems:** A number of studies show improvement in

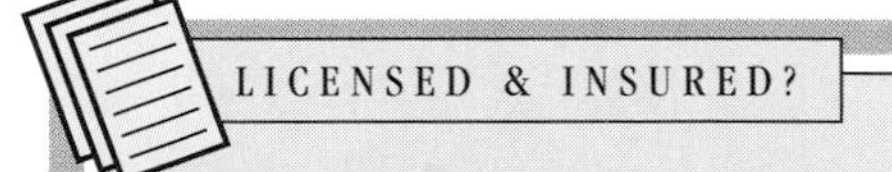

LICENSED & INSURED?

*There is no licensing procedure for guided imagery therapists, but many professionals who use or teach these methods are licensed in other fields of healthcare. Some health insurance companies may reimburse patients for training in guided imagery as a part of therapy for certain disorders.*

### CAUTION

**Guided imagery and hypnosis can be used as diagnostic tools in certain kinds of emotional therapy, sometimes involving the recovery of so-called repressed memories. In a number of cases, however, these memories, though seemingly quite real to both patient and therapist at the time of recovery, have been found to be false. This is an area where it pays to be careful and move slowly.**



CONTINUED

some immune reactions following imagery training. Sometimes guided imagery is combined with other mind/body techniques to boost the effectiveness of the immune system.

- **Cancer:** Guided imagery is often used by cancer patients in an effort to mobilize their immune system against the disease. There is no direct evidence that imagery alone can improve the prognosis, but people often report that imagery makes them better able to cope with cancer. Studies have shown that imagery can also ease nausea and promote weight gain in cancer patients undergoing treatments that interfere with their eating habits.
- **Irritable bowel syndrome:** Using guided imagery to visualize a soothing scene or activity can help relieve the symptoms of IBS.
- **Asthma:** Guided imagery may help asthma patients relax and assume better control of their breathing.

*Preparations/Techniques* • Guided imagery can be used actively—as when a cancer patient imagines immune cells attacking malignant cells—or receptively, allowing the mind to form images that might shed light on a particular ailment or condition. Techniques for both approaches can be learned on your own from a book or an audiotape, or under the guidance of a trained therapist.

Taking the time to concentrate on observing the world around you helps your mind create more convincing images. Clarity is important for healing, because the more vivid the image, the more "real" it seems and the greater its effect on the nervous system. While conjuring "pictures" is perhaps the easiest form of imagery, it is also possible—and equally relaxing—to imagine soothing sounds, sensations of touch, and smells. For chronic conditions, guided imagery is most beneficial when practiced for 15 or 20 minutes once or twice every day. You may want to keep a journal of your sessions and your symptoms to help you evaluate the results. Guided imagery for relaxation can be used regularly or on the spur of the moment—to handle a tense situation or cope with sudden pain, for example.

*Visiting a Professional* • Many kinds of therapists use guided imagery, and some teach individuals or groups how to continue its use on their own. It may take several sessions with a professional and some time working on your own before you notice results. Ask your healthcare provider for a referral to a therapist, or contact the Academy for Guided Imagery *(see For More Info, left).*

*Wellness* • Guided imagery can help you picture well-being or success in any number of endeavors. Using imagery to take minivacations throughout the day can keep you relaxed and help prevent or tone down the stress response.

**FOR MORE INFO**

Following is a list of organizations you can contact to learn more about guided imagery:

**The Academy for Guided Imagery**
PO Box 2070
Mill Valley, CA 94942
(800) 726-2070
fax: (415) 389-9342

**The Institute of Transpersonal Psychology**
744 San Antonio Road
Palo Alto, CA 94303
(415) 493-4430
fax: (415) 493-6835

# Mind/Body Medicine

## Hypnotherapy

*Healers have used hypnotism to induce trance states in patients since ancient times. Although the practice has largely fallen out of favor among mainstream physicians, over the last few decades a number of healthcare practitioners in various fields have begun to harness the power of hypnotherapy to treat an array of conditions.*

*What It's Good For* • Hypnotherapy aims to induce a state of focused concentration, described as neither sleep nor wakefulness, during which a willing subject is open and responsive to suggestion. (An unwilling subject cannot be hypnotized.) Hypnotherapy is most effective when used to treat ailments involving stress or anxiety. There are also reports of success with hypnotherapy in helping people break bad habits, such as bedwetting in children, or establish good ones.

- **Skin problems:** Hypnotherapy has been used successfully to treat warts and ichthyosis (fish skin disease), a severe genetic disorder.
- **Pain:** Some doctors, dentists, and childbirth attendants use hypnotherapy to counteract the fear and anxiety that can heighten pain, complicate healing, and slow labor in pregnant women. Clinical trials also show that hypnotherapy can help burn patients deal more effectively with pain.
- **Hemophilia:** Research shows that hypnotherapy may help reduce bleeding in people with this disorder, which interferes with the blood's ability to form clots.
- **Anxiety:** Hypnotherapy can help people overcome certain phobias, including stage fright, or cope with distressing situations such as hospitalization.

*Visiting a Professional* • A trained therapist can guide you through the steps of hypnosis or teach you how to perform the techniques yourself. Ask your healthcare provider for a referral to a qualified therapist, or contact a national organization *(far right).*

*Wellness* • Hypnosis is thought to bring about physiological changes similar to those induced by other relaxation techniques. It also offers the same potential for increased overall well-being and helps prevent or reduce the intensity of the stress response.

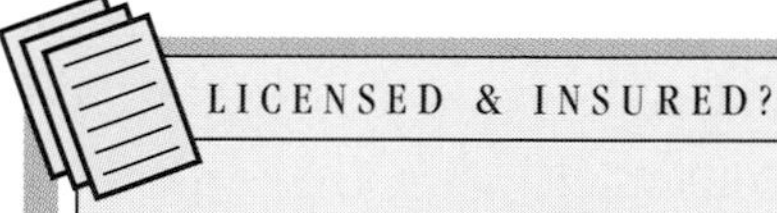

**LICENSED & INSURED?**

*States do not regulate hypnotherapists, but many of these practitioners are licensed in other fields of medicine and certified by the American Board of Hypnosis or the American Council of Hypnotist Examiners. Depending on the ailment, some health insurance companies will reimburse patients for hypnotherapy sessions performed by a licensed healthcare professional.*

### CAUTION

**Hypnotic suggestions can be very powerful. Before undergoing hypnotherapy, make sure that your practitioner is qualified and has experience in treating your particular condition.**

### FOR MORE INFO

Following is a list of organizations you can contact to learn more about hypnotherapy:

**American Council of Hypnotist Examiners**
1147 East Broadway, Suite 340
Glendale, CA 91205
(818) 242-5378
fax: (818) 247-9379

**American Society of Clinical Hypnosis**
2200 East Devon Ave., Suite 291
Des Plaines, IL 60018
(847) 297-3317
fax: (847) 297-7309

**Milton H. Erickson Foundation**
3606 North 24th Street
Phoenix, AZ 85016
(602) 956-6196
fax: (602) 956-0519



CONTINUED

## Meditation

*Many cultures throughout the world have recognized the calming, therapeutic effect of quiet contemplation. Most types of meditation practiced today, however, come from ancient Eastern or other religious traditions. Almost all of these methods share a few simple steps: Students are instructed to sit quietly, usually with eyes closed, and focus the mind on a single thought, allowing all other thoughts to float away. Some forms are more active or complex, meant to be performed while walking or chanting, for example.*

*One of the most famous methods is transcendental meditation, or TM, a simplified variation of ancient yoga that was brought to the United States by Maharishi Mahesh Yogi in the 1960s. Another type is known as the relaxation response (pages 138-139). A traditional Buddhist method called vipassana, or mindfulness meditation, has been practiced in the East for 2,500 years but only recently become known to the Western world. Students of mindfulness meditation are taught simply to focus on the present moment. The goal is to face and accept all aspects of life, thereby achieving a deeper sense of balance that contributes to overall well-being.*

*What It's Good For* • Meditation is commonly thought of as a spiritual endeavor, but it has frequently demonstrated physical effects as well. Most forms of meditation promote regular quiet relaxation, which in itself can help alleviate symptoms of stress-related ailments ranging from headaches to high blood pressure.

- **Chronic pain:** Use of TM or mindfulness meditation has been shown to reduce the suffering associated with chronic pain, possibly by helping people examine and sort out the negative thoughts commonly generated during intense discomfort.
- **High blood pressure:** Studies have shown a decrease in blood pressure among regular practitioners of TM. This evidence is so persuasive that cardiologists sometimes recommend meditation to their patients to help lower stress-related hypertension.
- **Stress:** TM has been used in treating posttraumatic stress disor-

### CAUTION

**Some people experience disorientation and anxiety when beginning to meditate. To overcome feelings like these, try keeping your eyes open and focusing your attention on a picture or an object. You can also learn to meditate while walking. Discuss such problems with your instructor, therapist, or healthcare provider.**

### LICENSED & INSURED?

*There are no licensing procedures for teachers of meditation, although sometimes the technique is taught in affiliation with a hospital, clinic, or medical practice. Under certain circumstances, some health insurance providers cover the costs of training in meditation techniques.*

der. Recent studies suggest a connection between meditation and a decrease in the levels of harmful stress-induced chemicals in the brain. Mindfulness meditation has been shown to reduce anxiety, depression, and other symptoms associated with chronic stress.

- **Panic disorders:** Mindfulness meditation can help people prone to panic attacks control their breathing and reactions, thereby forestalling full attacks.
- **Headaches:** The relaxation achieved through meditation can help reduce or eliminate headaches brought on by stress or muscle tension.
- **Respiratory problems:** For some patients with emphysema, asthma, or other lung ailments, mindfulness meditation can reduce the frequency and severity of attacks of breathlessness.

*Preparations/Techniques* • Meditation seems simple, but learning to stop the usual stream of conscious thoughts flowing through your mind takes practice. First, you must find a quiet place with as few distractions as possible. Sit quietly in a comfortable position, preferably with your back straight. Focus your mind on your breath or on a silently repeated sound, word, or phrase (called a mantra), or on a stationary object such as a flower or candle flame. If other thoughts intrude, take notice of them, but then let them go and return your focus to the phrase or object. Gently refocus as many times as necessary. Practice this for 15 to 20 minutes twice a day; meditating at the same time every day helps reinforce the habit.

For mindfulness meditation, begin the same way, using a single point of concentration to achieve calm. When thoughts or feelings surface, observe them without intention or judgment; don't try to decide if your thoughts are right or wrong, just be aware of them. The goal of this form of meditation is acceptance of the reality of the moment. For a technique known as the body scan, performed while seated or lying down, concentrate on moving your attention through your body, taking note of any sensations or impressions as you go along.

Although it is possible to learn to meditate on your own with the help of instruction books or courses on audiotape or videotape, it is best to begin with a qualified instructor. Classes and retreats in the various methods are widely available; many people, in fact, find that the support of others in a group setting provides the motivation necessary for developing the proper meditation skills.

*Wellness* • Many who practice meditation say that the relaxation and focus provided by regular sessions positively affects every aspect of life. Mindfulness meditation, in particular, appears to foster a sense of connection that promotes general good health and may actually bring about beneficial changes in specific areas of the body, including the cardiovascular system.

**FOR MORE INFO**

Following is a list of organizations you can contact to learn more about meditation:

**Institute for Noetic Sciences**
475 Gate Five Road, Suite 300
Sausalito, CA 94965
(415) 331-5650
fax: (415) 331-5673

**Insight Meditation Society**
1230 Pleasant Street
Barre, MA 01005
(508) 355-4378
fax: (508) 355-6398

**Vipassana Meditation Center**
PO Box 24
Shelbourne Falls, MA 01370
(413) 625-2160



CONTINUED

# Mind/Body Medicine CONTINUED

## Relaxation Techniques

*In the late 1960s, Harvard cardiologist Herbert Benson became intrigued by the incidence of high blood pressure in patients who were under stress. While researching this phenomenon, he noticed that blood pressure levels were lower in people who meditated than in those who didn't. Eventually, he identified a mechanism in the body that helps reduce stress. This mechanism, which Benson called the relaxation response, can be invoked in a number of ways. Yoga (pages 182-183), t'ai chi (pages 172-173), and qigong (pages 165-166), for example, are excellent techniques for promoting relaxation and reducing stress. Others include the relaxation methods listed below in "Preparations/Techniques." These simple techniques can be used virtually anywhere at any time, and most of them need no special training, just practice.*

*What It's Good For* • Relaxation is the goal of mind/body medicine because it helps reduce the negative effects of stress, which has been linked to many serious and chronic diseases, including cancer, heart disease, and depression. Summoning the relaxation response also lowers the respiration rate and relaxes muscle tension. One researcher found that regular use of relaxation techniques makes the body less responsive throughout the day to the effects of norepinephrine, a stress hormone that increases blood pressure and heart rate. Relaxation training may also be helpful after surgery or other medical procedures: Research suggests that using these techniques may speed healing, reduce bleeding and other complications, decrease pain and reliance on medications, and perhaps allow a quicker return to full function.

- **Insomnia:** Learning to evoke the relaxation response can help many people with chronic insomnia improve their ability to fall asleep. A technique referred to as progressive muscle relaxation (opposite) is a particularly beneficial way to promote deep, all-body relaxation and to overcome sleeplessness.

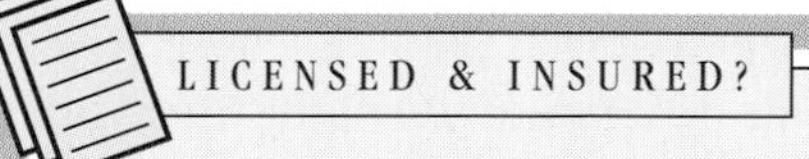


*Relaxation therapists are not licensed as such, but a number of medical professionals who are licensed in other fields—physicians, psychologists, and social workers, for example—offer training in these techniques, as do many hospitals and clinics. In some cases health insurance companies cover the costs of relaxation therapy for certain conditions. Check with your therapist or insurance carrier.*

### CAUTION

**Relaxation methods can reduce your need for certain medications. Whatever technique you decide to use, keep your healthcare provider informed so he or she can make any necessary adjustments in dosage.**

# Mind/Body Medicine

- **Premenstrual syndrome:** Symptoms of PMS were significantly reduced in women who practiced relaxation techniques twice a day for three months.
- **Immune problems:** Studies show an increase in immune cell activity after relaxation training.
- **High blood pressure:** Relaxation techniques are very effective in lowering elevated blood pressure in cases of stress-related hypertension.
- **Infertility:** Stress can interfere with the normal hormonal cycle of the reproductive process in women, sometimes resulting in infertility. In one study, a group of women thought to be infertile participated in relaxation training, and a third of them became pregnant. Relaxation techniques can also help alleviate the stress associated with the experience of infertility or its treatment.

*Preparations/Techniques* • Herbert Benson suggests the following technique for triggering the relaxation response: Sit comfortably in a place with minimal distractions. Close your eyes and relax your muscles. Breathe naturally; as you exhale, silently repeat a word or phrase you have chosen that has meaning to you—this is your "focus word." Many people use "peace" or "love," a short prayer, or the name of a religious figure as a focus word. Remain passive; when other thoughts intrude, let them go and return to your focus word. Continue to concentrate for 10 to 20 minutes, then open your eyes and sit quietly for a moment before you get up. Practice this technique once or twice a day.

Another method, which is called progressive muscle relaxation, involves concentrating on each muscle group in the body, one at a time, and moving progressively from one end of the body to the other. Inhale and clench your muscles for five seconds, then exhale and relax. Repeat for each area of your body until your entire body is relaxed.

A technique called autogenic training combines relaxation with self-hypnosis and guided imagery. Autogenic training involves the repetition of meaningful phrases to yourself while focusing on a sense of heaviness and warmth in the limbs, breathing calmly, and keeping the muscles limp and relaxed.

A number of relaxation techniques, including yoga and moving meditation, focus on the breath. Deep breathing can release tension and speed delivery of oxygen to the body and relax the nervous system. Breathing exercises can be done anywhere at any time and are easily combined with most other relaxation methods.

*Wellness* • Habitual use of relaxation techniques rests and recharges the body, thereby strengthening it against daily or unusual stress. Quieting the mind may also promote greater concentration and receptivity to information, suggesting that relaxation techniques can foster good health and boost overall well-being.

**FOR MORE INFO**

Contact the following organization to learn more about relaxation techniques:

**The Mind/Body Medical Institute**
Deaconess Hospital
1 Deaconess Road
Boston, MA 02215



CONTINUED

# Mind/Body Medicine CONTINUED

## Spiritual Healing and Prayer

*Almost every culture, society, and religious tradition throughout history has acknowledged the healing power of faith and prayer.*

*What It's Good For* • Religious belief and prayer bring comfort, hope, and relaxation to the faithful of all backgrounds. Studies have shown that regular spiritual observance, prayer, and religious ritual are beneficial to overall health.

- **Heart problems:** In one study showing the power of intercessory prayer, a group of heart patients for whom strangers had secretly prayed were found to have fewer complications than another group of patients who did not receive the prayers of others.
- **Addiction:** Many treatment programs use the concept of a "higher power" to help people refrain from substance abuse or other bad habits.
- **Terminal illness:** Spirituality and religion help dying patients cope with the prospect of death, especially as they search for meaning in their lives and in their suffering.

*Preparations/Techniques* • People of various faiths pray in different ways, and the style of prayer can differ vastly even among people who attend the same place of worship. Believers do not need a deity to pray, nor does prayer require words; certain feelings, such as compassion, and even silent contemplation of the infinite are also considered types of prayer. For some, it may be best to surrender health problems to a higher power and trust in the outcome, rather than to pray for a specific result.

*Wellness* • Spiritual belief can help people transcend sickness or pain and achieve a sense of health and well-being. To experience the healing effects of spirituality does not require religious adherence, though religious commitment can have positive effects. Rather, it demands nothing more than an ability to love, to forgive, and to seek meaning and purpose beyond the circumstances of the moment. ■

### LICENSED & INSURED?

*Spiritual healers are not licensed as such, but a number of licensed medical professionals use prayer, therapeutic touch, or related techniques in conjunction with other treatments. While insurance companies may provide coverage for the services of these licensed professionals, spiritual therapy itself is usually not covered. On the other hand, the healthcare services of practitioners of Christian Science, a church that rejects all medical methods and teaches that only religious belief can overcome illness, are covered by some insurance companies.*

### CAUTION

**Beware of any healer who promises a complete cure of a serious illness without the use of conventional diagnostic or therapeutic methods. Faith and prayer can be powerful medicine, but for many diseases their role should be considered supportive or complementary.**

### FOR MORE INFO

Following is a list of organizations you can contact to learn more about spiritual healing:

**National Institute for Healthcare Research**
6110 Executive Blvd., Suite 908
Rockville, MD 20852
(301) 984-7162
fax: (301) 984-8143

**Center for Mind-Body Medicine**
5225 Connecticut Ave. NW, Suite 414
Washington, DC 20015
(202) 966-7338
fax: (202) 966-2589

**The Interfaith Health Program**
The Carter Center
One Copenhill
Atlanta, GA 30307
(404) 614-3757
fax: (404) 420-5158

# Naturopathic Medicine

*Naturopathic medicine aims to provide holistic, or whole-body, healthcare by drawing from numerous traditional healing systems. At its core is the idea of vis medicatrix naturae—the healing power of nature. Naturopathic doctors believe that the body naturally strives for health and that the physician's role is to support the body's efforts. To achieve this, naturopathic physicians follow seven basic principles: Help nature heal, do no harm, find the underlying cause, treat the whole person, encourage prevention, recognize wellness, and act as a teacher.*

*A naturopathic doctor, or ND, may pay considerable attention to a patient's lifestyle, since naturopathic theory holds that physical, psychological, and even spiritual elements can all contribute to disease. In treating patients the naturopathic practitioner might use a number of alternative therapies, including homeopathy, herbal remedies, Chinese medicine, spinal manipulation, nutrition, hydrotherapy, massage, and exercise.*

## *Origins*

Although its origins trace to ancient times, naturopathy as a modern system of healing began in 1902, when German immigrant Benedict Lust founded the American School of Naturopathy in New York City. Having been cured of a debilitating condition by hydrotherapy, Lust became convinced that "nature cures" were the best approach to wellness. His school grew rapidly, and by 1919 the American Naturopathic Association, also founded by Lust, was incorporated in 19 states. The movement flourished in the twenties and thirties, with thousands of practitioners attending national conventions and naturopathic journals and books gaining a growing

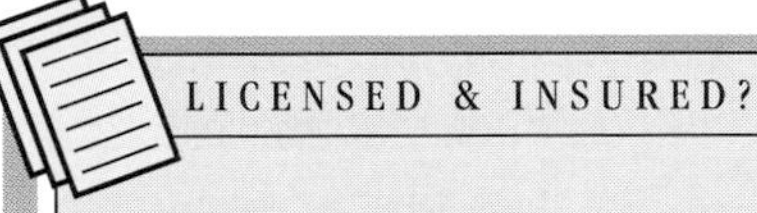


*At present naturopathic doctors are licensed to practice in 11 states: Alaska, Arizona, Connecticut, Hawaii, Maine, Montana, New Hampshire, Oregon, Utah, Vermont, and Washington. They have a legal right to practice in the District of Columbia and Idaho, and the majority of other states allow them to practice in limited ways. Naturopathic practice is regulated by state law, which dictates the therapies and prescriptive rights of NDs. Naturopathic doctors are eligible for malpractice insurance.*

*Some, but not all, insurance plans cover care by a naturopathic physician. In most cases the NDs are viewed as primary, preventive-care doctors within physician provider plans. Patients who are under the care of conventional physicians or HMOs will rarely be referred to naturopaths, however, unless they specifically request such a referral.*

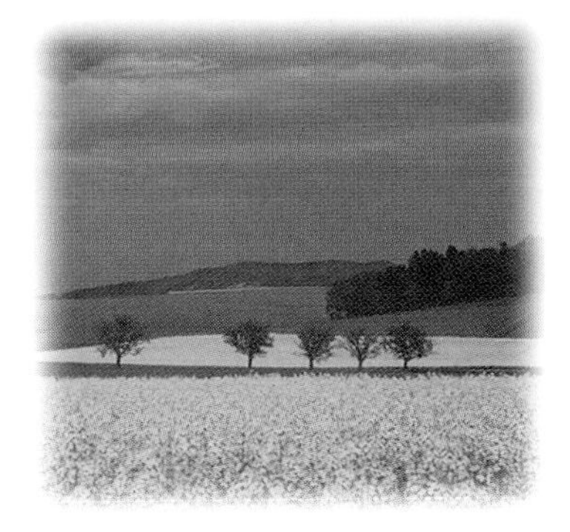

### Target Ailments

- Allergies
- Arthritis
- Asthma
- Back Problems
- Cholesterol Problems
- Constipation
- Depression
- Headache
- Heartburn
- High Blood Pressure
- Insomnia
- Menstrual Problems
- Nausea
- Pain, Chronic
- Stress

*See Common Ailments, beginning on page 194.*



CONTINUED

# Naturopathic Medicine CONTINUED

audience. By the 1990s many of naturopathy's practices regarding diet, exercise, and lifestyle had become accepted by the wider medical community.

### *What It's Good For*

Because of its emphasis on whole-body health, and with its wide range of techniques, naturopathy may be used for almost all basic healthcare. Patients visit naturopathic doctors for preventive care or for alternative therapies when conventional approaches have been unsatisfactory. Naturopathic physicians have reported success with conditions such as chronic infections, fatigue, and menstrual and menopausal problems. Diseases that are strongly affected by lifestyle and environment are among those most commonly treated by naturopaths. In a typical case of high blood pressure, for example, an ND might suggest a multifaceted approach involving changed diet, vitamin and mineral supplements, herbal medicines, and lifestyle modifications. For an arthritis sufferer, the primary treatments could include diet, homeopathic medicines, acupuncture, hydrotherapy, and massage. Naturopathic doctors also provide counseling for emotional and mental problems, such as depression and anxiety.

### *Visiting a Professional*

Naturopathic doctors are usually office-based primary-care providers. Their approaches and treatments depend on their background and philosophy. Some stick to a strict "natural" regimen of diet, detoxification, and hydrotherapy; others may differ from conventional doctors only in using herbal medicines instead of synthetic drugs. Some naturopathic doctors specialize in a particular form of alternative medicine such as homeopathy or acupuncture; others are generalists.

A first visit might take an hour,

OF SPECIAL INTEREST

#### Educational Background

*In states without licensing requirements, the naturopathic doctor's credentials may vary, although most will maintain an active license in one of the states that allow it. Most NDs licensed in recent years will have a degree from one of the three accredited naturopathic schools in the U.S.: National College of Naturopathic Medicine, Bastyr University, or the Southwest College of Naturopathic Medicine and Health Sciences. These physicians have undergone conventional premed training, followed by four years of graduate school. Their studies include standard subjects—anatomy, histology, pharmacology, pathology, and the like—as well as naturopathic philosophy, Chinese medicine, nutrition, hydrotherapy, and other alternative therapies. After learning standard diagnostic procedures, they will have worked with a licensed naturopath in a clinical setting before gaining an ND degree themselves.*

during which the doctor conducts a standard physical exam, possibly including conventional laboratory tests and radiology. In addition, the physician will spend considerable time taking a patient history, assessing every aspect of the person's lifestyle, including diet, exercise, stress, and mental, emotional, and spiritual issues.

After the initial evaluation, doctor and patient work together to establish a treatment program. Because naturopathy emphasizes noninvasive therapies, the doctor will probably suggest ways the patient can change disease-promoting habits, help set realistic, progressive goals, and identify the causes of unhealthy behavior.

If the patient has a specific complaint, the doctor may prescribe any one of many natural treatments or a combination of those treatments. These could include nutrition, homeopathic remedies, massage, botanical medicines, physical medicine (bodywork), hydrotherapy, acupuncture, or psychological and family counseling. Depending on state law, the naturopath may also prescribe conventional drugs, give vaccinations, or perform outpatient surgery. In general, though, the aim of naturopathy is not only to cure a particular ailment but also to aid the body in sustaining lifelong good health.

### *Wellness*

Wellness is what naturopathic medicine is all about. Naturopathic physicians believe that the body has an innate intelligence that strives for health; the role of both patient and doctor is to work with the body to help it promote its own well-being. Health, therefore, is more than the absence of disease; it is a vital state that needs encouragement and the proper environment. These physicians point out, for instance, that the substantial decline in deaths from heart attacks in recent decades is due not to improved coronary surgery but to public education regarding nutrition, exercise, and stress. In naturopathy, doctor and patient together will not only correct imbalances and states of disease but also plan a lifelong course of diet, exercise, and mental attitude that is designed to support the body's natural processes and fend off chronic disease and the debilitation normally associated with aging.

### *What the Critics Say*

Many members of the conventional medical establishment criticize naturopathy as being overly vague, too dependent on nutritional counseling and untested herbal remedies, and not subject to the scientific methods of experimentation and peer review. They say that the placebo effect is responsible for many of naturopathy's positive results. Because most states do not provide licensing for naturopathic doctors, critics also point out that almost anyone can get a mail-order naturopathy degree. Accredited NDs also acknowledge this danger and are attempting to persuade the government to establish standards for naturopathic physicians in all states. ■

**FOR MORE INFO**

Following is a list of organizations you can contact to learn more about naturopathy:

**American Association of Naturopathic Physicians**
2366 Eastlake Avenue East, Suite 322
Seattle, WA 98102
(206) 323-7610

**National College of Naturopathic Medicine**
11231 SE Market Street
Portland, OR 97216
(503) 255-4860

**Bastyr University**
14500 Juanita Drive, NE
Bothell, WA 98011
(206) 523-9585

**Southwest College of Naturopathic Medicine and Health Sciences**
2140 East Broadway, Suite 703
Tempe, AZ 85251
(602) 858-9100

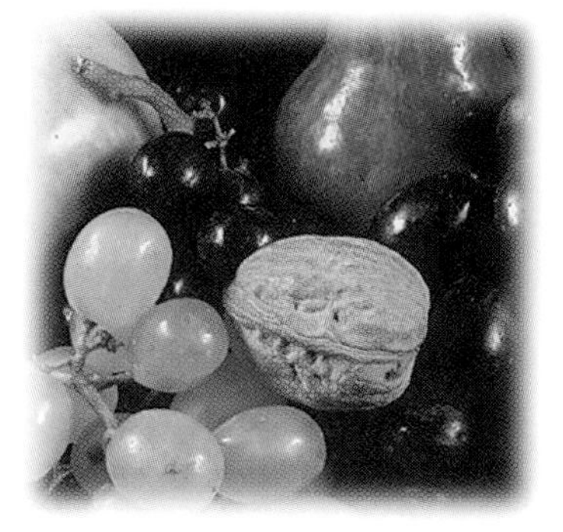

# Nutrition and Diet

*Eating a balanced diet is a major factor in a healthy lifestyle. Your body requires more than 40 nutrients for energy, growth, and tissue maintenance. Water, as the most plentiful component in the body, is also crucial to survival. It is the medium for bodily fluids, and it transports nutrients into cells and carries waste products and toxins out.*

*Conventional and alternative practitioners alike acknowledge the importance of a healthful diet. Alternative practitioners, however, place more emphasis on dietary intervention in some conditions where conventional medicine would turn first to drugs or even surgery. Treatment of atherosclerosis, for example, may take the form of an extremely low-fat diet with a program of meditation, exercise, and support-group therapy.*

## Basic Nutrition

Carbohydrates, proteins, and fats—macronutrients or "energy nutrients"—provide fuel in the form of calories. Carbohydrates, the body's main energy source, are divided into two types: Simple carbohydrates are sugars, such as cane sugar and molasses; complex carbohydrates include starches, such as those found in potatoes and whole grains.

Proteins support tissue growth and repair, and help produce antibodies, hormones, and enzymes, which are essential for all the body's chemical reactions. Protein sources include meat, fish, dairy products, poultry, dried beans, nuts, and eggs.

Dietary fat protects internal organs, provides energy, insulates against cold, and helps the body absorb certain vitamins. There are three kinds of fats: saturated, found in meat, dairy products, and coconut oil; monounsaturated, in canola, olive, and peanut oils; and polyunsaturated, in corn, cottonseed, safflower, sesame, soybean, and sunflower oils.

Your diet also supplies the important micronutrients we call vitamins and minerals. They are needed only in trace amounts, but the absence or deficiency of just one can cause major illness. With a few exceptions, the body does not manufacture micronutrients and so must obtain them from food.

Thirteen vitamins and some twenty minerals are considered essential for health. The Food and Nutrition Board of the National Research Council, National Academy of Sciences, has determined a recommended dietary allowance (RDA)—an appropriate range of intake with built-in margins to allow for variations in individual needs. Essential nutrients that do not yet have RDAs are assigned a safe and adequate daily intake or an estimated minimum daily requirement (EMDR). *(See pages 152-162 for information on specific vitamins and minerals.)*

# Nutrition and Diet

Your body also needs dietary fiber, the indigestible part of plant foods. A high-fiber diet reduces the risks of various gastrointestinal problems, promotes cardiovascular health, and may help decrease the risk of breast cancer and colon cancer.

## Diet Planning

In general, Americans eat more fat, protein, cholesterol, sugar, and salt than they need. Official diet guidelines, established jointly by the U.S. Departments of Agriculture and Health and Human Services, include some basic recommendations:

- **Eat a variety of foods.** This will help ensure that you get the calories, protein, fiber, vitamins, minerals, and other nutrients you need.
- **Control your weight.** Keep within recommended weight limits for your age, sex, and build.
- **Eat a low-fat, low-cholesterol diet.** Ideally, no more than 30 percent of your daily calories should come from fat, and no more than 10 percent should come from saturated fat.
- **Eat plenty of vegetables, fruits, and grains.** More than half of your daily calories should come from carbohydrates, rich in nutrients and low in fats; 80 percent of those calories should be from complex carbohydrates.
- **Eat sugar and salt in moderation.** Sugar is high in calories and promotes tooth decay. Too much salt may increase the risk of developing high blood pressure. Prepared foods are notoriously high in salt or other forms of sodium, so check labels.
- **If you drink alcohol, do so in moderation.** Alcohol

OF SPECIAL INTEREST

### Butter, Margarine, or Olestra?

*There is little question that limiting your intake of fat to 30 percent of your daily calories or less is good for your health. But what kind of fats should you use? For decades, margarine has been recommended to replace butter and lard, which contain saturated fats. But margarine contains what are called trans fatty acids, which can contribute to a higher risk of heart disease. Olestra is a fat substitute that provides no calories at all; however, there are some concerns that olestra and other fat substitutes could interfere with the body's absorption of some nutrients or drugs. Manufacturers put informational labels on products containing olestra, indicating that it may cause abdominal cramping and other problems in certain individuals. Because of these concerns, some practitioners now recommend small amounts of butter instead of either margarine or olestra.*

*Remember that some fat is essential to a well balanced diet. Choose monounsaturated oils over saturated fats whenever possible.*



CONTINUED

provides calories but no nutrients, and too much is harmful. However, some studies indicate that moderate consumption of red wine may actually lower the risk of heart disease. "Moderation" generally means one drink a day for women or two drinks for men.

### *Nutritional Supplements*

If you consistently eat a well-balanced diet of fresh fruits, vegetables, grains, and some animal protein, you probably don't require a nutritional supplement. Multinutrient supplements offer insurance for those times when eating well is a challenge—and can be indispensable during pregnancy or when you are ill, injured, or under great mental or physical strain.

Generally, vitamins and minerals are recommended for daily use as a preventive measure. Supplements do, however, figure in the dietary recommendations of many therapies. Orthomolecular medicine, a form of nutrient therapy, uses combinations of vitamins, minerals, and amino acids normally found in the body to treat specific conditions such as asthma, heart disease, depression, and schizophrenia. Such therapy can also be used to maintain general good health.

Taking vitamins or minerals in excess can upset the natural balance of nutrients. The fat-soluble vitamins—A, D, E, and K—can be retained in your body and may be toxic in high amounts. The rest are water soluble and are unlikely to be toxic; excess amounts are excreted in the urine. Always take supplements in moderation; they are safe in doses at or below RDAs, but higher doses may be harmful and should be taken only under the guidance of a doctor or a registered dietitian.

Supplement doses are measured by weight in milligrams (mg), or thousandths of a gram; in micrograms (mcg), or millionths of a gram; or in a universal standard known as international units (IU).

### *Food Allergies and Sensitivities*

Some people cannot tolerate certain foods or food additives; the most common culprits include dairy products, soybeans, peanuts, wheat, eggs, and shellfish. Allergic reactions can be very severe, even causing death, whereas sensitivities can cause troublesome symptoms such as rashes or bloating. Food intolerance may even be a factor in hyperactivity and many chronic diseases such as rheumatoid arthritis.

An elimination diet can help you pin down what food or foods are causing the reaction, and banning the offenders from your diet is one way to deal with this problem. A controversial method called desensitizing aims to train the body to accept foods it would otherwise not tolerate. One fairly common intolerance, that for milk sugar, can be addressed by adding a specific enzyme to the diet or by limiting the intake of dairy products to those, such as yogurt, that are more easily digested.

**FOR MORE INFO**

Following is a list of organizations you can contact to learn more about nutrition and diet:

**American Dietetic Association**
216 W. Jackson Blvd., Suite 800
Chicago, IL 60606
(800) 366-1655
(Consumer Nutrition Hotline)

**Nutrition Education Association, Inc.**
3647 Glen Haven
Houston, TX 77025
(713) 665-2946

**U.S. Department of Agriculture Center for Nutrition Policy and Promotion**
1120 20th Street, NW
Suite 200, North Lobby
Washington, DC 20036
(202) 418-2312

**American Association of Naturopathic Physicians**
2366 Eastlake Avenue East
Suite 322
Seattle, WA 98102
(206) 323-7610
fax: (206) 323-7612

# Nutrition and Diet

The Food Guide Pyramid—developed on the advice of nutritional scientists—makes healthy eating easier by showing how much of each type of food you should eat for good nutrition. Each of the groups provides some of the nutrients you need each day; no one group provides them all. Variety within and among groups is key.

The foundation of the pyramid is grain-based foods, which provide complex carbohydrates, vitamins, minerals, and fiber. On the next level are fruits and vegetables, which are rich in vitamins, minerals, and fiber but low in fat. The next two groups are critical sources of protein, calcium, iron, zinc, and other nutrients, but many of these foods are also high in fat and cholesterol. Fats, oils, and sweets occupy the tip of the pyramid and should be eaten sparingly.

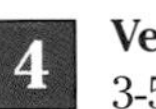

The pyramid suggests a range of daily servings for each group. Your actual needs depend on your daily caloric requirements. Experts recommend about 1,600 calories for older adults and sedentary women; 2,200 calories for children, teenage girls, active women, and sedentary men; and 2,800 calories for teenage boys, active men, and very active women.

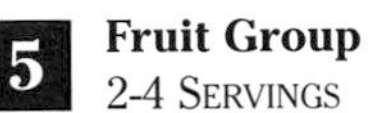

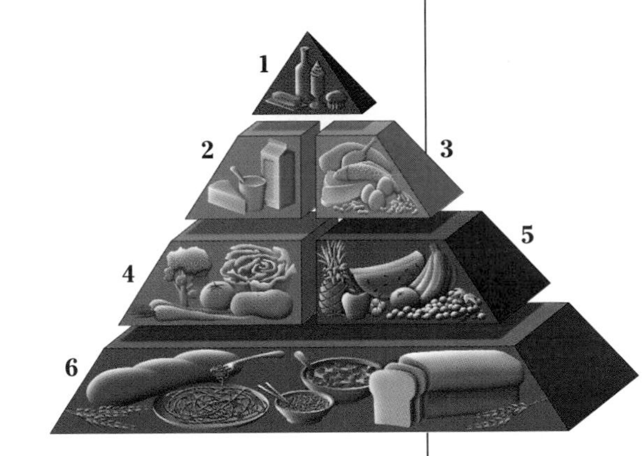


**1 Fats, Oils, & Sweets Group**
USE SPARINGLY
*One teaspoon of butter, oil, or margarine is a single serving.*

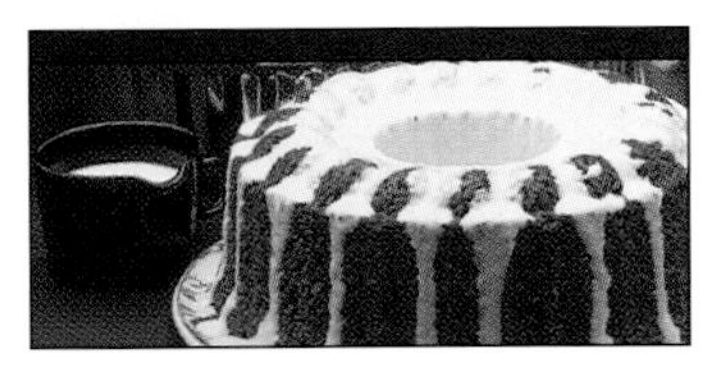

**2 Milk, Yogurt, & Cheese Group**
2-3 SERVINGS
*One serving equals 1 cup of milk or yogurt, 1½ oz of natural cheese, or 2 oz of processed cheese.*

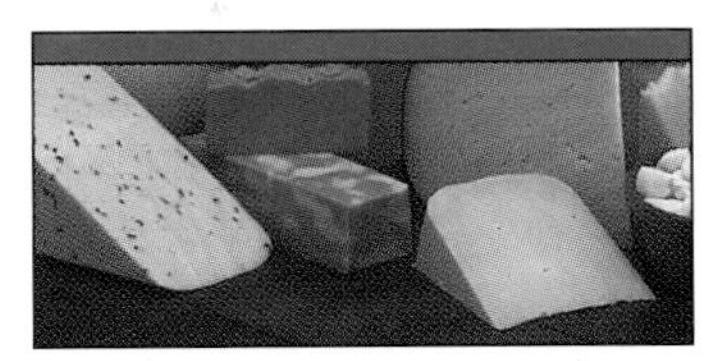

**3 Meat, Poultry, Fish, Dried Beans, Eggs, & Nuts Group** 2-3 SERVINGS
*One serving is 2 to 3 oz of cooked lean meat, poultry, or fish. An ounce of meat equals one egg or ½ cup cooked dried beans.*

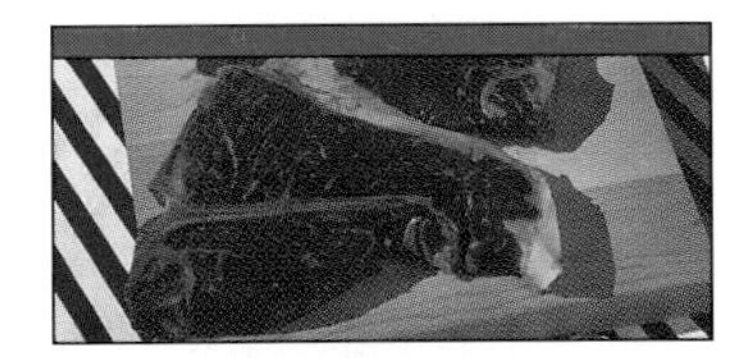

**4 Vegetable Group**
3-5 SERVINGS
*One serving equals 1 cup of raw leafy greens, ½ cup of other vegetables, or ¾ cup of vegetable juice.*

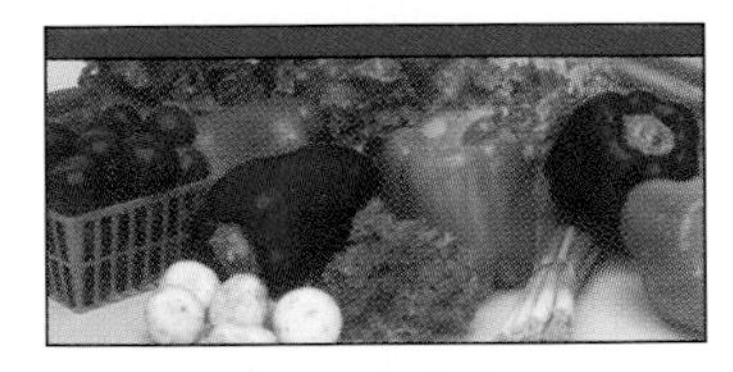

**5 Fruit Group**
2-4 SERVINGS
*One serving from the fruit group is equal to one apple, orange, or banana; ½ cup of chopped, cooked, or canned fruit; or ¾ cup of fruit juice.*

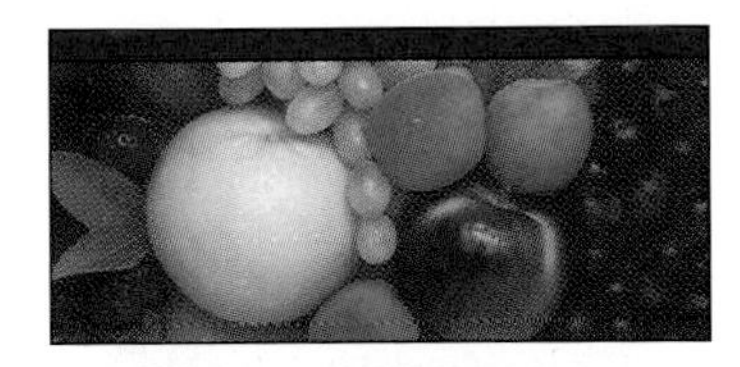

**6 Bread, Cereal, Rice, & Pasta Group**
6-11 SERVINGS
*One serving equals one slice of bread; half a bun, bagel, or muffin; 1 oz of dry cereal; or ½ cup of cooked cereal, rice, or pasta.*

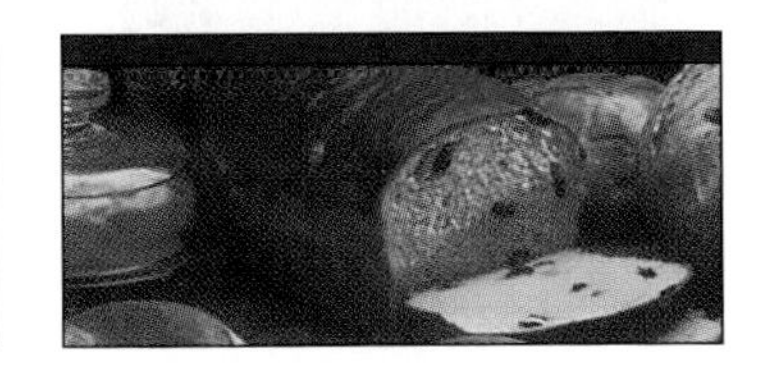



CONTINUED

# *Nutrition and Diet* CONTINUED

*Below and on the following pages are descriptions of four diets, two of which (Asian and Mediterranean) are based on the traditional eating habits of certain cultures. All four plans are reported to have specific health benefits and may be recommended to help treat or prevent specific ailments.*

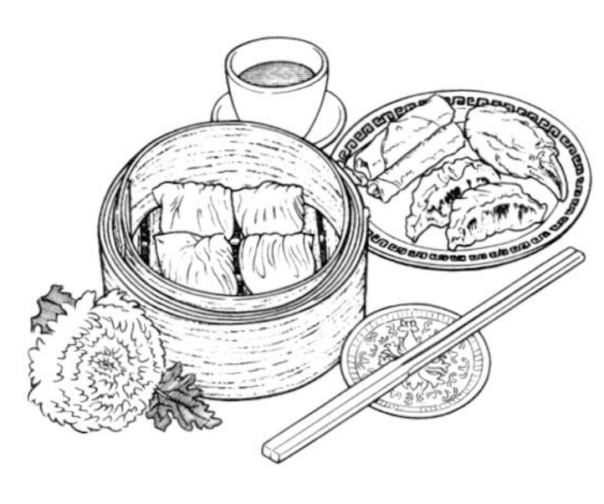

## *Asian Diet*

People in Japan, Korea, Southeast Asia, and China have traditionally eaten a diet largely composed of rice, soybean products, and fresh vegetables, with little meat or dairy products. This diet is low in fat and high in complex carbohydrates.

### *What It's Good For*

Besides generally avoiding saturated fats, the traditional Asian diet promotes good health in other ways.

- **Cancer:** Rice, a staple of the Asian diet, is high in protease inhibitors, substances believed to retard cancer. High consumption of rice is linked to low rates of some cancers, including colon, breast, and prostate. Soybeans also contain protease inhibitors; a study showed that consumption of one bowl a day of miso (soybean paste) soup lowered risk of stomach cancer by almost a third.

  Sea vegetables are also included in the Japanese diet, and they appear to have anticancer properties as well. Oriental green tea exhibits antimutagenic properties and lowers rates of stomach cancer in people who drink it regularly.
- **Atherosclerosis:** Regular consumption of soy foods confers many health benefits, including lower blood cholesterol levels and less risk of atherosclerosis.

### *Preparations/Techniques*

A diet based on Asian practices would include lots of rice—especially steamed—and soybean foods, commonly tofu and miso; fresh vegetables and seaweed, steamed or stir-fried; fresh fruit; moderate amounts of fish; and very little red meat or other animal products, including dairy products. Important seasonings are garlic, ginger, and soy sauce.

### *What the Critics Say*

As with all diets that minimize animal proteins, a wide variety of foods and attention to menu planning are essential.

# Nutrition and Diet

## Macrobiotic Diet

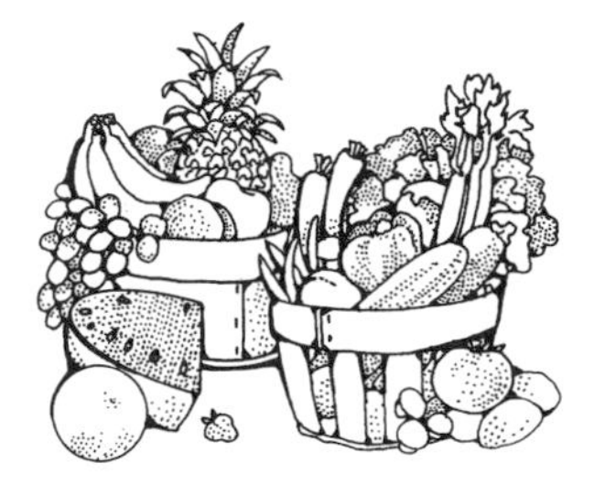

From the Greek words for "long" and "life," the macrobiotic diet is based on a system taught by Japanese educator and philosopher George Ohsawa in the early 20th century. The diet eliminates all animal products except a small amount of fish, and emphasizes whole grains and cooked vegetables. Foods are described as *yin* (contractive) or *yang* (expansive), with a balance sought between the two. Foods that are excessively one or the other are excluded.

### What It's Good For

Studies suggest that this diet's emphasis on whole grains and vegetables, and its elimination of processed foods, may have healthful effects on the body.

- **Heart disease:** Low in fat and high in complex carbohydrates and fiber, the macrobiotic diet promotes cardiovascular health.
- **Cancer:** There is evidence that a macrobiotic diet may lower the risk of breast cancer, and indeed the diet includes foods, such as soybean products and sea vegetables, that contain cancer-fighting compounds. Use of a macrobiotic diet to help treat cancer is, however, controversial *(see What the Critics Say, below)*.

### Preparations/Techniques

A macrobiotic diet prescribes deriving about 50 percent of the diet from whole cereal grains; 20 to 30 percent from vegetables; 5 to 10 percent from beans and sea vegetables; and 5 to 10 percent from soups. Occasional foods include fish—white-meat fish such as flounder and sole are recommended—fruits, and nuts.

Foods to be avoided include potatoes, peppers, meat products, eggs, warm drinks, hot spices, and any refined, mass-produced, or artificially treated food.

### What the Critics Say

While a low-fat, high-carbohydrate diet is widely considered healthful, some experts worry that a strict macrobiotic diet does not have enough variety, especially for children and pregnant women. Iron, calcium, and some vitamins are particular concerns on such a limited diet. Extremely restrictive versions that rely almost solely on grains could be dangerously low in protein and other nutrients for anyone.

Research is being conducted to determine the effect of macrobiotic food on the progress of some cancers. However, even some of those who support the diet and its avoidance of processed foods and saturated fats caution that there is so far no good evidence that any diet alone can cure disease.



CONTINUED

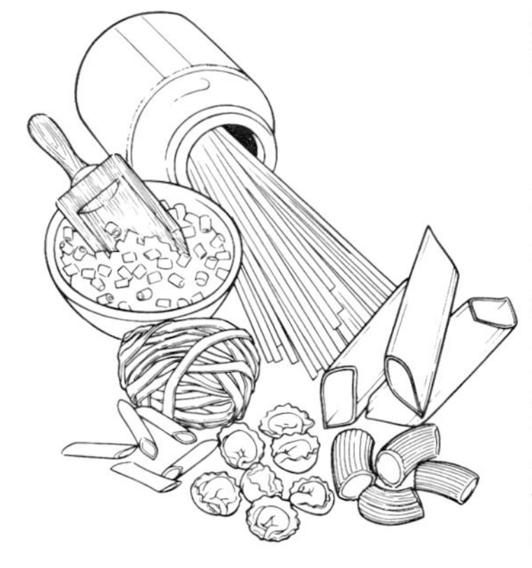

## Mediterranean Diet

The populations of 15 countries on three different continents live near the Mediterranean Sea, and despite variations from culture to culture, they share a remarkably similar traditional diet. Staples include grains, potatoes, pasta, legumes, vegetables, garlic, and olive oil. Sweets and most animal products are limited. Some fish is consumed, mostly of the oily varieties, such as mullet and tuna.

### *What It's Good For*

Quantities of complex carbohydrates and fresh vegetables align this diet with the Food Guide Pyramid's recommendations.

- **Heart disease:** The Mediterranean diet is quite high in fat, but it is mostly monounsaturated fat from olive oil, which has been shown to reduce the "bad" kind of cholesterol (low-density lipoprotein, or LDL) without lowering the amount of "good" cholesterol (high-density lipoprotein, or HDL) in the body—and so may help protect against heart disease.

  Omega-3 fatty acids present in oily fish seem to help lower blood cholesterol levels, and the vitamins and beta carotene present in brightly colored vegetables can protect the body against heart disease. Large amounts of garlic may be effective in lowering blood pressure.

  Mediterranean cultures traditionally consume red wine with meals. Some studies indicate that moderate consumption of red wine may help reduce the risk of heart disease for certain individuals.
- **Diabetes:** A high level of monounsaturated fats in the diet has been shown to help control blood sugar levels in the adult-onset type of diabetes.
- **Cancer:** The diet's emphasis on complex carbohydrates may help protect against colon cancer.

### *Preparations/Techniques*

Specifics of the Mediterranean diet vary from culture to culture, and recipes are widely available. Two simple ways to get some of the benefits of this diet are to substitute olive oil for other fats, and to add more vegetables and garlic to your meals.

### *What the Critics Say*

Olive oil is not a cure-all; you still must ensure enough variety in your diet to get all the nutrients you need.

# Nutrition and Diet

## Vegetarian Diet

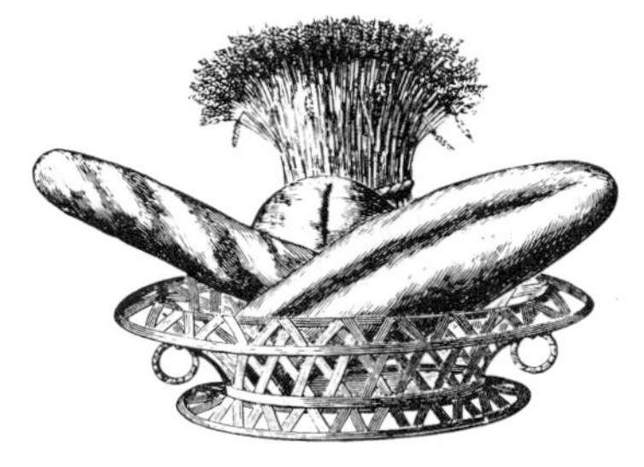

Many cultures have a longstanding tradition of avoiding the consumption of some or all animal products. The several forms of vegetarianism are among the most popular alternatives to a standard diet in the U.S. today. Some people believe that humans are physically better suited to digesting grains, beans, vegetables, and fruits than meat and other animal products; others avoid meat for philosophical or ecological reasons. In general, vegetarians enjoy a diet lower in fat and higher in complex carbohydrates than one with a lot of red meat and other animal products

### What It's Good For

Cutting your fat intake from animal products can be beneficial in many ways.

- **Heart disease:** Lower amounts of saturated fats and higher intake of polyunsaturated fats and fiber may help lower blood pressure and prevent heart disease.
- **Digestive disorders:** Higher consumption of fiber-rich foods may help vegetarians avoid diverticular disease and colon cancer.

### Preparations/Techniques

Vegans eat no animal foods at all. Lactovegetarians consume dairy products but no eggs or meat. Lacto-ovo-vegetarians eat eggs and milk products but no meat. Others exclude only red meat; some also abstain from either poultry or fish.

Take care to get enough variety to ensure proper nutrition. Protein is available from beans, grains, and some vegetables. Vitamin $B_{12}$ is a special worry on a vegetarian diet because there is no good plant source—supplements are necessary. Other micronutrients to be concerned about are vitamin D (available from egg yolks, fortified milk, or adequate sunshine); calcium (milk, fortified soybean milk, and dark green vegetables except spinach and chard); riboflavin (dark green vegetables, legumes, and whole grains); and iron (use iron cookware, eat soybeans, and ensure a plentiful intake of foods containing ascorbic acid to boost absorption of iron).

### What the Critics Say

Nutrition experts generally warn pregnant or lactating women to be very careful to assure adequate nutrition on this diet. Also, there is concern for children; rapid growth requires plenty of protein and adequate amounts of several micronutrients that can be in short supply in a totally vegetarian diet. A dietitian or nutritionist can help safeguard your well-being. For most adults who make wise food choices, vegetarianism can supply a healthful diet. ■

# The 32 Most Common Vitamins and Minerals

## Vitamins

### Biotin • VITAMIN $B_7$, VITAMIN H

**EMDR:**
30 mcg to 100 mcg

Along with other B vitamins, biotin helps convert food to energy and is required for the synthesis of carbohydrates, proteins, and fatty acids. Biotin is especially important for maintaining the health of hair, skin, and nails.

Among the types of food that are good dietary sources of biotin are cheese, kidneys, salmon, soybeans, sunflower seeds, nuts, broccoli, and sweet potatoes. Biotin deficiency is rare, and supplements are unnecessary. People can become biotin deficient through long-term use of antibiotics or by regularly eating raw egg whites, which contain avidin, a protein that blocks the body's absorption of biotin.

Because breast milk contains little biotin, infants who are breast-fed can suffer biotin deficiency, although this is uncommon. Signs of biotin deficiency include a scaly, oily skin rash; hair loss; nausea; vomiting; muscle pain; loss of appetite; a red, inflamed tongue; and fatigue. Research has not revealed a toxic level for biotin. ■

### Folic Acid • VITAMIN $B_9$

**RDA:**
**Men:** 200 mcg
**Women:** 180 mcg
**Women of childbearing age:** 400 mcg

Healthy hair, skin, nails, nerves, mucous membranes, and blood all depend on folic acid—sometimes called vitamin $B_9$, folacin, or folate. A critical component of RNA and DNA—the genetic material that controls the growth and repair of all cells—folic acid supports immune function and may help deter atherosclerosis as well as some cancers of the mucous membranes.

Sources of folic acid include liver, kidneys, avocados, beans, beets, celery, eggs, fish, green leafy vegetables, nuts, seeds, peas, orange juice, and vitamin-fortified breakfast cereals. A healthy diet should provide adequate folic acid, but the need increases during pregnancy, with injury, with some diseases—especially cancer—and with long-term use of drugs such as aspirin and oral contraceptives. Supplements taken during pregnancy may help deter the birth defects spina bifida and cleft palate. For this reason, experts now recommend that all women of childbearing age consume 400 mcg daily. High doses of folic acid are not toxic but may mask the symptoms of vitamin $B_{12}$ deficiency. Therefore, it's best to increase folic acid intake through diet or a multivitamin that contains a low dose of folic acid, rather than through individual supplements, which have to be prescribed by a doctor.

Extreme vitamin $B_9$ deficiency may cause megaloblastic anemia, a disease characterized by red blood cells that are too few in number and malformed. Symptoms include pallor; fatigue; loss of appetite; insomnia; diarrhea; and a red, inflamed tongue. Those who are most susceptible to folic acid deficiency include alcoholics, people with gastrointestinal diseases, adolescents who subsist mainly on junk food, women taking oral contraceptives, and pregnant women who are not taking supplements. ■

### Niacin • VITAMIN $B_3$

**RDA:**
**Men:** 19 mg
**Women:** 15 mg
**Pregnant women:** 17 mg

Niacin contributes to more than 50 vital bodily processes: It helps convert food into energy; build red blood cells; synthesize hormones, steroids, and fatty acids; maintain the skin, nerves, and blood vessels; support the gastrointestinal tract; stabilize mental health; and detoxify certain drugs and chemicals in the body. In addition, it helps insulin regulate blood sugar levels. Niacin is also a powerful drug, capable of lowering blood cholesterol and triglycerides, dilating blood vessels to improve circulation, and alleviating depression, insomnia, and hyperactivity.

Niacin-rich foods include liver, poultry, lean meats, fish, nuts, peanut butter, and enriched flour. If you get enough protein, you are probably getting enough niacin. If adequate vitamin $B_6$ is present, the body can also produce niacin from the amino acid tryptophan, found in milk, eggs, and cheese. Signs of niacin deficiency include indigestion, diarrhea, muscle weakness, appetite loss, dermatitis made worse by sunlight, mouth sores, an inflamed tongue, headaches, irritability, anxiety, and depression. Pregnant or breast-feeding women, the elderly, alcoholics, and people with hyperthyroidism are most likely to be niacin deficient. Extreme deficiency results in pellagra, characterized by diarrhea, dermatitis, and mental illness. Pellagra was common until the discovery that niacin was a cure; the disease is now virtually nonexistent in the U.S. thanks to niacin-enriched flour and other foods. Multivitamin supplements can raise niacin levels safely. Vitamin $B_3$ is toxic in high amounts, so take megadoses only under a doctor's supervision. Nausea, which often prevents further intake, is the first symptom; continued overuse may cause a rash, itchy skin, and liver damage. ■

## Vitamin A • BETA CAROTENE, RETINOL

**RDA:**
**Men:** 5,000 IU (or 3 mg beta carotene)
**Women:** 4,000 IU (or 2.4 mg beta carotene)

The first vitamin ever discovered, vitamin A is essential for good vision—especially in dim light—and for healthy skin, hair, and mucous membranes of the nose, throat, respiratory system, and digestive system. This vitamin is also necessary for the proper development of bones and teeth. It stimulates wound healing and is used to treat some skin disorders. Beta carotene, the precursor to vitamin A, is a carotenoid, a type of pigment found in plants. Your skin stores beta carotene and your body metabolizes it to produce vitamin A as needed. Excess beta carotene, along with other carotenoids, acts as an antioxidant and supports immune function, so it increases your resistance to infection; it may help prevent some cancers and vision problems such as night blindness. Beta carotene may also help lower cholesterol levels and reduce the risk of heart disease.

Vitamin A is present in orange and yellow vegetables and fruits; dark green leafy vegetables such as mustard greens and kale; whole milk, cream, and butter; and organ meats. Because it is fat soluble, vitamin A is stored in the body for a long time, and supplements are generally not recommended. Too much vitamin A can cause headaches, vision problems, nausea, vomiting, dry and flaking skin, or an enlarged liver or spleen. Other names for vitamin A are retinol, retinene, retinoic acid, and retinyl palmitate. ■

## Vitamin B Complex

**RDA:**
See individual vitamin entries

As its name implies, vitamin B complex is a combination, or mixture, of eight essential vitamins. Although each is chemically distinct, the B vitamins coexist in many of the same foods and often work together to bolster metabolism, maintain healthy skin and muscle tone, enhance immune and nervous system function, and promote cell growth and division—including that of the red blood cells that help prevent anemia.

Foods rich in B-complex vitamins include liver and other organ meats, fish, poultry, brewer's yeast, eggs, beans and peas, dark green leafy vegetables, whole-grain cereals, and dairy products. B vitamins, which are water soluble, are dispersed throughout the body and must be replenished daily; any excess is excreted in urine. People susceptible to vitamin B deficiency include pregnant women, nursing mothers, vegetarians, alcoholics, "sugarholics," the elderly, and people who have malabsorption conditions or who take certain antibiotics over a long period of time; the symptoms include oily and scaly skin, upset stomach, headaches, anxiety, moodiness, and heart arrhythmias. A deficiency of one B vitamin usually means that intake of all B vitamins is low. If your doctor suggests you need more B vitamins, take a daily multivitamin or B-complex supplement rather than individual B-vitamin supplements. Most B vitamins are nontoxic unless taken in excessively large amounts. ■

## Vitamin $B_1$ • THIAMINE

**RDA:**
**Men:** 1.5 mg
**Women:** 1.1 mg

Thiamine, sometimes called the energy vitamin because it is needed to metabolize carbohydrates, fats, and proteins, helps convert excess glucose into stored fat. Vitamin $B_1$ also ensures proper nerve-impulse transmission and contributes to maintaining normal appetite, muscle tone, and mental health. In the 1930s thiamine was discovered to be the cure for the crippling and potentially fatal disease beriberi.



CONTINUED

Now that rice, flour, and bread are generally enriched with thiamine, beriberi is relatively rare.

A diet that regularly includes lean pork, milk, whole grains, peas, beans, peanuts, or soybeans generally provides enough thiamine. Athletes, laborers, pregnant women, and others who burn lots of energy may require more than the adult RDA of thiamine. Mild deficiency may cause fatigue, loss of appetite, nausea, moodiness, confusion, anemia, and possibly heart arrhythmias. Alcohol suppresses thiamine absorption; for this reason and because of typically poor diets, alcoholics are likely to be deficient in thiamine and other nutrients. To increase thiamine levels, try changing your diet or taking a multivitamin rather than thiamine supplements. Large doses up to 100 mg of thiamine may alleviate itching from insect bites; otherwise, megasupplements are not known to be either harmful or helpful. ■

## Vitamin $B_2$ • RIBOFLAVIN

**RDA:**
**Men:** 1.7 mg
**Women:** 1.3 mg
**Pregnant women:** 1.6 mg

Like other members of the vitamin B complex, riboflavin helps produce energy from carbohydrates, fats, and proteins. Riboflavin also promotes healthy skin, hair, nails, and mucous membranes; aids the production of red blood cells, corticosteroids, and thyroid hormones; and is required for the proper function of the nerves, eyes, and adrenal glands. It is often used to treat acne, anemia, cataracts, and depression.

A well-balanced diet provides most people with adequate riboflavin, although athletes and others who need a great deal of energy may require more than the RDA. Lean organ meats, enriched bread and flour, cheese, yogurt, eggs, almonds, soybean products such as tofu, and green leafy vegetables—especially broccoli—are good sources. Store these foods in the dark, because vitamin $B_2$ breaks down in sunlight. Alcoholics and elderly people are susceptible to riboflavin deficiency: The signs include oily, scaly skin rash; sores, especially on the lips and corners of the mouth; a swollen, red, painful tongue; sensitivity to light; and burning or red, itchy eyes. Although vitamin $B_2$ supplements are available, they provide far more riboflavin than anyone needs. Diet changes are better, or take a multivitamin supplement. It is best to take the supplements with food, which increases their absorption tremendously compared with tablets alone. ■

## Vitamin $B_5$ • PANTOTHENIC ACID

**EMDR:**
4 mg to 7 mg

The Greek term *pan* in *pantothenic acid* means "everywhere," indicating this vitamin's abundance. Along with other B vitamins, pantothenic acid is required for converting food to energy; building red blood cells; making bile; and synthesizing fats, adrenal gland steroids, antibodies, and acetylcholine and other neurotransmitters—chemicals that permit nerve transmission. Pantothenic acid in dexpanthenol lotions and creams relieves the pain of burns, cuts, and abrasions; reduces skin inflammation; and speeds the healing of wounds.

Vitamin $B_5$ is abundant in organ meats, dark turkey meat, salmon, wheat bran, brewer's yeast, brown rice, lentils, nuts, beans, corn, peas, sweet potatoes, and eggs. Excess pantothenic acid may cause diarrhea. A deficiency in this vitamin does not seem to occur naturally in humans and is likely only with extreme starvation. A pantothenic acid supplement, calcium pantothenate, is available. ■

## Vitamin $B_6$ • PYRIDOXINE

**RDA:**
**Men:** 2 mg
**Women:** 1.6 mg
**Pregnant women:** 2.2 mg

Vitamin $B_6$ encompasses a family of compounds that includes pyridoxine, pyridoxamine, and pyridoxal. This vitamin supports immune function, transmission of nerve impulses (especially in the brain), energy metabolism, and synthesis of red blood cells. Prescribed as a drug, it can sometimes alleviate carpal tunnel syndrome, infant seizures, and PMS.

A healthy diet provides enough vitamin $B_6$ for most people. Brown rice, lean meats, poultry, fish, bananas, avocados, whole grains, corn, and nuts are rich in vitamin $B_6$. People most likely to be at risk for vitamin $B_6$ deficiency include anyone with a malabsorption problem such as lactose intolerance or celiac disease; diabetic or elderly people; and women who are pregnant, nursing, or taking oral contraceptives. Severe deficiency is rare. Mild deficiency may cause acne and inflamed skin, insomnia, muscle weakness, nausea, irritability, depression, and fatigue. A daily multivitamin supplement is usually recommended to boost low vitamin $B_6$ levels. Taking too much or too little vitamin $B_6$ can impair nerve function and mental health. If high levels (2,000 mg to 5,000 mg) are taken for several months, vitamin $B_6$ can become habit forming and may induce sleepiness as well as tingling, numb hands and feet. These symptoms will most likely disappear when the vitamin $B_6$ intake is reduced, and there is usually no permanent damage. ■

## Vitamin $B_{12}$ • COBALAMIN

**RDA:**
**Adults:** 2 mcg
**Pregnant women:** 2.2 mcg

The largest and most complex family of the B vitamins, Vitamin $B_{12}$ includes several chemical compounds known as cobalamins. Cyanocobalamin, the stablest form, is the one most likely to be found in supplements. Like other B vitamins, $B_{12}$ is important for converting fats, carbohydrates, and protein into energy, and assisting in the synthesis of red blood cells. It is critical for producing the genetic materials RNA and DNA, as well as myelin, a fatty substance that forms a protective sheath around nerves. Unlike other B vitamins, vitamin $B_{12}$ needs several hours to be absorbed in the digestive tract. Excess vitamin $B_{12}$ is excreted in urine, even though a backup supply can be stored for several years in the liver.

Vitamin $B_{12}$ is not produced by plants but is supplied through animal products such as organ meats, fish, eggs, and dairy products. Dietary deficiency is uncommon and is usually limited to alcoholics, strict vegetarians, and pregnant or nursing women—who should take supplements. More often, deficiency stems from an inability to absorb the vitamin, a problem that may occur for years before symptoms show; it tends to affect the elderly, those who have had stomach surgery, or people who have a disease of malabsorption, such as colitis.

Lack of calcium, vitamin $B_6$, or iron may also interfere with the normal absorption of $B_{12}$. Signs of vitamin $B_{12}$ deficiency include a sore tongue, weakness, weight loss, body odor, back pains, and tingling arms and legs. Severe deficiency leads to pernicious anemia, causing fatigue, a tendency to bleed, lemon yellow pallor, abdominal pain, stiff arms and legs, irritability, and depression.

Without treatment, pernicious anemia can lead to permanent nerve damage and possibly death; the disease can be controlled, although not cured, with regular $B_{12}$ injections. Vitamin $B_{12}$ is considered nontoxic, even when taken at several times the RDA. ■

## Vitamin C • ASCORBIC ACID

**RDA:**
**Adults:** 60 mg
**Pregnant women:** 70 mg

Vitamin C is well known for its ability to prevent and treat scurvy, a disease that causes swollen and bleeding gums, aching bones and muscles, and in some cases even death. It is also essential to the healing of wounds, burns, bruises, and broken bones because collagen, the substance that constitutes the body's connective tissue, depends on vitamin C for its production. As a powerful antioxidant and immune system booster, vitamin C may alleviate the pain of rheumatoid arthritis, protect against atherosclerosis and heart disease, and help prevent some forms of cancer; and has the reputed potential capacity (yet unproved) to prevent the common cold. More than the RDA may be needed under conditions of physical or emotional stress.

Sources of vitamin C include citrus fruits, rose hips, bell peppers, strawberries, broccoli, cantaloupes, tomatoes, and leafy greens. Vitamin C breaks down faster than any other vitamin, so it is best to eat fruits and vegetables when fresh and to cook them minimally or not at all. Slight vitamin C deficiency is rather common, although severe deficiencies are rare in the United States today. Symptoms of deficiency include weight loss, fatigue, bleeding gums, easy bruising, reduced resistance to colds and other infections, and slow healing of wounds and fractures.

Because it is water soluble, excess vitamin C is excreted in the urine, so large amounts of it may usually be taken without fear of toxicity. Doses larger than 1,000 mg a day have been suggested for preventing cancer, infections such as the common cold, and other ailments. In some people, large doses may induce such side effects as nausea, diarrhea, reduced selenium and copper absorption, excessive iron absorption, increased kidney stone formation, and a false-positive reaction to diabetes tests. ■



CONTINUED

# The 32 Most Common Vitamins and Minerals

## Vitamin D • CHOLECALCIFEROL, ERGOCALCIFEROL

**RDA:**
**Adults:**
200 IU (5 mcg)
**Children, adolescents, and pregnant women:**
400 IU (10 mcg)

Vitamin D not only promotes healthy bones and teeth by regulating the absorption and balance of calcium and phosphorus, but also fosters normal muscle contraction and nerve function. Vitamin D prevents rickets, a disease of calcium-deprived bone that results in bowlegs, knock-knees, and other bone defects. Vitamin D supplements may help treat psoriasis and slow or even reverse some cancers, such as myeloid leukemia.

Fatty fish such as herring, salmon, and tuna, followed by dairy products, are the richest natural sources of this nutrient. Few other foods naturally contain vitamin D, but 10 minutes in midday summer sun enables the body to produce about 200 IU of it. Milk, breakfast cereals, and infant formulas are fortified with vitamin D. In adults, vitamin D deficiency can cause nervousness and diarrhea, insomnia, muscle twitches, and bone weakening, and it may worsen osteoporosis. Too much vitamin D raises the calcium level in the blood, which in turn may induce headaches, nausea, loss of appetite, excessive thirst, muscle weakness, and even heart, liver, or kidney damage as calcium deposits accumulate in soft tissue. Vitamin D is fat soluble; excess amounts of it are stored in the body. Because of its potentially toxic effects, vitamin D should not be taken in supplements of more than 400 IU daily unless prescribed by a doctor. ■

## Vitamin E

**RDA:**
**Women:** 12 IU (8 mg)
**Men and pregnant or nursing women:**
15 IU (10 mg)

Vitamin E encompasses a family of compounds called tocopherols, of which alpha-tocopherol is the most common. It is required for proper function of the immune system, endocrine system, and sex glands. As a potent antioxidant, it prevents unstable molecules known as free radicals from damaging cells and tissues. In this capacity, vitamin E deters atherosclerosis, accelerates wound healing, protects lung tissue from inhaled pollutants, and may reduce risk of heart disease and prevent premature aging of skin. Researchers suspect that vitamin E has other beneficial effects ranging from preventing cancer and cataracts to alleviating rheumatoid arthritis and a skin disorder associated with lupus.

Most people get enough vitamin E through their diet and don't need supplements. Vegetable oils, nuts, dark green leafy vegetables, organ meats, seafood, eggs, and avocados are rich food sources. Symptoms of vitamin E deficiency, such as fluid retention and hemolytic anemia, are rare in adults but are sometimes seen in premature infants. Because of its many suggested therapeutic roles, vitamin E is popular as an oral supplement and an ingredient of skincare products. Although it is fat soluble, vitamin E is considered nontoxic because it does no harm except in extremely high doses. ■

## Vitamin K • MENADIONE, PHYTONADIONE

**RDA:**
**Men:** 80 mcg
**Women:** 65 mcg

Vitamin K is needed in a small but critical amount to form certain proteins essential mainly for blood clotting but also for kidney function and bone metabolism. Vitamin K exists in two natural forms that require some dietary fat for absorption.

Bacteria living in the intestines produce about half the body's needs; the rest comes from diet. Good food sources include spinach, cabbage, broccoli, turnip greens, or other leafy vegetables; beef liver; green tea; cheese; and oats. Vitamin K deficiency is extremely rare in adults but may occur in newborns until their intestinal bacteria begin producing the vitamin. To enhance blood-clotting ability in a newborn, the mother may take vitamin K supplements before delivery, and infants usually receive them after birth. Otherwise, supplements are neither necessary nor recommended. Megadoses higher than 500 mcg can be toxic or cause an allergic reaction and must be prescribed by a doctor. Large doses of vitamin E may interfere with vitamin K's blood-clotting effects. ■

# The 32 Most Common Vitamins and Minerals

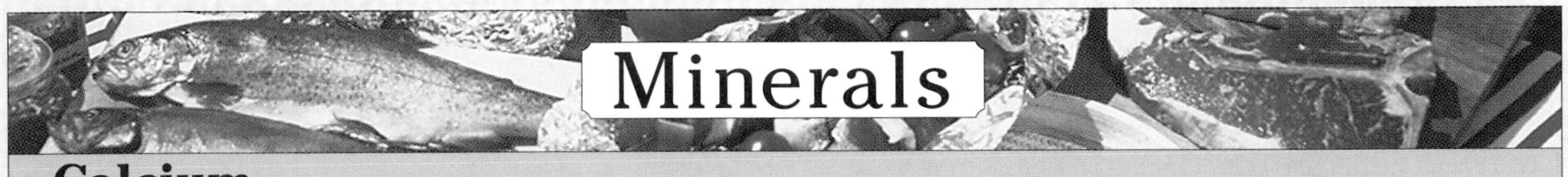


## Calcium

**RDA:**
**Adults:** 800 mg
**Pregnant women and young adults:** 1,200 mg

Calcium, the most abundant mineral in the body, is essential for the growth and maintenance of bones and teeth. It enables muscles, including the heart, to contract; it is essential for normal blood clotting, proper nerve-impulse transmission, and connective-tissue maintenance. It helps keep blood pressure normal and may reduce the risk of heart disease; taken with vitamin D, it may help lessen the risk of colorectal cancer. It helps prevent rickets in children and osteoporosis in adults.

Good sources include dairy products, dark green leafy vegetables, sardines, salmon, and almonds. Calcium is needed in varying amounts by different people. Too much calcium can lead to constipation and to calcium deposits in soft tissue, causing damage to the heart, liver, or kidneys. For calcium to be properly absorbed, the body must have sufficient levels of vitamin D and of hydrochloric acid in the stomach and a balance of other minerals, including magnesium and phosphorus. A sedentary lifestyle and consuming too much alcohol, dietary fiber, and fat can interfere with calcium absorption; too much protein and caffeine results in calcium being excreted in urine. Supplemental calcium is available in many forms; the form that is best absorbed by the body is calcium citrate-malate. ■

## Chloride

**EMDR:**
**Adults:** 750 mg

A natural salt of the mineral chlorine, chloride works with sodium and potassium to help maintain the proper distribution and pH of all bodily fluids and to encourage healthy nerve and muscle function. Independently, chloride contributes to digestion and waste elimination. It is a key component of hydrochloric acid, one of the gastric juices that digest food.

A diet of unprocessed natural foods provides more than enough chloride for human health. Just a pinch of table salt contains about 250 mg, one-third of the EMDR. Chloride deficiency is extremely rare and is usually due to illness. Excessive vomiting can reduce the stomach's chloride level, upsetting its pH balance and causing sweating, diarrhea, loss of appetite, slow and shallow breathing, listlessness, and muscle cramps. Although toxic in large amounts, excess chloride is excreted in urine, preventing potentially dangerous accumulation. ■

## Chromium

**EMDR:**
**Adults:** 50 mcg to 200 mcg

As a component of a natural substance called glucose tolerance factor, chromium works with insulin to regulate the body's use of sugar and is essential to fatty-acid metabolism. Its contribution to metabolism makes chromium a helpful supplement in weight-loss programs. Additional evidence suggests that chromium may help deter atherosclerosis and reduce risk of cardiovascular disease. Inadequate chromium can result in alcohol intolerance, elevate blood sugar levels, and possibly induce diabetes-like symptoms such as tingling in the extremities and reduced muscle coordination.

Trace amounts of chromium are found in many foods, including brewer's yeast, liver, lean meats, poultry, molasses, whole grains, eggs, and cheese. Chromium is not absorbed well, so the body must take in far more than it actually uses. Most people do not get enough dietary chromium, and some may benefit from a multinutrient supplement, such as chromium citrate or chromium picolinate. Supplemental chromium may be used to treat some cases of adult-onset diabetes, to reduce insulin requirements of some diabetic children, and to relieve symptoms of hypoglycemia. Taken regularly in supplements greater than 1,000 mcg, however, chromium inhibits insulin's activity and can be toxic. ■



CONTINUED

# The 32 Most Common Vitamins and Minerals

## Cobalt

**RDA/EMDR:**
Not established

The mineral cobalt is a constituent of cobalamin (vitamin $B_{12}$). Cobalt helps form red blood cells and maintain nerve tissue. Consuming large amounts of inorganic cobalt stimulates growth of the thyroid gland and may lead to the overproduction of red blood cells, a disorder known as polycythemia.

To be biologically useful, cobalt must be obtained from foods such as liver, kidneys, milk, oysters, clams, or sea vegetables, or from vitamin $B_{12}$ supplements. Inorganic cobalt has no nutritional value but is sometimes added to beer as an antifoaming agent. ■

## Copper

**EMDR:**
**Adults:** 1.5 mg to 3 mg

Copper is indispensable to human health. Its many functions include the following: helping to form hemoglobin in the blood; facilitating the absorption and use of iron so that red blood cells can transport oxygen to tissues; assisting in the regulation of blood pressure and heart rate; strengthening blood vessels, bones, tendons, and nerves; promoting fertility; and ensuring normal skin and hair pigmentation. Some evidence suggests that copper helps prevent cardiovascular problems such as high blood pressure and heart arrhythmias and that it may help treat arthritis and scoliosis. Copper may also protect tissue from damage by free radicals, support the body's immune function, and contribute to preventing cancer.

Most adults get enough copper from a normal, varied diet. Seafood and organ meats are the richest sources; blackstrap molasses, nuts, seeds, green vegetables, black pepper, cocoa, and water passed through copper pipes also contain significant quantities. Supplemental copper should be taken only on a doctor's advice. Common supplemental forms are copper aspartate, copper citrate, and copper picolinate. Excess calcium and zinc will interfere with copper absorption, but a true copper deficiency is rare and tends to be limited to people either with certain inherited diseases that inhibit copper absorption, such as albinism, or with acquired malabsorption ailments, such as Crohn's disease and celiac disease. The deficiency may also occur in infants who are not breast-fed and in some premature babies. Symptoms of copper deficiency include brittle, discolored hair; skeletal defects; anemia; high blood pressure; heart arrhythmias; and infertility. Taking more than 10 mg of copper daily can bring on nausea, vomiting, muscle pain, and stomachaches. Women who are pregnant or taking birth-control pills are susceptible to excess blood levels of copper. Some research suggests that high levels of copper and iron may play a role in hyperactivity and autism. ■

## Fluoride

**EMDR:**
**Adults:** 1.5 mg to 4 mg

Fluoride, a natural form of the mineral fluorine, is required for healthy teeth and bones. It helps form the tough enamel that protects the teeth from decay and cavities, and increases bone strength and stability. Since the 1950s, many U.S. cities have added fluoride to municipal drinking water at a ratio of about 1 part per million (ppm), or 1 mg per liter. Many believe this practice is responsible for the 40 to 70 percent reduction in tooth decay that dentists have since observed. Fluoride's decay-reducing effects are strongest if children are exposed to the mineral while their teeth are forming. Fluoride toothpaste is helpful, but it is not nearly as effective as regularly ingested fluoride.

Fluoridated water provides most individuals with at least 1 mg of fluoride per day; other dietary sources are dried seaweed, seafood—especially sardines and salmon—cheese, meat, and tea. Nursing babies and children who do not regularly drink fluoridated water should be given supplements, but only as prescribed by a dentist or doctor, because excess fluoride can have adverse effects: At levels of 2 ppm to 8 ppm, the teeth may soften and discolor; at over 8 ppm, fluoride toxicity can depress growth, harden ligaments and tendons, make bones brittle, and induce degeneration of major body systems; 50 ppm may cause fatal poisoning. The low fluoride levels in fluoridated drinking water, however, pose no harmful effects to health. ■

## Iodine

**RDA:**
**Adults:** 150 mcg
**Pregnant women:** 175 mcg

Iodine was one of the first minerals recognized as essential to human health. For centuries, it has been known to prevent and treat goiter—enlargement of the thyroid gland. As part of several thyroid hormones, iodine strongly influences nutrient metabolism; nerve and muscle function; skin, hair, tooth, and nail condition; and physical and mental development. Iodine may also help convert beta carotene into vitamin A.

Kelp, seafood, and vegetables grown in iodine-rich soils are good sources of this mineral. More than half of all the salt consumed in the U.S. is iodized, supplying sufficient iodine in a regular diet. Supplements are usually unnecessary, but pregnant women should take in enough iodine for themselves and their babies to prevent potential mental retardation or cretinism, a form of dwarfism in infants. Iodine deficiency is now uncommon; besides goiter, its effects include weight gain, hair loss, listlessness, insomnia, and some forms of mental retardation. Most excess iodine is excreted, but extremely high intake may cause nervousness, hyperactivity, headache, rashes, a metallic taste in the mouth, and goiter—in this case due to thyroid hyperactivity. ■

## Iron

**RDA:**
**Adults:** 10 mg
**Premenopausal women:** 15 mg
**Pregnant women:** 30 mg

Iron is found in hemoglobin, the protein in red blood cells that transports oxygen from the lungs to body tissues. It is also a component of myoglobin, a protein that provides extra fuel to muscles during exertion.

Dietary iron exists in two forms: heme iron, found in red meat, chicken, seafood, and other animal products; and nonheme iron, found in dark green vegetables, whole grains, nuts, dried fruit, and other plant foods. Many flour-based food products are fortified with iron. Heme iron is easier to absorb, but eating foods containing nonheme iron along with foods that have heme iron or vitamin C will maximize iron absorption.

Coffee, tea, soy-based foods, antacids, and tetracycline inhibit iron absorption, as do excessive amounts of calcium, zinc, and manganese. Lack of iron deprives body tissues of oxygen and may cause iron deficiency anemia; warning signs include fatigue, paleness, dizziness, sensitivity to cold, listlessness, irritability, poor concentration, and heart palpitations. Because iron strengthens immune function, iron deficiency also may increase susceptibility to infection. Women need more iron before menopause than after, because menstruation causes iron loss each month. People who have special iron intake needs include menstruating or pregnant women, children under two years of age, vegetarians, anyone with bleeding conditions such as hemorrhoids or bleeding stomach ulcers, and anyone taking the medications listed above.

On a doctor's recommendation, adults can augment their iron intake by means of a multinutrient supplement; straight iron supplements should be taken only under a doctor's supervision. Excess iron inhibits absorption of phosphorus, interferes with immune function, and may increase your risk of developing cancer, cirrhosis, or heart attack. Symptoms of iron toxicity include diarrhea, vomiting, headache, dizziness, fatigue, stomach cramps, and weak pulse. Though uncommon, severe iron poisoning can result in coma, heart failure, and death. Children should never be given adult iron supplements, which can easily poison them. If your pediatrician recommends an iron supplement, make sure it is a specific, child-formulated variety. ■

## Magnesium

**RDA:**
**Men:** 350 mg
**Women:** 280 mg
**Pregnant women:** 320 mg

Magnesium contributes to health in many ways. Along with calcium and phosphorus, it is a main constituent of bone. A proper balance of calcium and magnesium is essential for healthy bones and teeth, reduces the risk of developing osteoporosis, and may minimize the effects of existing osteoporosis. Calcium and magnesium also help regulate muscle activity: While calcium stimulates contraction, magnesium induces relaxation. Magnesium is essential for metabolism—converting food to energy—and for building proteins. Adequate blood levels of magnesium protect the body from cardiovascular disease, heart arrhythmias, and possibly, stroke due to blood clotting in the brain.



CONTINUED

On average, people get enough (or nearly enough) magnesium in their diet. Fish, green leafy vegetables, milk, nuts, seeds, and whole grains are good sources. Many over-the-counter antacids, laxatives, and analgesics contain magnesium, but these medications should not be used as magnesium supplements. A multinutrient supplement is a relatively safe way to augment your magnesium intake. Take specific magnesium supplements only under a doctor's supervision. Of the supplemental forms, magnesium citrate-malate is the easiest to absorb, while magnesium glycinate is the least likely to cause diarrhea at high doses.

The body's need for magnesium increases with stress or illness. Administered as a supplement, magnesium may successfully treat insomnia, muscle cramps, premenstrual syndrome, and cardiovascular problems including high blood pressure, angina due to coronary artery spasm, and leg pain and cramping due to insufficient blood flow. Studies indicate that giving magnesium immediately to a heart attack patient greatly increases the chance of survival.

The body processes magnesium efficiently; the kidneys conserve it as needed and excrete any excess, so both severe deficiency and toxicity are rare. These conditions are dangerous when they do occur, however. Magnesium deficiency may cause nausea, listlessness, muscle weakness, tremor, disorientation, and heart palpitations. Toxicity can induce diarrhea, fatigue, muscle weakness, and in extreme cases, severely depressed heart rate and blood pressure, shallow breathing, loss of reflexes, coma, and possibly death. People who abuse laxatives or experience kidney failure are the most vulnerable to magnesium poisoning. ■

## Manganese

**EMDR:**
2.5 mg to 5 mg

Manganese is essential for the proper formation and maintenance of bone, cartilage, and connective tissue; it contributes to the synthesis of proteins and genetic material; it helps produce energy from foods; it acts as an antioxidant; and it assists in normal blood clotting.

Most people get enough manganese through their diet alone; for example, a breakfast consisting of orange juice, a 1-oz serving of bran cereal, and a banana provides just over 2.5 mg of manganese. Other food sources include brown rice, nuts, seeds, wheat germ, beans, whole grains, peas, and strawberries. Manganese citrate, a supplement, may help repair damaged tendons and ligaments. Excess dietary manganese is not considered toxic, and manganese deficiency is extremely rare. ■

## Molybdenum

**EMDR:**
**Adults:** 75 mcg to 250 mcg

The obscure mineral molybdenum is an enzyme component. It helps generate energy, process waste for excretion, mobilize stored iron for the body's use, and detoxify sulfites—chemicals used as food preservatives. As such, molybdenum is essential to normal development, particularly of the nervous system. It is also a component of tooth enamel and may help prevent tooth decay.

Molybdenum is present in peas, beans, cereals, pastas, leafy vegetables, yeast, milk, and organ meats. People generally get enough through diet; deficiency is virtually nonexistent. Toxicity is also rare. Molybdenum is available in supplement form as molybdenum picolinate; however, prolonged intake of more than 10 mg daily can cause gout-like symptoms such as joint pain and swelling. ■

## Phosphorus

**RDA:**
**Adults over 25 years old:** 800 mg
**Young adults and pregnant women:** 1,200 mg

Phosphorus is the second most plentiful mineral in the body and is found in every cell. Like calcium, phosphorus is essential for bone formation and maintenance; more than 75 percent of the body's phosphorus is contained in bones and teeth. Phosphorus stimulates muscle contraction and contributes to tissue growth and repair, energy production, nerve-impulse transmission, and heart and kidney function.

Phosphorus exists to some degree in nearly all foods, especially meats, poultry, eggs, fish, nuts, dairy products, whole grains, and soft drinks. Deficiency is rare—most people take in far more phosphorus than they need—but may be induced by long-term use of antacids or anticonvulsant drugs that contain aluminum hydroxide. Symptoms of phosphorus deficiency include general weakness, loss of appetite, bone pain, and increased susceptibility to bone fracture. Excess phosphorus in the bloodstream promotes calcium loss, which may weaken bones. Extreme phosphorus toxicity is rare, except in the event of kidney disease. ■

## Potassium

**EMDR:**
**Adults:** 2,000 mg

Potassium is the third most abundant mineral in the body. It works closely with sodium and chloride to maintain fluid distribution and pH balance and to augment nerve-impulse transmission, muscle contraction, and regulation of heartbeat and blood pressure. It is also required for protein synthesis, carbohydrate metabolism, and insulin secretion by the pancreas. Studies suggest that people who regularly eat potassium-rich foods are less likely to develop atherosclerosis, heart disease, and high blood pressure, or to die of a stroke.

Dietary sources include lean meats, raw vegetables, fruits—especially citrus fruits, bananas, and avocados—and potatoes. Many Americans may get only marginal amounts of potassium, but supplements, such as potassium aspartate, are best taken only under a doctor's guidance. Marginal potassium deficiency causes no symptoms but may increase the risk of developing high blood pressure or aggravate existing heart disease. More severe deficiency can result in nausea, diarrhea, muscle cramps and muscle weakness, poor reflexes, poor concentration, heart arrhythmias, and rarely, death due to heart failure. Acute potassium toxicity may have similar effects, including possible heart failure. However, acute toxicity is rarely linked to diet and tends to occur only in the event of kidney failure. ■

## Selenium

**RDA:**
**Men:** 70 mcg
**Women:** 55 mcg
**Pregnant women:** 65 mcg

An antioxidant, selenium protects cells and tissues from damage wrought by free radicals. Because its antioxidant effects complement those of vitamin E, the two are said to potentiate, or reinforce, each other. Selenium also supports immune function and neutralizes certain poisonous substances such as cadmium, mercury, and arsenic that may be ingested or inhaled. Although its full therapeutic value is unknown, adequate selenium levels may help combat arthritis, deter heart disease, and prevent cancer.

Whole grains, asparagus, garlic, eggs, and mushrooms are typically good sources, as are lean meats and seafood. Very little selenium is required for good health, and most people get adequate amounts through diet alone. High-dose supplements such as selenium citrate and selenium picolinate should be taken only if prescribed by a doctor. Selenium can be toxic in extremely high doses, causing hair loss, nail problems, accelerated tooth decay, and swelling of the fingers, among other symptoms. Some multinutrients contain selenium, but always in small, safe amounts. ■

## Sodium

**EMDR:**
**Adults:** 500 mg

All bodily fluids—including blood, tears, and perspiration—contain the mineral sodium. Together with potassium and chloride, sodium maintains fluid distribution and pH balance; with potassium, sodium also helps control muscle contraction and nerve function.

Most of the sodium in the American diet is from table salt. Among many other sources are processed foods, soft drinks, meats, shellfish, condiments, snack foods, food additives, and over-the-counter laxatives. Americans generally consume far too much sodium. A single teaspoon of salt contains 2,000 mg—four times the daily minimum—but average daily consumption in the United States ranges from 3,000 mg to 7,000 mg.

Keeping sodium intake within reasonable limits is critical to maintaining long-term health. When sodium levels are persistently elevated, the body loses potassium and retains water, making blood pressure rise. Adopting a low-sodium



CONTINUED

diet can reduce high blood pressure and correct a potassium deficiency. Overexertion, particularly in the hot sun, can induce temporary sodium deficiency, which is characterized by nausea, dehydration, muscle cramps, and other symptoms of heatstroke and exhaustion. Drinking several glasses of water with a pinch of salt added replaces the sodium and eases the symptoms. ■

## Sulfur

**RDA/EMDR:**
Not established

Accounting for some 10 percent of the body's mineral content, sulfur is part of every cell, especially in the protein-rich tissues of hair, nails, muscle, and skin. It assists in metabolism as a part of vitamin $B_1$, biotin, and vitamin $B_5$; helps regulate blood sugar levels as a constituent of insulin; and helps regulate blood clotting. Sulfur is also known to convert some toxic substances into nontoxic ones that can then be excreted, and therefore is used to treat poisoning from aluminum, cadmium, lead, and mercury.

Any diet that provides sufficient protein is also providing adequate sulfur. Meat, fish, poultry, eggs, dairy products, peas, and beans are rich in both nutrients. Neither sulfur deficiency nor toxicity occurs naturally in humans. Inorganic sulfur ingested in large amounts can be harmful, but excess organic sulfur from food is readily excreted. ■

## Vanadium

**RDA/EMDR:**
Not established

Vanadium is a trace mineral whose role in nutrition is uncertain but possibly essential. Evidence suggests that it lowers blood sugar levels in some people and inhibits tumor development, perhaps protecting against diabetes and some cancers. It also may contribute to cholesterol metabolism and hormone production. Vanadium exists in whole grains, nuts, root vegetables, liver, fish, and vegetable oils. Because symptoms of its deficiency are unknown, it is assumed that humans need only a small amount, which diet apparently provides. ■

## Zinc

**RDA:**
**Adults:** 15 mg
**Pregnant women:** 30 mg

The mineral zinc is integral to the synthesis of RNA and DNA, the genetic material that controls cell growth, division, and function. In various proteins, enzymes, hormones, and hormonelike substances called prostaglandins, zinc contributes to many bodily processes, including bone development and growth; cell respiration; energy metabolism; wound healing; the liver's ability to remove toxic substances such as alcohol from the body; immune function; and the regulation of heart rate and blood pressure. An adequate zinc intake enhances the ability to taste, promotes healthy skin and hair, enhances reproductive functions, and may improve short-term memory and attention span. As an anti-inflammatory agent, zinc is sometimes used to treat acne, rheumatoid arthritis, and prostatitis. Taking supplemental zinc may boost resistance to infection, especially in the elderly, and stimulate wound healing.

Zinc is most easily obtained from lean meat and seafood, but it is also found in eggs, soybeans, peanuts, wheat bran, cheese, oysters, and other foods. Many American diets are slightly low in zinc. Young children, pregnant women, vegetarians, and elderly people are the most susceptible to zinc deficiency. Loss of taste is usually the first warning; other symptoms are hair loss or discoloration, white streaks on the nails, dermatitis, loss of appetite, fatigue, and poor healing of wounds. In children, zinc deficiency can retard growth and stunt sexual development in boys. On the other hand, ingesting extreme amounts of zinc daily can impair immune function and cause nausea, headaches, vomiting, dehydration, stomachaches, poor muscle coordination, fatigue, and possibly kidney failure. Experts recommend increasing zinc levels by increasing the zinc-rich foods in your diet or by taking a multinutrient supplement that includes zinc chelate, zinc picolinate, or zinc aspartate, the three most easily absorbed forms. If zinc is used for more than three to six months to treat a chronic condition, it is essential to consult a nutritionist to avoid creating a mineral imbalance. Zinc ointment, which contains zinc oxide, is the most common topical form, and is useful for treating skin disorders, burns, and other wounds. ■

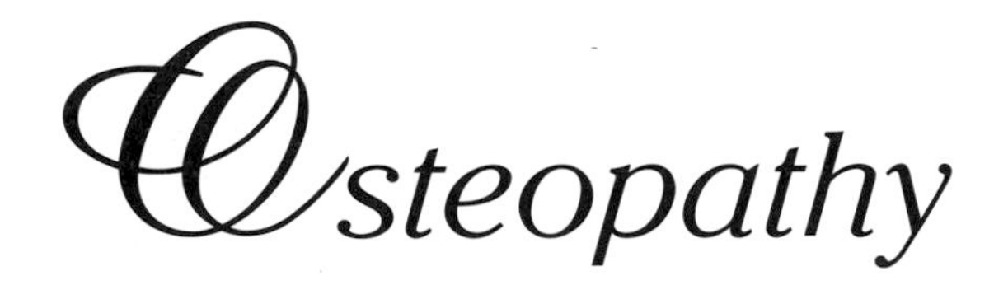

# Osteopathy

*Osteopathic medicine is a system of healing and health maintenance that focuses on the musculoskeletal system in order to improve the overall functioning of the body. To restore structural balance and thus help a patient regain health, an osteopathic physician will combine manipulation of the joints and soft tissues with instruction in proper posture, body mechanics, and exercise. Because osteopathic care is holistic, or targeted to the whole person, the doctor also considers psychological factors, lifestyle, and diet in addressing an illness or developing a plan for maintaining health.*

## Origins

Manipulation of muscles and joints was used to treat illness as far back as the days of the pharaohs of ancient Egypt. But the specific techniques and theoretical underpinnings of osteopathy were not developed until the late 19th century, by an American physician named Andrew Taylor Still. After losing three of his children to a spinal meningitis epidemic in 1864, Still became disillusioned with conventional medicine—particularly the use of drugs—and began a personal search for a better way of treating disease and restoring health. He eventually concluded that the entire body had to be considered when treating an illness and that the musculoskeletal system played a central role in both health and disease.

## What It's Good For

Founded as it is on holistic principles, osteopathic medicine is used to diagnose and treat virtually all types of ailments, from viral infections to sports injuries; the list at right is a representative sample of conditions treated by osteopathic physicians. As well as employing techniques specific to osteopathy, practitioners incorporate both conventional and other therapies into their care of patients. For example, osteopathic physicians are licensed to prescribe antibiotics and other drugs, to deliver and care for babies, and to perform surgery, including brain and heart surgery.

LICENSED & INSURED?

**YES!** *Osteopathic physicians must complete four years of medical training at an accredited college of osteopathic medicine, followed by a one-year internship in primary care (family practice, internal medicine, pediatrics, or obstetrics and gynecology). Many also complete a residency in one of 120 medical specialties, ranging from dermatology to neurosurgery. Osteopathic physicians are licensed in all 50 states as full physicians and are authorized to prescribe medication and to practice the specialties for which they are qualified. Insurance coverage is the same as for MDs.*

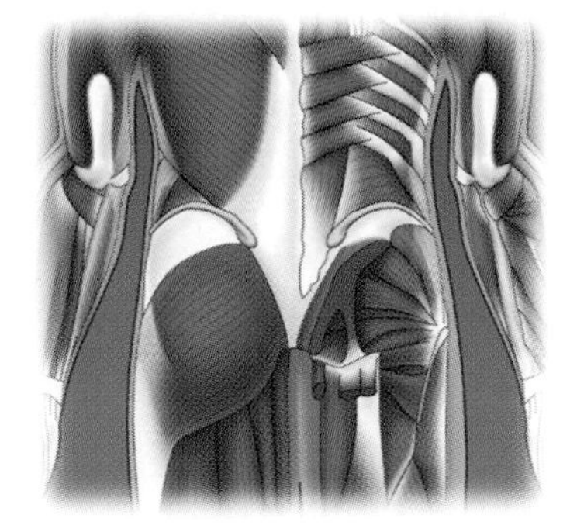

### Target Ailments

- Arthritis
- Asthma
- Athletic Injuries
- Back Problems
- Bronchitis
- Bursitis
- Carpal Tunnel Syndrome
- Constipation
- Earache
- Endometriosis
- Flu
- Headache
- Hearing Problems
- Heartburn
- Hemorrhoids
- Menstrual Problems
- Muscle Cramps
- Pain, Chronic
- Prostate Problems
- Sinusitis
- Varicose Veins

*See Common Ailments, beginning on page 194.*



CONTINUED

# Osteopathy CONTINUED

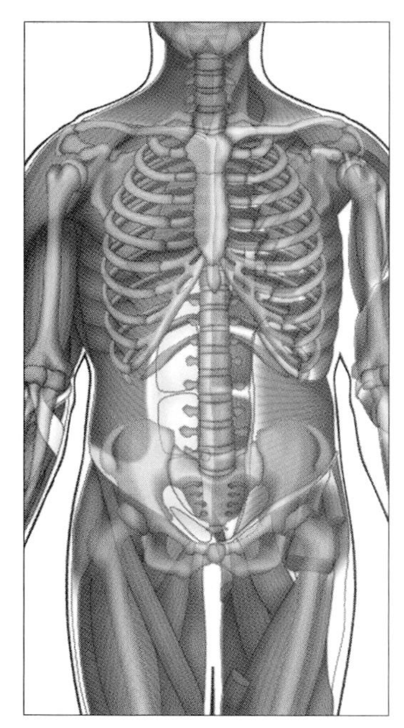

***Muscle and bone*** • *In osteopathic medicine, both diagnosis and treatment involve manipulation of the muscles, bones, and joints of the musculoskeletal system.*

## Preparations/Techniques

What sets osteopathic medicine apart from other healing approaches is its use of a diagnostic and treatment system known as osteopathic manipulative therapy, or OMT. Literally a hands-on approach to medical care, OMT involves various forms of massage, muscle pressure, and joint realignment. The purposes of manipulation are threefold: to relieve tension in the affected muscles and ligaments and to restore them to their proper position; to improve circulation and stimulate the nervous system; and to improve body mechanics, such as posture. Osteopathic manipulative therapy is thus designed to treat the underlying mechanical dysfunction that is presumed to be causing or contributing to a disease, rather than simply the disease itself.

## Visiting a Professional

When you visit an osteopathic physician, you will receive a complete physical exam, including, if your condition warrants it, standard blood tests, urine tests, and imaging techniques such as x-rays. Your osteopathic physician will also give you a so-called structural exam, which begins with an assessment of your posture, spine, and balance. The various muscles, tendons, and ligaments of your body will be gently pressed for indications of tenderness, tension, and weakness. Your joints will also be examined to discover whether their movement is restricted or causes pain. If a structural abnormality is found to be the source of your illness or injury, your physician will then apply the techniques of osteopathic manipulative therapy to treat the problem. It is possible that more than one treatment session will be recommended.

## Wellness

Osteopathic medicine has always emphasized preventive medicine. At the core of its philosophy is the belief that the body is inherently capable of healing itself. Osteopathic physicians thus work closely with their patients to help them develop healthier lifestyles. Preventive techniques recommended by osteopathic practitioners vary, but may include nutritional counseling, acupressure, medicinal herbs, yoga, and other forms of alternative medicine.

## What the Critics Say

Although once ridiculed and shunned by conventional practitioners, osteopathic medicine has gained considerable favor from the medical mainstream in recent years, primarily because of its holistic approach to treatment and its emphasis on prevention of illness and maintenance of a healthy lifestyle. ■

**FOR MORE INFO**

Following is a list of organizations you can contact to learn more about osteopathy:

**American Osteopathic Association**
142 East Ontario Street
Chicago, IL 60611
(800) 621-1773
e-mail: www.am.osteo.assn.org

**The American Academy of Osteopathy**
3500 DePauw Boulevard, Suite 1080
Indianapolis, IN 46268-1139
(317) 879-1881

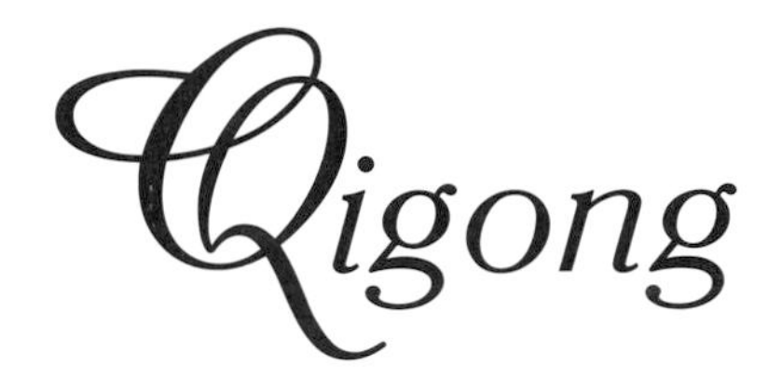

# Qigong

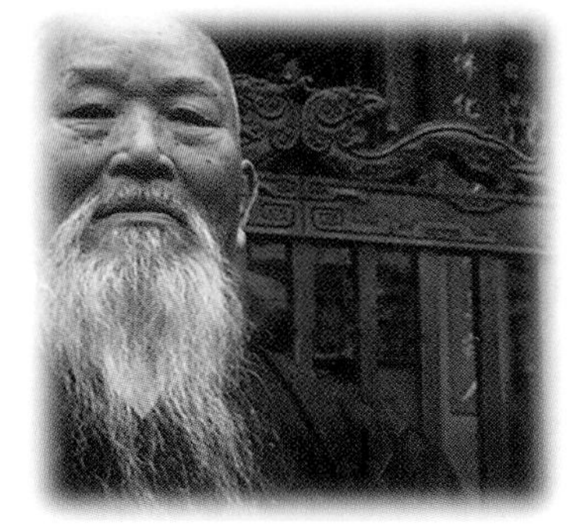

*Qigong ("chee-goong") is an ancient Chinese discipline that uses breathing exercises, movement, and meditation to balance and strengthen the body's vital energy (chi, sometimes spelled "qi"). Several of the martial arts, including t'ai chi (pages 172-173) and kung fu, are derived from qigong, but qigong itself is oriented more toward healing and less toward self-defense than these related practices.*

*Qigong, meaning "energy cultivation," is intended to manipulate two forms of energy: internal chi and external chi. Internal chi can be developed by the repetition of qigong's ritual exercises and by meditation, a practice that is believed to balance the body's energies and promote internal wellness. Some qigong masters are said to be able to emit external chi, energy transmitted from one person to another for healing purposes.*

## Target Ailments

- Back Problems
- Carpal Tunnel Syndrome
- Circulatory Problems
- Depression
- Hay Fever
- High Blood Pressure
- Insomnia
- Menopause
- Neuralgia
- Pain, Chronic
- TMJ Syndrome

*See Common Ailments, beginning on page 194.*

### *Origins*

Like many other forms of Chinese medicine, qigong dates back thousands of years. The modern practice of strengthening chi through ritual exercise and meditation contains strands of Buddhist, Taoist, and Confucian philosophy developed over millennia. The Buddhist approach concentrates on freeing the self through awareness; the Taoist focuses on connection with the natural world; and the Confucian philosophy is more concerned with the place of the individual in society. Together they form the balance of inner and outer awareness that marks qigong today.

During China's Cultural Revolution in the 1960s and 1970s qigong was banned, but it later became clear that the discipline had millions of proponents in its native country. By the 1990s qigong was gaining popularity in the West as well.

### *What It's Good For*

Qigong's supporters say that the practice can greatly improve overall health and even help cure a wide variety of ailments. In the years since the Cultural Revolution, China has hosted a number of medical conferences devoted to the healing effects of qigong. Papers presented at these meetings claim beneficial effects for ailments ranging from allergies and asthma to diabetes, hypertension, liver disorders, and even paralysis and cancer. In more serious diseases, patients usually employ qigong along with conventional medical care to speed recovery and alleviate pain.

### *Preparations/Techniques*

Those wishing to practice qigong should begin by studying with a teacher. The exercises are deceptively simple and need to be performed over and over again under



CONTINUED

the guidance of an expert before the student begins to feel their effects. There are literally thousands of qigong exercises, but the techniques can be divided into standing, sitting, lying, and walking. Students may stand with legs apart and breathe from the diaphragm in a particular pattern while performing ritual movements with arms and legs; or they may sit and roll objects between their palms to stimulate energy points. Walking may be slow and regular, or more random and free. Students may also practice meditation techniques, focusing the mind on an energy point while counting breaths.

Between classes (which are taken once or twice a week), students go through the movements every day for about 30 minutes, morning and evening. Those who have particular medical problems may practice movements specific to their ailments for longer daily periods.

Some patients want to take the next step and visit a qigong master to experience the reputed healing power of external chi. These masters, more commonly found in China than in the United States, believe that energy emitted from their hands passes into the patient's body, helping it to balance its own chi and heal its ailments. Such a master might touch or press specific "chi points" on the body, or might pass his or her hands several inches above the body. Even these masters, however, will encourage patients to learn to develop internal chi so that they can take charge of their own health.

### *Wellness*

Qigong, say its supporters, is a way of life. When practiced every day, it is supposed to boost chi circulation and enhance overall health. Although people do turn to it for specific ailments, it is most properly used as a daily approach to wellness.

### *What the Critics Say*

Because the medical research on qigong's health benefits is almost entirely Chinese, and critics claim that much of it does not conform to Western scientific standards, the Western medical establishment does not give much credence to qigong's reputed cures. The concept of external chi comes in for special criticism as being unlikely and unscientific. As with any form of medicine, conventional doctors urge the public to be extremely cautious of any practitioner making claims for "miracle cures." ■

**LICENSED & INSURED?**

*Although some practitioners of qigong may have licenses in other specialties, such as acupuncture, qigong itself is not subject to licensing, and only in rare cases has it been covered by insurance companies.*

**FOR MORE INFO**

Following is a list of organizations you can contact to learn more about qigong:

**Qigong Institute**
**East West Academy of Healing Arts**
450 Sutter Place, Suite 2104
San Francisco, CA 94108
(415) 788-2227
fax: (415) 788-2242

**World Natural Medicine Foundation**
College of Medical Qi Gong
9904 106 Street
Edmonton, AB T5K 1C4 Canada
(403) 424-2231
fax: (403) 424-8520

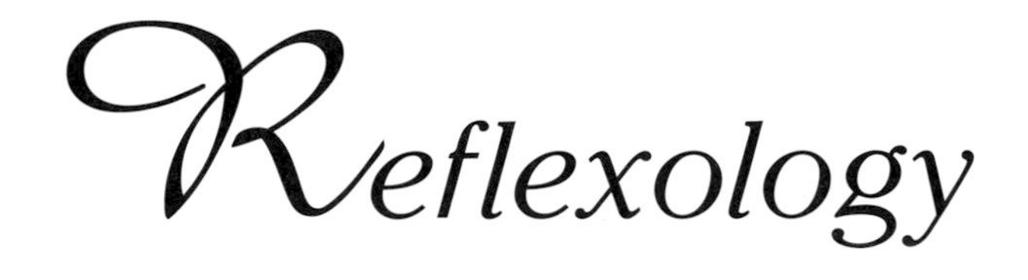

# Reflexology

Reflexology involves the manipulation of specific areas on the feet—and sometimes on the hands or limbs—with the goal of bringing the body into homeostasis, or balance. According to reflexologists, distinct regions of the feet correspond to particular organs or body systems. Stimulating the appropriate region with a thumb or finger is intended to eliminate energy blockages thought to produce pain or disease in the associated structures. The arrangement of reflexology areas on the feet mirrors the organization of the body, to the extent that organs on the right side of the body are represented on the right foot, and so with the left.*

## Origins

The precise beginnings of reflexology are obscure, but the practice seems to have its roots in ancient Egypt as well as in Chinese medicine *(pages 57-60),* with its belief in energy pathways and body zones. Around 1900, American physician William Fitzgerald, who had worked with European practitioners, introduced foot reflexology and the related practice of hand reflexology into the United States. These therapies were then described in such books as *Stories the Feet Can Tell,* written by Eunice Ingham in 1938.

## What It's Good For

The overall goal of reflexology is to balance the body's vital energies and thus promote overall health. Reflexologists maintain that their therapy helps improve blood supply, normalize overactive or underactive glands, unblock nerve impulses, and relieve stress. Although prevention, rather than cure, is the primary aim of reflexology, practitioners use it to relieve a wide variety of ailments, including headaches, sinus problems, constipation, and insomnia.

## Preparations/Techniques

Patients who want to try reflexology can visit a certified reflexologist for treatment. However, most people can also perform reflexology at home after studying the reflex areas and the techniques for working them.

Reflexologists divide the body into 10 longitudinal zones running from the head to the soles of the feet. By working a particular zone on the foot, proponents claim, you are affecting an organ within the corresponding zone in the upper body. The foot is further subdivided into specific reflex areas that relate to particular organs and structures, such as the eyes, liver, and kidneys. Reflexologists recognize nearly 30 areas on the sole of each foot *(see the illustration on page 169).*

Reflexology features techniques that can be performed either by yourself or by

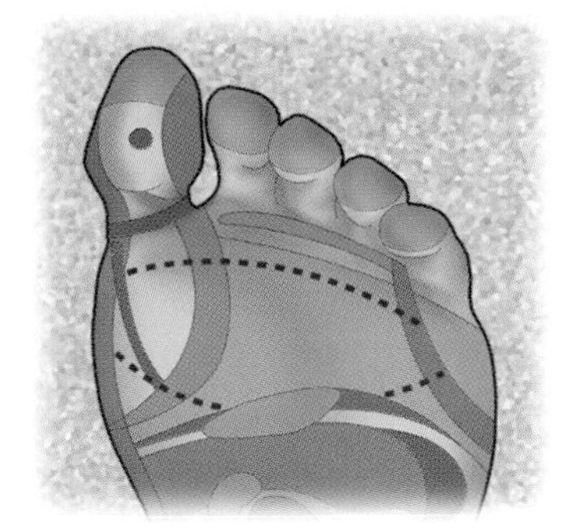

### Target Ailments

- Anemia
- Arthritis
- Back Problems
- Carpal Tunnel Syndrome
- Constipation
- Gout
- Hay Fever
- High Blood Pressure
- Ménière's Disease
- Motion Sickness
- Premenstrual Syndrome
- Stress
- Thyroid Problems

*See Common Ailments, beginning on page 194.*



CONTINUED

a partner. The basic thumb technique uses the inside edge of the thumb pad (the side away from the fingers) to "walk" along reflex areas; walking consists of a forward, creeping movement, with the first joint of the thumb bending and unbending slightly as the digit inches ahead. The finger technique uses the same walking motion but with the edge of the index finger next to the thumb. When working an area, one hand should work and the other should hold the foot in a comfortable position with the sole flat and the toes straight. As they work each reflex area, reflexologists feel for tension or minute grainy spots, or "crystals," beneath the skin, believing that these are signs of blockages or pain in the relevant part of the body. The thumb and finger techniques aim to remove the tension and these crystals.

Some reflexologists also teach that the hands and other so-called referral areas can be worked in the same way. In hand reflexology, the thumb of one hand works the palm of the other; the index finger works the areas between the fingers and the V between the thumb and the index finger of the opposite hand. Referral areas are places on the body thought to have an anatomical similarity to the afflicted area. For instance, the elbow would be the referral area for the knee, the wrist for the ankle. If a patient sprained a right ankle, a reflexologist might work the right wrist in addition to, or in place of, the corresponding area on the foot.

## Wellness

Reflexologists view their therapy as preventive maintenance: Daily practice of its techniques, they say, can keep the body running smoothly. Like the ancient physicians who went before them, reflexologists believe that a person who pursues wellness by balancing the body's energies and relaxing stress and tension will rarely fall sick.

## What the Critics Say

Many conventional medical practitioners dismiss reflexology as an example of "magical thinking"—the belief that objects can be influenced simply by thinking about them. Skeptics also point out that reflexologists have not established any scientific basis for asserting that the feet or hands are connected in a therapeutic way with other parts of the body. To some critics, in fact, reflexology treatments are nothing more than glorified foot massages. Proponents, however, maintain that the health benefits of reflexology are extensive and well documented. ■

**LICENSED & INSURED?**

*Reflexology is not recognized as a valid treatment by the medical establishment, and therefore reflexologists are unlikely to be licensed or insured. However, practitioners who have completed formal instruction in reflexology may be certified by the International Institute of Reflexology.*

**FOR MORE INFO**

Following is a list of organizations you can contact to learn more about reflexology:

**International Institute of Reflexology**
PO Box 12642
St. Petersburg, FL 33733
(813) 343-4811

**Reflexology Research**
PO Box 35820
Station D
Albuquerque, NM 87176
(505) 344-9392

# Reflexology

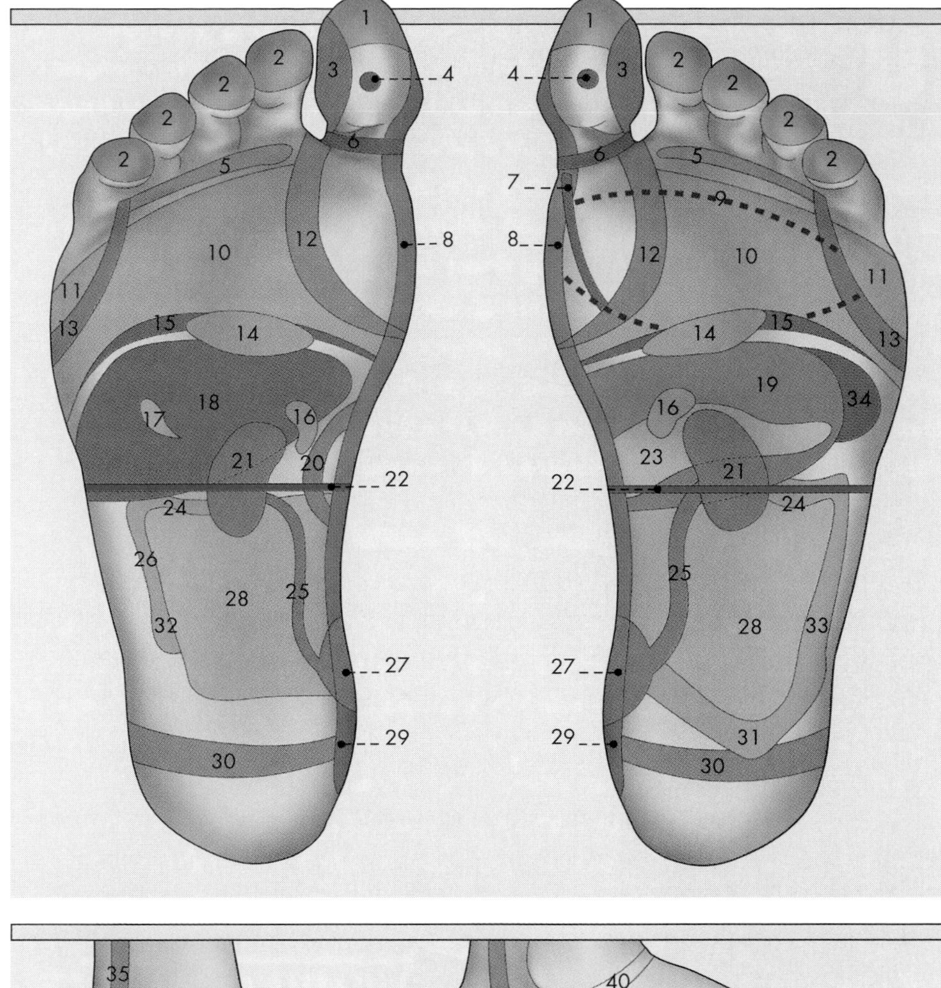


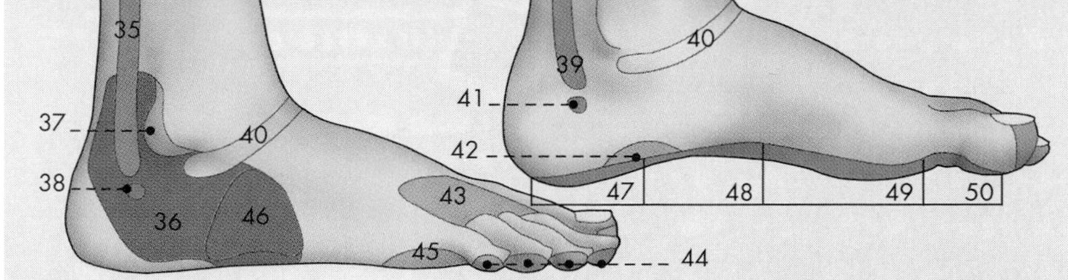


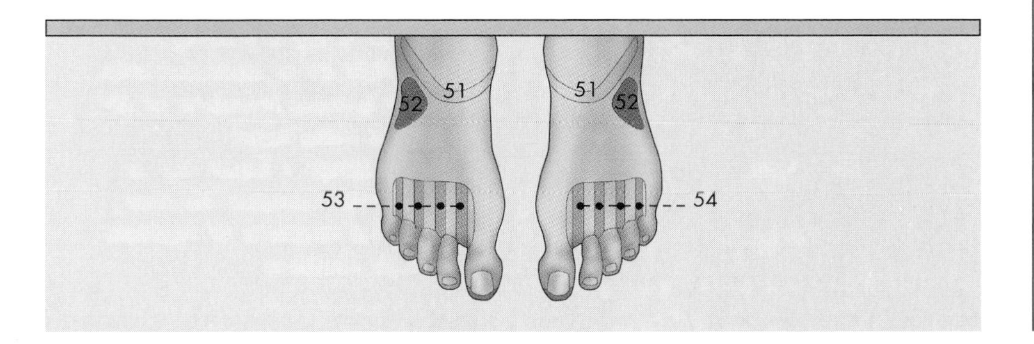


**REFLEXOLOGY AREAS**

***Right and Left Bottom***

1. Brain
2. Sinus, Head, Brain
3. Side, Neck
4. Pituitary, Pineal
5. Eyes, Ears
6. Throat, Neck, Thyroid
7. Esophagus
8. Thymus
9. Heart
10. Lung, Breast
11. Arm
12. Thyroid, Bronchi
13. Shoulder
14. Solar Plexus
15. Diaphragm
16. Adrenal Glands
17. Gallbladder
18. Liver
19. Stomach
20. Duodenum
21. Kidneys
22. Waistline
23. Pancreas
24. Transverse Colon
25. Ureter Tubes
26. Ascending Colon
27. Bladder
28. Small Intestine
29. Sacrum, Coccyx
30. Sciatic
31. Sigmoid Colon
32. Ileocecal Valve, Appendix
33. Descending Colon
34. Spleen

***Right Outside, Left Inside***

35. Sciatic
36. Pelvic Area
37. Hip, Back, Sciatic
38. Ovary, Testicle
39. Prostate, Uterus, Rectum, Sciatic
40. Lymph, Groin, Fallopian Tube
41. Uterus, Prostate
42. Bladder
43. Breast, Lung
44. Sinus, Head, Brain
45. Arm, Shoulder
46. Lower Back
47. Sacrum, Coccyx
48. Lumbar
49. Thoracic
50. Cervical

***Right and Left Top***

51. Lymph, Groin, Fallopian Tube
52. Knee, Leg, Hip, Lower Back
53. Chest, Lung, Breast, Back
54. Chest, Lung, Breast, Back, Heart

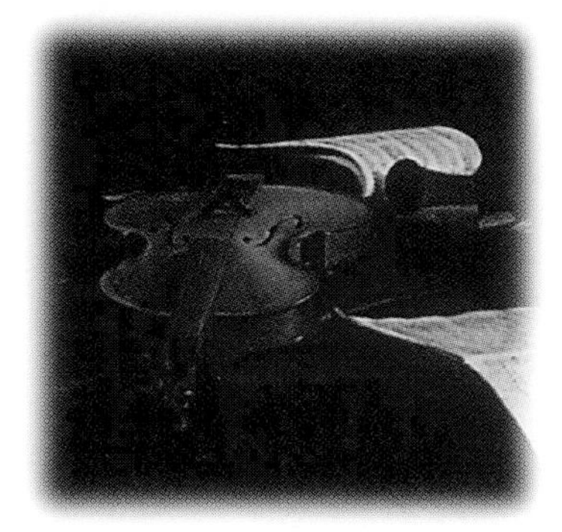

## Target Ailments

- Cancer
- Chronic Fatigue Syndrome
- Depression
- Headache
- Heart Problems
- High Blood Pressure
- Immune Problems
- Insomnia
- Irritable Bowel Syndrome
- Menopause
- Pain, Chronic
- Premenstrual Syndrome
- Stomach Ulcers
- Stress

*See Common Ailments, beginning on page 194.*

# Sound Therapy

*Using sound to soothe is as natural as singing a lullaby to a cranky baby. This notion has developed into the complex system of healing known as sound therapy, the two major elements of which are the related practices of music therapy and sound healing. Both approaches are designed to foster physical, psychological, and social health. In music therapy, patients listen to or perform music—anything from Mozart to rhythmic drumming—with the goal of addressing specific problems or ailments. In sound healing, a practitioner projects nonmusical sound directly onto a part of the patient's body, a technique based on the belief that the body contains its own interlocking system of vibrations that can be brought into balance by sound waves.*

### Music and Sound

Music therapy is as eclectic as music itself, encompassing both classical and popular forms, ancient folk music, and even pure percussion. Those who have apparently benefited include a diverse array as well: people with chronic pain, autistic children and adults, Alzheimer's sufferers, and patients undergoing surgery. Depending on the ailment, therapists may ask patients to listen to music, perform it, move to its rhythms, or react to the memories it might evoke.

Sound healing, in contrast, uses the physical vibrations of sound waves to promote health. Many different methods exist, based on different theories about the inner workings of the body. One sound healer might train the patient to project nonverbal sounds inward to balance the body's energy fields. Another might use a tuning fork or a computerized sound generator, held near the body, to restore the normal vibration of systems and organs. Others might "read" the patient's body or energy by singing a series of tones and detecting areas of resistance, or they might ask patients to listen to a specific range of tones in order to restore frequencies missing from the patient's life.

> **LICENSED & INSURED?**
>
> *A music therapist must hold a degree in music therapy, complete an internship, and pass a national examination in order to be board certified by the Certification Board for Music Therapists. The United States currently has more than 80 degree-granting programs. There are no established certification or licensing procedures for other kinds of sound healers.*
>
> *Music therapy is usually not covered by health insurance, but some insurers will reimburse for treatment for specific conditions.*

### Origins

Some forms of sound healing are ancient, such as the use of Tibetan

# Sound Therapy

singing bowls, sacred instruments said to produce healing sounds. Others, especially those that use computerized equipment, developed only recently. Music therapy dates from the 1940s, when music was used to rehabilitate soldiers returning from war.

## *What It's Good For*

Music therapists and sound healers alike seek to improve health and reduce dysfunction, heal emotional and psychological disorders, and enhance creativity, energy, and brain function. Music therapy has been shown to ease headaches, improve gait in stroke patients, enhance memory among those with Alzheimer's disease, encourage learning in children with autism or learning disabilities, and ease anxiety and pain during surgery and labor. Sound healing addresses similar problems, including chronic pain and stress, with a particular emphasis on physical functioning, body alignment, and energy balancing.

## *Preparations/Techniques*

Informal music therapy can be as easy as playing upbeat tunes when energy is low. Seriously ill patients and their families often gain comfort from listening to music together. Soothing music can augment guided imagery, or visualization, techniques, strengthening the relaxation response. *(See Mind/Body Medicine, pages 133-134.)* Music therapists work in many kinds of treatment facilities and schools, and in private practice. Some specialize in areas such as stroke recovery, pain management, or mental health. Consult with a board-certified music therapist for information on the application of music therapy in particular health issues.

Some kinds of sound healing can be learned and practiced anywhere; others require tapes or other special equipment. Sound healers from many backgrounds use different methods to analyze conditions and promote healing. Some offer therapeutic sessions; others teach methods that can be used independently.

## *Wellness*

Music can promote relaxation and reduce stress. Advocates of sound healing assert that regular use of sound can bolster energy and empower the body's self-healing mechanisms.

## *What the Critics Say*

Although music therapy is well supported by scientific study, there is little scientific evidence to support many claims of sound healers. These practices are often based on longstanding non-Western approaches to health such as Chinese or Ayurvedic medicine. Critics urge caution when deciding to use an unconventional therapy. Ask potential healers about their training, methods, and experience. ■

### FOR MORE INFO

Following is a list of organizations you can contact to learn more about sound therapy:

**National Association for Music Therapy**
8455 Colesville Road, Suite 1000
Silver Spring, MD 20910
(301) 589-3300
e-mail: info@namt.com
(can provide list of music therapists by area and informational brochures)

**Institute for Music, Health, and Education**
3010 Hennepin Avenue South, #269
Minneapolis, MN 55408
(800) 490-4968
e-mail: imhemn@pressenter.com
(offers training in sound-healing techniques)

**Sound Healers Association**
PO Box 2240
Boulder, CO 80306
(303) 443-8181
(can provide a directory of members)

**Sound Healers Colloquium**
219 Grant Road
Newmarket, NH 03857
(distributes books and tapes on sound healing)

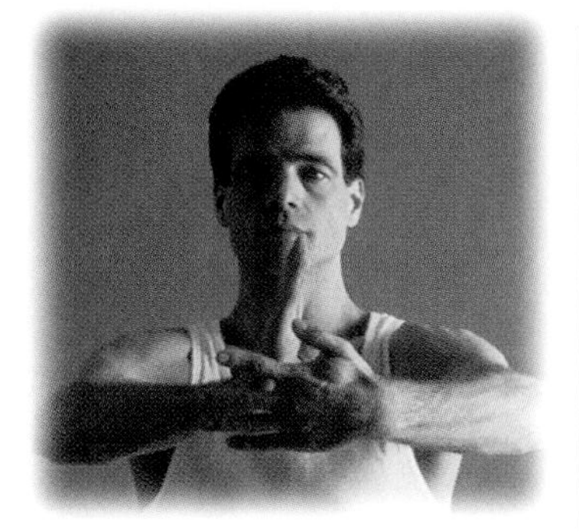

## Target Ailments

- Arthritis
- Back Problems
- Bronchitis
- Cholesterol Problems
- Depression
- Gas and Gas Pains
- Hay Fever
- Headache
- Insomnia
- Neuralgia
- Osteoporosis
- Pain, Chronic
- Stress
- Tendinitis

*See Common Ailments, beginning on page 194.*

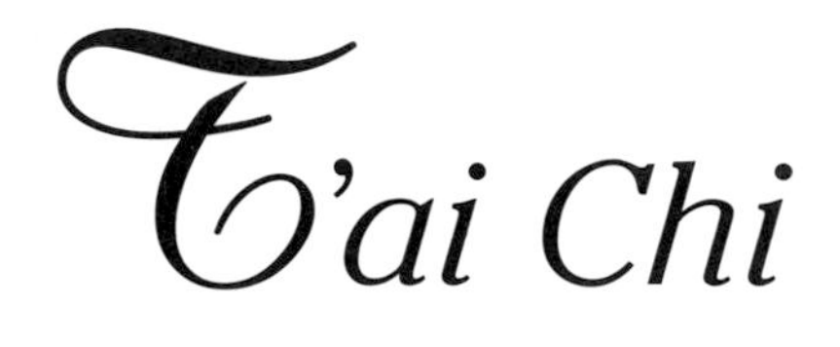

# T'ai Chi

*T'ai chi ch'uan—commonly known as t'ai chi—is an ancient Chinese practice that combines martial arts, exercise, and meditation in one graceful, slow-motion art. Every morning in parks across Asia, and increasingly in America and Europe as well, practitioners of t'ai chi perform what appears to be a trancelike, controlled dance. This dance is in fact a combination of t'ai chi "forms"—ritual movements intended to promote the flow of internal energy, increase self-awareness, and strengthen and relax the body.*

*Though often considered more a martial art than a therapeutic technique, t'ai chi provides many health benefits, including improved strength, flexibility, and relaxation. The ritual movements are meant to move the body's energy (chi—sometimes spelled "qi") to its natural center, called the tan t'ien, about two inches below the navel. The energy is then said to circulate throughout the body, correcting existing conditions and preventing illness.*

### Origins

T'ai chi's roots reach down thousands of years to the origins of Eastern philosophy itself. Many of its principles are found in the *Tao Tê Ching,* traditionally written by the sage Lao-tzu (604-531 BC). Taoist philosophy holds that *tao*—"the way"—is the force that gives shape and energy to all things, and that to understand tao one must understand one's place in the natural world. Chinese physicians and martial artists alike incorporated Taoist and then Buddhist views into their practices, developing ritual exercises that mimicked the natural movements of animals such as the horse, the tiger, and the crane.

By the 19th century, the modern forms of t'ai chi were brought to Beijing, where they quickly became popular. Chinese immigrants then took the art to America. In recent years t'ai chi has gained a considerable following in the United States.

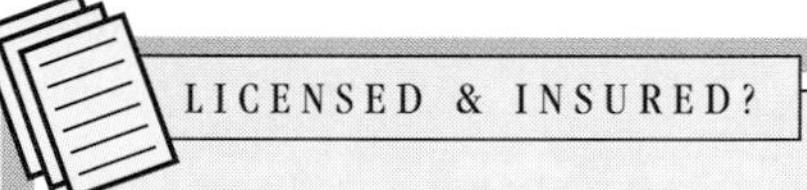

LICENSED & INSURED?

*T'ai chi is not a medical art but a martial one. Although some of its teachers may also have specialties in Chinese therapies such as acupuncture, in general those who teach t'ai chi will have varying credentials and will not be licensed. Experts advise students to check their teacher's credentials as they would with any provider of services: Ask for the teacher's background and experience, visit a class, and talk to students.*

### What It's Good For

Advocates of t'ai chi discourage its use as a remedy for specific ills. Instead, they say, the art is intended to

# T'ai Chi

correct imbalances in one's life and to strengthen inner energy, so that those who practice it feel calm, harmonious, and invigorated. The positive effects of this slow, intense exercise include improved muscle strength, particularly in the lower body, better flexibility, better posture and balance, and relaxation. Proponents say the exercise may also prevent sleeplessness, backache, and the pain of arthritis. Because it is slow and can be practiced so as not to stress joints, t'ai chi is good exercise for children and the elderly. In fact, older people are among its devoutest followers.

### *Preparations/Techniques*

Newcomers to t'ai chi are advised to study the art with an experienced teacher. Classes can be found through local YMCAs, health clubs, Taoist centers, and in the yellow pages under "Martial Arts." A class might begin with meditation and warm-ups, proceed to work on specific forms, and end with a cooldown. The slow, lissome movements look deceptively easy; in fact, they require serious concentration and control, and participants will work up a sweat. Progress takes time. Although some of the forms can be learned in a few weeks, students typically need one or two years to achieve the state of relaxed alertness and control of detail that t'ai chi requires.

Students should attend class at least once a week and then practice at home every day. The movements require only a modest amount of flat, open space. Many people like to practice in the morning, when they are alert and fresh, or in the evening, as a way to unwind after a stressful day. Experts recommend exercising in the open air, if possible; the fresh air and tranquillity are conducive to a peaceful state of mind, and some advocates feel that energy travels more freely in a natural setting.

T'ai chi forms are combinations of stances that flow continuously into one another. "Short forms" might have as few as 24 postures; a "long form" would have up to 88. The following eight pages show basic stances that might be used in a 30-movement short form.

### *Wellness*

T'ai chi, like other Chinese arts, is devoted to wellness. Incorporating physical, mental, and spiritual exercise, t'ai chi's mission is to invigorate both body and mind and clear the flow of energy. In that way, proponents claim, t'ai chi practitioners can live into old age strong and free of disease.

### *What the Critics Say*

The concept of chi—energy flowing through channels in the body—is not accepted by everyone. Critics note that there is no scientific evidence for such an energy flow. But even critics acknowledge that t'ai chi exercises are unlikely to do harm—and, like any exercise, quite probably do some good. ■

**FOR MORE INFO**

Following is a list of organizations you can contact to learn more about t'ai chi:

**Qigong Institute**
**East West Academy**
**of Healing Arts**
450 Sutter Place, Suite 2104
San Francisco, CA 94108
(415) 788-2227
fax: (415) 788-2242

**Taoist T'ai chi Society of USA**
1060 Bannock Street
Denver, CO 80204
(303) 623-5163
fax: (303) 623-7908

# Gallery of T'ai Chi Positions

## Learning a "Form"

Mastering t'ai chi requires a knowledgeable teacher, who will instruct you in what are known as t'ai chi forms—a series of movements and positions that are performed in sequence, without stopping. The images here and on the following pages depict stances that might be components of a short form; they represent key transitional moments in the continuous flow through the various positions. Whenever you perform t'ai chi, stay relaxed, yet alert; note the position of your hands and feet, and keep your back straight. With a teacher's guidance and everyday practice, you may begin to experience the long-term health benefits that t'ai chi can provide.

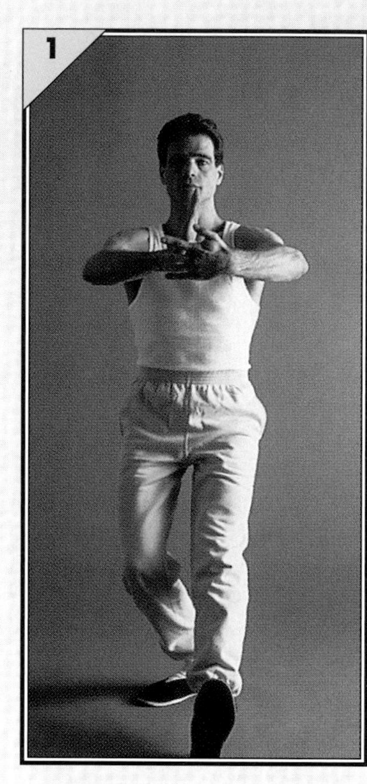

### Salutation to the Buddha

*Start out standing erect. Turn your right foot out 45 degrees and sink down slightly on your right leg. Shift all your weight onto that leg and extend your left leg, flexing your foot and crossing your hands in front of your chest.*

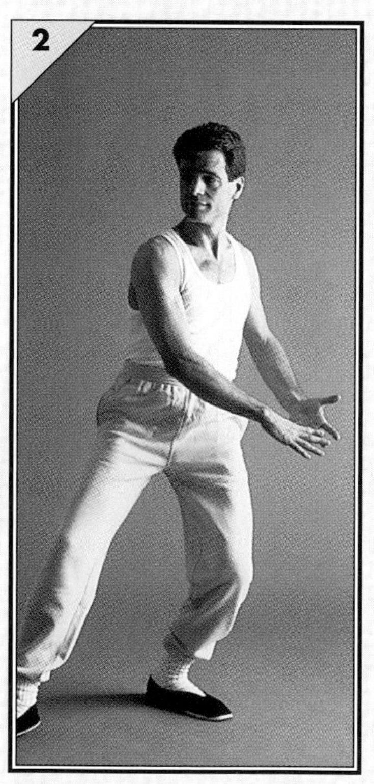

### Grasp Bird's Tail

*Step back onto your left foot, turning it out, then move your hands to waist level as you shift your weight onto your left leg.*

# Gallery of T'ai Chi Positions

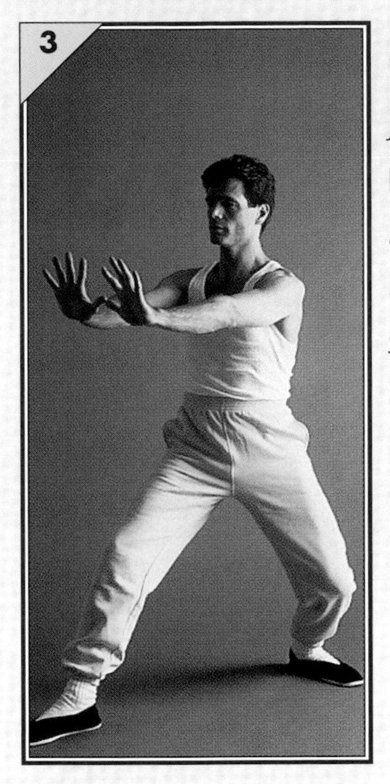

3

## Grasp Bird's Tail

*Swing your arms to the right and press forward, shifting some of your weight onto your right leg.*

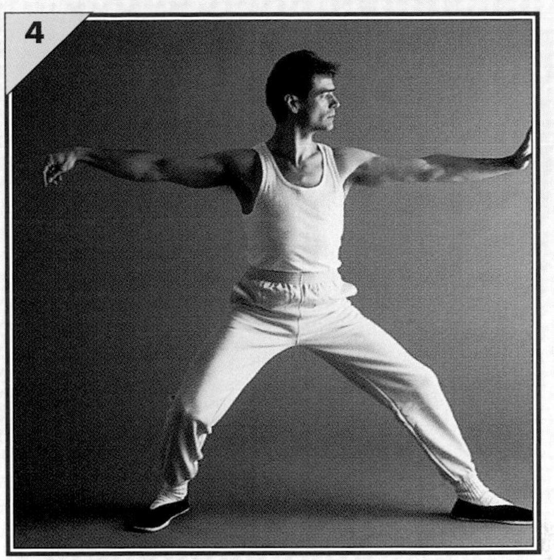

4

## Single Whip

*Pivot left, shifting your weight to your right leg, bringing your left foot around, and opening your arms.*

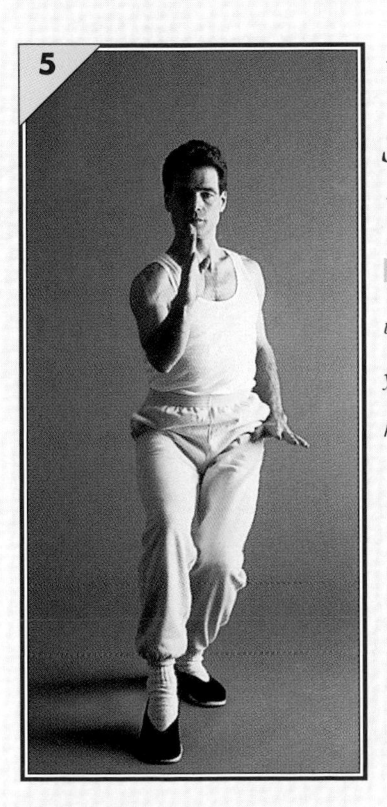

5

## White Crane Spreads Its Wings

*Step forward, leading with your right leg. Align your right hand, elbow, knee, and toes.*

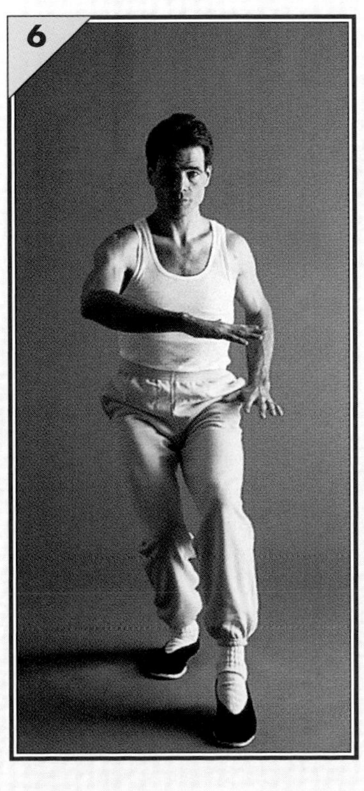

6

## White Crane Spreads Its Wings

*Slide your left foot forward and move your right arm so that it is parallel to the floor.*



CONTINUED

# Gallery of T'ai Chi Positions

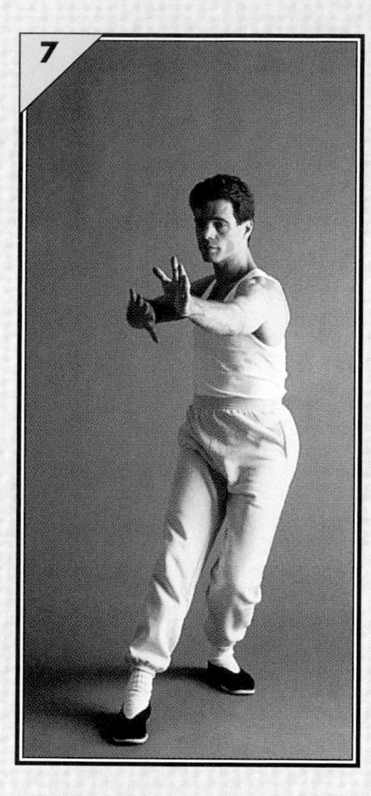

7

## Brush, Knee, Twist, Step

Step back onto your left foot as you raise your left hand and twist to the right.

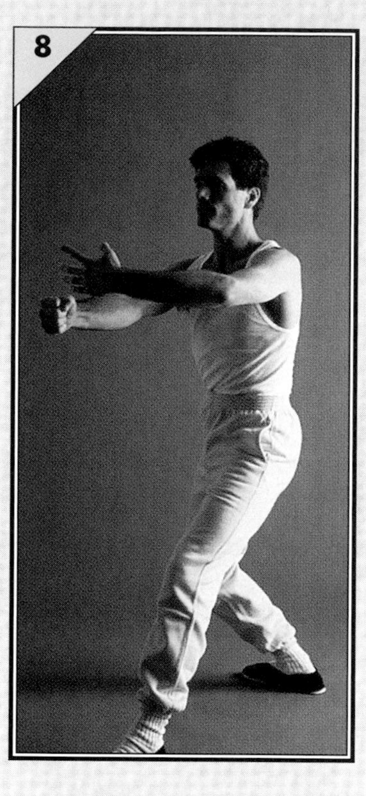

8

## Parry, Punch

Step back onto your right foot, and change the position of your hands as shown.

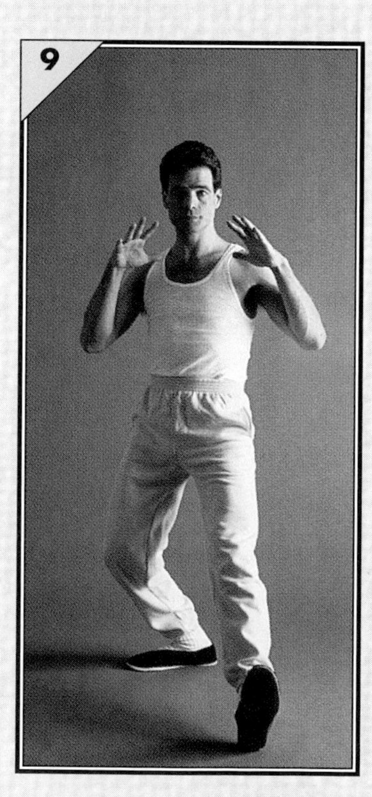

9

## Closing

Parry with your left arm and punch with your right. Rock back onto your right leg and bring your arms up.

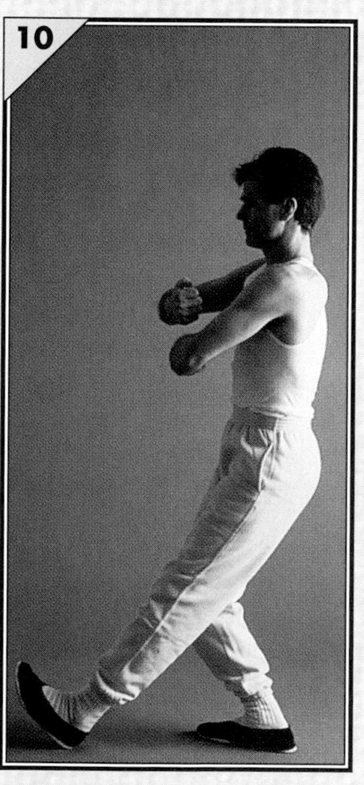

10

## Embracing Tiger

Pivot 90 degrees to the right, crossing your arms in front of you.

# Gallery of T'ai Chi Positions

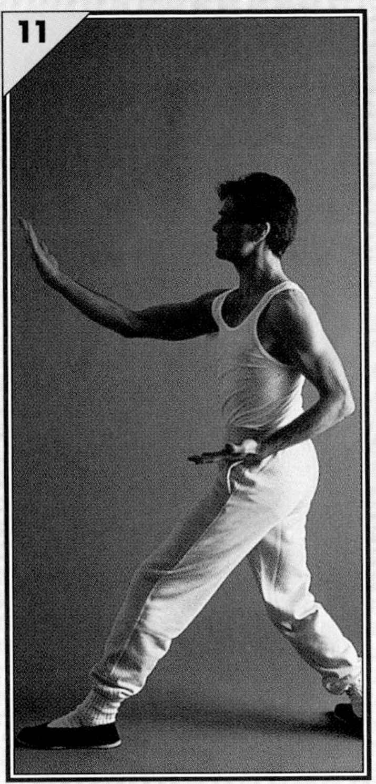

## Fist under Elbow

Slide forward, dropping your left hand to waist level and extending your right hand.

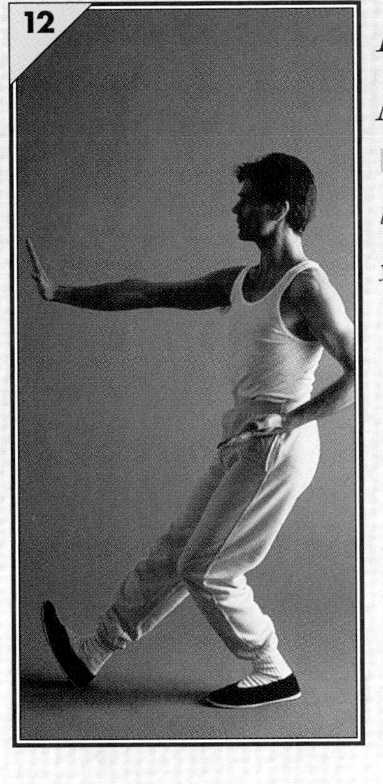

## Repulse Monkey

Step back with your left foot and straighten your right leg and arm.

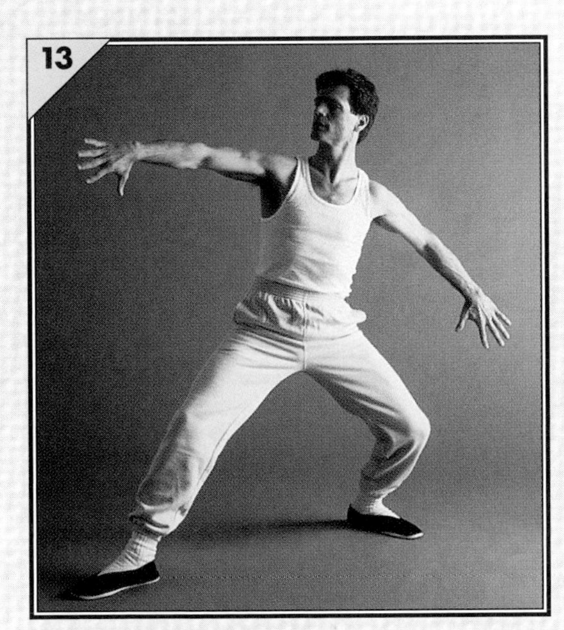

## Diagonal Flying

Pivot on your left foot, and step out with your right, opening your arms.

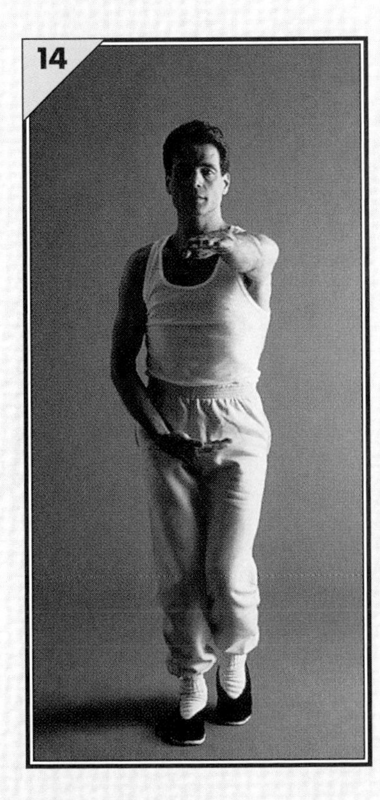

## Raise Left Hand

Come forward, shifting your weight to your right leg, and extend your left arm.



CONTINUED

# Gallery of T'ai Chi Positions

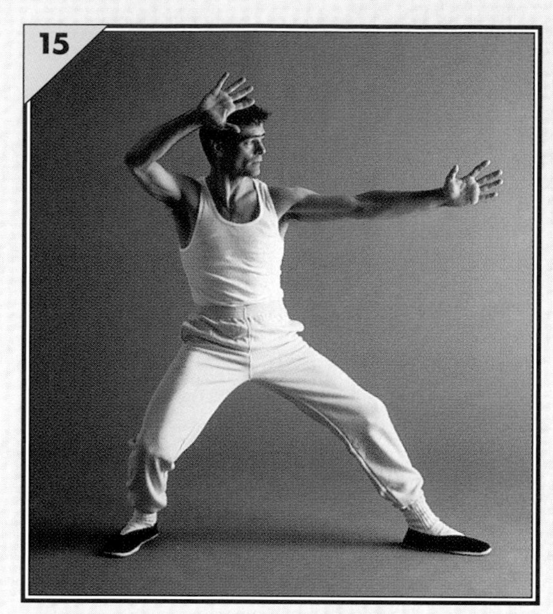

15

## Fan through the Arms

Pivot and step out with your left foot, moving your right hand up to your temple.

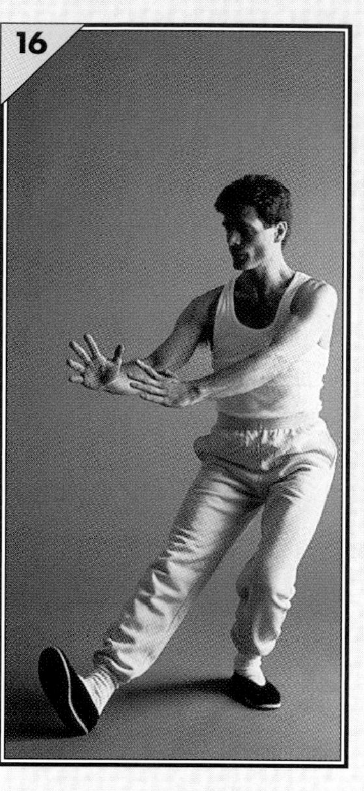

16

## Green Dragon Dropping Water

Pivot right, changing the position of your legs and arms as shown.

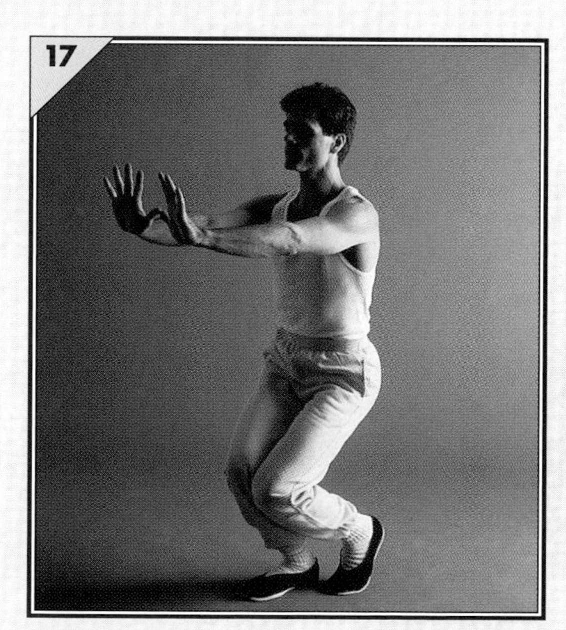

17

## Step Up and Push

Step up, with knees bent, and push out with hands flexed.

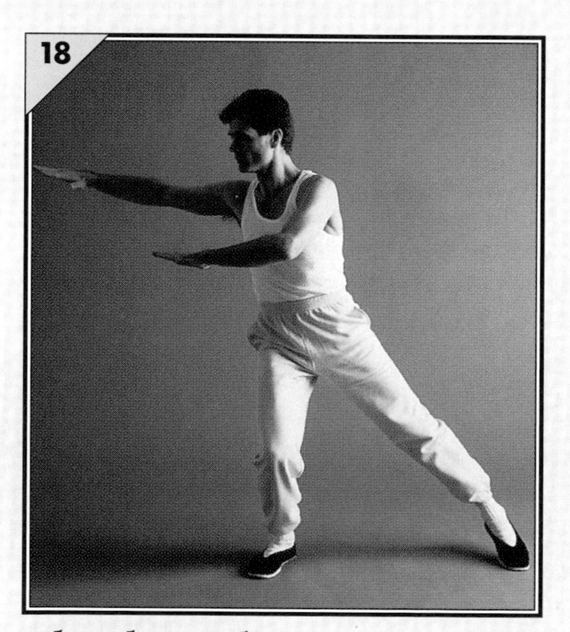

18

## Cloud Hands

Pivot right, and extend your left leg out as your arms and torso rotate right.

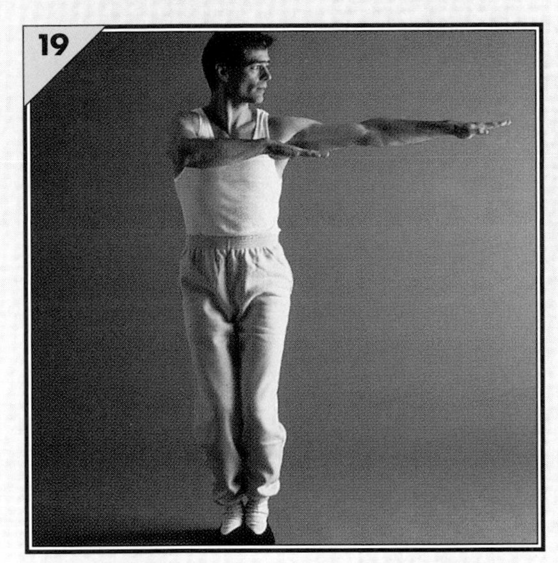


## Cloud Hands

*Rotate to the left as you bring your feet together and move your arms as shown.*

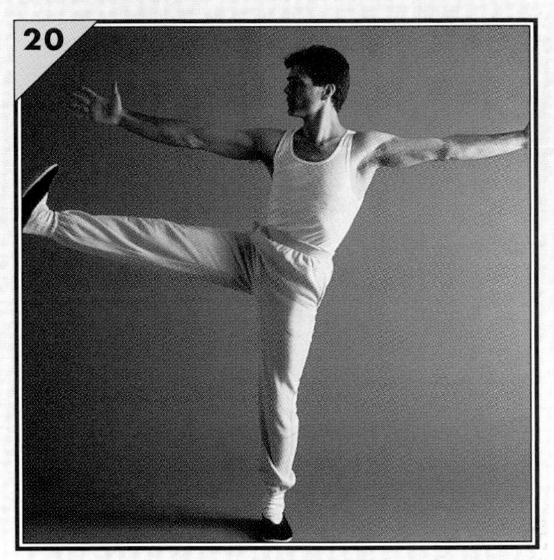


## Separation of Legs

*Rotate right, then left, four times, ending in a Single Whip (step 4). Rotate your torso right and kick your right leg straight out as you open your arms.*

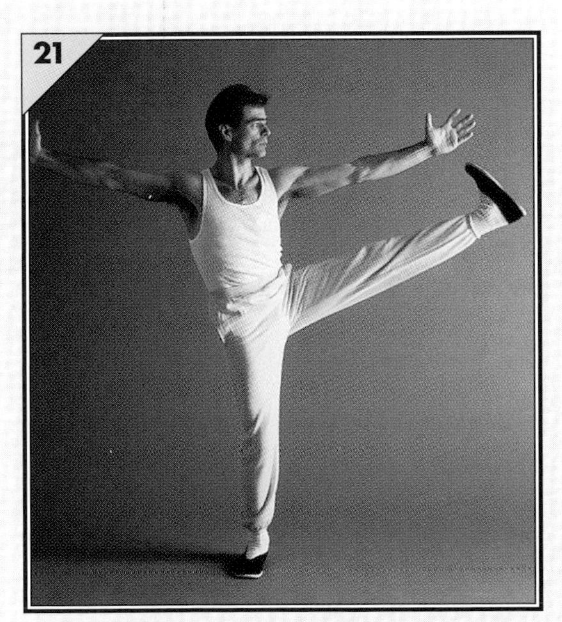


## Separation of Legs

*Shift your weight to your right leg and kick with your left.*

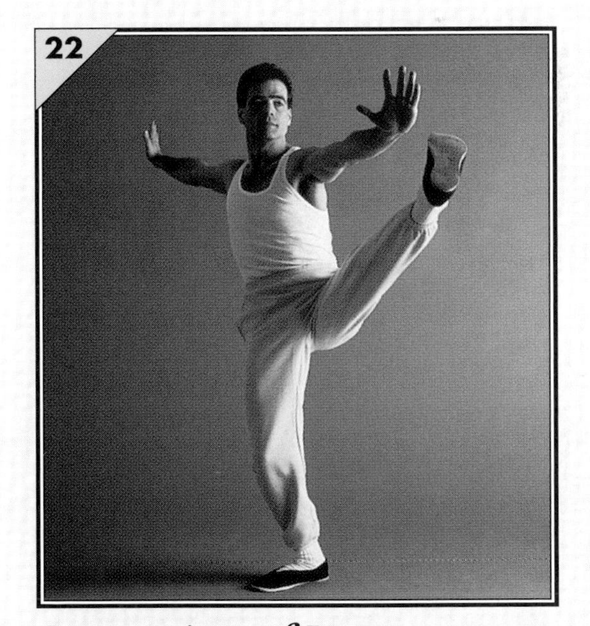


## Separation of Legs

*Lower your leg almost to the floor, turn your right foot out, and kick again with your left leg.*



CONTINUED

# Gallery of T'ai Chi Positions

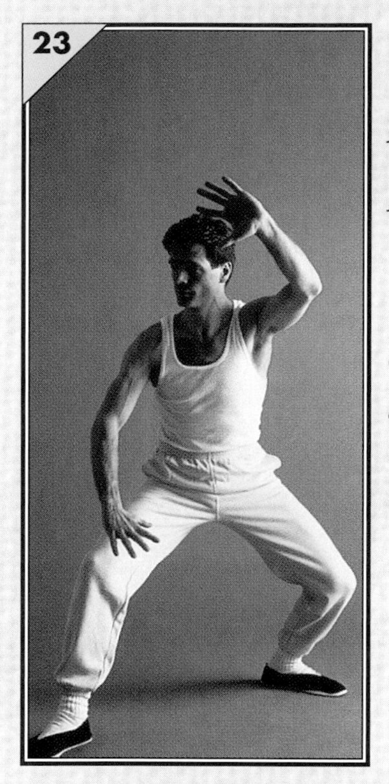

23

## Wind Blowing Lotus

*Drop your left leg back, shift your weight onto it, and parry high and low with your arms.*

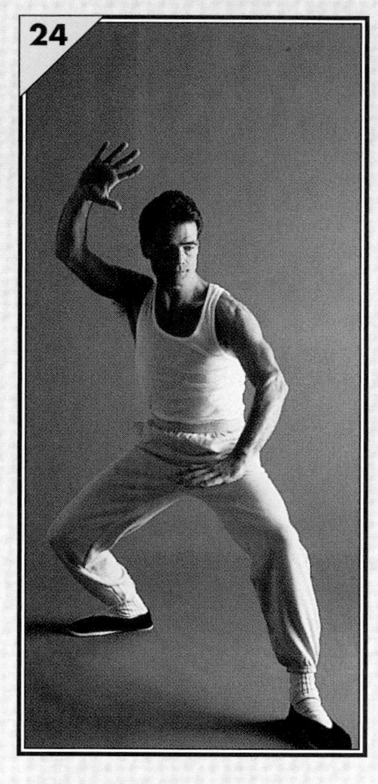

24

## Wind Blowing Lotus

*Pivot on your left foot and switch the position of your hands.*

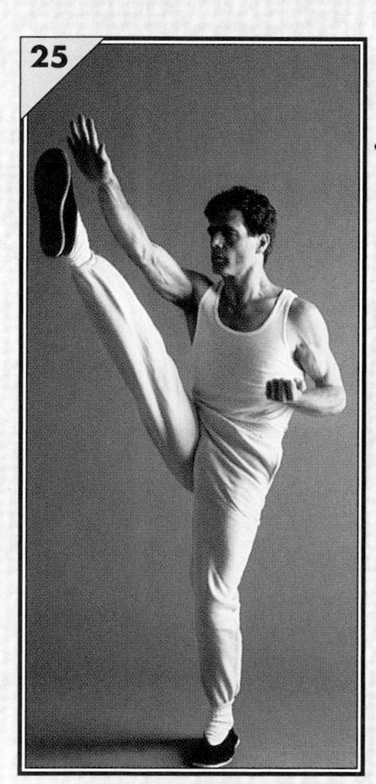

25

## Double Jump Kick

*Pivot on your right foot, jump onto the left, and kick your right leg—without straining—toward your extended right arm.*

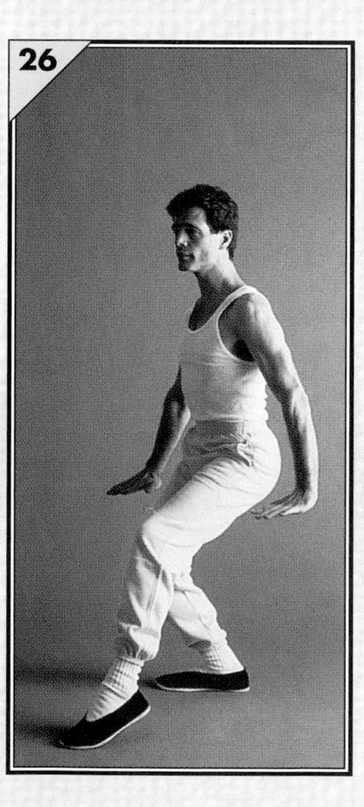

26

## Step Back, Hands to the Side

*Step back on your right leg, drop your arms, then shift backward onto your left foot.*

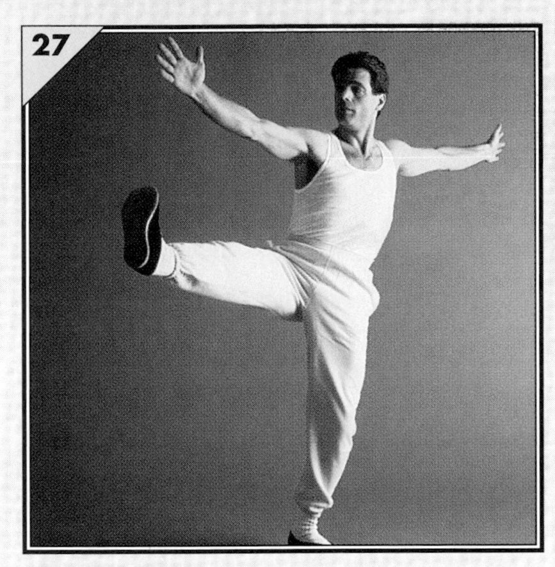


## Kick with the Sole

*Pivot on your left foot until you complete a full circle, coming around to stand on your left leg, and kick with your right.*

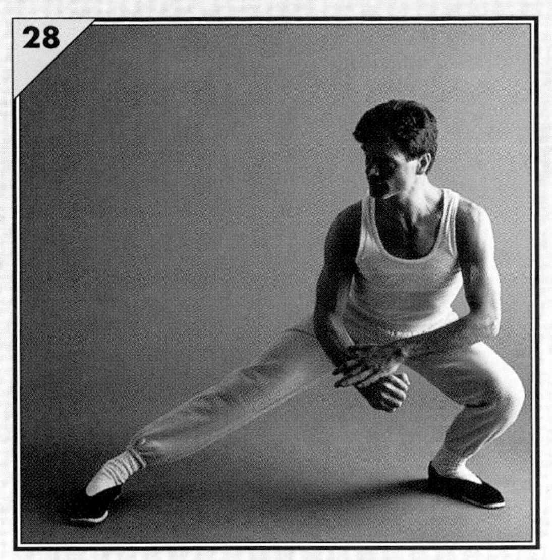


## Clap Opponent with Fist

*Drop down on your left leg, keeping your right leg straight and your feet parallel; cover your right wrist with your left palm.*

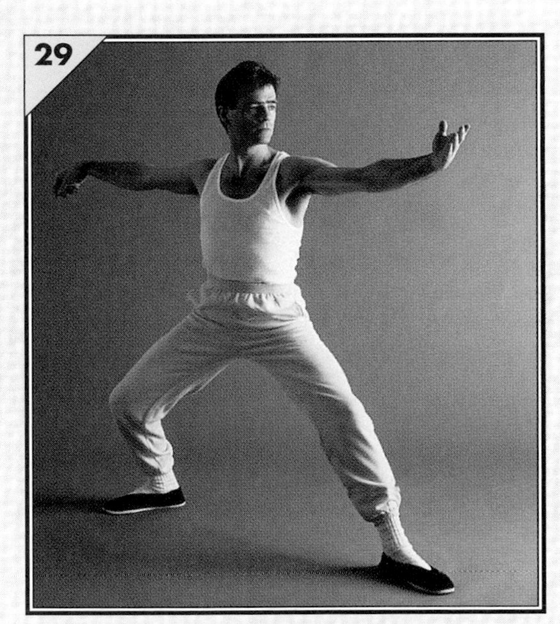


## Diagonal Single Whip

*Swing your right leg back while you open your arms.*

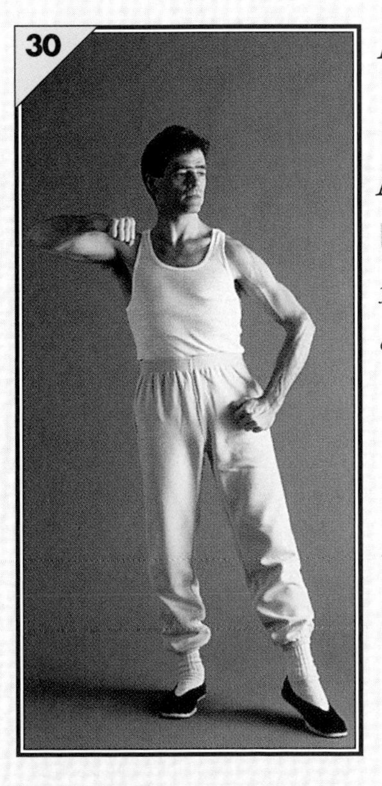


## Parting of Wild Horse's Mane

*Step forward, moving your fists to your chest and hip.*

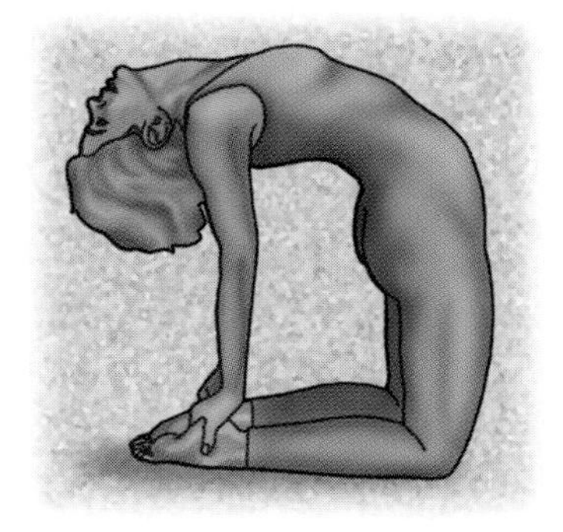

## Target Ailments

- Asthma
- Athletic Injuries
- Back Problems
- Cancer
- Chronic Fatigue Syndrome
- Depression
- Diabetes
- Headache
- Heart Problems
- High Blood Pressure
- Indigestion
- Irritable Bowel Syndrome
- Menstrual Problems
- Mononucleosis
- Pain, Chronic
- Premenstrual Syndrome
- Sore Throat
- Stress

*See Common Ailments, beginning on page 194.*

# Yoga

*Yoga is an ancient philosophy of life developed in India over the course of thousands of years. The word "yoga" is derived from the Sanskrit "yuj," which means union. Practitioners of yoga believe that by following its precepts, which include ethical principles, dietary restrictions, and physical exercise, they can unite—or bring into equilibrium—the mind, the body, and the spirit. According to yoga teaching, physical illness is a sign that these elements are out of balance.*

*There are many different forms of yoga. Hatha-yoga, widely practiced in the West, consists of a series of body positions and movements, known as asanas, and breathing exercises, called pranayama. Many Western practitioners also include relaxation and meditation in their daily yoga routine.*

## *Origins*

No one knows exactly when people in India began practicing yoga, but small stone carvings of figures in yogic postures, thought to be more than 5,000 years old, have been excavated in the Indus Valley. In the third century BC, the sage Patanjali wrote the Yoga Sutras, verses that describe eight steps to spiritual enlightenment. The postures and breathing techniques in the Yoga Sutras form the foundation of the modern practice of hatha-yoga.

## *What It's Good For*

Yoga is thought to be a powerful health enhancer, helping the body become stronger and more resilient against disease and injuries. The postures stretch and strengthen muscles, massage internal organs, relax nerves, and increase blood circulation. Because yoga can work every muscle, nerve, and gland in the body, it is used to treat and prevent a wide array of conditions and illnesses.

- **Athletic injuries.** Athletes from long-distance runners to professional football players use yoga stretches to keep the body agile and the muscles injury free.
- **Back problems.** Because yoga postures flex, tone, and strengthen muscles, they are often prescribed for chronic back problems.
- **Heart problems.** Studies have shown that performing yoga can

> LICENSED & INSURED?
>
> *There is no nationally recognized standard for the certification of yoga instructors. Although some organizations grant certification, their requirements vary widely. Health insurance companies in several states offer discounts on yoga classes.*

# Yoga

help the heart work more efficiently. It can also aid in lowering blood pressure and cholesterol levels.

- **Stress.** Regular yoga practice has been found to reduce feelings of anxiety, anger, fatigue, and depression.

### Preparations/Techniques

Yoga can be performed with an instructor or alone. Experts recommend that you set aside at least half an hour each day, preferably in the morning or late evening, primarily because the postures should be done on an empty stomach. Choose a clean, warm area with a level floor. Wear loose clothing.

Begin with a few minutes of deep breathing to draw energy and oxygen into your body and help calm your mind. Follow with a few warmup exercises, then practice the postures you have chosen for that day's session *(see pages 184-193 for recommended postures).* Go slowly and gently; no posture should cause extreme or increased pain. End each session with the Corpse pose *(page 186)* and five to 10 minutes of relaxation.

### Visiting a Professional

To find an instructor, check the phone book to see if your community has a yoga center. Yoga classes are also offered in many health clubs, hospitals, and community centers. When choosing a yoga teacher for class or individual instruction, find one who practices yoga daily and who studies regularly with a teacher of his or her own. Your teacher should also be knowledgeable about major muscle groups and body systems and should tailor yoga techniques to your individual capability.

### Wellness

Daily yoga practice offers a gentle and effective way of achieving good health and staying well. Practitioners believe that because yoga calms the mind as well as the body, it can prevent many chronic stress-related diseases and conditions.

### What the Critics Say

Although acknowledging yoga's many beneficial effects, critics worry that people will injure themselves by jumping into yoga too enthusiastically and attempting advanced postures for which they have not adequately prepared their body. They are also concerned that people will use yoga instead of, rather than as a complement to, conventional medicine for serious conditions such as cancer and diabetes. Most yoga experts share these concerns and stress that beginners should start with easy postures and gradually work toward more difficult ones. They also advise people with preexisting conditions to check with their doctor before trying any postures. ■

### CAUTION

**Some of the more advanced, upside-down yoga postures, such as headstands, can be dangerous for people with high blood pressure or eye problems. Pregnant women should avoid postures that compress or strain the abdomen or back.**

### FOR MORE INFO

Following is a list of organizations you can contact to learn more about yoga:

**The American Yoga Association**
513 South Orange Avenue
Sarasota, FL 34236-7598
(800) 226-5859
e-mail: AmYogaAssn@aol.com

**International Association of Yoga Therapists**
20 Sunnyside Avenue
Suite A243
Mill Valley, CA 94941
(415) 868-1147
e-mail: IAYT@yoganet.com

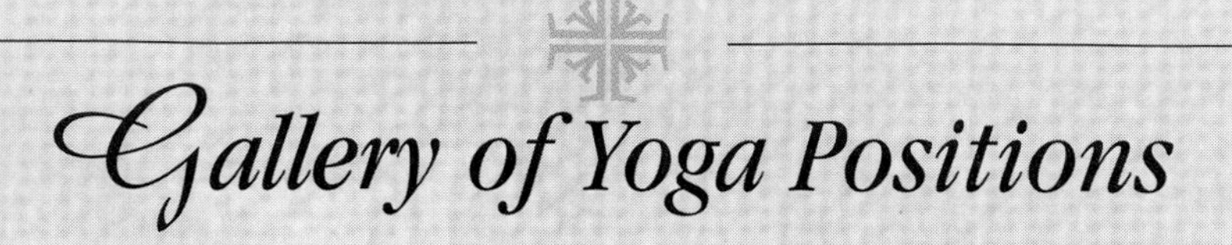

# Gallery of Yoga Positions

## Abdominal Massage

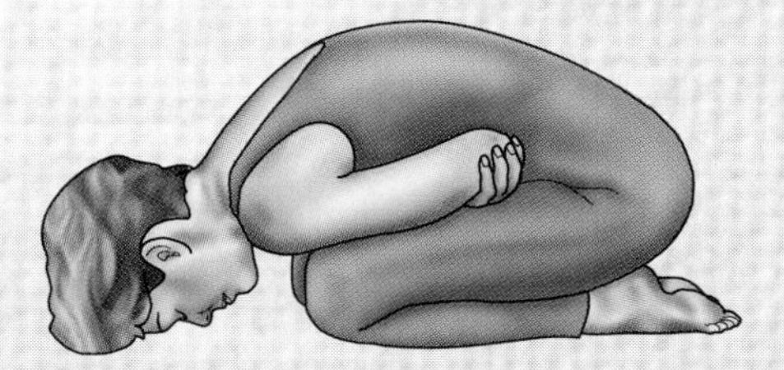

*Kneel upright and fold your arms, placing your left fist on the right side of your belly and your right hand over your left elbow. Bend at the hips and lower your forehead toward the floor. Raise your torso slowly, then switch arm positions and repeat.*

## Boat

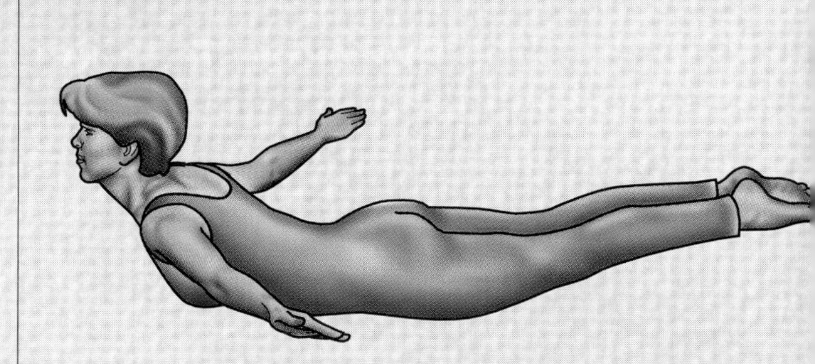

*Lie on your stomach with your arms at your sides and lift your head, chest, arms, and legs off the floor. Stretch and hold your arms behind you, then relax back onto the floor.*

## Bow

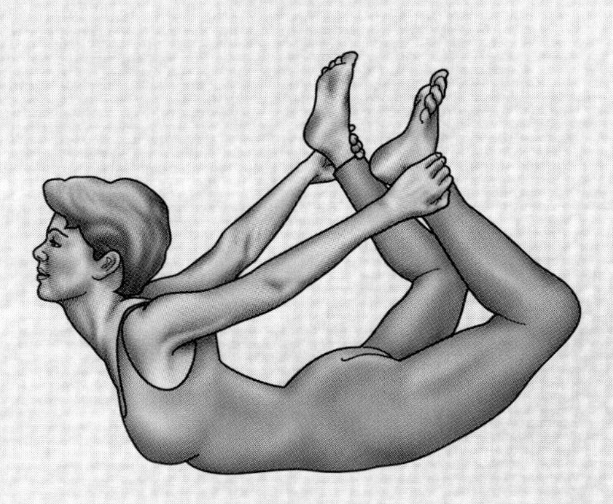

*Lie on your stomach and grasp both ankles. While inhaling, squeeze your buttocks and slowly raise your head, chest, and thighs off the floor, pressing your ankles outward. Exhale and breathe slowly, then release.*

## Bridge

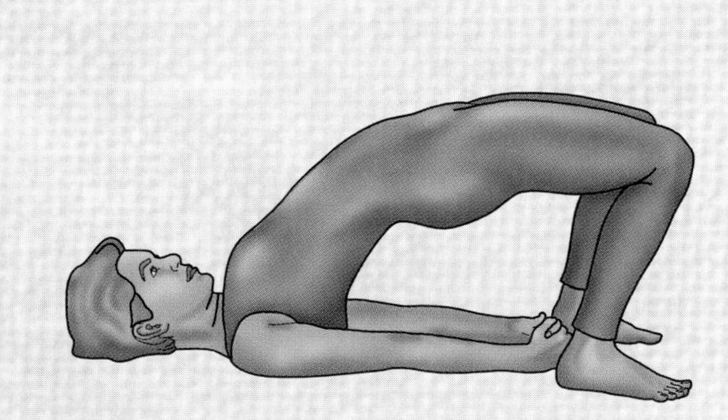

*Lie on your back, knees bent, palms on the floor. Tense your buttocks and slowly raise your pelvis. Clasp your hands, arching as you press your shoulders to the floor. Hold this position, then unclasp your hands and slowly lower your pelvis to the floor.*

# Gallery of Yoga Positions

## C

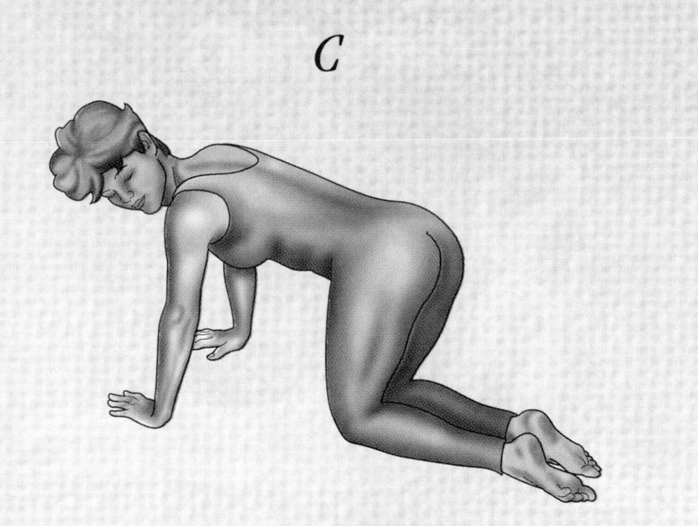

On your hands and knees, exhale and swing your head and buttocks as far to the left as you can. Inhale as you slowly straighten your back, and then do the same movement to the right.

## Camel

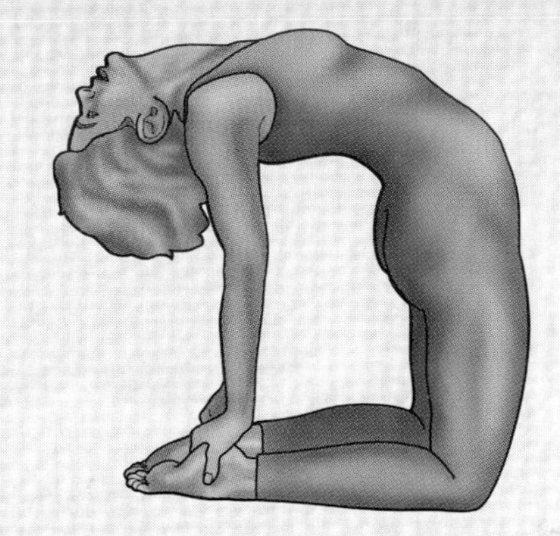

From an upright kneeling position, bend your head backward. Exhale and arch your back, placing your right hand on your right heel, your left hand on your left heel. Then slowly straighten up, breathing evenly. Relax, sit back on your heels, and lift your head.

## Cat

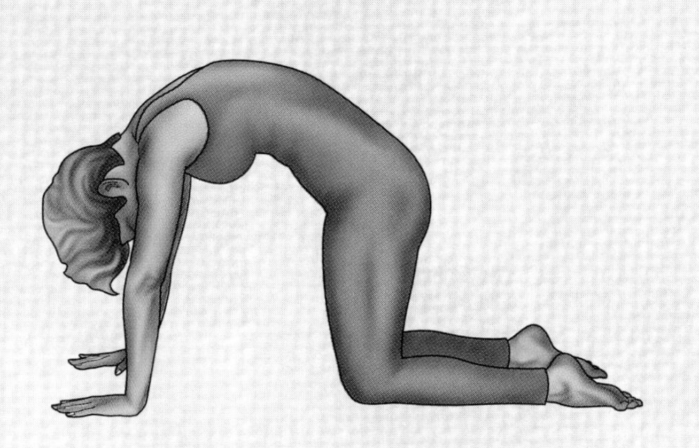

On your hands and knees, exhale as you arch your back, stretching your shoulder, neck, and back muscles. Inhale and bring your back to the horizontal.

## Child

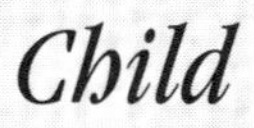

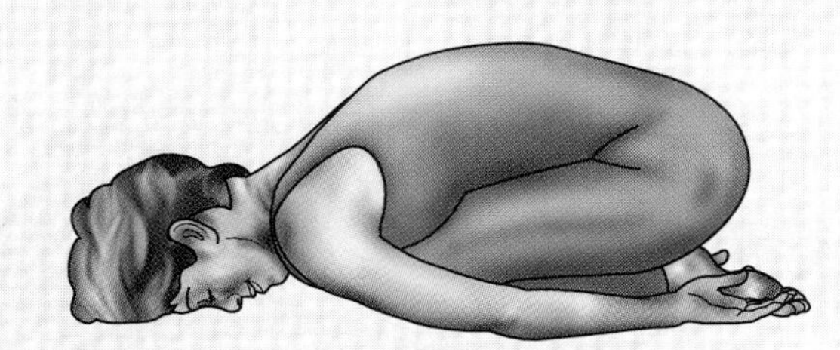

Sit on your heels, knees together. With your arms at your sides, palms up, bend from the hips and extend your upper body over your knees, bringing your forehead toward the floor. Then slowly sit up.



CONTINUED

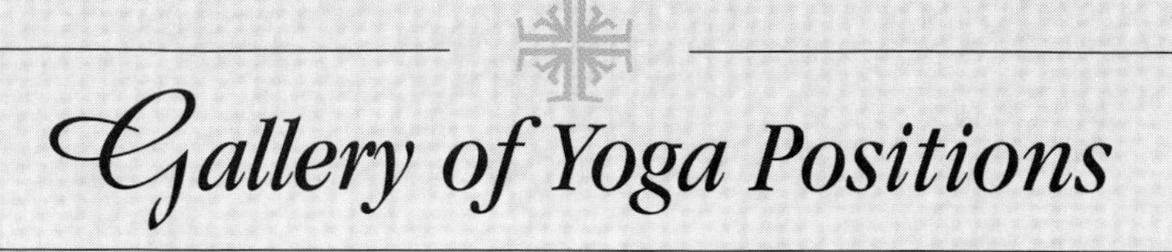

# Gallery of Yoga Positions

## Cobra

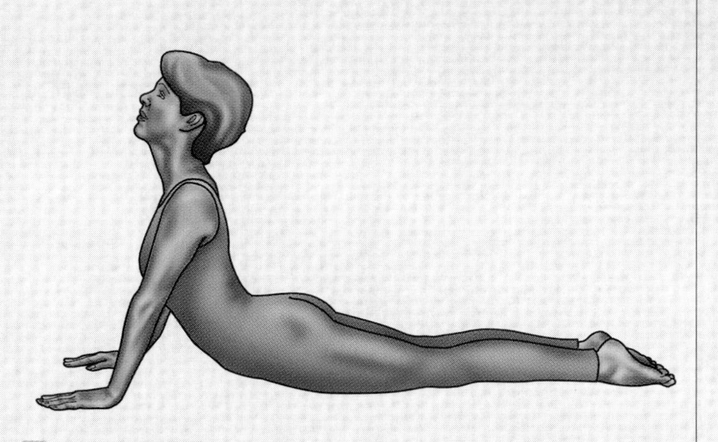

*Place both forearms on the floor, elbows directly under your shoulders. Slowly straighten your arms and arch your back until your abdomen is off the ground. Relax and slowly uncurl, lowering your torso back to the floor.*

## Cobra (Half)

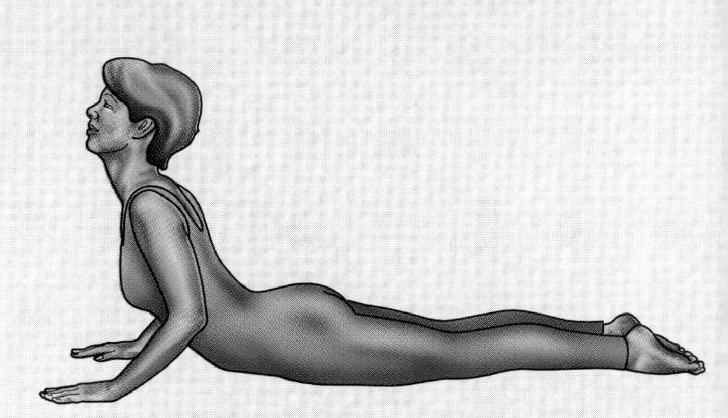

*Begin as you would for the Cobra. Press your pelvis and palms against the floor to raise your chest. Keep your arms bent as you arch your back, stopping just before your navel comes off the floor. Lower your torso to release.*

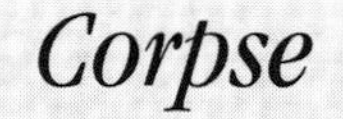

## Corpse

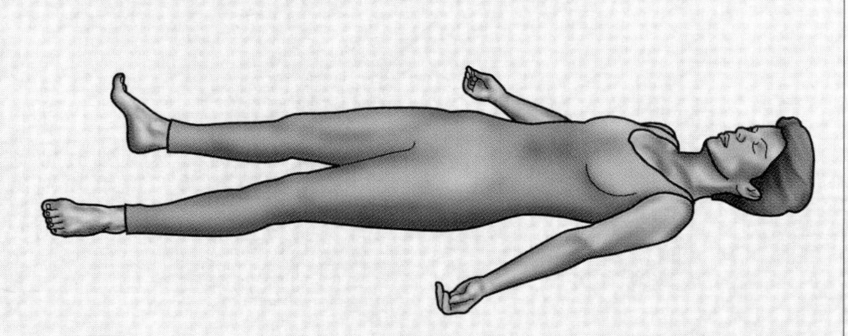

*Lie on your back, with your feet about 18 inches apart and turned out slightly. Place your hands about 6 inches from your hips, palms up. Close your eyes and breathe deeply.*

## Dog

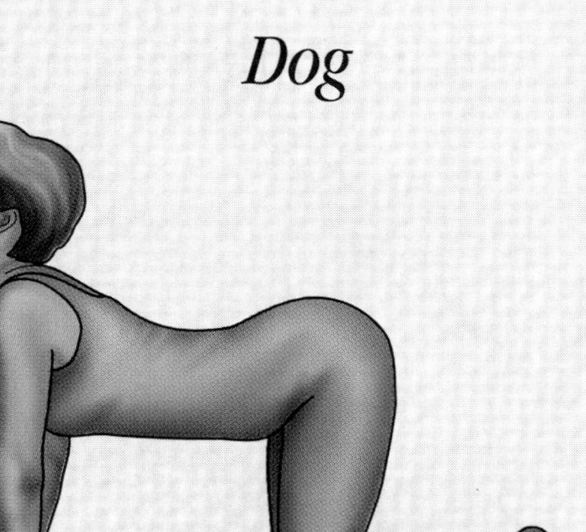

*While on your hands and knees, inhale as you dip your back, bringing your head and buttocks up. Exhale as you return your back to the horizontal.*

# Gallery of Yoga Positions

## Downward Dog

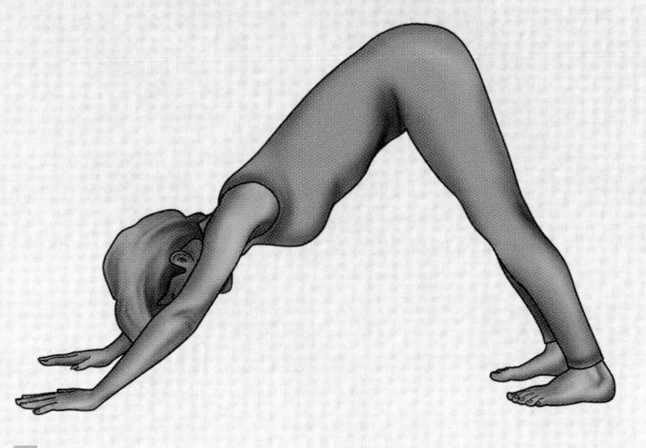

Get on your hands and knees. Inhale and raise your pelvis to form an inverted V, with knees slightly bent. Press your palms and heels against the floor as you breathe deeply. Hold for 20 to 30 seconds. Exhale as you return to the starting position.

## Half-Moon

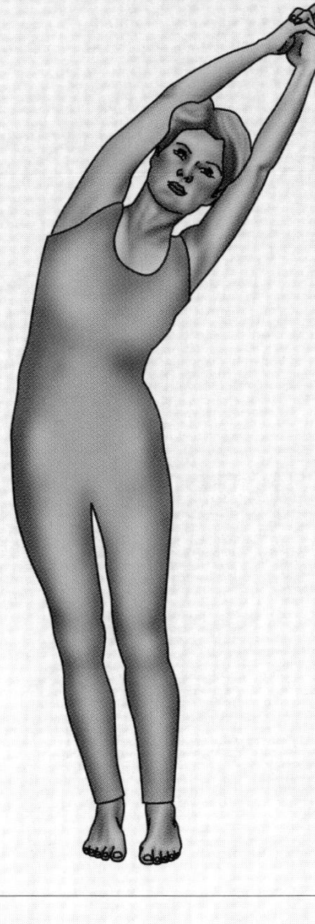

Inhale and clasp your hands over your head. Exhale and stretch to the left, pushing out your right hip. Breathe deeply, keeping your shoulders and hips in the same plane. Inhale and return to the center. Repeat on the right side.

## Hand and Thumb Squeeze

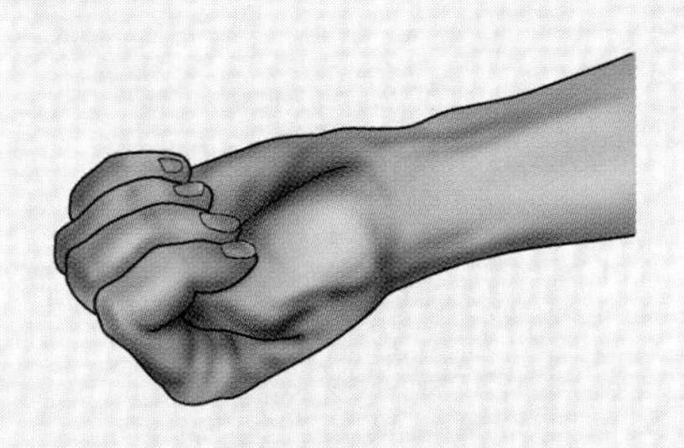

To loosen finger joints, curl your fingers into a fist around your thumb and gently squeeze. Then release slowly. Do this 10 times with each hand.

## Head to Knee

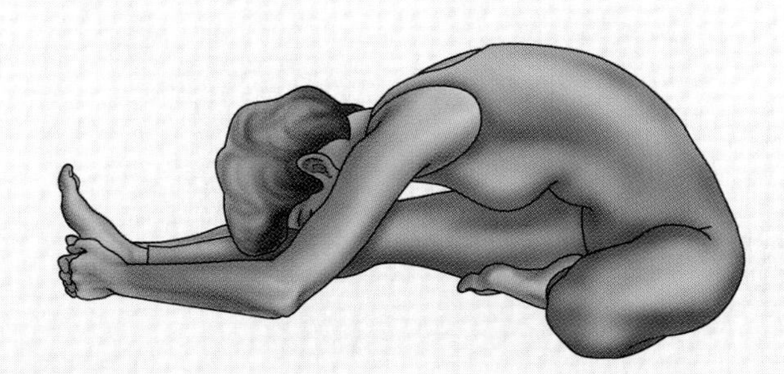

Sit with your right leg out, the sole of your left foot against your right thigh. Raise your arms overhead, then bend forward from the hips and clasp your right foot with both hands, pressing your forehead to your knee. Release and repeat on the other side.



CONTINUED

# Gallery of Yoga Positions

## Hero

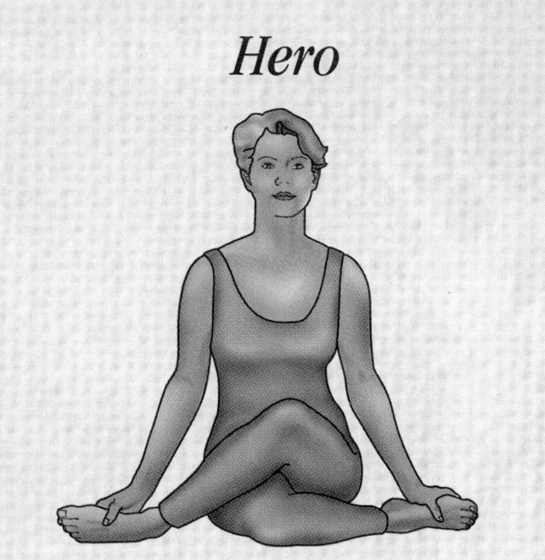

*While on hands and knees, cross your left knee in front of your right knee. Keep your knees in place as you sit back between your heels. With your back straight, place your palms on the soles of your feet, then slowly release. Repeat on the other side.*

## Knee Down Twist

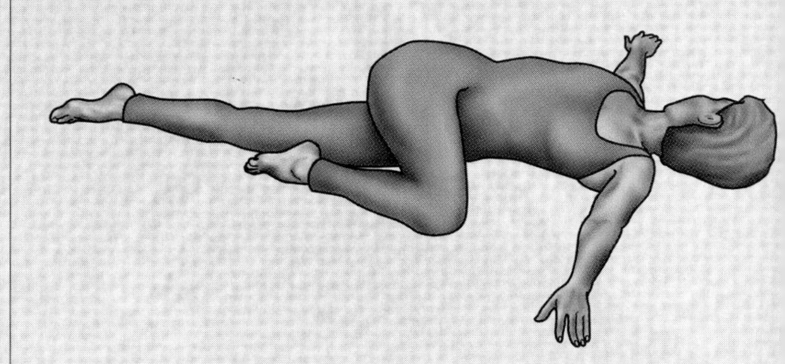

*Lie on your back with your arms out. Inhale and place your right foot on your left knee. Exhale, then turn your head to the right and bring your right knee toward the floor to your left (above). Release slowly, then repeat on the other side.*

## Locust (Full)

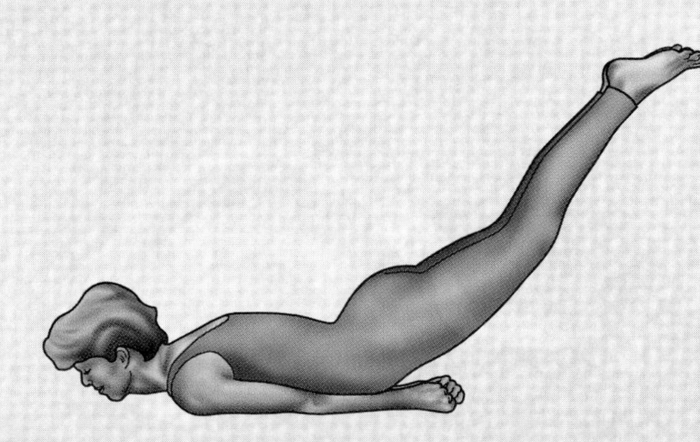

*Lie on your stomach, arms under your body. Squeeze your buttocks as you press down with your arms. Raise your legs, keeping them straight as you press outward through the toes and heels. Slowly lower legs to release.*

## Locust (Half)

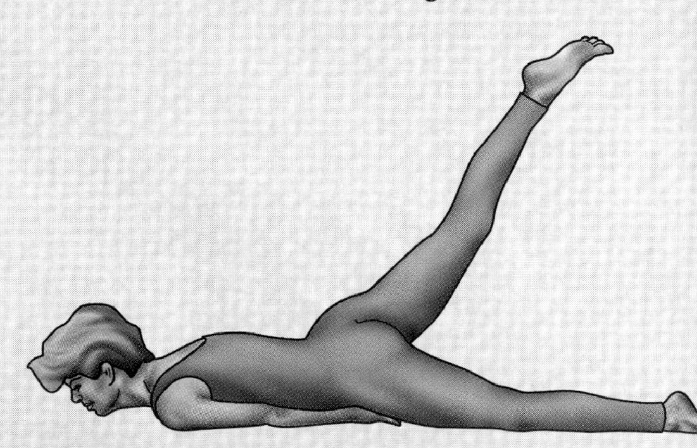

*While on your stomach, put your arms under your body. Squeeze your buttocks as you press down with your arms. Raise your right leg, keeping it straight as you press outward through the toes and heel. Release slowly and do the same with the left leg.*

# Gallery of Yoga Positions

## Lotus (Half)

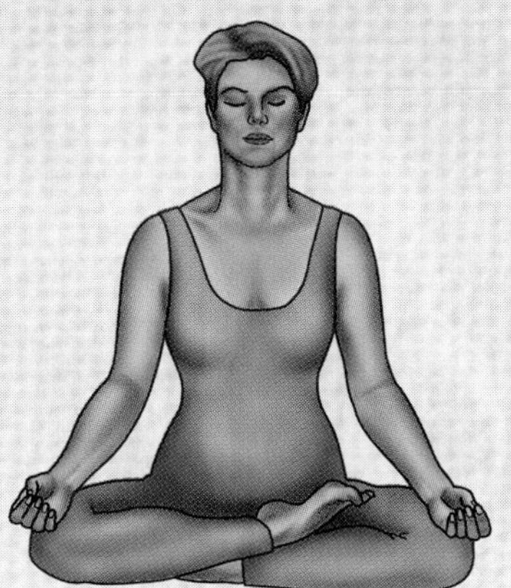

*Sit with your legs in a V, spine straight. Bend one leg and bring the foot close to your body. Bend the other leg and place the foot high on the opposite thigh. Ideally, your knees should touch the floor. (For full Lotus, place each foot on the opposite thigh.)*

## Mountain

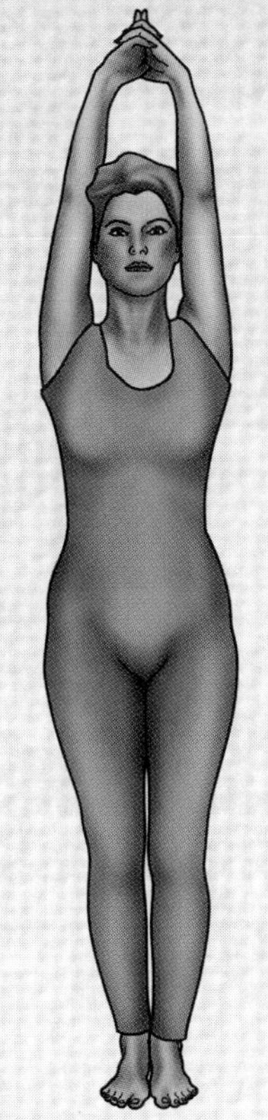

*Stand with your feet together. Inhale and raise your arms straight out from your sides, then join them over your head. To release, exhale and slowly lower your arms.*

## Pigeon

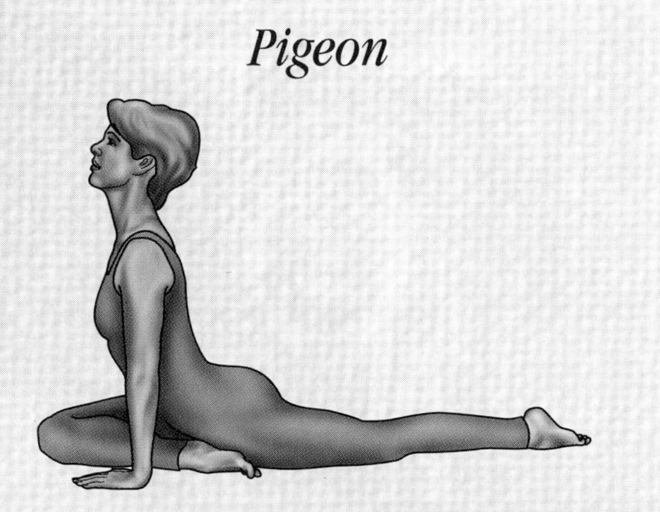

*From a kneeling position, slide your left leg straight behind you and place your right knee between your hands. Inhale and stretch up through your torso while arching your back slightly. Release, then repeat on the other side.*

## Plow

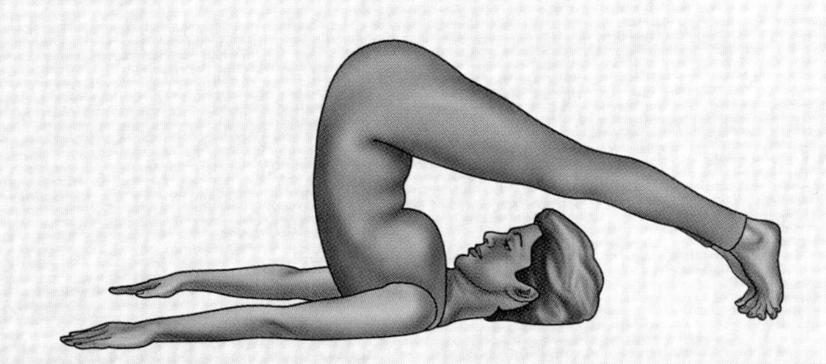

*While on your back, inhale and raise both legs, using your hands to support your hips. Exhale as you try to touch the floor behind you with your toes. Stretch out your arms on the floor, then place your hands back on your hips and slowly lower your legs.*



CONTINUED

# Gallery of Yoga Positions

## Posterior Stretch

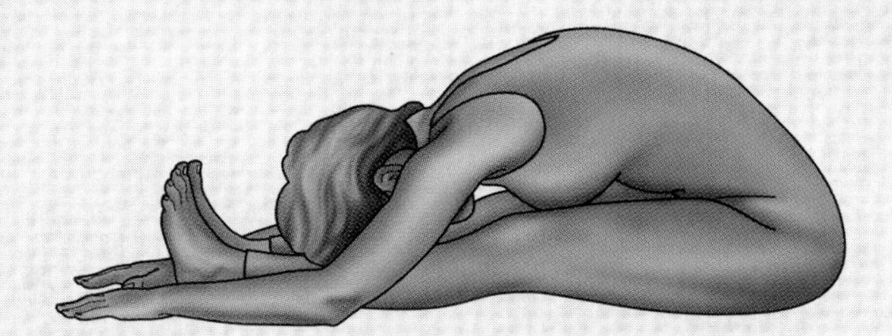

Sit with legs extended and feet together. Raise your arms overhead, then bend forward from the hips and place your hands on your ankles or on the floor beside your feet. Move your head as close to your toes as possible. Slowly raise your torso as you inhale.

## Rag Doll

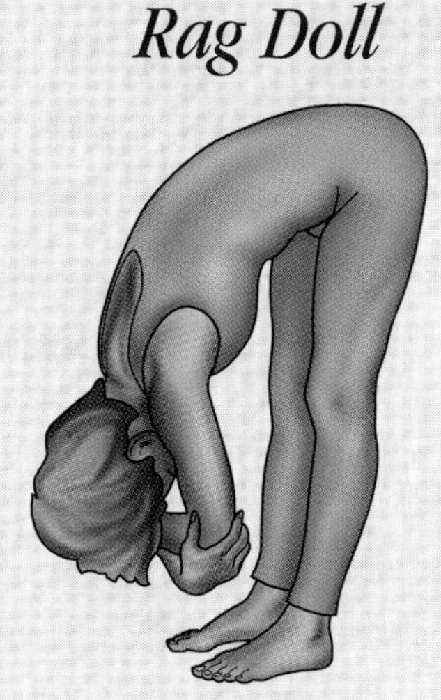

Standing with arms at your sides, exhale and bend forward from the hips, letting the top of your head drop toward the floor. Cup your elbows in your palms and breathe deeply. Slowly stand up, bringing your head up last.

## Seated Angle

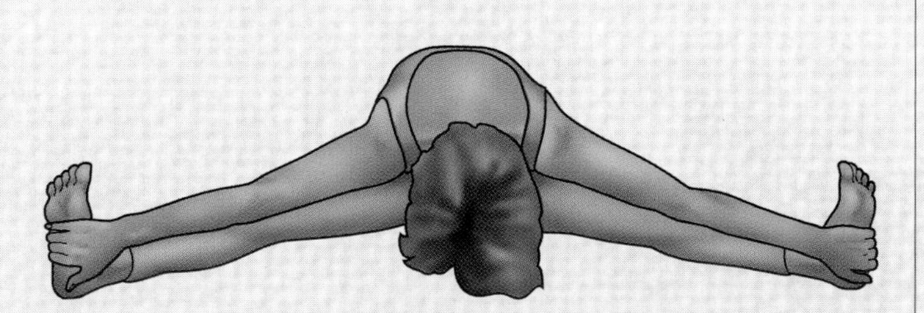

Sit with your legs in a V. Raise your arms over your head. Bending from the hips, extend your arms and grab your legs or feet. Move your head toward the floor. Release by lifting your arms back over your head, then slowly raise your torso.

## Shoulder Crunch

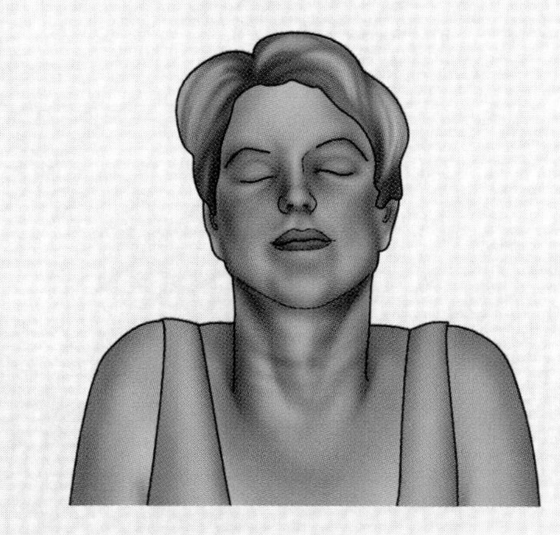

Straighten your back and relax your neck. Slowly lift your right shoulder, then lower it. Repeat with your left shoulder. Lift both shoulders together and slowly bring them down.

# Gallery of Yoga Positions

## Shoulder Stand

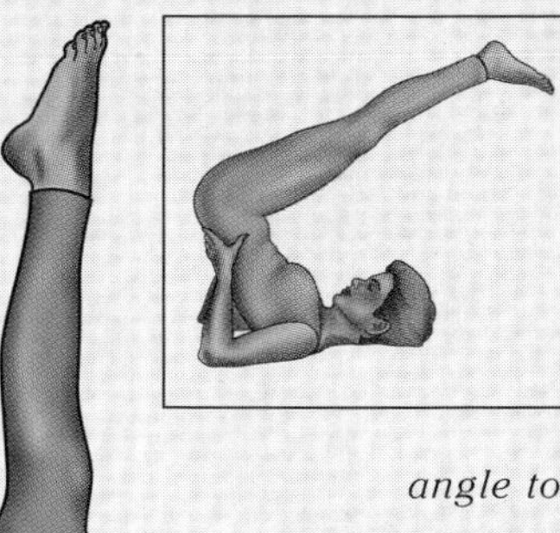

Lie on your back, hands at your sides. Lift both legs until they are at a right angle to your back. Supporting your hips with hands, inhale and extend your legs at the angle shown (inset) for the Half Shoulder Stand. Extend back and legs vertically for the full position (left). Slowly lower legs to release.

## Sphinx

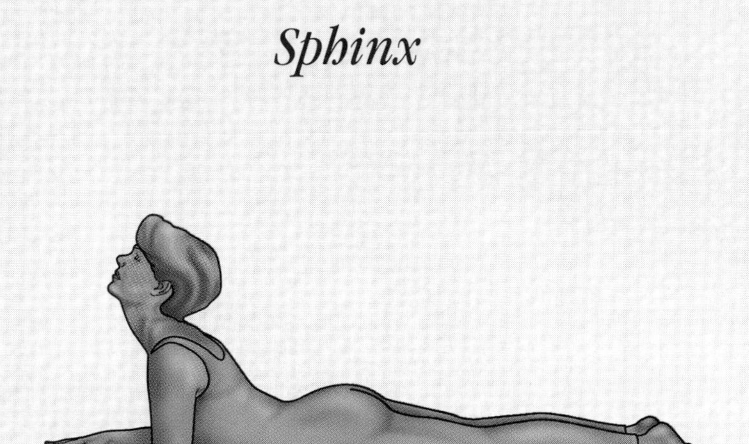

Lie on your stomach and place both forearms on the floor, palms down and elbows directly under your shoulders. Push your chest away from the floor as far as comfortably possible and look upward slightly. Lower your torso to release.

## Spider

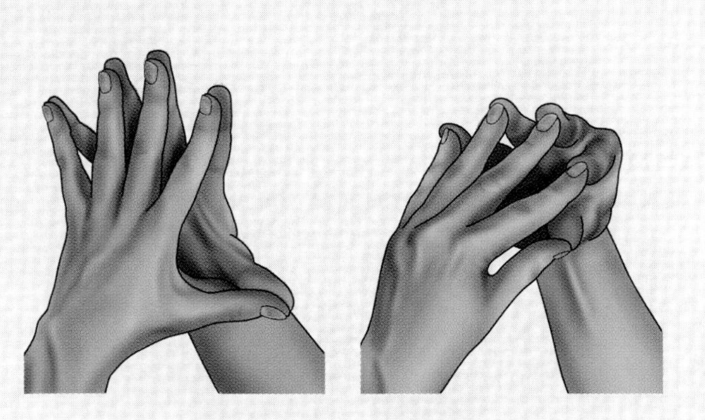

Press your fingertips together firmly, holding your palms two to three inches apart. Then push your palms toward each other (above, left) and with your fingertips still together move them apart (above, right). Relax, then repeat the push-up motion.

## Spinal Twist

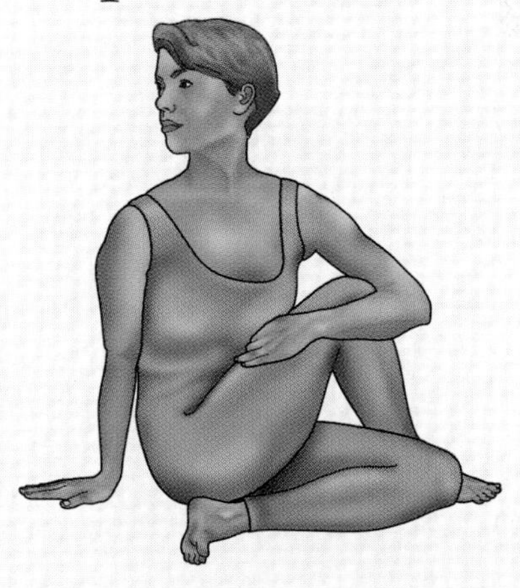

While sitting, place your right foot outside of the left knee. Grasp your right knee with your left arm and place your right hand on the floor behind you. Inhale, then exhale as you twist your torso slowly as far as you can to the right. Repeat on the other side.



CONTINUED

# Gallery of Yoga Positions

## Standing Angle

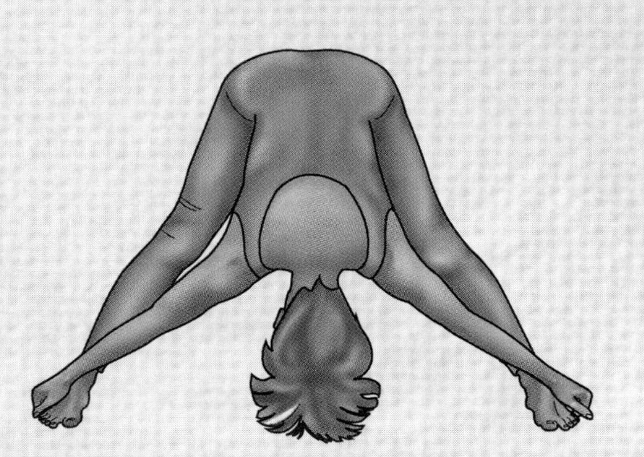

Inhale and step wide to your right with arms outstretched. Exhaling, bend forward at the hips and grasp your feet, moving the top of your head toward the floor. Rise slowly, keeping your back straight.

## Standing Yoga Mudra

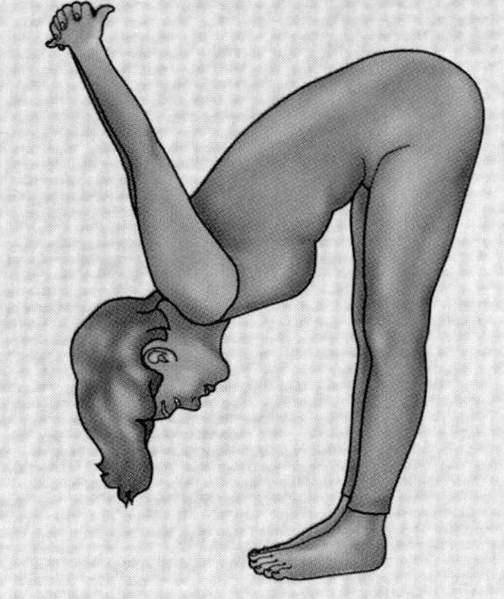

Stand with your arms at your sides. Inhale, raise your arms in front of you, then exhale and sweep them behind your back, squeezing the shoulder blades. Interlace your fingers and bend forward as you lift your arms. Raise your torso and drop your arms to release.

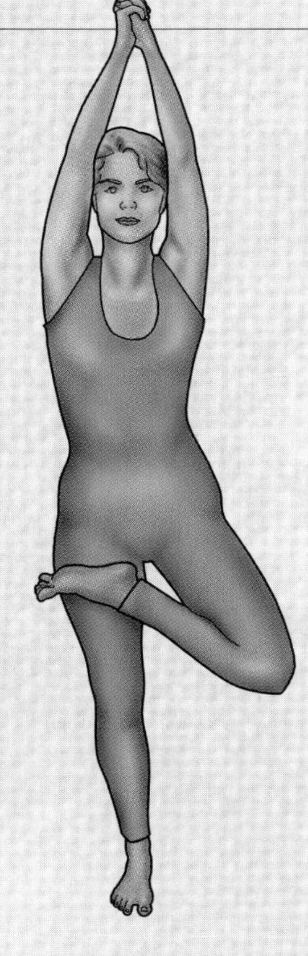

## Tree

Use your hands to lift one foot to the top of the opposite thigh. Place your palms together at heart level and raise your hands overhead; point the index fingers and interlace the others. Press your bent knee down and back without tilting your pelvis. Bring your hands back down to heart level and lower your leg. Repeat on the other side.

## Triangle

With arms parallel to the floor and feet apart, turn your right toes out and left toes forward. Bend to the right, moving your left arm up and right arm to the right leg. Look up at your raised palm. Return to the starting position and repeat on the other side.

# Gallery of Yoga Positions

## Upward Dog

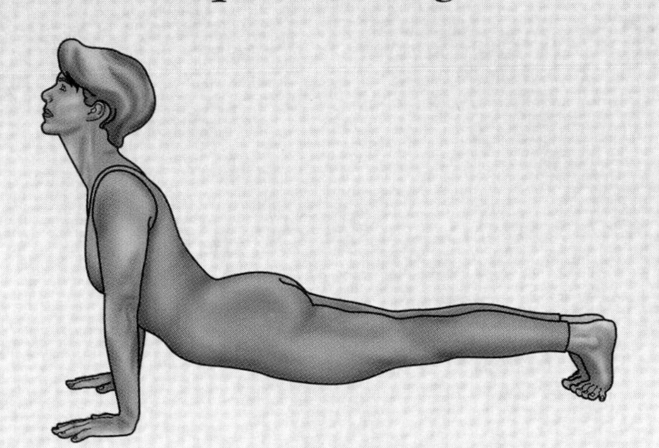

Lie facedown, palms at chest level and elbows close to the body. Spread your fingers, keeping the index fingers forward. Using your hands and toes, lift your torso, hips, and knees off the floor, arching your back slightly. Return to the starting position.

## Warrior 1

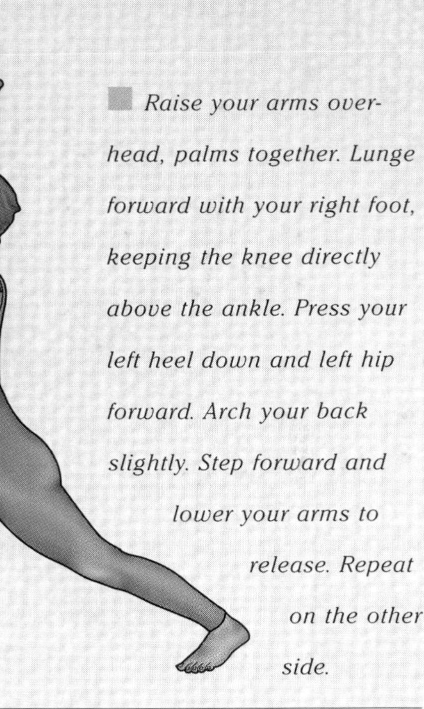

Raise your arms overhead, palms together. Lunge forward with your right foot, keeping the knee directly above the ankle. Press your left heel down and left hip forward. Arch your back slightly. Step forward and lower your arms to release. Repeat on the other side.

## Warrior 2

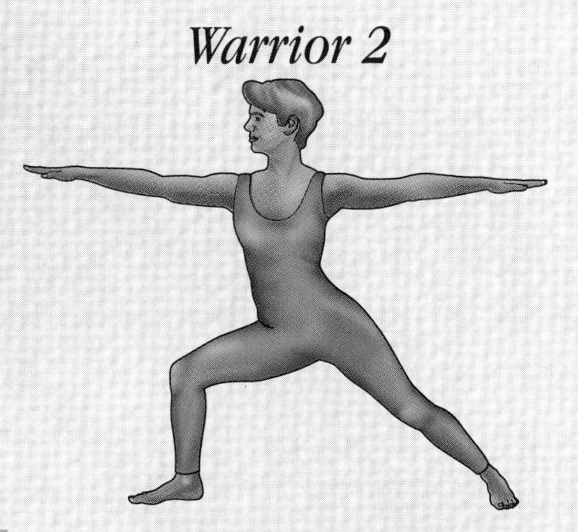

With arms parallel to the floor and feet apart, turn your right toes out and left toes forward. Bend your right knee and bring it above your right ankle, keeping your hips forward. Look over your right hand. Return to the starting position, then repeat on the opposite side.

## Yoga Mudra

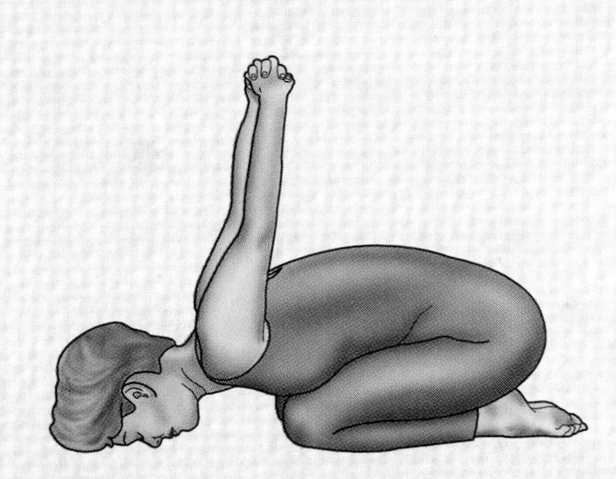

Sit on your heels, knees together, then follow the arm motion and stretch for Standing Yoga Mudra. Move your forehead to the floor and stretch your arms overhead. Breathe deeply, then exhale, bringing your arms back down. Inhale and slowly raise your torso.